INTRODUCTION TO MEDICAL BIOCHEMISTRY

1

9781779568144
AF734377

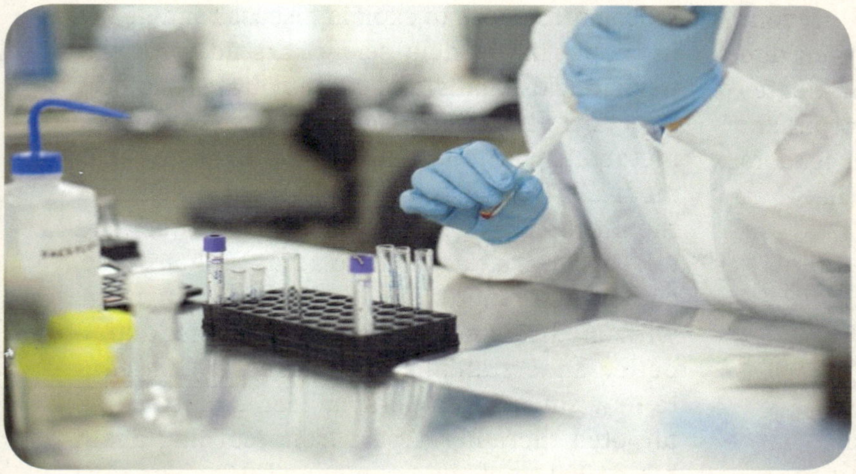

LEARNING OBJECTIVES

After studying this chapter, you will be able to:

1. Describe the biomolecules in medicine;
2. Know the metabolic pathways;
3. Understand the enzymes and enzyme kinetics;
4. Describe the genetic biochemistry;
5. Learn about hormones and signaling molecules;
6. Describe the clinical applications of medical biochemistry.

Introduction

It is through medical biochemistry that scientists discover how diseases occur at the molecular level and how this knowledge helps doctors. It is concerned with proteins, lipids, carbohydrates, and nucleic acids, which are vital for how cells work and their metabolism. It is important for doctors to know about biochemical processes when studying health and disease. For instance, knowing the biochemical stages of drug metabolism can help doctors give the right treatment to each patient. Pharmacogenomics is a useful example, since it examines how changes in genes can affect a person's reaction to drugs because of enzymes such as cytochrome P450. As a result, medical biochemistry plays a role in picking the best treatment for each patient. Medical biochemistry is easily viewed in clinical settings, especially when looking at pharmacology, through real case studies. Using datasets about cytochrome P450 genes in exercises shows how biochemistry is used in pharmacotherapy. For instance, through studying cases such as a breast cancer survivor struggling with pain management due to opioid metabolism variance, students can recognize the critical nuances in drug interactions and patient responses (Blevins et al., 2020). Studying such cases sharpens critical thinking and teaches people about the role of biochemistry in medical practice. Consequently, this exercise demonstrates that biochemistry plays a key role in helping medical professionals give excellent care to their patients. In addition, it is very important to maintain patient records accurately in medical biochemistry. Properly identifying patients is necessary to prevent any negative outcomes that could happen due to errors in healthcare. Research indicates that numerous factors, from incorrect patient registration to erroneous testing, can lead to significant harms if not addressed (Lippi et al., 2017).

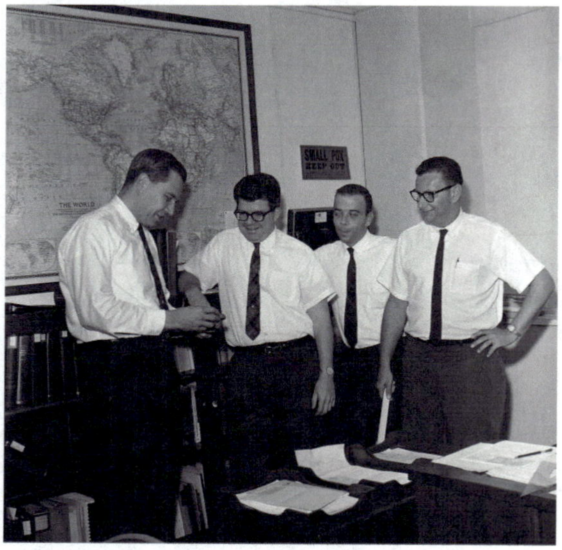

Figure 1.1. Medical biochemistry.

Source: By CDC/ Dr. John J. Witte - CDC PHIL #13230, Public Domain, https://commons.wikimedia.org/w/index.php?curid=15461811

Seeing the biochemical reasons behind identification errors proves that quality care is necessary in healthcare. With the help of recent technology, healthcare staff can accurately identify patients and safely treat them. Paying close attention indicates that medical biochemistry is essential for improving healthcare, which underlines the importance of more education and new answers to healthcare issues (Figure 1.1).

Definition and Scope of Medical Biochemistry

In biochemistry, medical biochemistry is important because it uses molecular and biochemical ideas to explain diseases and health in people. In this field, scientists study proteins, nucleic acids, lipids, and carbohydrates and how they take part in biological processes. Analyzing metabolic pathways and enzymatic reactions in medical biochemistry helps doctors understand the biochemistry behind several disorders and take appropriate actions to address them. Also, combining genetic and molecular knowledge with medical biochemistry gives scientists a better understanding of diseases, which leads to new advances in personalized medicine and targeted therapies. Apart from learning about biological molecules, medical biochemistry covers laboratory medicine, which is important in the healthcare system. Thanks to the careful use of laboratory methods, medical biochemistry helps doctors and improves patient outcomes. To give an example, the results of diagnostic tests rely on analyzing biochemical samples from the body, which helps doctors decide on treatments. As a result of the connection between laboratory medicine and medical biochemistry, finding disease markers and metabolic problems becomes easier, which helps improve both diagnosis and treatment. This connection underscores the importance of leadership in laboratory settings to ensure high-quality services and promote innovations as outlined in the principles of optimal laboratory practice (Beastall, 2013). The connection between medical biochemistry and research and clinical practice is very important for healthcare. Work done in this area can result in new drugs, tests, and ways to prevent many health problems.

The regular connection between lab results and their use in the clinic encourages the medical field to learn and adapt. When evidence-based practices are applied in biochemistry research, the quality of healthcare is improved, proving that science plays a key role in healthcare. Consequently, medical biochemistry serves both a fundamental scientific purpose and a critical clinical function, affirming its indispensable role within the broader spectrum of health sciences (Marzolla, 2016) (Figure 1.2).

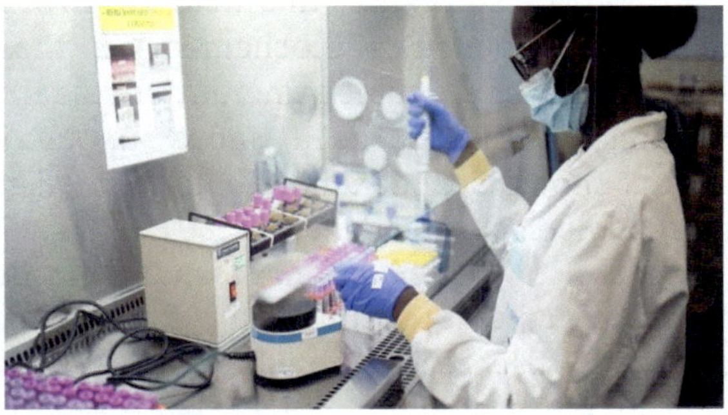

Figure 1.2. Laboratory scientist handling blood samples in a biosafety cabinet.

Source: https://comonline.unn.edu.ng/media/files/school-slider-images/Bio1.jpg.

Importance in the Field of Medicine

It is especially important to highlight the role of medical biochemistry in helping with disease understanding and diagnosis. The field of medical biochemistry provides the information needed for clinical decisions by studying how biochemical processes control cell functions. For instance, looking into metabolic pathways has allowed scientists to find biomarkers important for diagnosing and predicting cancer and diabetes. They increase the accuracy of diagnosis and also make it possible to choose treatments that improve the outcomes for patients. Moreover, having knowledge of biochemical changes connected to diseases enables healthcare providers to choose effective treatments that address the main issues instead of just treating the symptoms. So, medical biochemistry acts as a key area in modern medicine that links research done in the lab with its use in medical care. Additionally, medical biochemistry's use is crucial in drug design and therapeutic interventions. The subject is important for pharmacokinetics and pharmacodynamics since it describes how drugs are processed and how they can affect human biochemistry. Because of biochemistry, scientists are able to create drugs that target certain molecules, making personalized medicine more popular in today's medicine. Animal models are used a lot here, as they give details about how effective and safe a drug may be before it is tested on people. As noted earlier, animal models have been highly relevant in biochemistry and the discovery of vaccines, besides drug discovery, as they reflect biological responses that are critical for effective therapy to take place (Costa-Pinto et al., 2016). For this reason, the way medical biochemistry and drug development work together is very important for progress in medicine. Medical biochemistry is important for public health and epidemiology, mainly when it comes to monitoring and controlling disease outbreaks. Tracking infectious agents and their ways of spreading depends on the use of biochemical assays. Researchers use biochemical markers in different populations to find out about disease trends and create strategies to address health-related issues. Altimetric data has added a new way to look at the evaluation of biomedical research. Just like the measures being studied now, social media measures are linked to citation measures. This means that engaging with the public will increase the spread of crucial health information (Aljohani et al., 2017). This shows that biochemists and researchers should be involved in sharing their knowledge, which makes their research more important for public health activities. Because medical biochemistry plays many roles, it clearly contributes to medicine and can be used in various medical activities.

Historical Development and Milestones

The study of medical biochemistry was formed in the early 19th century as scientists started to understand chemical reactions within the body. Thanks to William Beaumont's work on gastric digestion, the first important ideas for the field were established. In the 20th century, biochemistry made significant progress, including when Watson and Crick determined the structure of DNA in 1953. This important discovery showed the molecular reason behind heredity and started a series of studies that related genetics to biochemistry. Thanks to these developments, it became easier to study complex biochemical processes, and medical research was greatly affected, showing how biochemistry affects clinical practices. In the late 20th century, biochemistry made another important step forward by using computational methods. When globalization and technology improved, countries started using computational biology to analyze a lot of biological data. Programs in computational methods being launched in Greece and Cyprus show that this field is growing internationally. The results of a study suggest that the progress in medical biochemistry in these countries is hopeful and shows a positive trend. The expectation of a doubled amount of research publications reflects how biochemistry is gaining attention globally and needs more support in terms of resources and finances. This dynamic environment showcases the adaptability of medical biochemistry as it embraces novel technologies and methodologies (Chasapi et al., 2019). Now in the 21st century, important developments in medical biochemistry are being made, mainly in the fields of personalized medicine and new types of treatment. The complete sequencing of the Human Genome by genomics has boosted our understanding of many diseases at the molecular level. By mapping the entire human genome, healthcare providers can now provide treatment that is tailored to each person's genetic information, which is a big change from the old approach. Moreover, biochemists, medical experts, and technologists working together have sped up the development of new drugs and tools for testing diseases. As these developments emerge, the field acknowledges the collective contributions from both historical and contemporary milestones, shaping the future trajectory of medical biochemistry (Graduate School of Biomedical Sciences, 2013) (Figure 1.3).

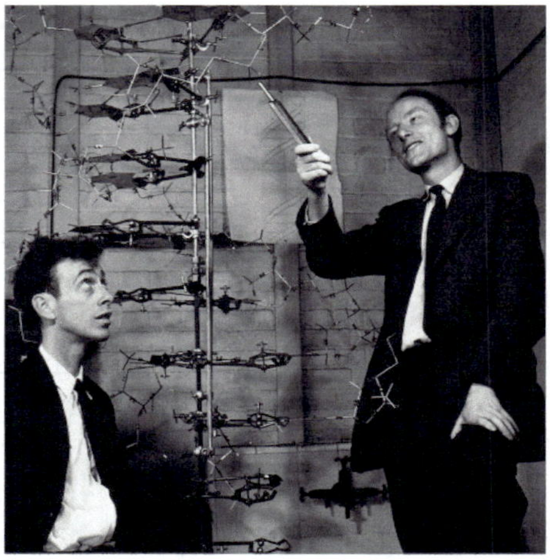

Figure 1.3. James Watson and Francis Crick with their DNA model at the Cavendish Laboratories in 1953.

Source: https://www.sciencehistory.org/wp-content/uploads/2023/04/watson-crick-dna-model_crop3.jpg.

1.1. Biomolecules in Medicine

Learning Outcome

1. Describe the structure and function of proteins;
2. Understand the role of carbohydrates in health and disease;
3. Understand the significance of lipids and nucleic acids.

The importance of biomolecules in medicine is very high, especially when it comes to diagnosing and controlling diseases. The most prominent advance in this respect is the application of biomarkers for tracking acute myocardial infarction (AMI). Studies have confirmed that cardiac troponin, which is found in the heart muscle, is a main sign that someone has coronary disease. Within hours of an AMI, the level of troponin in the blood increases a lot and stays high for 4 to 10 days, giving doctors enough time to diagnose the problem. Such a long period gives professionals enough time to intervene and choose the best treatment for each patient. The improvement of the sensitivity of the detection methods for cardiac troponin has significantly improved the reliability of diagnoses, which eventually contributes to better clinical outcomes for those patients at risk of cardiac events (Abdolrahim et al., 2015). Traditional medicine provides a lot of important information about how plant-based biomolecules can be used in modern medicine. For example, the Euphorbia genus, which contains many different chemicals, has attracted attention because of its many biological activities. Scientists are studying sesquiterpenes and flavonoids from such plants to see if they might treat diseases such as inflammation, cancer, and microbial infections. The presence of many phytochemicals in Euphorbia species demonstrates that they can be used as the basis for making new medicines. Having been used traditionally for centuries, continued studies on the bioactive potential of these compounds reflect the significance of biomolecules in the discovery of new therapeutic agents in the field of medicine (Adedoyin et al., 2019). Biomolecules are expected to bring major changes to both diagnosing and treating diseases in medicine. Because of progress in biomolecule research, it is now possible to provide personalized medicine that matches each patient's unique biology. This way of working makes interventions more precise and effective, mainly in oncology, where treatments are chosen based on the tumor's molecular features. The study of proteins and their roles in the body through proteomics is making it easier to understand how diseases happen. With further research revealing the details of biomolecule interactions, medicine is expected to change a lot and introduce precision medicine based on what we know about medical biochemistry (Figure 1.4).

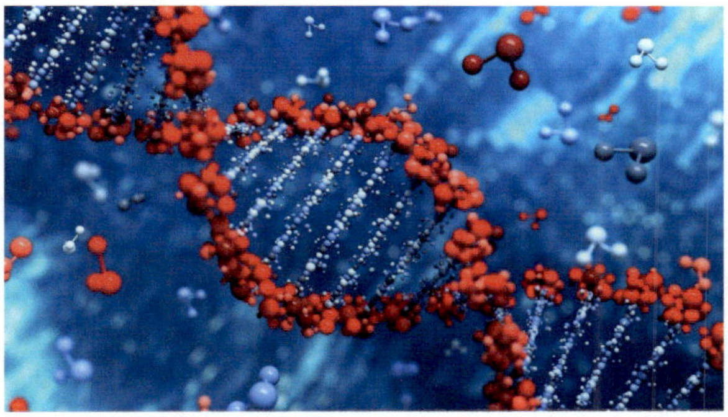

Figure 1.4. 3D illustration of a DNA double helix structure with surrounding molecules.

Source: https://media.licdn.com/dms/image/v2/D5612AQGTO1AVhfGWCQ/article-cover_image-shrink_720_1280/article-cover_image-shrink_720_1280/0/1687097465424?e=2147483647&v=beta&t=r6NuSms4z-iewXfo7E_neGxFdqm5vOODL5Ar6H1Tcrk.

1.1.1. Structure and Function of Proteins

How proteins are built and how they function is very important in medical biochemistry. The way proteins are folded into three-dimensional shapes using amino acids determines what they do in the body. Proteins are known to function as enzymes that help with biochemical reactions and also as parts of the cell's structure. Protein folding and its ability to interact with other biomolecules are mostly influenced by the way amino acids are arranged in the protein's primary sequence. Essentially, a protein's conformation is a sophisticated manifestation of its primary sequence, emphasizing that even minor alterations can lead to significant functional changes, as evidenced by mutations in proteins such as DUSP5 that impact their activity and role in cellular signaling pathways (Nayak et al., 2014). Researching the importance of certain amino acids in proteins shows more details about their actions. In globular proteins, the hydrophobic parts are found inside to stay away from water, but the polar and charged parts are found outside, interacting with the water and other polar substances. It helps hold the protein structure steady and also supports the interactions that are important for the protein's function. Notably, studies have shown a correlation between the presence of polar residues in core positions and protein stability, suggesting that these residues contribute to a well-defined three-dimensional conformation crucial for biological activity (Bolon et al., 2001). So, both hydrophobic and polar interactions are necessary for proteins to keep their structure and function, proving that structure and function are closely linked. Besides, using advanced approaches like molecular modeling and enzymatic assays has helped us learn more about how proteins function. For example, scientists have studied DUSP5 to learn that the S147P mutation can influence how the protein operates and impacts various body functions. Mutational analyses combined with computational simulations have revealed that even subtle changes can lead to hypoactivity, fundamentally altering the signaling pathways dependent on DUSP5 activity (Nayak et al., 2014). They not only explain how proteins work but also encourage scientists to develop treatments for proteins that are not working properly. So, understanding protein structure and function is very important in medical biochemistry, since it helps us target diseases and create new treatments based on what we know about these important molecules (Figure 1.5).

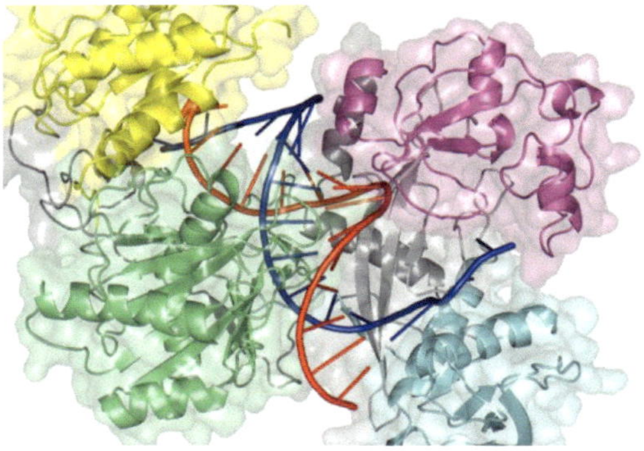

Figure 1.5. Protein structure and function.

Source: https://www.wur.nl/upload_mm/2/7/3/76810f20-cf40-400c-8252-1e314f8de543_Daan_84cacd95_750x400.jpg.

1.1.2. Role of Carbohydrates in Health and Disease

Carbohydrates are necessary for our health and are used by the body as the main source of energy. Biochemical pathways related to carbohydrate metabolism in medical biochemistry show how they can be involved in health and disease. Whenever we consume carbohydrates, they are broken down to glucose and are needed to maintain the body's energy balance. Eating too many refined carbohydrates can cause problems with insulin and lead to being overweight. Such conditions are linked to an issue with glucose control that makes it more likely for someone to get type 2 diabetes. The interactions that exist between carbohydrate intake and insulin sensitivity make carbohydrates of central importance for the development of strategies for the promotion of health or the prevention of metabolic disorders, requiring a balanced diet that involves complex carbohydrates as an essential source of energy and nutrition (Sarmidi, 2012). Carbohydrates affect health in more ways than giving energy; they are also important for cellular signaling and regulation. For example, carbohydrates take part in making glycoconjugates that help cells communicate and respond to infections. Problems with carbohydrate metabolism may cause major health concerns. Since high levels of glycated hemoglobin point to long-term high blood sugar, controlling blood sugar is very important in diabetic patients. Oxidative stress plays a key role in this condition, as reactive oxygen species (ROS) harm cells and this process is affected by how much sugar the body has and how it uses it. Research shows that elevated lipid peroxidation correlates with high glycated hemoglobin levels, indicating the oxidative stress suffered by tissues in the context of carbohydrate imbalances (Bhat et al., 2011). It demonstrates that it is important to understand the details of carbohydrate metabolism to lower disease risks and improve health. Also, dietary carbohydrates play a significant role in managing inflammation and diseases that last a long time. It is known that chronic low-grade inflammation is related to conditions like cardiovascular disease (CVD) and metabolic syndrome (MS). Eating many refined carbs can lead to more inflammation, whereas whole grains and fibers help reduce it. Biochemical processes include the way carbohydrates affect the microbiota in the gut, which then changes the level of systemic inflammation. It is well known from research that fiber from complex carbohydrates acts as a prebiotic, helping to increase the number of helpful microbes that are good for metabolic health. Therefore, integrating nutrient-dense carbohydrates is essential not just for energy, but for their protective effects against disease through the modulation of inflammation and improvement of gut health (Sarmidi, 2012). Knowing about these interactions will help develop dietary advice and public health plans to decrease the number of carbohydrate-related diseases (Figure 1.6).

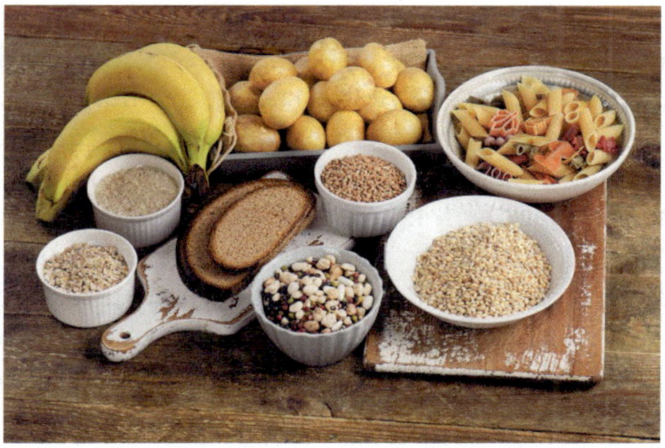

Figure 1.6. The role of carbohydrate in health and disease.

Source: https://taitalksnutrition.com/wp-content/uploads/2021/03/p1_carbs_ml0618_gi613046884.jpg?w=720.

1.1.3. Significance of Lipids and Nucleic Acids

Lipids are very important in medical biochemistry since they influence many biological activities in the human body. Lipids, for example, triglycerides (TGs), phospholipids, and cholesterol, provide energy and also work as parts of cellular membranes. Because they have amphipathic properties, they can create lipid bilayers needed for the stability and flexibility of cell membranes. Besides, a few lipids work as signals, affecting the way cells communicate and metabolic processes function. The effects of lipid metabolism can be seen clearly in hyperlipidemia since problems with lipid levels can result in CVDs. Recent research has established a link between dietary components, such as vitamin B4, and lipid metabolism, highlighting how nutritional interventions can modify lipid levels and related health outcomes (Buang, 2010). Nucleic acids, primarily deoxyribonucleic acid (DNA) and ribonucleic acid (RNA), are integral to the storage and transmission of genetic information, thereby underpinning all biological life. Nucleic acids are important in medical biochemistry because they take part in making proteins and controlling how genes are expressed. The use of transcription and translation on RNA intermediates helps the DNA's genetic code be expressed as proteins that have many functions in the body. If nucleic acid metabolism is not normal, it can result in genetic disorders and diseases, for example, cancer, since mutations in DNA can interfere with regular cell functioning. It is important to know the biochemical pathways of nucleic acids to design gene therapy and other treatments for genetic problems. The relationship between lipids and nucleic acids emphasizes their role in medical biochemistry, mainly regarding diseases and treatments. Lipid molecules have an effect on nucleic acids, as seen when lipid carriers are used in gene delivery. The use of lipids in this application allows the application to carry nucleic acids across cellular membranes and improves the results of gene therapies. The modification of lipid profiles, as indicated by studies showing increased triglyceride and phospholipid levels following dietary interventions, reinforces the idea that lipids can impact nucleic acid functions in various biological contexts (Buang, 2010). Exobiologists also focus on studying biomolecules in various conditions, because the basic roles of lipids and nucleic acids in life could vary from one ecosystem to another, therefore highlighting their importance in biology.

Test Your Knowledge

1. hat is the function of the proteins?
2. What is the role of carbohydrates in health and disease?

1.2. Metabolic Pathways

Learning Outcome

1. Give an overview of catabolic and anabolic pathways;
2. Describe the key metabolic pathways in human health;
3. Understand the regulation of metabolism and its clinical implications.

Metabolic pathways are made up of many enzymatic reactions that oversee the chemical processes happening in living organisms. The pathways are essential for keeping the body's balance and for cells to react well to changes around them. Every pathway consists of a particular group of substrates, enzymes, and intermediates that help control how metabolites change and move. As an illustration, catabolic reactions break down big molecules and release energy from their bonds, whereas anabolic reactions use energy to build important macromolecules. To understand both normal and abnormal functions in the body, learning these processes is very important. This basic understanding prepares you to study specific topics in medical biochemistry since it points out the role of metabolic pathways in health and disease. A significant part of studying metabolic pathways is looking at how certain transporters handle metabolites, for example, URAT1. Since URAT1 is the main way uric acid is reabsorbed by the kidneys, it is now clear that it plays a key role in gout and cardiovascular disorders. It has been shown by recent studies that URAT1 not only moves uric acid but also works with other organic anions and can impact several metabolic pathways. For example, studies in mice lacking the URAT1 ortholog uncovered substantial alterations in plasma and urinary levels of various small molecules, which are biomarkers of generalized changes in metabolism (Eraly et al., 2015). It shows that metabolic pathways are linked and URAT1 plays a key part in balancing the body's metabolic state. Besides transporters, metabolic pathways are also being significantly affected by redox mechanisms, most notably with regard to the issue of multidrug resistance (MDR) in cancer treatment. MDR is partly caused by the redox state of tumor cells, which manages how much chemotherapy drugs enter the cells and how they are metabolized. Furthermore, the interplay between redox mechanisms and various metabolic enzymes facilitates rapid detoxification of cytotoxic metabolites produced during chemotherapy (Cort et al., 2016). They show that metabolic pathways are complex and can adjust to treatment, so it is important to study how redox regulation affects both the success and failure of drugs. More study of these processes by scientists could lead to new treatments that help overcome MDR and improve chemotherapy's effectiveness (Figure 1.7).

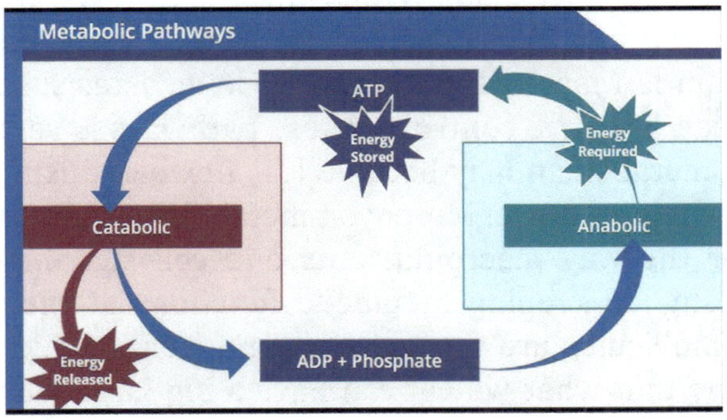

Figure 1.7. Metabolic pathways.

Source: https://i.ytimg.com/vi/m61bQYio9ys/hq720.jpg?sqp=-oaymwEhCK4FEIIDSFryq4qpAxMIARUAAAAAGAElAADIQj0AgKJD&rs=AOn4CLBN18ehEDx8-Jqm7hueyu2sIY6dVg.

1.2.1. Overview of Catabolic and Anabolic Pathways

For medical biochemistry, it is necessary to understand catabolic and anabolic pathways to describe how cells metabolize. Catabolic pathways mainly help in breaking down molecules to supply the energy needed for different body functions. The process of breaking down carbohydrates, lipids, and proteins into simpler parts in metabolism helps the cell make ATP, which is its main energy source. In addition, the processes of catabolism help produce metabolic intermediates that are used by anabolic pathways. It is also important to control these catabolic routes, as incorrect activation can bring about health problems. Therefore, knowing about catabolism well gives the basic understanding needed to explore new therapies for metabolic control. On the other hand, anabolic pathways take in simple molecules and create more complex ones, which usually need energy from ATP made during catabolic reactions. Cells depend on these pathways for growth and repair, as they are important for maintaining a stable metabolism. A good example is the process of osteogenesis, where anabolic activity helps bones form and this process is boosted when the transcription factor Nmp4 is missing. In studies involving $Nmp4^{-}/^{-}$ mesenchymal stem/progenitor cells, it was discovered that this genetic alteration boosts the anabolic capacity of these cells by promoting higher levels of glycolysis and enhanced collagen synthesis, both of which are crucial for bone matrix formation and overall structural integrity of bone tissue (Adaway et al., 2019).

It is clear from the balance between catabolic and anabolic pathways that nutrition is very important for metabolic processes, especially in cases of wound healing. Evidence suggests that general nutritional support and the administration of anabolic agents can bolster the healing process by increasing lean body mass and enhancing protein synthesis, both vital for tissue repair (Demling et al., 2011). Injury adds to the body's stress, and this makes it necessary to use a well-planned diet to lessen the dangers of malnutrition. So, knowing both catabolism and anabolism allows clinicians and biochemists to plan effective strategies for handling metabolic health and achieving good results in different medical situations (Figure 1.8).

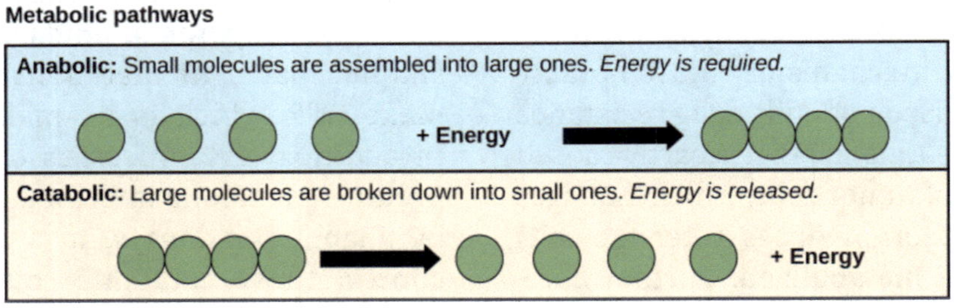

Figure 1.8. Anabolic pathways are those that require energy to synthesize larger molecules. Catabolic pathways are those that generate energy by breaking down larger molecules. Both types of pathways are required for maintaining the cell's energy balance.

Source: https://s3-us-west-2.amazonaws.com/courses-images/wp-content/uploads/sites/110/2016/05/02235219/Figure_06_01_03.jpg.

1.2.2. Key Metabolic Pathways in Human Health

Metabolic pathways are very detailed and make sure that humans remain healthy by controlling many essential functions in cells. Most important of these pathways is glycolysis, the citric acid cycle, and oxidative phosphorylation, which are central to energy production and permit cells to generate adenosine triphosphate (ATP) from glucose and fatty acids. When these pathways are interfered with, it may result in metabolic disorder and can be recognized as obesity, diabetes, or CVD. In this way, anabolism-catabolism equilibrium is responsible for energy homeostasis, so when we consume more calories, we may gain extra fat. Effective control of these pathways is very important for health, mainly in older adults, as their metabolism may become less flexible, raising the risk of health problems and making it harder for them to move. Moreover, metabolic pathways are important for energy production as well as for the way macronutrients and cell signaling interact. Foods and nutrition are extremely important for keeping metabolic functions at their best. All the important biomolecules and signaling molecules are formed using nutrients, which are amino acids, carbohydrates, and lipids. They show that what we eat can have a big impact on our metabolism and the chances of developing metabolic disorders. As has been discussed in the literature, nutritional strategies predicated upon a biochemical understanding may aid in achieving cellular homeostasis and health, and a holistic approach to nutrition is suggested to function to heighten metabolic resilience (Sarmidi, 2012). As people age, the consequences of altered metabolism become clearer, as is seen in sarcopenia, where muscles are lost and there is more body fat. As time goes by and a person grows older, the shifting of adipose tissue to non-adipose areas like the skeletal muscle leads to a reduction in muscle function and quality. Because the muscle fibers are close to adipose tissue, there is a risk that lipotoxicity will harm the muscles. Such changes should be dealt with by understanding how biological factors influence muscle contraction and metabolism. Studies indicate that cellular machinery susceptible to lipid-induced stress must be addressed in order to enhance conditions when aging impacts physical performance (Carter et al., 2019). Therefore, it is necessary to use medical biochemistry together when designing strategies to improve healthy aging by influencing major metabolic routes.

1.2.3. Regulation of Metabolism and Its Clinical Implications

Metabolism is regulated in many ways, and this plays a key role in ensuring human health by using biochemical pathways to keep cells stable. Thanks to these pathways, nutrients are used to produce energy, which affects the body's functions and metabolism. Understanding how foods are processed by the body can show the links between diet, metabolic problems, and health. For example, having a balanced mix of macronutrients can help the body function properly and lower the chance of getting obesity and diabetes. Moreover, the integration of biochemistry and human physiology reveals that disruptions in metabolic regulation can lead to significant health challenges, emphasizing the importance of maintaining proper dietary habits and metabolic function in achieving and sustaining metabolic balance and overall well-being (Sarmidi, 2012). Metabolic regulation has important effects on how diseases such as cancer are treated. Changes in how cells metabolize are commonly linked to cancer, since these changes allow tumor cells to grow more and resist treatment. Specifically, MDR has been linked to redox mechanisms that enable cancer cells to evade the cytotoxic effects of chemotherapeutic agents. This situation shows that knowing more about metabolic control in cancer is important, as how drugs affect cellular metabolism can determine how effective the treatment is.

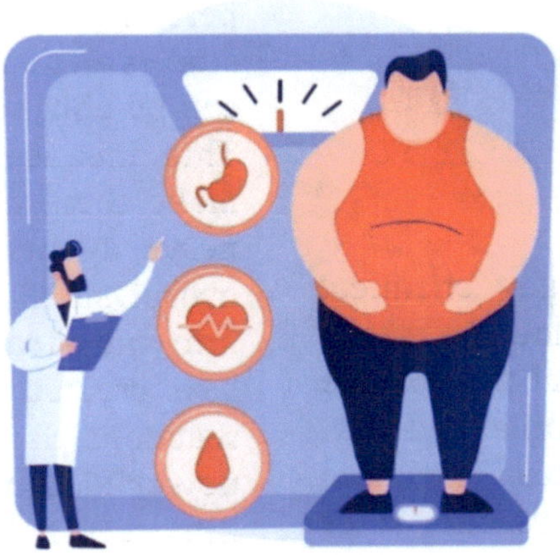

Figure 1.9. Illustration of obesity-related health risks and medical consultation.

Source: https://img.freepik.com/free-vector/obesity-problem-overweight-man-medical-consultation-diagnostics-negative-impact-obesity-humans-health-internal-organs-vector-isolated-concept-metaphor-illustration_335657-1305.jpg?semt=ais_hybrid&w=740.

The development of innovative treatments, such as redox-active drugs or inhibitors targeting the antioxidant defense systems of tumor cells, promises to enhance the effectiveness of existing chemotherapy options and improve patient outcomes by overcoming MDR associated with various malignancies (Cort et al., 2016). Also, since chronic diseases are often made worse by problems in metabolism, it is important to regulate metabolism properly. When people have CVD, MS, or type 2 diabetes, their metabolism is not properly controlled and they do not react well to the body's needs. Scientists in medical biochemistry explain how metabolic pathways are affected by genetic, environmental, and lifestyle factors, which gives ideas for prevention and treatment. Working on pathways linked to energy production and inflammation, doctors may be able to reduce or stop the effects of chronic metabolic diseases. This perspective highlights the importance of personalized medicine approaches and the need for effective public health strategies that promote metabolic health through lifestyle modifications and dietary interventions (Sarmidi, 2012) (Figure 1.9).

Test Your Knowledge

1. What is an anabolic pathway and a catabolic pathway?
2. What is the regulation of metabolism?

1.3. Enzymes and Enzyme Kinetics

Learning Outcome

1. Describe the enzyme structure and function;
2. Know the factors affecting enzyme activity;
3. Understand the clinical significance of enzyme assays.

They speed up the rate of many chemical reactions in living organisms by a lot. The reason catalytic efficiency happens is that the enzyme and its substrates connect to each other and form enzyme-substrate (ES) complexes. The main idea of kinetics of enzymes is that reaction rates can be explained with established models such as the Michaelis–Menten model. Under substrate excess conditions, the reaction rate levels off to an optimum velocity (V_{max}), which involves saturation kinetics. Since medical biochemistry is concerned with enzyme regulation, learning about kinetics is important for scientists to discover new treatment strategies. As an example, drug therapies that change the activity of certain enzymes involved in diseases use enzyme inhibition protocols to change the way metabolic pathways function. Studies on enzymes also focus on how things such as pH and temperature can change their ability to catalyze reactions and how stable they are. Every enzyme works best in certain conditions, and any change from these can lead to big changes in its activity. In some cases, mutations in enzymes can make them bind to different substrates or work at different rates, which may affect a person's chances of getting a disease. Recent studies also show that the properties of enzymes can be enhanced to better deal with toxicants. This means changing carboxylesterases to make them active against organophosphorus nerve agents by breaking them down with hydrolysis. By integrating strategic mutations into the structure of the enzyme, scientists have created variants that are able to catalyze reactions that reduce the risk posed by such powerful inhibitors of acetylcholinesterase, illustrating the applied nature of enzyme kinetics in therapeutic applications (Andrew et al., 2010). Besides, enzyme-based reactions are often closely linked to understanding the processes in living systems. As an example, oxidative chloroperoxidase reactions are key in biochemical pathways for biotransformations. Such reactions are described by kinetics that indicate the formation of an ES complex. It has been found through experiments that changes in temperature and the environment around the reaction can control the rate constants a lot, which explains how enzymes work in different conditions. For instance, cryo-kinetic studies of the generation mechanism of short-lived reactive species in an oxidation process facilitated further understanding of how such enzymatic processes would support metabolic defense mechanisms against stress from the environment (Bennett et al., 2010). For this reason, the relationship between an enzyme's structure, its function, and the environment is still significant for medical biochemistry (Figure 1.10).

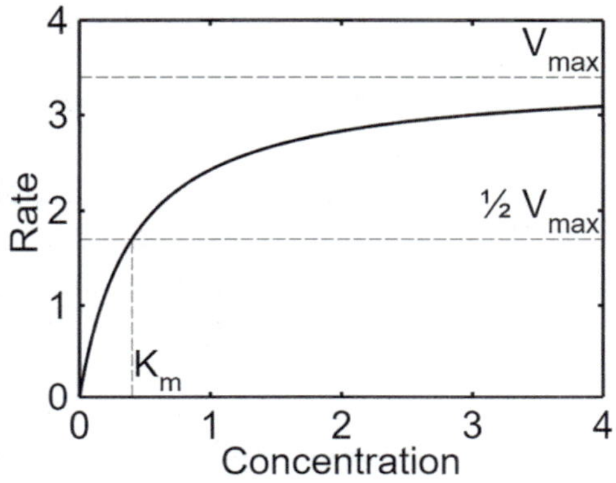

Figure 1.10. Michaelis–Menten saturation curve of an enzyme reaction. Parameter values used are V_{max} = 3.4 and K_m = 1.7.

Source: https://d2jx2rerrg6sh3.cloudfront.net/image-handler/ts/20170530074449/ri/673/picture/2017/5/Enzyme_kinetics_Michaelis_and_Menten_graph.jpg.

1.3.1. Enzyme Structure and Function

How enzymes work in biochemistry is mainly dependent on their structure and function. Most enzymes are proteins that boost the speed of biochemical reactions by lowering the energy needed for them to take place. How amino acids are arranged in an enzyme result in a three-dimensional shape with a special active site that is designed to hold substrates. Many times, this specificity is referred to as the lock and key model, where the substrate is held perfectly by the enzyme, much like a key fit into a lock. Moreover, modifications to amino acid residues in the active site can significantly impact enzyme reactivity and stability, affecting overall catalytic efficiency, as highlighted by investigations into chorismite mutase variants which demonstrated how secondary active-site residues can influence enzymatic activity (Kast et al., 2007). Along with the classic understanding of ES interactions, recent studies point out that additional protein motions are important for enzymes. In particular, the enzyme's structure is flexible enough to allow for changes needed for binding the right substrate and catalyzing reactions. As an illustration, when a substrate binds to an enzyme, the enzyme structures can change to help the catalysis process. New computational methods have highlighted this idea since scientists are now altering secondary active-site residues to find out their role in catalysis. The ability to tolerate amino acid substitutions without detrimental effects on function demonstrates the robustness of certain enzymes, indicating pathways toward optimizing or even creating novel enzymes with enhanced properties through guided mutation studies (Kast et al., 2007). New methods in enzyme engineering help us learn more about enzymes and also have major uses in medicine. For example, changing human carboxylesterase 1 so it can break down organophosphorus nerve agents is a good case of enzyme redesign to fight toxicity. In this way, using special amino acids made the enzyme more efficient at catalysis and still able to bind to nerve agents, which helps in creating useful antidotes. They demonstrate that biochemists are able to modify enzymes to get the desired results, which helps with drug design, fighting toxins, and using biotechnology in several ways. In medical biochemistry, research on enzymes is important since it provides knowledge about diseases and how to treat them (Figure 1.11).

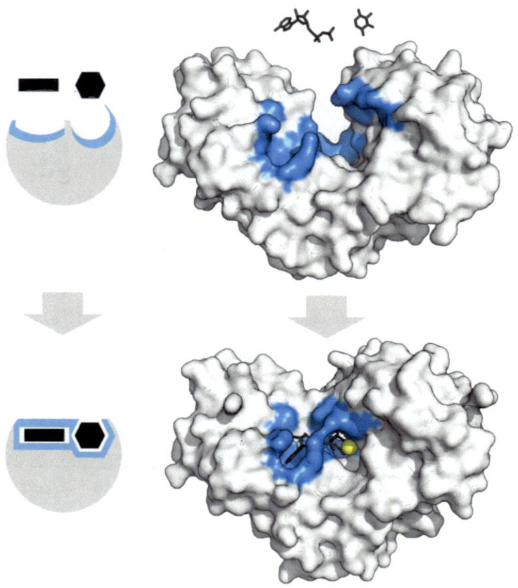

Figure 1.11. (a) According to the lock-and-key model, the shape of an enzyme's active site is a perfect fit for the substrate. (b) According to the induced fit model, the active site is somewhat flexible and can change shape in order to bond with the substrate.

Source: By Thomas Shafee - Own work, CC BY 4.0, https://commons.wikimedia.org/w/index.php?curid=45801557

1.3.2. Factors Affecting Enzyme Activity

Various things decide how active enzymes are, and each of these can either help or hinder the enzyme's ability to work. The temperature is a major factor that impacts enzymes since every enzyme has its own temperature range for maximum activity. Mostly, when temperatures rise, the movement of molecules goes up, which causes enzymes and substrates to collide more often. Yet, when temperatures get very high, the structure of the enzymes is altered, which makes them less functional. The temperature function demonstrates that the conditions of the environment, guided by thermodynamics and molecular biology, are very important for biochemical reactions in medicine. It is especially important to understand these dynamics since they are used in therapy to control drugs and metabolism by affecting enzymes. Another important thing that affects enzymes is pH, as it changes the ionization of amino acids at the active site. Every enzyme is most active at a certain pH range; if the pH changes from this range, the enzyme may become less active or stop working completely. Pepsin, for example, works well in the strongly acidic stomach, whereas alkaline phosphatase is best at work in the intestines, which are less acidic. In medical biochemistry, the dependence on pH is very important since keeping the body's pH within normal ranges is vital for metabolic processes. Understanding how enzymes react to pH changes also gives information about diseases of metabolic pathways and possible treatments.

If pH is adjusted in treatment plans, it can help enzymes work better and lead to better health results for patients. The concentration of the substrate in the solution is a major factor that affects how much an enzyme works. The Michaelis–Menten model says that when substrate levels increase, the rate of reaction goes up until it reaches its highest value, after which the enzyme is saturated. This point demonstrates that both the amount and strength of an enzyme play a key role in its reactions. Maintaining the right substrate levels is often important in treating conditions where metabolism is disturbed. In diabetes, the levels of glucose in the body are important because they can control the activity of main enzymes in glycolysis and gluconeogenesis. Besides, some drugs are made to act like substrates and change the activity of enzymes, which shows the interesting role of substrate analogs in therapeutic development. It improves the way enzymes and biochemical regulation affect disease and health management (Figure 1.12).

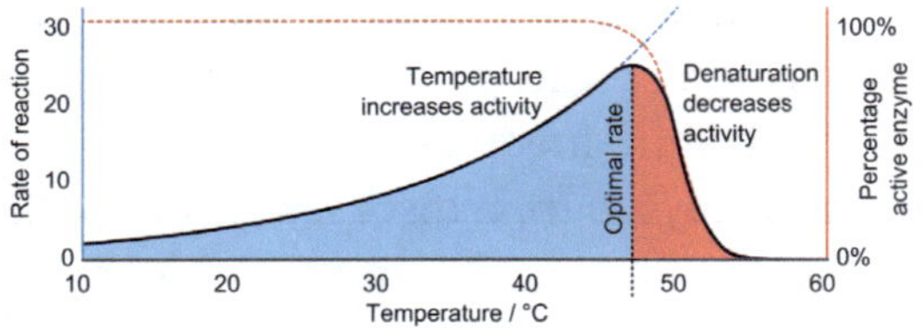

Figure 1.12. Factors affecting enzyme activity.

Source: By Thomas Shafee - Own work, CC BY 4.0, https://commons.wikimedia.org/w/index.php?curid=47436421

1.3.3. Clinical Significance of Enzyme Assays

Enzyme assays in medical biochemistry are important because they give information about many conditions, not only for diagnosis. Enzymes are important in metabolic reactions, and their levels may show signs of tissue damage, inflammation, or different diseases. For instance, the assessment of liver enzymes such as alanine aminotransferase (ALT) and aspartate aminotransferase (AST) is crucial in diagnosing hepatic conditions. If these enzymes are found in higher amounts, it indicates that the liver is damaged by hepatitis, steatosis, or cirrhosis, making it possible to act quickly and handle the condition. In this situation, using enzyme assays is crucial for diagnosis and checking the effectiveness of treatments, which shows how important they are in clinical work. Moreover, enzyme assays give a special insight into how diseases, especially cancers, develop. The measurement of lactate dehydrogenase (LDH) activity, for example, has emerged as an important biomarker in various cancers, including endometrial carcinoma. In the study, LDH activity in the tissues of endometrial carcinoma was found to be higher than in normal uterine tissues, suggesting that it may be useful for diagnosis. The LDH assays' high levels of sensitivity and specificity make them important in oncology. Notably, combining LDH assays with other biomarkers, such as the proteolytic activity of dipeptidyl peptidase III (DPP III), can enhance diagnostic accuracy, thereby aiding in early detection and management of malignancies. This research points out that enzyme assays are important for both medical diagnosis and studying the biology and growth of tumors. Lastly, enzyme assays play an important part in checking oxidative stress, which is related to diseases that result from a mismatch between ROS and antioxidants. Checking biomarkers of oxidative stress in both enzymatic and nonenzymatic antioxidant systems can give us information about diseases and the benefits of antioxidants. Still, the methods used to measure these markers can introduce biases, which means their clinical importance should be reviewed. It is suggested to develop indices that measure different oxidative stress markers, as this would give a better understanding of its clinical role. This integration of enzyme assays into clinical practice not only facilitates better disease evaluation but also underscores the dynamism and evolving nature of medical biochemistry in addressing complex health challenges (Abramić et al., 2008; Marrocco et al., 2017).

Test Your Knowledge

1. What are the factors affecting enzyme activity?
2. What is the clinical significance of enzyme assays?

1.4. Genetic Biochemistry

Learning Outcome

1. Describe the DNA structure and replication;
2. Describe the RNA synthesis and protein translation;
3. Know the genetic mutations and their biochemical consequences.

It explains how diseases happen and provides a base for designing treatments. Genetic material and its expression are based on molecules that are important for health. The spotlight on such enzymes, including farnesyl diphosphate synthase, has revealed information about metabolic disorders and possible drugs that can treat them. Recent progresses in drug discovery through the use of virtual-screening approaches, including Cao et al.'s (2011), indicate that inhibitors targeting key enzymes in metabolic pathways are highly promising for anti-infective as well as anticancer indications. Thanks to these biochemical events, researchers can develop more precise medical treatments that consider a person's unique genes, which is better for personalized medicine and patients. Apart from chronic diseases, genetic biochemistry helps explain the challenges and ethical issues of biopiracy and using genetic resources. One-World Medicine points out that using Indigenous knowledge by pharmaceutical companies brings up many ethical concerns. The framework seeks to merge traditional medicine with modern medicine, allowing Indigenous groups to receive benefits and making it possible for scientists to advance their studies. Legislative initiatives like the Nagoya Protocol, discussed by Abdelfatah et al. (2019), illustrate the shifting landscape toward a more equitable model of benefit-sharing in genetic research. Besides dealing with challenges using traditional knowledge, these initiatives also help develop medical biochemistry that includes various medicinal practices to improve health solutions across the globe. Including genetic biochemistry in medical biochemistry helps create new ways to treat diseases. As researchers use both traditional and alternative medical methods, biochemistry plays an even bigger role. Evaluating the efficacy of complementary and alternative medicine (CAM) requires rigorous scientific methodology to establish safety, efficacy, and quality, an area where genetic biochemistry can contribute significantly. For example, knowing how herbal remedies affect biochemical pathways can help improve care for patients in hospitals. Moreover, the need for established standards in herbal product production, as mentioned by Abdelfatah et al. (2019), emphasizes the necessity for a robust framework that can guide the integration of genetic insights into practical medical solutions. It will improve therapy results and guarantee that every medical biochemistry method is safe and effective for different people (Figure 1.13).

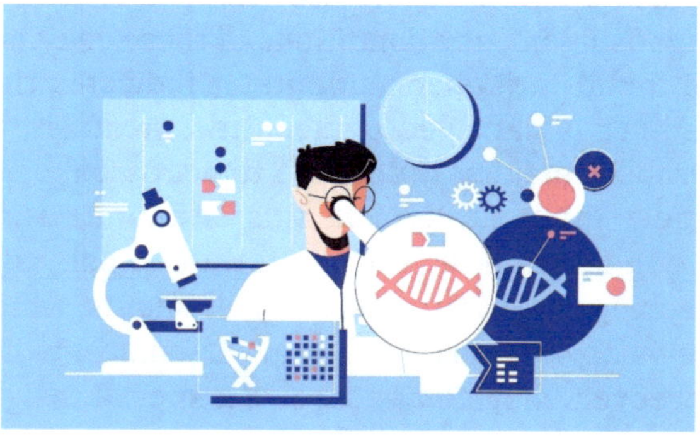

Figure 1.13. Illustration of a scientist analyzing genetic data and DNA sequencing.

Source: https://d2jx2rerrg6sh3.cloudfront.net/images/Article_Images/ImageForArticle_22413_16508965894669618.jpg.

1.4.1. DNA Structure and Replication

DNA's structure is important for its function in biology because it outlines how proteins are made. It is made up of two long strands that twist around each other to become a double helix, and every strand contains nucleotides. The smallest part of DNA, called a nucleotide, has a sugar, a phosphate group, and a nitrogenous base. Adenine, thymine, cytosine, and guanine arranged in a sequence hold the genetic code. Correct replication and transcription happen because adenine pairs with thymine and cytosine pairs with guanine. It supports the stability and structure of the cell while also making it possible for the genetic code to have redundancies, which are necessary for repairing damage and therefore maintaining cellular health and function as a basis for medical biochemistry. The process of replicating DNA is very important and carefully organized to allow cells to divide and maintain their genes. At certain points on the DNA called origins of replication, helicase enzymes separate the two strands of the DNA to form replication forks. After that, DNA polymerase is brought in to make a new strand by adding matching nucleotides to the original one. This process goes in both directions, so both strands act as templates, resulting in the formation of two identical DNA molecules from one double helix. Additionally, the presence of single-stranded DNA (ssDNA)-binding proteins, such as *Escherichia coli* ssDNA binding protein (SSB), is critical in stabilizing the unwound DNA during replication, preventing the strands from re-annealing, or forming secondary structures (Bell et al., 2015). These mechanisms point out the great care and accuracy needed to keep the genome intact, which is very important in medical biochemistry. Maintaining accuracy in DNA replication is necessary to stop mutations that could cause diseases such as cancer. DNA is accurately replicated because many enzymes and proteins are involved in checking and repairing it. As an example, mismatch repair systems are turned on to repair mistakes that happen while DNA is being made. Besides, many chemicals that occur naturally or are used in medicine can interfere with DNA replication.

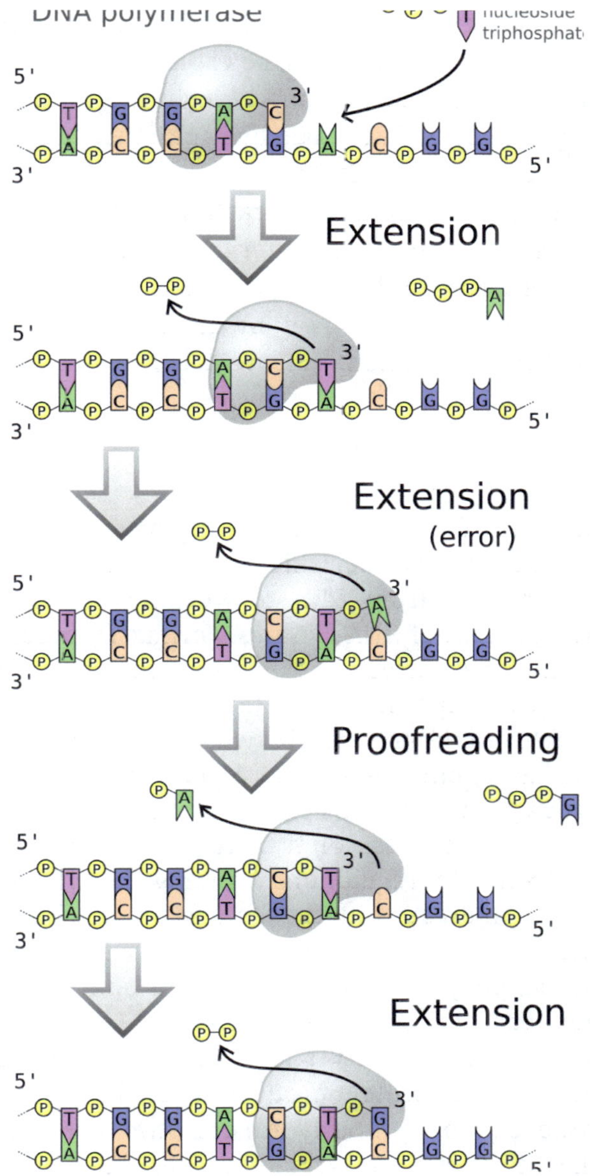

Figure 1.14. DNA replication. During the process of DNA replication, the original DNA molecule is uncoiled by DNA helicase, separating the two strands. Each then forms the template upon which DNA polymerase syntheses a new double helix, with complementary nucleotide pairs ensuring faithful replication of the original DNA sequence.

Source: By I, Madprime, CC BY-SA 3.0, https://commons.wikimedia.org/w/index.php?curid=2527732

Understanding the biocidal effects of agents like ozone on pathogens, as explored in recent studies on foodborne illnesses, highlights the dual importance of DNA structure and functionality (Anderson et al., 2003). Researchers use the study of these agents' interactions with nucleic acids to develop new therapy methods. The importance of DNA replication to medical biochemistry is shown by its influence on medical applications (Figure 1.14).

1.4.2. RNA Synthesis and Protein Translation

The basic steps in a cell are RNA synthesis and protein translation, which help move genetic information from DNA to working proteins. The process of RNA synthesis primarily occurs within the nucleus and is performed through the transcription of DNA into messenger RNA (mRNA). RNA polymerase, which is the enzyme in charge, binds to certain regions on the DNA called promoters and helps form single-stranded RNA. The process of transcription is closely controlled by regulations affecting the binding of polymerase and the activation of genes. After being synthesized, mRNA is modified by capping, polyadenylation, and splicing to get ready for translation. They are important for mRNA's stability and effectiveness in the next steps of protein production, so the genetic code can be properly turned into proteins that do various tasks in the cell. When RNA is synthesized, the next important process is protein translation, which occurs inside ribosomes found in the cytoplasm or attached to the endoplasmic reticulum (ER). The mRNA is used as a template for the construction of amino acids into polypeptides, where transfer RNA (tRNA) molecules deliver specific amino acids to the ribosome according to the sequence of codons. The anticodon present on tRNA matches with the mRNA codon, making sure amino acids are added to the protein in the right order. Errors in translation can result in unhealthy proteins in the cells. Besides, post-translational modifications (PTMs) can make changes to proteins, which help them function better, go to certain places, or be broken down. All these processes prove the complexity of the mechanisms that manage RNA synthesis and protein translation, which are key aspects of medical biochemistry. Moreover, disturbances in RNA synthesis and protein translation are linked to many diseases, which proves their importance in clinical medicine. It has been found that in Alzheimer's disease, problems with protein synthesis are related to the loss of brain cells. Research indicates that ER stress activates the unfolded protein response (UPR), with downstream effects on global protein synthesis and selective translation of proteins like activating transcriptor factor 4 (ATF4) associated with cellular stress responses (Diehl et al., 2016). Additionally, in conditions such as osteoporosis, transcription factors like Nuclear Matrix Protein 4 (Nmp4) significantly influence gene expression related to bone formation, affecting the outcomes of therapeutic interventions (Adaway et al., 2019). They highlight how RNA synthesis, protein translation, and disease mechanisms are closely connected and important for fighting different diseases.

1.4.3. Genetic Mutations and Their Biochemical Consequences

It is important to study genetic mutations and their effects on biochemistry to understand different metabolic disorders. Mutations can happen in the DNA inside the nucleus or in the mitochondria, and this can cause some enzymes needed for biochemical pathways to be defective. As an example, mitochondrial diseases usually occur when there are mutations in electron transport chain complexes, which results in less ATP and more oxidative stress. Recent advancements in techniques such as electron paramagnetic resonance (EPR) spectroscopy have enhanced our ability to detect and characterize these dysfunctions in vitro. By assessing changes in the redox state of mitochondrial components, EPR provides insight into the molecular mechanisms driving the pathology of these diseases, which is vital for developing targeted therapeutic strategies and diagnostic tools as outlined in recent studies demonstrating its application in mitochondrial disease models (Bennett et al., 2016). Disturbances in the way nucleotides are metabolized are a major factor in how diseases are expressed. Orotic aciduria, for example, is a disorder characterized by elevated orotic acid levels due to genetic defects in the bifunctional enzyme uridine monophosphate synthase (UMPS). Such a condition can result in megaloblastic anemia and delays in development, which happen due to the body's inability to synthesize pyrimidines for DNA and RNA. Those with orotic aciduria usually have symptoms that can be seen early in life, underlining the need for fast diagnosis. Effective treatment options such as Xuriden have emerged, underscoring how understanding the precise biochemical pathways altered by genetic mutations can lead to impactful therapeutic interventions (Fonteh, 2018). Even though genetic mutations may be the cause of metabolic disorders, their effects are seen throughout many cellular functions. In these situations, we can see how mutations in genes and changes in cellular chemistry affect the patient's health. As an example, in mitochondrial diseases, the inefficient ATP synthesis leads to more cellular damage by increasing the amount of ROS. Combining genetics and biochemistry will allow us to understand these interactions better, which may lead to new ways of treating patients. Once these mechanisms are clarified, they will be vital for creating personalized medicine that is based on each person's unique genes and the effects they have in the body from a biochemical point of view (Figure 1.15).

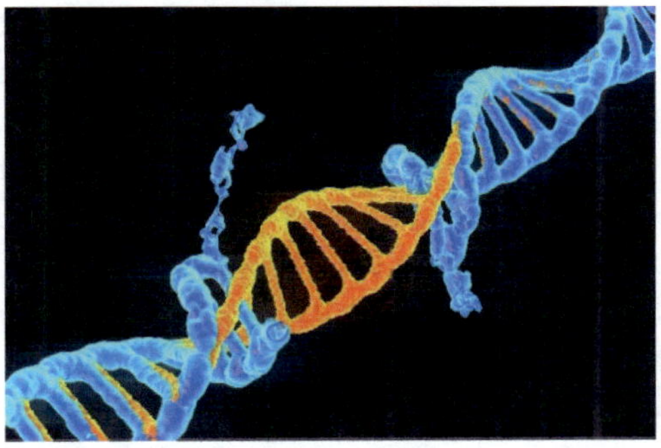

Figure 1.15. Colored 3D representation of a DNA double helix strand.

Source: https://www.health.com/thmb/IiTPaos2TQl21Pz6booXaJ7HfSQ=/1500x0/filters:no_upscale():max_bytes(150000):strip_icc()/GettyImages-1167533800-4661243613304c548ed0275a4943fb30.jpg.

Test Your Knowledge

1. What is the structure of the DNA?
2. What are genetic mutations and their consequences?

1.5. Hormones and Signaling Molecules

Learning Outcome

1. Describe the types of hormones and their functions;
2. Understand the mechanisms of hormone action;
3. Describe the hormonal imbalances and related diseases.

The functions of the body are supported by the complex system of cellular communication involving hormones and signaling molecules. Hormones, made by the endocrine glands, move in the blood to reach target organs or tissues, where they attach to certain receptors and cause reactions. They can include regulating metabolism as well as controlling growth and development, proving how vital hormones are for keeping the body stable. Hormones are either hydrophilic and work on the surface of the cell, or hydrophobic and enter the cell to attach to receptors inside, which affects genes and the cell's function. Different peptide hormones and their substrates prove that hormones have a wide range of specific functions. For example, dipeptidyl peptidase 4 (DPP4) cleaves several hormones such as glucagon-like peptide 1 (GLP-1) and glucose-dependent insulinotropic polypeptide (GIP), raising questions about their functions after cleavage. Experts have recently shown that DPP4-cleaved peptides do have activity, as they may behave differently and bind to various receptors than unmodified peptides. DPP4-cleaved GLP-1 has been found to work through receptors that are not the usual ones. This discovery emphasizes the need to revisit the biological functions of such peptides in order to appreciate their complete range of activities and related implications in metabolic disease so as to highlight the pivotal interface of hormones and signaling molecules in clinical biochemistry (Elmansi et al., 2019). Also, by better understanding DPP4 and its substrates, we can see how complicated hormone signaling is and identify useful areas for further research and treatment. The discovery of new evidence about the activity of DPP4-cleaved ligands has led more people to believe that these interactions can strongly affect the outcomes of diabetes and other metabolic diseases. So, it is important for clinicians to recognize both the whole and the broken-down forms of peptide hormones because of DPP4 inhibitors. It is very important to understand the actions of modified ligands in inflammation, immunology, and diseases when planning treatment. Therefore, hormone and signaling molecule exploration is not merely a scholarly endeavor but seeking to understand mechanisms that may result in novel therapies in different medical disciplines (Kumar & McEwan, 2012).

1.5.1. Types of Hormones and Their Functions

Hormones play a key role in the body by signaling different processes to take place. They are mainly classified as peptide hormones, steroid hormones, and amine hormones. Insulin and glucagon are examples of peptide hormones that consist of amino acids and function by binding to certain receptors in cells, which starts a series of reactions inside the cell. It helps to control metabolism and growth with great accuracy. Alternatively, steroid hormones, which come from lipids, can get into cells and connect with receptors inside the cell to influence gene activity. The fact that they take time to work is necessary for long-term changes in the body, as in puberty or when dealing with stress. Since hormones play many important roles in keeping the body stable and functioning well, studying their roles in medical biochemistry is necessary. Apart from peptide and steroid hormones, amine hormones, such as catecholamines including adrenaline, are also very important in hormone-mediated signaling. Cortisol and epinephrine are made from amino acids, mainly tyrosine and tryptophan, and they are mainly responsible for the body's quick reaction to stress. Amine hormones help the body change fast in response to changes in the environment. As an example, adrenaline helps the body use its energy by raising the heart rate and releasing glucose from its energy stores. Furthermore, the discovery of DPP4 as an exopeptidase has introduced a novel understanding of hormone interactions, particularly concerning its role in cleaving various peptide substrates. The cleaved forms of these hormones may exhibit distinct bioactivities, suggesting the complexity of hormonal regulation in health and disease (Elmansi et al., 2019). As a result, scientists look more closely into how these peptides can be used in therapy by changing the receptors they interact with. Because of these newly discovered complexities, scientists should now focus more on how hormones function, especially due to DPP4 cleavage. The lack of information in the literature points out the importance of carefully studying these cleaved peptides, since they could serve as different signaling pathways or new ways to treat diseases. For example, DPP4-cleaved GLP-1 has been shown to exhibit different receptor selectivity, suggesting that its biological activity may extend beyond traditional expectations. Moreover, the implications for diabetes care are significant, as medications like DPP4 inhibitors can alter the function of these ligands, thereby influencing metabolic outcomes (Arnold et al., 2001). Learning more about these mechanisms might help doctors create new treatments for obesity, heart diseases, and MS by using hormone-based therapies for patients (Figure 1.16).

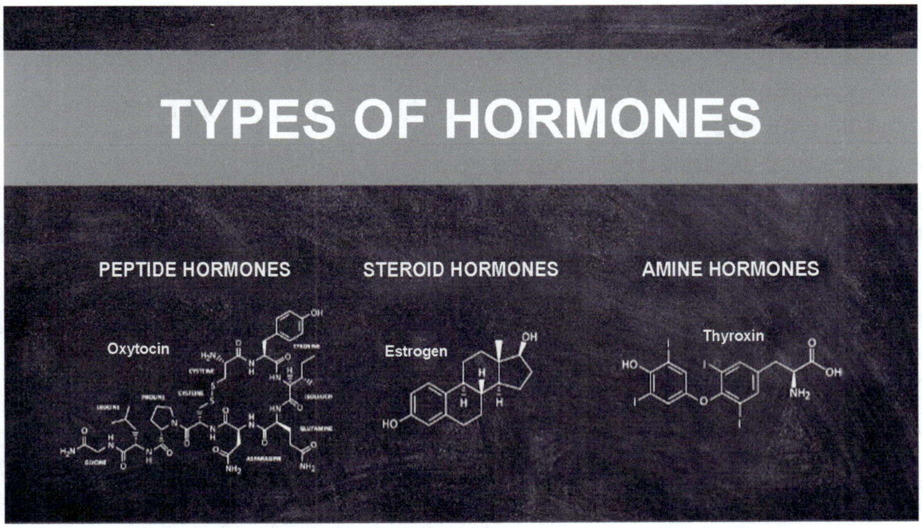

Figure 1.16. Types of hormones.

Source: https://i.ytimg.com/vi/zZjdMyQ9rVg/maxresdefault.jpg.

1.5.2. Mechanisms of Hormone Action

Hormones help the body remain stable and manage different functions. They mostly use two main ways to work: endocrine and paracrine signaling systems. Hormones are released into the bloodstream by the endocrine system and then go to target tissues to cause certain reactions. Paracrine signaling happens when hormones work on the nearby cells instead of on distant organs. This leads to quick changes in the local area because it acts on certain cells by interacting with receptors and triggering a series of signals inside these cells that increase the uptake of glucose. Understanding these pathways precisely is essential to medical biochemistry, where disruptions in hormonal signaling lead to metabolic disorders and other health problems; it is particularly important to advance further the mechanisms under study (Sarmidi, 2012). The way hormones work with their special receptors best shows how detailed and specific hormone action is. Their chemical features vary widely, so steroids can pass through cell walls, but peptide hormones need surface receptors to trigger actions in the cell. Such a distinction matters a lot because it determines the cellular reactions that happen. For example, steroid hormones, such as cortisol, can directly influence gene expression by binding to intracellular receptors, whereas peptide hormones initiate signaling cascades via G-protein coupled receptors (GPCRs).

They show that hormones use a variety of ways to control metabolism, growth, and homeostasis. A complex appreciation of these processes not only expands our appreciation for physiology but also guides the construction of therapeutic strategies designed to restore normal hormone function in disease states (Kumar & McEwan, 2012). Also, the way hormones connect with other biochemical pathways points to the fact that metabolism is regulated by several factors. Hormones work together with other cellular activities that depend on the body's nutritional status, the environment, and energy needs. For instance, insulin is linked with glucagon and other hormones that together manage the level of glucose in the body. In addition, the components found in food can change how hormones are received and processed by cells. These many interactions show that medical biochemistry needs to be studied using systemic and holistic methods. In understanding these relationships, one is better suited to devise a plan that ensures optimal metabolic health and possibly tackles disorders as a result of hormonal imbalances (Sarmidi, 2012) (Figure 1.17).

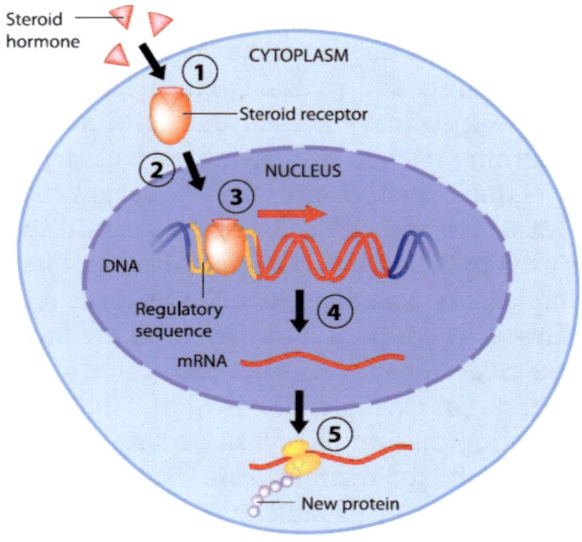

Figure 11.18: Mechanism of steroid hormone action

Figure 1.17. Mechanism of steroid hormone action.

Source: https://img.brainkart.com/imagebk34/Nz59OZr.jpg.

1.5.3. Hormonal Imbalances and Related Diseases

More and more, it is understood that hormonal imbalances play a major role in many diseases, mainly those involving the digestive system and reproductive organs. In disorders such as irritable bowel syndrome (IBS) and inflammatory bowel disease (IBD), fluctuations in hormonal levels can exacerbate symptoms like abdominal pain, bloating, and irregular bowel movements. It has been found in recent studies that hormones, mainly progesterone, could be responsible for these symptoms. Sometimes, surges in progesterone can lead to symptoms similar to IBS, proving how closely hormones and the gut are connected. Understanding these hormonal influences presents an opportunity for novel therapeutic strategies aimed at addressing the underlying causes of these debilitating conditions rather than merely alleviating symptoms, as indicated in recent studies exploring hormonal-based treatments (Linson et al., 2013). Many couples across the globe suffer from male infertility due to hormonal imbalances in the reproductive health field. The interplay between various hormones, including testosterone, luteinizing hormone (LH), and follicle-stimulating hormone (FSH), is crucial for maintaining male reproductive function. If the hormones are not at the right level, it can result in fewer and poorer sperm, which can harm a person's ability to have children. The latest findings point out that it is important to use detailed diagnostic methods to measure hormones in people with infertility. When these hormonal problems are recognized, healthcare providers can choose treatments that match the patient's unique needs. This comprehensive approach acknowledges the multifactorial nature of infertility, providing a pathway toward more effective management strategies (AlAsmi, 2025). Hormonal imbalances can cause more than gastrointestinal and reproductive problems, affecting the whole body. Diabetes and MS are closely related to hormonal problems, mainly because of insulin and glucagon. They demonstrate that metabolic hormones are responsible for keeping energy levels in balance and affecting a person's overall health. If hormones do not function properly, patients can develop insulin resistance, which increases their chances of becoming obese and suffering from heart diseases. Knowing about the biochemical pathways involved in hormone regulation may help create new treatments that bring hormone levels back to normal. As a result, these approaches reveal the key role of medical biochemistry since they show both the immediate body responses to hormonal changes and their effects on the health of the population (Figure 1.18).

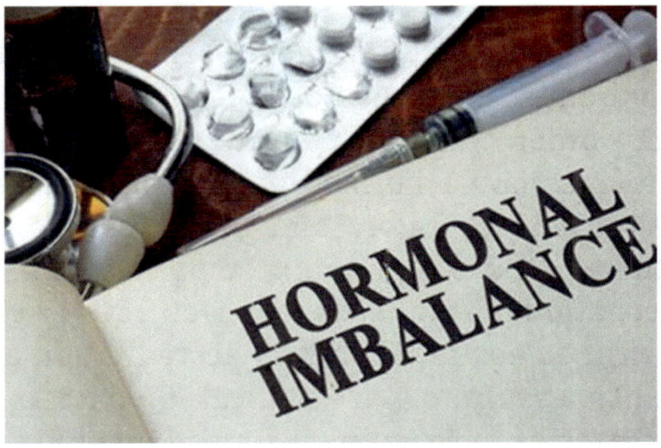

Figure 1.18. Hormonal imbalance.

Source: https://smb.ibsrv.net/imageresizer/image/article_manager/1200x1200/117000/606058/heroimage0.628870001653333959.jpg.

Test Your Knowledge

1. What are the three types of hormones?
2. What are the mechanisms of hormone action?

1.6. Clinical Applications of Medical Biochemistry

Learning Outcome

1. Describe the diagnostic techniques in biochemistry;
2. Understand role of biochemical markers in disease management;
3. Explore the therapeutic interventions based on biochemical principles.

Besides finding out the levels of biochemical compounds, medical biochemistry is used in many other clinical applications. Laboratory medicine should be incorporated into patient care to ensure safety and better results for patients. One of the main steps is to follow international standards, such as ISO 15189, when it comes to laboratory accreditation and quality assurance. If medical biochemistry laboratories focus on high service quality, they can help patients be managed more effectively through precise and prompt testing. Moreover, laboratory leadership plays a crucial role in harnessing the potential of these disciplines to "add value" in various domains, such as clinical effectiveness and cost-effectiveness, thereby enriching the overall healthcare system (Beastall, 2013). Properly identifying patients can be the main factor in making a clinical application in medical biochemistry efficient. Mistaken identifications cause significant problems because they result in wrong test results and can harm people's health. This is because there are many reasons like homonymy and wrong patient information, so laboratories need strong ways to identify patients. Innovative identifiers and new technology can lessen the risks that occur in laboratory procedures. The use of effective strategies and advanced technology in laboratories improves the quality of sample labels and the way results are sent. Such efforts are crucial not only for individual patient safety but also for the overall integrity of laboratory medicine (Lippi et al., 2017). Medical biochemistry makes it possible to give patients personalized medical care. By knowing the molecular reasons behind diseases, clinicians can choose the best treatment for each patient. In addition, it makes therapies more effective and less likely to cause dangerous side effects from drugs. The combination of biochemistry and methods like genomics and proteomics makes it possible to study how diseases work. In the end, medical biochemistry plays an important role in advancing precision medicine, as it helps doctors manage patients better and achieve better health results using personalized treatments.

1.6.1. Diagnostic Techniques in Biochemistry

Modern biochemistry has changed the way doctors and other medical staff handle the detection and management of diseases. At first, diagnostics relied on simple observations of the body and its parts, but now they go beyond just using doctors' intuition. Today's diagnostics make use of different biochemical tests that depend on certain biomarkers to detect and track diseases. As an example, the progress of serological tests for infectious diseases demonstrates how science has improved, making it easier and faster to detect pathogens by analyzing the immune system. By using high-throughput screening and automated laboratory systems, the process of testing has improved, giving doctors the key information they need to act fast. Furthermore, the adaptation of these approaches emphasizes the necessity for ongoing education and training, enabling health professionals to effectively utilize sophisticated diagnostic tools in practice (Galdames, 2024). A significant change in diagnostic biochemistry is the introduction of synthetic antibodies, which may be a better alternative to monoclonal antibodies. Even though monoclonal antibodies are known for their accuracy in targeting biomarkers, there are still ethical and financial issues that need to be dealt with. The development of synthetic antibodies that incorporate novel elements, such as 3,4-dihydroxy-l-phenylalanine (L-DOPA), demonstrates potential for enhanced binding capabilities while circumventing some limitations of monoclonal antibodies. As a result, new innovations might make it easier and less expensive for people to detect cancers, especially prostate cancer, which needs to be found early for successful treatment. By providing comparable specificity to existing diagnostic methods, synthetic antibodies represent a significant advancement within medical biochemistry, highlighting the importance of ongoing research in the field (Batiuk et al., 2017).

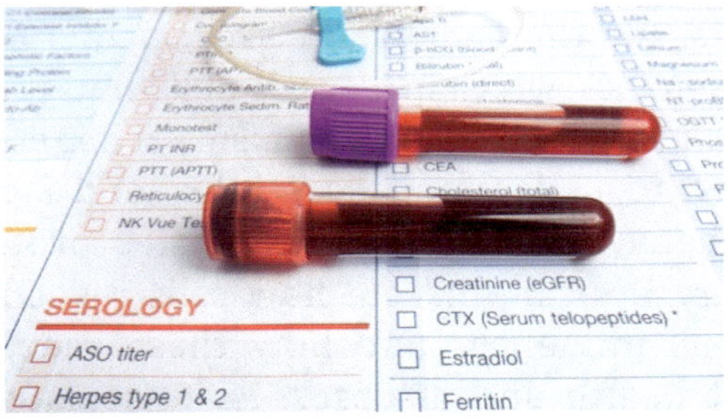

Figure 1.19. Serological tests.

Source: https://www.thomsonmedical.com/_next/image?url=https%3A%2F%2Fimages.contentstack.io%2Fv3%2Fassets%2Fblt5f400315f9e4f0b3%2Fblt3500a68e762d37ac%2F68104a0077bfb629074b6979%2Fscreening_serology-test_hero-image.png%3Fbranch%3Dprod&w=3840&q=75.

The incorporation of artificial intelligence (AI) into biochemical diagnostics further illustrates the transformative potential of technology in healthcare. AI systems help analyze large amounts of data and notice patterns that are not easy to see with traditional methods. As a result, tests are more accurate and can help develop personalized medicine that fits each person's needs. With the progress of healthcare, it will be necessary for medical professionals to blend their medical knowledge with skills in technology. Yet, since data privacy and algorithmic bias are ethically important, it is necessary to focus on what is best for patients. To cultivate this dual skill set, medical education must adapt, integrating digital literacy alongside traditional clinical training, preparing future physicians to navigate an increasingly digitized landscape of medical diagnostics (Galdames, 2024) (Figure 1.19).

1.6.2. Biochemical Markers in Disease Management

Biochemical markers are now more important in managing diseases in the field of medical biochemistry. They help healthcare providers spot different medical conditions, predict how the disease will progress, and check if the treatment is effective. The existence of certain biomarkers can point to the start or spread of a disease, as well as the patient's reaction to treatment, giving important information about their health. Even though biochemical markers have a huge potential, they are still not used widely or are misread in clinical settings, which is why it is necessary to make biomarker testing a regular part of patient care. This challenge arises from a mindset that often suggests the mere availability of tests warrants using them, disregarding judgment as necessary for actualist clinical decision-making (Buhagiar et al., 2005). The use of biochemical markers is very important in oncology and can be directly used to manage breast cancer. Even though serum markers are not helpful for early detection, they can identify if the disease has come back after a period of observation. For instance, monitoring is feasible with serum markers like CA 15.3 and carcinoembryonic antigen (CEA) in breast cancer. Also, markers found in tissue are crucial for designing the best treatment strategy. The estrogen and progesterone receptors are necessary for deciding whether hormone therapy is suitable. Besides, it is necessary to assess HER-2 status to decide who should get trastuzumab treatment. Therefore, the effective employment of these biomarkers not only aids in survival rates but also improves the quality of life as lived with cancer (Abraha et al., 2005). Standardization of using and interpreting the developed biomarkers is still a problem in different areas of medicine. That means that most of the biomarkers used in clinical settings are not very sensitive or specific, which makes their use in managing diseases difficult. On the other side, laboratories struggle to check the reliability of the new tests as they handle a lot of other tasks. Therefore, it is important for clinicians and laboratory workers to join forces, so that only necessary and useful tests are carried out. The advancement of biochemical markers in disease management necessitates ongoing education and a shift in the culture of laboratory utilization, promoting evidence-based practices that can ultimately lead to better clinical outcomes and rational healthcare spending (Buhagiar et al., 2005) (Figure 1.20).

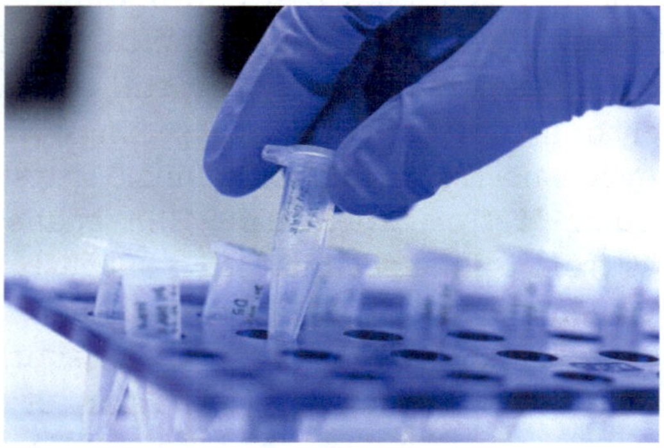

Figure 1.20. Gloved hand handling microcentrifuge tubes for PCR analysis.

Source: https://media.istockphoto.com/id/1186871650/photo/polymerase-chain-reaction-and-agarose-gel-electrophoresis-is-a-method-of-gel-electrophoresis.jpg?s=612x612&w=0&k=20&c=rfPDWYdGnJoEz_B65pgo0mXyGId8y11R6q05Zil3LSQ=.

1.6.3. Therapeutic Interventions Based on Biochemical Principles

In medical biochemistry, looking into treatments based on biochemical processes is very important. Researchers and clinicians can design drugs that address specific biochemical problems in diseases by knowing about cellular biochemical pathways. Therapies involving enzymes are being used more often, especially when it comes to treating genetic disorders that are caused by enzyme shortages. As a result, these interventions get the biochemistry back to normal in the affected areas and help ease the symptoms, which is good for the patient. Better understanding of how molecules and signals work has made it possible to design biopharmaceuticals that target particular disease processes more precisely, so patients get the best treatment with the fewest side effects. Another important area in therapy is optogenetics, which makes use of light to control cellular activity in living organisms. It has greatly helped to understand how cells send signals and behave. Using light-responsive proteins, researchers can find out how cells respond to various influences and how these reactions affect health and diseases. As articulated in recent studies, optogenetics promises to deepen our understanding of cellular perception and its regulatory role in normal and pathological functions, leading to refinements in therapeutic approaches for neurodegenerative diseases, cancers, and other conditions where cellular signaling is dysregulated (Bugaj et al., 2017). Combining light-based techniques with biochemistry opens up new ways to treat diseases, proving the flexibility of biochemistry in today's medicine. Besides, homeopathy uses a contrasting strategy for biochemical therapy and has been applied for more than two centuries. Even though traditional pharmacology follows well-known biochemical rules, homeopathy uses different concepts. According to detailed studies, many people use homeopathy as an alternative or in addition to regular treatments when the main treatments do not work. People continue to question homeopathy's credibility in the law and science, mainly because there is not enough biochemical evidence to show that it works.

Nonetheless, some veterinary surgeons and practitioners argue for its application, particularly in cases where patients exhibit resistance to standard treatments (Lees et al., 2017). The difference between drug-based pharmacology and homeopathy shows the need to base medical treatments on well-tested biochemical principles for better patient outcomes.

Test Your Knowledge

1. What are the different diagnostic techniques in biochemistry?
2. What is the role of biochemical markers in disease management?

SUMMARY

To sum up, medical biochemistry is vital for increasing our knowledge of different functions in the body and diseases. We have seen in this chapter that both biochemical pathways and molecular mechanisms are important for diagnosing and treating diseases, so it is essential to have thorough education in this area. The application of advanced analytical techniques, such as item response theory (IRT), illustrates the significance of refining assessment methodologies to ensure that student comprehension is accurately measured. With evidence of improved examination outcomes and enhanced educational standards presented in studies, a clear pathway emerges for integrating innovative teaching strategies into biochemistry curricula, ultimately empowering future healthcare professionals with the necessary knowledge and skills to navigate complex medical scenarios (Baharuddin et al., 2024). Furthermore, the investigations into enzyme activity, such as glutathione S transferase (GST), reveal the biochemical underpinnings of various physiological responses and the impacts of lifestyle choices, such as alcohol consumption. Before and after someone stops drinking alcohol, GST activity changes a lot, which suggests that the enzyme could be used to predict outcomes and guide patient care. Such insights reinforce the importance of medical biochemistry not only as a specialized field but also as an essential component in the broader context of public health and medicine (Bhandary et al., 2009). So, realizing how biochemical education and clinical practice are linked is necessary for training medical professionals ready to handle present-day health issues. When all the findings are put together, it is clear that advances in medical biochemistry play an important role in education and clinical work. The new ways of assessing students in medical education increase the quality of their education and help them give better care to patients. All in all, using IRT in education and studying GST shows a promising path for future research and medical care. It is through such integrative efforts that the field will continue to evolve, ensuring that medical professionals are adept in utilizing biochemical insights to inform patient care and enhance overall health outcomes (Bhandary et al., 2009; Baharuddin et al., 2024).

It is very important in medical biochemistry to grasp how different biochemical processes relate to diseases. The use of additional therapies to help improve patient care, mainly in dealing with serious diseases such as severe malaria, is a main priority. Recent studies indicate the potential of oral activated charcoal (oAC) in reducing mortality associated with experimental cerebral malaria (ECM) in mouse models. It is clear from the results that oAC helps patients live longer, as it affects the immune system and different markers related to ECM. This positions oAC as a promising candidate for further exploration in human clinical trials, given its low cost, accessibility, and safety profiles, thus underscoring its relevance in public health initiatives aimed at minimizing malaria-related mortality (de Souza et al., 2010). Also, medical biochemistry is giving more attention to how pharmacogenomics supports personalized medicine. The importance of genetic variability in drug metabolism is clear, especially for the cytochrome P450 enzyme system that helps metabolize a lot of medicines. Students in medicine are taught to consider how genetic information affects the decisions doctors make. For example, case studies of patients with different reactions to opioids and anticoagulants prove that genetics can play a big part in how drugs work and how safe they are. This highlights the necessity for future healthcare providers to integrate genetic insights into their practice to optimize pharmacotherapy (Blevins et al., 2020). Moreover, when biochemistry is combined with clinical practice, it helps people understand how drugs interact and what effects they have on patients. Exploring the use of oAC with standard treatments shows that new approaches can be used to fight serious diseases. At the same time, pharmacogenomics makes it possible for doctors to manage patients individually by selecting treatments that fit each patient's genetic information. They both point out the need for teamwork between biochemists and those working in healthcare. This comprehensive approach not only enhances treatment efficacy but also paves the way for advancements in medical research that can significantly influence patient outcomes in various healthcare settings (de Souza et al., 2010; Blevins et al., 2020).

KEY TERMS FROM THIS CHAPTER

- Biochemical analysis
- Biochemistry
- Drug interactions
- Leadership
- Novel therapeutic agents
- Personalized medicine
- Pharmacokinetics
- Targeted therapies
- Biochemical markers
- Breast cancer
- Evidence-based practices
- Medical biochemistry
- Patient identification
- Pharmacodynamics
- Sample labeling

CRITICAL THINKING QUESTIONS

1. **What is the primary role of biochemistry in medicine?**
   a. To study the structure of cells
   b. To diagnose and manage diseases through chemical processes
   c. To identify environmental toxins
   d. To analyze mechanical functions of organs
2. **Which of the following is a biomolecule?**
   a. Glucose
   b. Sodium chloride
   c. Carbon dioxide
   d. Oxygen
3. **What is the fundamental building block of proteins?**
   a. Fatty acids
   b. Amino acids
   c. Monosaccharides
   d. Nucleotides
4. **Which biomolecule serves as the main energy currency of the cell?**
   a. DNA
   b. ATP
   c. RNA
   d. Glucose
5. **What is the study of chemical reactions within living organisms called?**
   a. Biophysics
   b. Biochemistry
   c. Microbiology
   d. Pharmacology

Answers to Critical Thinking Questions

1. (b); 2. (a); 3. (b); 4. (b); 5. (b)

Short Answer Questions

1. Define the medical biochemistry.
2. Why is clinical biochemistry important in the medical field?
3. Who discovered the structure of the DNA?
4. What is the significance of biomolecules in the medical field?
5. What is a metabolic pathway?

REFERENCES

1. Lees, P., Pelligand, L., Whiting, M., Chambers, D., Toutain, P. L., & Whitehead, M. L. (2017). Comparison of veterinary drugs and veterinary homeopathy: part 1. *The Veterinary record, 181*(7), 170–176. https://doi.org/10.1136/vr.104278 (accessed on 11th June 2025).
2. Abdelfatah, S., Abu-Darwish, M. S., Banerjee, M., Bhakta-Guha, D., et al. (2019). Biopiracy *versus* one-world medicine–from colonial relicts to global collaborative concepts. https://core.ac.uk/download/228178415.pdf (accessed on 11th June 2025).
3. Abdolrahim, M., Alhosseini, S. N., Rabiee, M., Tahriri, M., et al. (2015). Development of optical biosensor technologies for cardiac troponin recognition. https://core.ac.uk/download/213059311.pdf (accessed on 11th June 2025).
4. Bräutigam, L., Zhang, J., Dreij, K., Spahiu, L., Holmgren, A., Abe, H., Tew, K. D., Townsend, D. M., Kelner, M. J., Morgenstern, R., & Johansson, K. (2018). MGST1, a GSH transferase/peroxidase essential for development and hematopoietic stem cell differentiation. *Redox biology, 17*, 171–179. https://doi.org/10.1016/j.redox.2018.04.013 (accessed on 11th June 2025).
5. Abraha, R. S., Andreasen, P. A., van Dalen, A., ASCO Expert Panel, Barak, V., Barnes, D. M., Baselga, J., et al. (2005). Tumor markers in breast cancer–European Group on Tumor Markers recommendations. https://core.ac.uk/download/16432224.pdf (accessed on 11th June 2025).
6. Abramić, M., Babić, D., Ilić-Forko, J., Osmak, M., et al. (2008). Total tissue lactate dehydrogenase activity in endometrial carcinoma. https://core.ac.uk/download/11699771.pdf (accessed on 11th June 2025).
7. Kumar, R., & McEwan, I. J. (2012). Allosteric modulators of steroid hormone receptors: structural dynamics and gene regulation. *Endocrine reviews, 33*(2), 271–299. https://doi.org/10.1210/er.2011-1033(accessed on 11th June 2025).
8. Lippi, G., Chiozza, L., Mattiuzzi, C., & Plebani, M. (2017). Patient and Sample Identification. Out of the Maze?. *Journal of medical biochemistry, 36*(2), 107–112. https://doi.org/10.1515/jomb-2017-0003 (accessed on 11th June 2025).
9. Adaway, M., Allen, M. R., Bidwell, J. P., Brustovetsky, T., et al. (2019). Loss of Nmp4 optimizes osteogenic metabolism and secretion to enhance bone quality. https://core.ac.uk/download/187423805.pdf (accessed on 11th June 2025).
10. Adedoyin, O., Aleksandrov, A., Bard, S., Barla, A., Baslas, N., Chanda, V., Colley, D., et al. (2019). *Euphorbia*-derived natural products with potential for use in health maintenance. https://core.ac.uk/download/232150563.pdf (accessed on 11th June 2025).
11. Beastall G. H. (2013). Adding value to laboratory medicine: a professional responsibility. *Clinical chemistry and laboratory medicine, 51*(1), 221–227. https://doi.org/10.1515/cclm-2012-0630(accessed on 11th June 2025).
12. Elmansi, A. M., Awad, M. E., Eisa, N. H., Kondrikov, D., Hussein, K. A., Aguilar-Pérez, A., Herberg, S., Periyasamy-Thandavan, S., Fulzele, S., Hamrick, M. W., McGee-Lawrence, M. E., Isales, C. M., Volkman, B. F., & Hill, W. D. (2019). What doesn't kill you makes you stranger: Dipeptidyl peptidase-4 (CD26) proteolysis differentially modulates the activity of many peptide hormones and cytokines generating novel cryptic bioactive ligands. *Pharmacology & therapeutics, 198*, 90–108. https://doi.org/10.1016/j.pharmthera.2019.02.005(accessed on 11th June 2025).

13. Ahmed, A., Batool, K., Bibi, A., Faiz, N., et al. (2017). Microbial β-glucosidase: Sources, production and applications. https://core.ac.uk/download/188825639.pdf (accessed on 11th June 2025).

14. Chasapi A, Aivaliotis M, Angelis L, Chanalaris A, Iliopoulos I, Kappas I, et al. (2019) Establishment of computational biology in Greece and Cyprus: Past, present, and future. PLoS Comput Biol 15(12): e1007532. https://doi.org/10.1371/journal.pcbi.1007532 (accessed on 11th June 2025).

15. AlAsmi, R. (2025). *Hormonal Dysfunction and Male Infertility: A Comprehensive Review of Current Treatment Options*. https://core.ac.uk/download/640070691.pdf (accessed on 11th June 2025).

16. de Souza, J. B., Okomo, U., Alexander, N. D., Aziz, N., Owens, B. M., Kaur, H., Jasseh, M., Muangnoicharoen, S., Sumariwalla, P. F., Warhurst, D. C., Ward, S. A., Conway, D. J., Ulloa, L., Tracey, K. J., Foxwell, B. M., Kaye, P. M., & Walther, M. (2010). Oral activated charcoal prevents experimental cerebral malaria in mice and in a randomized controlled clinical trial in man did not interfere with the pharmacokinetics of parenteral artesunate. *PloS one*, *5*(4), e9867. https://doi.org/10.1371/journal.pone.0009867 (accessed on 11th June 2025).

17. Aljohani, N. R., Bowman, T. D., Didegah, F., Gillani, N., et al. (2017). Measuring social media activity of scientific literature: An exhaustive comparison of Scopus and novel altimetric big data. http://arxiv.org/abs/1705.03258 (accessed on 11th June 2025).

18. Marrocco, I., Altieri, F., & Peluso, I. (2017). Measurement and Clinical Significance of Biomarkers of Oxidative Stress in Humans. *Oxidative medicine and cellular longevity*, *2017*, 6501046. https://doi.org/10.1155/2017/6501046(accessed on 11th June 2025).

19. Anderson, J. G., Goudie, A. C., MacGregor, S. J., Olateju, O. M., et al. (2003). Inactivation of pathogens on food and contact surfaces using ozone as a biocidal agent. https://core.ac.uk/download/9020578.pdf (accessed on 11th June 2025).

20. Arnold, B. S., Gross, T. S., McDonald, K., Spulveda, M. S., et al. (2001). Relations of environmental contaminants, algal toxins, and diet with the reproductive success of American alligators on Florida lakes. https://core.ac.uk/download/11016994.pdf (accessed on 11th June 2025).

21. Baharuddin, B., Handayani, L., & Rusli, R. (2024). Enhancing biochemistry assessment quality in medical education through item response theory (IRT). https://core.ac.uk/download/597535963.pdf (accessed on 11th June 2025).

22. Batiuk, E., Kiyohara, C., & Nguyen, T. (2017). Engineering synthetic antibody by expanded genetic code. https://core.ac.uk/download/84118620.pdf (accessed on 11th June 2025).

23. Bell, J. C., Kowalczykowski, S. C., & Liu, B. (2015). Imaging and energetics of single SSB-ssDNA molecules reveal intramolecular condensation and insight into RecOR function. https://core.ac.uk/download/323065735.pdf (accessed on 11th June 2025).

24. Bennett, B., Dimmock, D. P., Friederich, M. W., Geurts, J., et al. (2016). Potentially diagnostic electron paramagnetic resonance spectra elucidate the underlying mechanism of mitochondrial dysfunction in the deoxyguanosine kinase deficient rat model of a genetic mitochondrial DNA depletion syndrome. https://core.ac.uk/download/213064759.pdf (accessed on 11th June 2025).

25. Bennett, B., Fung, L. W. M., Horner, J. A., Newcomb, M., et al. (2010). Low temperature photo-

oxidation of chloroperoxidase compound II. https://core.ac.uk/download/213080479.pdf (accessed on 11th June 2025).

26. Bhandary, P. V., Kedage, V., Muttigi, M. S., Prabhu, K., et al. (2009). Glutathione S-transferase activity and total thiol status in chronic alcohol abusers before and 30 days after alcohol abstinence. https://core.ac.uk/download/pdf/87217.pdf (accessed on 11th June 2025)

27. Bhat, G. P., & Varashree, B. S. (2011). Correlation of lipid peroxidation with glycated hemoglobin levels in diabetes mellitus. https://core.ac.uk/download/pdf/13598630.pdf (accessed on 11th June 2025).

28. Blevins, A. E., Foster, E. D., Harrington, M. A., Pratt, S. D., et al. (2020). Introducing first year medical students to personalized medicine concepts in a small group activity. https://core.ac.uk/download/322846987.pdf (accessed on 11th June 2025).

29. Bolon, D. N., & Mayo, S. L. (2001). Polar residues in the protein core of *Escherichia coli* thioredoxin are important for fold specificity. https://core.ac.uk/download/4889512.pdf (accessed on 11th June 2025).

30. Buang, Y. (Yohanes) (2010). The effects of dietary food fortified with vitamin B4 on lipid profiles in serum and liver tissue. https://media.neliti.com/media/publications/148709-EN-the-effects-of-dietary-food-fortified-wi.pdf (accessed on 11th June 2025).

31. Bugaj, L. J., Lim, W. A., O'Donoghue, G. P. (2017). Interrogating cellular perception and decision making with optogenetic tools. https://core.ac.uk/download/323072710.pdf (accessed on 11th June 2025).

32. Buhagiar, G. (2005). Rationalization of the biochemistry laboratory: Which way forwards? https://core.ac.uk/download/46602008.pdf (accessed on 11th June 2025).

33. Cao, R., Durrant, J. D., Gorfe, A. A., Li, L., et al. (2011). Non-bisphosphonate inhibitors of isoprenoid biosynthesis identified via computer-aided drug design. https://core.ac.uk/download/323066371.pdf (accessed on 11th June 2025).

34. Carter, C. S., Justice, J. N., & Thompson, L. (2019). Lipotoxicity, aging, and muscle contractility: Does fiber type matter? https://open.bu.edu/bitstream/2144/40625/7/carter_justice_thompson_Lipotoxicity_paper_04302019.pdf (accessed on 11th June 2025).

35. Cort, A., De Luca, C., Korkina, L., Ozben, T., et al. (2016). Redox control of multidrug resistance and its possible modulation by antioxidants. https://core.ac.uk/download/74320865.pdf (accessed on 11th June 2025).

36. Costa-Pinto, A., Neves, N. M., Reis, R. L., Santos, M. I., et al. (2016). Testing natural biomaterials in animal models. https://core.ac.uk/download/155248253.pdf (accessed on 11th June 2025).

37. Demling, R. H. (2011). Nutrition, anabolism, and the wound healing process: An overview. https://core.ac.uk/download/28936579.pdf (accessed on 11th June 2025).

38. Devincenzi, D. L., & Pleasant, L. G. (2025). *Publications of the Exobiology Program for 1979: A Special Bibliography*. https://core.ac.uk/download/pdf/42863116.pdf (accessed on 11th June 2025).

39. Diehl, J. A., Lewko, D., Majsterek, I., Nowak, M., et al. (2016). The role of the amyloid precursor protein mutations and PERK-dependent signaling pathways in the pathogenesis of Alzheimer's disease. https://core.ac.uk/download/80535082.pdf (accessed on 11th June 2025).

40. Eraly, S. A., Jamshidi, N., Liu, H. C., Nigam, S. K., et al. (2015). Transcriptome-based reconstructions from the murine knockout suggest involvement of the urate transporter, URAT1 (*slc22a12*), in novel metabolic pathways. https://core.ac.uk/download/323080180.pdf (accessed on 11th June 2025).

41. Fonteh, Aliah L. (2018) "Orotic Aciduria," *Fidei et Veritatis: The Liberty University Journal of Graduate Research*: Vol. 2: Iss. 1, Article 1. Available at: https://digitalcommons.liberty.edu/fidei_et_veritatis/vol2/iss1/1(accessed on 11th June 2025).

42. Nayak, J., Gastonguay, A. J., Talipov, M. R., Vakeel, P., Span, E. A., Kalous, K. S., Kutty, R. G., Jensen, D. R., Pokkuluri, P. R., Sem, D. S., Rathore, R., & Ramchandran, R. (2014). Protein expression, characterization and activity comparisons of wild type and mutant DUSP5 proteins. *BMC biochemistry, 15*, 27. https://doi.org/10.1186/s12858-014-0027-0(accessed on 11th June 2025).

43. Graduate School of Biomedical Sciences, University of Texas Health Science Center at Houston/M.D. Anderson Cancer Center. (2013). *GSBS News, Spring 2015*. https://core.ac.uk/download/46720056.pdf (accessed on 11th June 2025).

44. Hemmert, A. C., Cadieux, C. L., Edwards, C. C., Cerasoli, D. M., Rodrigues-Lima, F., Cashman, J. R., Edwards, J. S., et al. (2010). Nerve agent hydrolysis activity designed into a human drug metabolism enzyme. https://core.ac.uk/download/4888755.pdf (accessed on 11th June 2025).

45. Kast, P., Keeffe, J. R., Lassila, J. K., Mayo, S. L., et al. (2007). Exhaustive mutagenesis of six secondary active-site residues in *Escherichia coli* chorismite mutase shows the importance of hydrophobic side chains and a helix N-capping position for stability and catalysis. https://core.ac.uk/download/4890557.pdf (accessed on 11th June 2025).

46. Linson, E. A. (2013). *The Interplay Between Hormones and Irritable Bowel Disease*. https://open.bu.edu/bitstream/2144/12149/6/Linson_Elyse_2013_nosig_nocv.pdf (accessed on 11th June 2025).

47. Marzolla, M. (2016). Assessing evaluation procedures for individual researchers: The case of the Italian National Scientific Qualification. http://arxiv.org/abs/1507.04720 (accessed on 11th June 2025).

48. Sarmidi, Mohamad Roji (2012) *Food is our medicine*. In: Professorial Inaugural Lecture «Food is Our Medicine», 26 September 2012, Senate Hall, Universiti Teknologi Malaysia, Johor Bahru. (accessed on 11th June 2025).

49. Suazo Galdames, I. (2024). *De La Anatomía Al Algoritmo: Alcance De Las Competencias Diagnósticas Asistidas Por Inteligencia Artificial En La Educación En Ciencias De La Salud*. https://core.ac.uk/download/630469681.pdf (accessed on 11th June 2025).

BIOMOLECULES

2

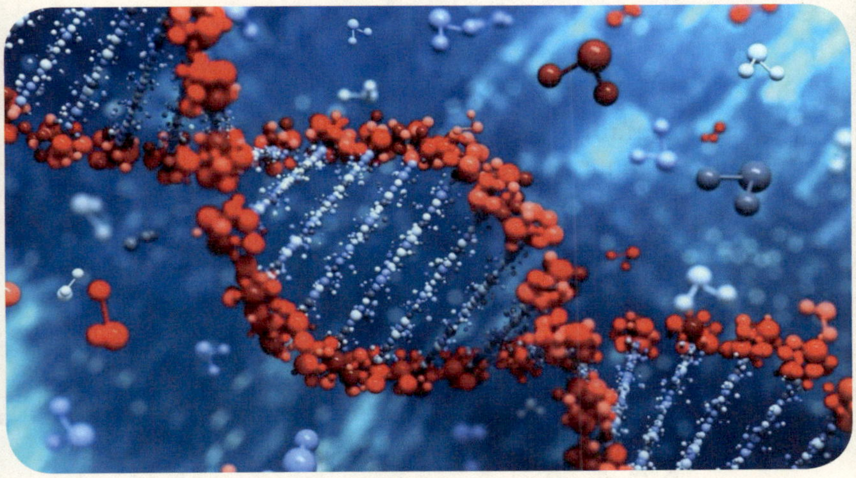

LEARNING OBJECTIVES

After studying this chapter, you will be able to:

1. Describe the four primary biomolecules: carbohydrates, proteins, lipids, and nucleic acids;
2. Understand the metabolism of biomolecules;
3. Describe the biomolecules in health and disease.

Introduction

In biology, biomolecules are the main focus, and they assist in explaining the molecular nature of life. Proteins, nucleic acids, carbohydrates, and lipids are important for the structure and function of cells. All of these groups help the cell by taking part in energy storage, signaling molecules, and genetic information, which supports and enables transport processes. Basically, knowing more about these biomolecules is crucial for understanding how biological systems work. Nevertheless, it is very challenging to classify and characterize proteins, which are among the important biomolecules. As discussed, protein functions cannot be ascertained from their amino acid sequence or three-dimensional structure alone; rather, multiple attributes are needed to establish a full ontology of protein functions (Kumar & Smith, 2003). Being aware of this is important because it provides the background for more research on the complex networks found in biological organisms. During the past decade, new developments in computational biology have allowed us to learn more about biomolecules using fresh approaches. Using algebraic topology and other novel approaches has improved our understanding of biomolecular complexes and helped see the geometric features involved in them. For instance, multicomponent persistent homology retains crucial chemical and biological information within the topological simplification process of these molecules (Cang et al., 2017).

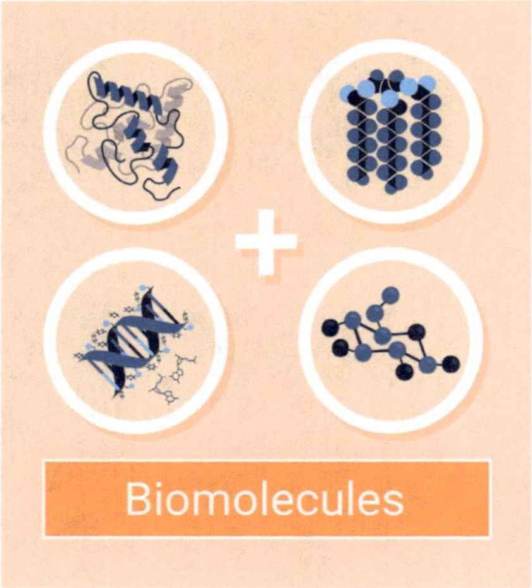

Figure 2.1. Biomolecules.

Source: https://conductscience.com/wp-content/uploads/2021/07/Biomolecules.png.

With this refinement, it is easier to explain the important interactions between and within molecules involved in biochemical processes. By using topological methods together with machine learning, scientists can find out if molecules have similar structures and functions, which improves how they model and predict biological processes. As we learn more about biomolecules, advanced analytical tools have more opportunities to connect how biological functions and interactions work. Having partial charge details in topological analyses is helping biology and chemistry come together, which in turn makes the models more accurate in predicting binding affinity. This strategy has proven its effectiveness in large-scale numerical simulations, surpassing other machine learning techniques in different applications like protein-ligand binding affinity prediction (Cang et al., 2017). The discovery shows how important it is to use different approaches in biomolecular research and indicates that the field will keep developing. As we venture deeper into the realm of biomolecules, it's obvious that sustained innovation and interdisciplinary collaboration will be the key to deciphering the codes of life and improving biomedical outcomes (Figure 2.1).

Definition of Biomolecules

Biomolecules are important to all living organisms because they help form and function the cells in the body. They are mainly organized into four groups: carbohydrates, proteins, lipids, and nucleic acids. Every type of biomolecule has a special structure and a particular function. Carbohydrates help the body store and move energy, while proteins help reactions in the body and form structures in cells. Membrane integrity and energy are maintained by lipids, whereas DNA and RNA, which are nucleic acids, hold and transmit genetic data. It highlights the variety of functions that biomolecules play, proving how certain combinations of them are necessary for life at both cellular and organism levels. Because these biomolecules rely on each other, the body can function normally and respond to different situations. To give an example, proteins need their polypeptide chains to fold properly, which is affected by the lipids and carbohydrates nearby. Also, proteins are made according to the genetic information in nucleic acids, affecting the body's metabolism and cellular activities. It proves that life emerges because biomolecules work together and not by themselves. When we study these interactions further, it becomes obvious that biomolecules play a key role in biotechnology and medicine, as working with them can bring new solutions to treating and stopping diseases. Lately, scientists have used ideas from evolutionary biology and structural bioinformatics to better study how biomolecules function. For instance, topological methods are used in modern studies to show and describe how biomolecules interact and behave. Methods such as multicomponent persistent homology and electrostatic persistence make it easier to study biomolecules and how they interact, which supports predictive modeling in biochemistry. These methods have proven to be effective, surpassing the traditional ones in predicting protein-ligand binding, which helps us create new drugs. The more research is done, the more it becomes clear that biological systems are both very complex and highly adaptable, showing why it is important to keep exploring this area (Figure 2.2).

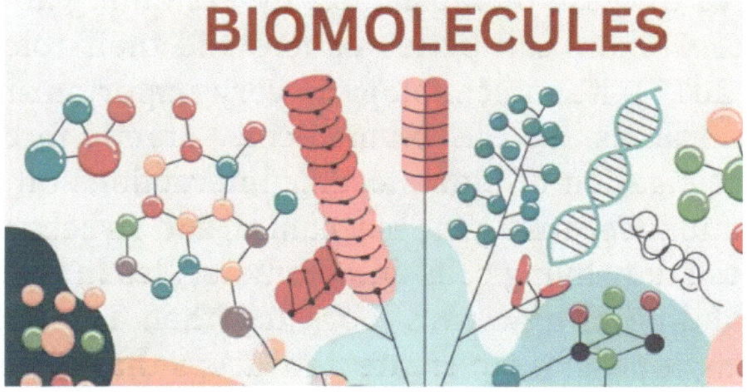

Figure 2.2. Definition of biomolecules.

Source: https://cache.careers360.mobi/media/article_images/2024/10/3/Biomolecules%20(1).jpg.

Importance in Biological Systems

The importance of biomolecules in living organisms is clear because they help make possible the important biochemical reactions needed for life. Biomolecules are important because they help with metabolic reactions and also maintain the structure of cells. The compatibility of various computational methods, particularly density functional theory (DFT), enhances our understanding of these interactions, allowing researchers to investigate large biomolecules in intricate biological contexts. Thanks to progress in DFT, scientists can now examine weak van der Waals forces that are important in biomolecular binding and the way they control key biological activities. By accurately modeling these weak interactions, researchers can glean insights into the stabilization of protein structures and the dynamics of molecular recognition, ultimately elevating our comprehension of biological systems and their underlying mechanisms (Kolb & Thonhauser, 2012). Moreover, the methods used to see biomolecules have advanced a lot, helping us greatly in understanding cells. Although traditional fluorescence microscopy has helped a lot, it cannot detect small biomolecules well because the large fluorescent labels disrupt the system. Because small biomolecules are important in metabolism and signaling, it is important to use techniques that cause the least disturbance and still detect them well. The advent of bio-orthogonal chemical imaging represents a breakthrough in this field, incorporating technologies like stimulated Raman scattering (SRS) microscopy with tiny vibrational probes. This innovative approach enhances specificity and sensitivity for observing small biomolecules in real-time, thus allowing researchers to monitor their dynamics within live biological systems, which is vital for understanding metabolic processes in health and disease (Chen et al., 2016). All in all, biomolecules are important in many ways within living organisms because they play various key roles. Thanks to advanced computational tools and latest imaging systems, researchers can study and observe biomolecules with great precision. Improvements in methods that deal with the weaknesses of traditional techniques allow us to understand biological processes better. As well as giving us new insights into cells, these advancements help create new treatments that target the interactions of biomolecules in different diseases. With more research, scientists hope to understand how biomolecules play a key role in life at both the molecular and cellular levels.

Overview of Types of Biomolecules

The main types of biomolecules, which make up life, are carbohydrates, proteins, nucleic acids, and lipids. Groups of molecules are necessary for biological activities, including keeping energy and passing on genetic information. Energy in the body is partly supplied by carbohydrates, which are found in sugars and starches. They are made of carbon, hydrogen, and oxygen and provide energy as well as structure for cells. Proteins made from amino acids are called enzymes and help control almost all the body's functions. It is necessary to understand biomolecular scaffolds in biochemistry and molecular biology since the interactions between the molecules control how cells and their functions work. Apart from the main types, biomolecules are also organized by their detailed three-dimensional structures, which have a big impact on their function. For instance, the shape of a protein is necessary for it to function well, as any wrongly folded protein can cause serious illnesses. Lately, new technologies have provided new knowledge about the structures of biomolecules. Methods like X-ray crystallography and nuclear magnetic resonance (NMR) spectroscopy enable scientists to see the spatial arrangement of proteins and nucleic acids to previously unimagined levels of detail. Besides, algebraic topology methods, such as multicomponent persistent homology, have helped describe and define the geometric features of these biomolecules. By examining how different biomolecules interact and are structured, researchers can better understand their roles and develop new therapeutic strategies (Cang et al., 2017). Nanotechnology is very important in helping us learn more about and use biomolecules in areas such as biomedicine. Atomic force microscopy (AFM) instruments give the facility of investigation of biomolecular interactions on a nanoscale so that scientists can make enormous observations regarding the mechanical and structural nature of biological specimens. AFM allows scientists to study living cells and biomolecules in their natural environment, giving a more serious understanding of how cells work together. The link between biomolecular science and technology is making it possible to create new drugs that target specific areas and help with healing. The fusion of knowledge between biomolecular research and technological advancements is a promising new area in biological research, which translates into tangible advances in health care and disease management (Canetta & Adya, 2011) (Figure 2.3).

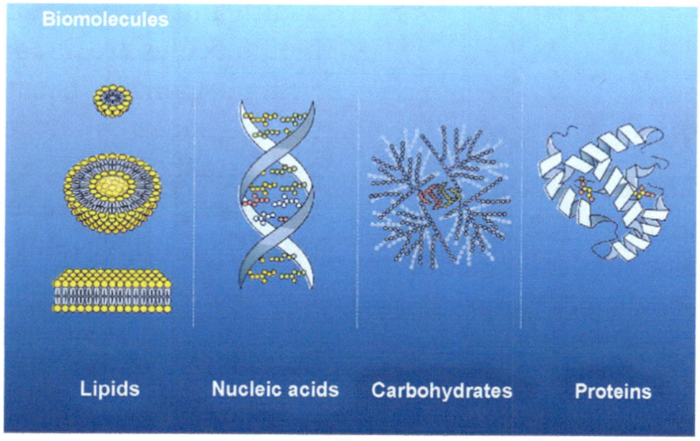

Figure 2.3. Types of biomolecules.

Source: https://www.datocms-assets.com/117510/1722396859-adele_art-01-catalysing_chemical_reactions_with_enzymes_biomolecules.png.

2.1. Carbohydrates

Learning Outcome

1. Understand the structure and classification of biomolecules;
2. Describe the functions of living organisms;
3. Describe the examples of carbohydrates in nature.

The structure and energy metabolism of living things depend greatly on carbohydrates as one of the main biomolecules. Sugars called monosaccharides and more complex types such as disaccharides and polysaccharides are both part of carbohydrates. Glucose and fructose are monosaccharides that supply energy right away to cells, but starch and cellulose are polysaccharides that are used for energy storage and building structures. The many ways carbohydrates can be arranged with glycosidic bonds make them useful in many ways. Besides, they are involved in key processes, such as cellular respiration and photosynthesis, which demonstrate their central role in energy transfer and storage needed for life to work. Carbohydrates are important for cell recognition as well as for sending and receiving signals. When carbohydrates bond with proteins and lipids, the resulting glycoproteins and glycolipids are necessary for communication among cells, their adhesion, and immune responses. Such carbohydrates have an impact on how the body functions, since their shape affects how cells communicate with their surroundings. As an example, the unique oligosaccharide chains on cells may determine whether immune cells or pathogens recognize them, highlighting their effect on health. Consequently, carbohydrates are important in regulating the body's systems as well as providing energy. With new tools and methods, the study of carbohydrates has progressed a lot. Techniques such as Raman optical activity (ROA) spectroscopy have enhanced our understanding of carbohydrate structures in solution, as well as their interactions with proteins and other biomolecules (Barron et al., 2015). Such developments make it possible to analyze how carbohydrates are shaped, which is important for finding out what they do in the body. Furthermore, the integration of programming in biomolecular education, as demonstrated through platforms like PyMol, enables students to visualize and model carbohydrate structures alongside protein architectures, fostering a more comprehensive understanding of biomolecular interactions (Nusz, 2014). As studies continue, it is becoming more obvious that carbohydrates have a strong impact on health, diseases, and biotechnology (Figure 2.4).

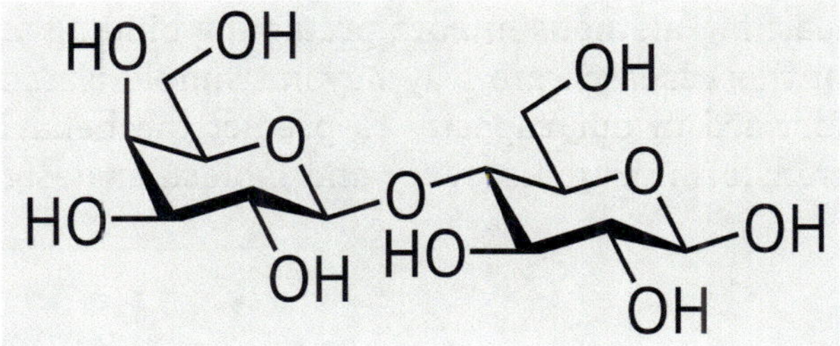

Figure 2.4. Carbohydrates.

Source: By Calvero. - Own work using: ChemDraw, Public Domain, https://commons.wikimedia.org/w/index.php?curid=1670221

2.1.1. Structure and Classification

To understand how biomolecules work in living organisms, it is necessary to know their structure and how they are grouped. Proteins can have different structures related to their jobs, and this means they should be grouped in a unified way. Most often, proteins are grouped by their amino acid sequence or shape, but this approach does not show the whole picture of their function. It is possible to build a useful ontology of protein functions by considering different traits, for example, structural features, positions that are conserved in evolution, and biochemical aspects. According to Kumar & Smith (2003), it requires a meticulous top-level ontological classification analysis of the classifications to reconcile different databases in order to better enable us to describe protein functions and their relationships in diverse biological contexts effectively. Among the growing field of biomolecular analysis, topological data analysis gives us a better way to use multicomponent persistent homology. It helps to find chemical and biological details without losing their geometry and can help sort biomolecules by their topological features and the forces that affect their interactions. Also, multi-level persistent homology adds detailed explanations of both intramolecular and intermolecular interactions needed for studying biomolecular behavior. Using electrostatic persistence, scientists can use charge-related data to improve the classification, giving a more complete picture of how molecules interact. From using these methods on various datasets, which are backed by a lot of research, it is obvious that they can help improve the structure and classification of biomolecules. The use of algebraic topology along with machine learning is very significant in biomolecular classification. If Wasserstein distance is used with machine learning, scientists will be able to identify similarities between biomolecules and so improve predictions in these fields. When topological approaches and data-driven models are used together, it can help us learn more about protein-ligand interactions and biomolecular complexes. Many simulations of protein-ligand complexes have proved that topological methods outperform classical machine learning methods in both predicting binding affinity and discriminating ligands. Such implications of this research are way beyond simple classification because it ultimately indicates a large step forward in our capacity to predict the behavior and interaction of molecules, with potential to transform drug discovery and molecular design, as suggested by Cang et al. (2017) (Figure 2.5).

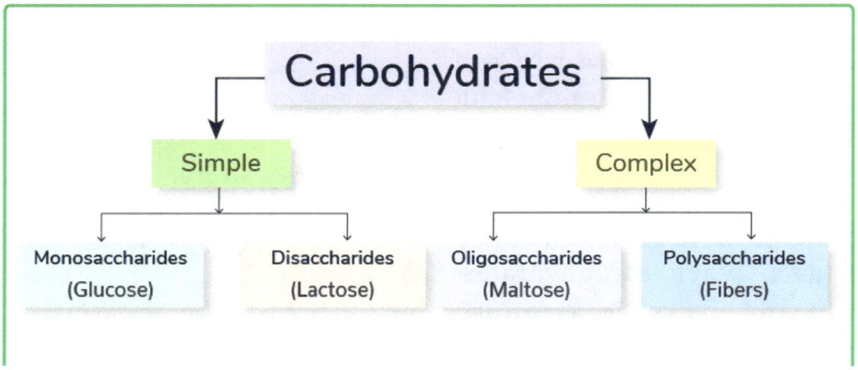

Figure 2.5. Classification of carbohydrates.

Source: https://cdn.entrance360.com/media/uploads/2024/09/23/carbo.png.

2.1.2. Functions in Living Organisms

Living organisms carry out their functions mainly because of the biomolecules that make them up. Proteins, nucleic acids, carbohydrates, and lipids are important at the molecular level for life to exist. Apart from being part of the body's structure, proteins also help speed up biochemical reactions by acting as enzymes. They increase the speed of many cell activities, which proves how important the structure of proteins is for their function. In the same way, DNA and RNA, types of nucleic acids, hold the genetic code needed for the growth and reproduction of organisms, underlining their importance in heredity and evolution. The precise and detailed features of biomolecules are needed for the balanced functioning of metabolic processes in living organisms. It is especially interesting that biomolecules are able to communicate and express information in living creatures. Genes carry the information that is used to make the proteins needed for cell functions and growth of the organism. In addition, epigenetics is involved in inheritance since it changes how genes work without changing the DNA itself. Because of this connection between genes and epigenetics, living things can adjust better to changes in their environment, showing that different inheritance systems help each other in biological functions. While the genetic system remains paramount in evolution, the significance of epigenetic regulation suggests a more dynamic view of heredity, where environmental interactions can shape the genetic landscape over generations, thus impacting organismal functions and survival strategies (Griffiths et al., 2017). In addition, biology is shifting towards using more numbers and analytical methods, just like what is happening in physics and mathematics. It is not only a new method but also a sign of better understanding of the biomolecular side of life. When mathematical models are used on biological data, predictions about biological outcomes become more accurate. Population genetics and evolutionary biology are other fields where such quantitative approaches help us learn more about living systems. As the study of biomolecules and their functions becomes increasingly intertwined with computational methods and data analysis, a clearer picture of the interdependencies among various biological processes emerges, enriching our comprehension of life itself (Wei, 2017).

2.1.3. Examples of Carbohydrates in Nature

Carbohydrates are found everywhere in nature and support energy storage, provide structure, and take part in cell communication. Simple sugars such as glucose and fructose are familiar examples and act as main sources of energy for living things. Monosaccharides combine to make disaccharides, such as sucrose and lactose, which add more types of carbohydrates. Plants depend on starch as energy stored in their bodies, and glycogen is the same for animals. Plant cell walls are made rigid by cellulose, another polysaccharide, which allows carbohydrates to perform many functions in the environment. Because of their different chemical structures, carbohydrates are important in evolution and affect both metabolism and interactions between cells in many types of living things. It is clear from looking at carbohydrates' structure that how they are arranged determines their functionality. Because carbohydrates can exist in different three-dimensional forms, they can take part in important interactions with other biomolecules. ROA spectroscopy has emerged as a powerful tool for elucidating these structural properties, providing insights into the solution structure of carbohydrates in various states. Examining the way polarized light is scattered by such molecules allows researchers to learn more about carbohydrates and their effects on biological processes.

This knowledge is necessary when we think about how carbohydrates take part in cell recognition, signaling, and diseases. So, the detailed structure of carbohydrates makes it clear how important they are for life and how closely they are connected to living systems. Also, carbohydrates play a role in how living things sense and communicate, and this area is becoming a main focus for research. Cell surface receptors that recognize carbohydrates allow important interactions that play a role in both getting nutrients and responding to infections. Many artificial sensors use ideas from how carbohydrates are recognized in nature, and these show great potential for new innovations. By using different and precise detection methods, researchers are trying to make sensors that can precisely detect and measure biomolecules. Because of these developments, diagnostics and treatments could improve, proving that carbohydrates are important for both energy use and biotechnology. Examples like these prove how carbohydrates play many roles in nature, increasing their importance in the overall structure of biomolecules (Figure 2.6).

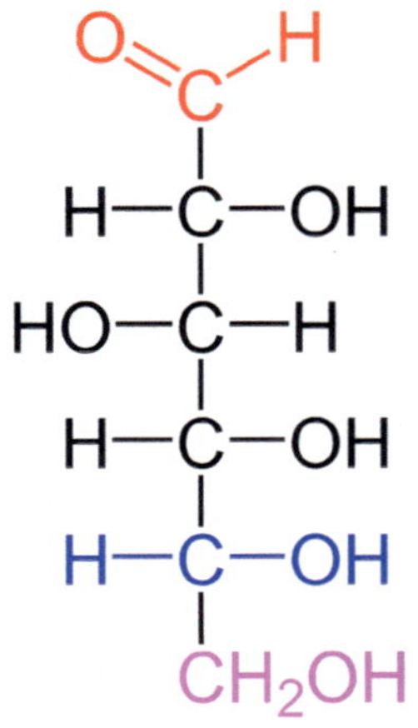

Figure 2.6. Examples of carbohydrates.

Source: By ClockworkSoul at English Wikipedia - Transferred from en.wikipedia to Commons., Public Domain, https://commons.wikimedia.org/w/index.php?curid=3534327

Test Your Knowledge

1. What is the structure of a biomolecule?
2. What is the function of the living organism?

2.2. Proteins

Learning Outcome

1. Describe the amino acids and protein structure;
2. Understand the role of proteins in cellular functions;
3. Describe the enzymes as biological catalysts.

Among all the biomolecules, proteins are special due to their wide range of roles and complex shapes. Long chains of amino acids form proteins, and these proteins fold into special three-dimensional shapes needed for their work. It matters a lot that proteins are built as expected, as changes in amino acids can result in either useful or useless proteins. The determination of protein structures is predominantly achieved through sophisticated techniques, such as X-ray crystallography and NMR spectroscopy. These methods provide invaluable insights into protein dynamics and interactions, with NMR particularly adept at studying transient protein-protein interactions, thus revealing the intricacies of biological pathways, and signaling processes vital for maintaining cellular homeostasis (Hameed et al., 2012). Proteins help regulate the cell by acting as main agents in biochemical reactions. Enzymatic proteins, in particular, support metabolic pathways by quickening reactions that are important for energy and molecule synthesis. Proteins are important for more reasons than enzymes; some proteins keep cells and tissues strong, while others help move molecules across cell membranes. Also, the study of post-translational modifications (PTMs), for example phosphorylation or ubiquitination, further increases our knowledge of protein function. Such changes may impact how stable, where located, and what functions proteins have, which impacts main cellular activities. Mass spectrometry has emerged as a pivotal technology in this regard, allowing for the identification and characterization of protein modifications rapidly and accurately (Hameed et al., 2012).

It has been discovered in recent studies that DIS3 is important in conditions like cancer. DIS3 is an enzyme that helps break down RNA and its mutations have been related to multiple myeloma, a cancer that impacts plasma cells. Although we know how DIS3 helps RNA decay, its mutations and their possible links to cancer are not well understood. Using model organisms has helped us see how DIS3 is important for the cell cycle and microtubule formation. This area of study emphasizes the need for more research on how changes in proteins can lead to cancer, proving once again the key role of proteins in both healthy and unhealthy conditions (Figure 2.7).

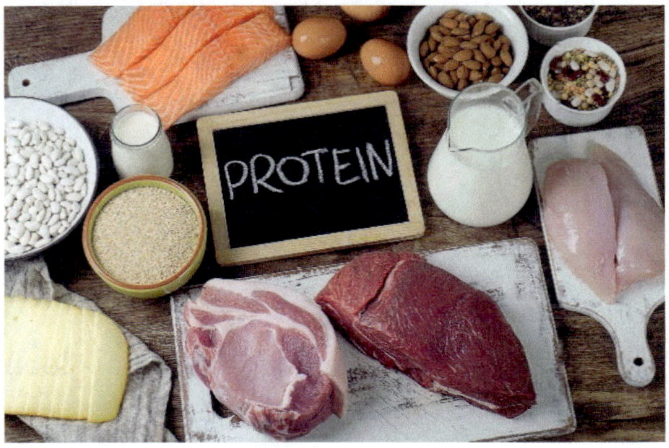

Figure 2.7. Protein.

Source: https://content.dhhs.vic.gov.au/sites/default/files/2022-01/protein_0.jpg.

2.2.1. Amino Acids and Protein Structure

Proteins are made up of amino acids, which are important biomolecules needed for millions of biological activities. All 20 common amino acids have a different side chain, or R group, which determines how they act and what they do in a protein. The arrangement of amino acids in a protein determines its shape in three dimensions, which is important for the protein's function. The difficulty of this folding process is also shown by Levinthal's paradox, which points out that proteins must find their right shape out of many possible ones in a short period. Such complexities of protein structures require more knowledge of the interactions of amino acids and their contribution towards the development of such a complex architecture of proteins (Sargoytchev et al., 2017).

Even though the way proteins fold is determined by the amino acid sequence, the cell environment also plays a role, mainly during the translation process. Studies done recently indicate that ribosomes help proteins begin to fold as they are being made. The way this process happens depends on the space inside the ribosome and the characteristics of the polypeptide. While the protein is still being made, early stages of compaction guided by the ribosome's environment can play a big role in determining whether the protein folds correctly or not. The case is the same with the folding pathway of multidomain proteins because each of the domains affects the stability and structural resilience of the whole protein (Liutkute et al., 2020). How amino acids affect the structure of proteins is important for both cell activity and evolution. Different properties of amino acids and their teamwork in a protein environment are what makes them useful in various biological processes. Protein interactions may alter how enzymes function, how receptors bind to other substances, and how cells are structured.

Studying this topic improves our knowledge of proteins and also makes us wonder about the changes in proteins that allowed them to have so many different functions in nature. It turns out that amino acids are more important than just building blocks, since they help form the basic structure of life (Figure 2.8).

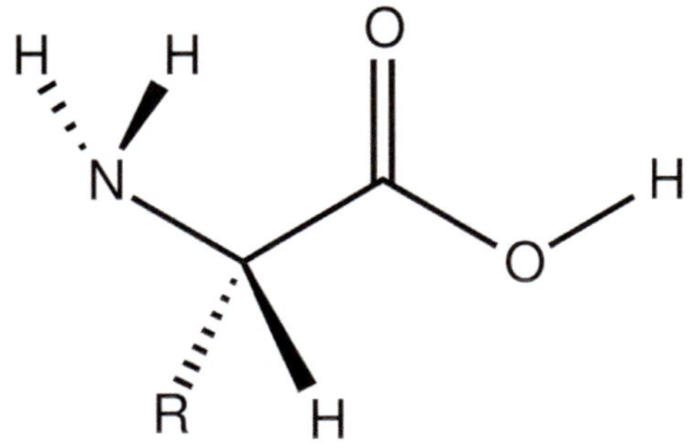

Figure 2.8. Amino acids.

Source: By Smokefoot - Own work, Public Domain, https://commons.wikimedia.org/w/index.php?curid=106539890

2.2.2. Role of Proteins in Cellular Functions

Proteins are vital for many cell activities as they help with important reactions and support the cell's structure. Enzymes, being proteins, help speed up certain chemical reactions in the body. Because each enzyme is specific, it helps control metabolic processes so that energy production and biosynthesis happen smoothly. Also, proteins called collagen and keratin help maintain the structure and shape of cells and tissues in the body. The changes in protein function and activity brought by phosphorylation and ubiquitination emphasize their key role in cellular activities, since these changes respond to the cell's environment. Besides being important for building and breaking down substances, proteins also take part in cellular communication and reactions to different stimuli. On the cell membrane, receptor proteins receive hormones and neurotransmitters from the outside and trigger changes inside the cell that keep the body stable. It is important that proteins change shape when they bind to ligands, as this helps them send messages in the cell and affect activities such as cell division, differentiation, and apoptosis. In addition, problems in these signaling pathways, caused by mutated or misfolded proteins, can result in diseases, for example, cancer. The study of such dysfunctional proteins, such as the mutation of DIS3 linked to multiple myeloma, highlights not only the importance of proteins in normal cellular function but also their critical roles in pathophysiological conditions (Carazo-Salas et al., 2015). This interaction also demonstrates that proteins are involved in several ways to preserve the health of cells. For instance, the unfolded protein response (UPR) is a protective mechanism activated in response to the accumulation of misfolded proteins, particularly within the endoplasmic reticulum (ER).

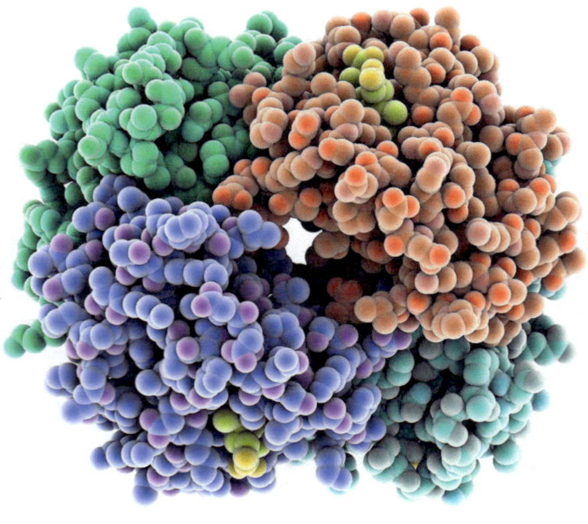

Figure 2.9. Molecular model of a hemoglobin protein structure.

Source: https://www.thoughtco.com/thmb/Xw8aZYFwT4YMmyrXXDCiO4ctzsw=/1500x0/filters:no_upscale():max_bytes(150000):strip_icc()/protein-hemoglobin-58a222955f9b58819ca8f902.jpg.

When this response is activated, several signaling pathways are used to help the body recover and get rid of damaged proteins by activating autophagy. Recent studies have shown that misfolded proteins, such as mutant p53 variants, can disrupt cellular homeostasis, promoting aggressive tumor behavior and therapy resistance (Cirone et al., 2020). For this reason, learning about the connections between proteins and cell functions helps us understand basic biology and also offers ideas for treating diseases that happen due to protein abnormalities (Figure 2.9).

2.2.3. Enzymes as Biological Catalysts

Enzymes play a critical role in cellular activities. They help speed up different biochemical reactions that are important for living things. The way they help is by decreasing the energy needed for a reaction, which leads to much faster metabolic processes than would happen without their help. That is why speed is important for the cells to maintain their proper functions and allow even the most complex biochemical pathways to work smoothly. Because enzymes are very specific, they usually help with just one or a few reactions, which allows the cell's metabolism to be controlled. The way an enzyme is folded in three dimensions usually provides the best spot for substrate to attach. Enzymes are essential to the proper working of different metabolic networks since they affect both energy production and the creation and breakdown of important biomolecules. The progress of enzymes may suggest how life started on Earth and how early metabolic processes could have formed. It has been found that before genetically encoded enzymes existed, other simpler ways of catalysis might have been used with small molecules or minerals. As an illustration, the idea of proto-metabolism is that early reactions handled by simple catalysts could develop into more advanced enzymatic reactions with time. Using both network-based algorithms and knowledge of chemistry and physics, researchers have tried to explain how early metabolic functions could have arisen in conditions such as temperature and pH. Particularly, this review has identified that certain proto-metabolic networks would be able to survive without essential constituents like fixed nitrogen, which implies early biochemical pathways were very adaptable to changing environmental pressures (Goldford et al., 2019). In addition, the biochemical information of ancient organisms can be found in the structures of today's enzymes. Researchers have discovered that a thioester-based metabolism could have existed before enzymes were invented. According to the recent study, the most important metabolic pathways could function even if phosphate were not involved in present-day biochemical processes. The most recent discovery about this old network is that enzymes use iron-sulfur clusters, which may have led to new biosynthesis processes that were not known before. According to these findings, the first catalysts in life interacted with each other, which led to the appearance of advanced cellular machinery. The insights derived from these biochemical ventures not only shed light on the past but also hold potential in comprehending the flexibility and resilience of life molecular systems (Goldford et al., 2017).

Test Your Knowledge

1. What is the role of proteins in cellular functions?
2. Why are enzymes important for cellular function?

2.3. Lipids

Learning Outcome

1. Describe the types of lipids and their structures;
2. Know the functions of lipids in the body;
3. Describe the lipids in energy storage and membrane formation.

Lipids, which are hydrophobic biomolecules, are important for the organization and function of cells. They are organized into several groups, for example, fatty acyls, glycerolipids, glycerophospholipids, sphingolipids, sterol lipids, and polyketides, and each one carries out a distinct role in the body. The presence of lipids in cellular membranes helps the membrane form a bilayer that is needed for maintaining the cell's shape and for allowing only certain substances to enter or leave the cell. It is mainly because of their amphipathic nature that glycerophospholipids play a key role in forming lipid bilayers that support both the insertion of proteins and the initiation of signaling pathways. Their unique properties enable lipids to modulate membrane fluidity, supporting various processes such as transport, signal transduction, and cell-to-cell communication (Macabuhay et al., 2021). Apart from their structural duties, lipids are used as messengers in the body and as sources of energy. They participate in different metabolic processes and regulation, affecting the body's reactions to changes in the environment. For instance, lipid-derived molecules such as jasmonates and phosphatidic acid act as secondary messengers in plant defense mechanisms against pathogens (Goldford et al., 2017). Cholesterol and similar sterol lipids are important for the creation of lipid rafts, which play a role in organizing receptors and cell communications. Changes in the structures of lipids allow cells to react quickly to outside stimuli, showing how important lipid metabolism is for maintaining balance and flexibility. As a result, lipids are important for cell structure and also take part in signaling and energy control, showing how important they are in biology. For cells to work properly and carry out metabolic activities, lipids and proteins must interact. Lipid rafts are particular regions of the membrane that have a high concentration of cholesterol and sphingolipids and help arrange membrane proteins. These microdomains contribute to various signaling pathways by clustering receptors and facilitating their interactions with downstream effectors (Goldford et al., 2017). Besides, the type of lipids in membranes helps control the activities of enzymes and the movement of proteins between parts of the cell, which is important for endocytosis and exocytosis. Since lipids play many roles in cells, scientists must keep studying them to understand their functions. When scientists understand the roles of various lipids, they will gain more insight into how these biomolecules coordinate the functioning and response of cells in different organisms (Figure 2.10).

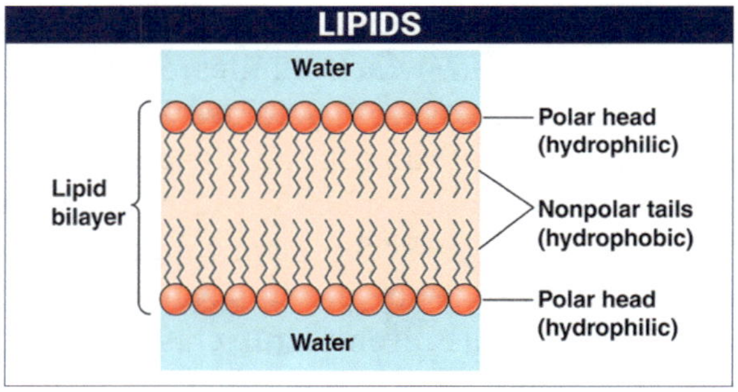

Figure 2.10. Lipids.

Source: https://www.learninsta.com/wp-content/uploads/2021/07/Biomolecules-of-Lipids-img-1.png.

2.3.1. Types of Lipids and Their Structures

To know how lipids work in different ways, it is important to classify them. There are several types of lipids, for example, TGs, phospholipids, and sterols, and every type has a unique structure that matches its functions. Since TGs are made of glycerol and three fatty acids, they act as energy storage molecules and are hydrophobic, which makes them a strong source of energy. Meanwhile, phospholipids, made of glycerol, two fatty acids, and a phosphate group, are needed to form the structure of the membrane. Because of their amphipathic nature, lipid bilayers are formed and cells become divided into compartments. Being flexible in structure is why lipids are important for storing energy, forming cell membranes, and taking part in signaling. Phospholipids differ from other lipids since they have complex structures and are important for membrane movement. Bilayers are formed by phospholipids due to their tails being hydrophobic and their heads being hydrophilic. This setup offers both strength to cells and selective control over the things that enter or leave the cell. Also, having unsaturated fatty acids in some phospholipids adds bends to the membrane, which affect its fluidity. Such changes in lipid composition may greatly affect how proteins are arranged and how cell membranes fuse. The way phospholipids are structured is essential for the proper functioning of biological membranes in any cell and situation. Sterols are important lipids, as they are built with several rings that allow cell membranes to be both stiff and flexible. Cholesterol is present in cells in greater numbers than other sterols and affects the fluidity of the membrane. It goes into the lipid bilayer and binds to phospholipids to maintain the shape of the membrane, especially when temperatures change. Besides, cholesterol is needed to make steroid hormones, vitamin D, and bile acids, making it more important than just keeping cells strong. How cholesterol and other lipids in the membrane interact is vital for maintaining balance in the cell and for passing on signals. Knowledge of the different classes of lipids and the fine detail of their structure therefore gives better insights into their function in cellular processes and general biological functions within organisms, as well as implications for health and disease (Ivankin et al., 2016; Kallepitis et al., 2017) (Figure 2.11).

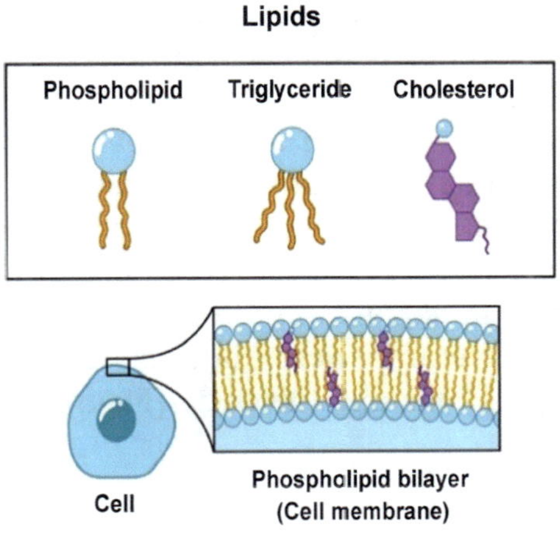

Figure 2.11. Lipids are useful chemical compounds in all of your body's cells.

Source: https://my.clevelandclinic.org/-/scassets/images/org/health/articles/24425-lipids.

2.3.2. Functions of Lipids in the Body

Among all the biomolecules that are important in biology, lipids are unique because they are involved in many physiological processes. Primarily, lipids serve as critical energy storage molecules. Fats are able to store more energy in a single gram than carbohydrates or proteins, so they are preferred by the body when there is no food for a long time or during hard exercise. It is partly because of their chemical structure that lipids are advantageous; fatty acids in lipids have long hydrocarbon chains that generate a lot of energy when they are oxidized. In addition, adipocytes store TGs, which are made of glycerol and three fatty acids, which shows that lipids play a part in both energy storage and balancing energy in the body. As well as storing energy, lipids are important parts of cell membranes. The lipid bilayer of cell membranes is mainly made possible by phospholipids. With the bilayer, the cell is able to keep its interior different from the outside and allows only some substances to enter or leave. Besides, having cholesterol in cell membranes is necessary; it helps the membrane remain stable and flexible as temperatures change. Cells need the different lipids to work together to support communication, signaling, and homeostasis, which proves that they play an active role in cell function. In addition, lipids are important in signaling pathways because they become precursors to signaling molecules. Some phospholipids are split by enzymes to produce secondary messengers that take part in processes such as inflammation and cellular growth. Lipids such as sphingolipids and eicosanoids have shown the ability to affect how cells react to outside signals. The functional diversity of lipids is exemplified through metabolites produced during lipid metabolism which can influence metabolic pathways in tissues, as observed in studies on Drosophila melanogaster, where specific lipids were identified in correlation to tissue function (Kamleh et al., 2013). So, lipids are not only important for structure and energy but also take part in the many biochemical processes that control the stability of cells and the body (Figure 2.12).

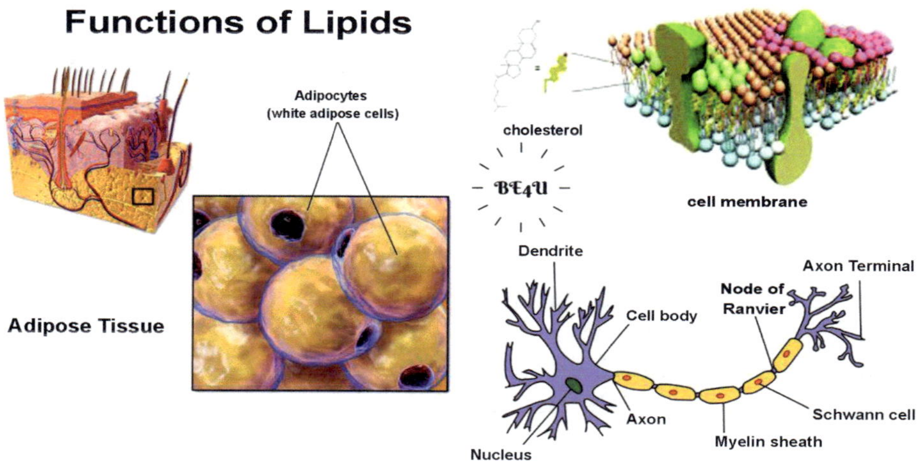

Figure 2.12. Functions of lipids.

Source: https://blogger.googleusercontent.com/img/b/R29vZ2xl/AVvXsEjAXfTpiZM5eH2VQp2QB_CtSk9_lrMukhmzZkkJntMQT8qwlsQpOsDL_ZimOjyILUi39U678-JNDsfMxwLeYDJhMCXxSKYXS8MIe6XlCDRwTJ0VtNnaua0ki9GZSfrbG3GZGlkPCkZMhhcJJhi2sq8_gXfdGQnNdyFx2RxZIHz2YQmXt2IyMRong4A/s1024/lpids%20functions%20(1).jpg.

2.3.3. Lipids in Energy Storage and Membrane Formation

Lipids are important for cells, as they help store energy and are part of membranes, which proves their importance in the body. Several kinds of lipids, including TGs, phospholipids, and sterols, have different functions in different biological systems. In adipose tissue, TGs are the main kind of energy storage and are efficient because they hold a lot of energy. When energy is required, lipids are broken down into fatty acids that can be converted to give energy to cells. The structure of lipids decides their properties and the way they help store energy, showing how different their functions can be. In addition to energy, lipids are important for forming the cell membrane and its structure.

Because phospholipids have water-loving heads and water-repelling tails, they automatically form a double layer that gives shape to cell membranes. This special structure acts as a barrier that allows some molecules to pass through and maintain the proper conditions inside the cell. The presence of cholesterol in cell membranes helps them remain flexible and steady, which supports the active processes of cell signaling and movement of materials. The complex way in which membrane proteins and lipids interact hints that lipids are involved in all types of cellular signaling, showing that they play an important role in organizing and running the cell. In addition, research on novel lipid signaling molecules has revealed some interesting details about their roles in development and stress in living beings. Nitrated fatty acids have become important in signaling between cells, mainly in plants. They are responsible for several processes in the plant and are included in the systems that guide plant development. The way storage lipids are changed into useful forms at different times in life demonstrates that lipids have more functions than just storing energy. Studies have demonstrated that lipid modifications influence membrane dynamics and protein interactions, further underscoring the complexity of lipid functions within biological systems (Harris et al., 2010; Aranda-Caño et al., 2022). As our knowledge grows, it keeps shaping our view of biomolecules and their key roles in life sciences.

Test Your Knowledge

1. What are three types of lipids?
2. What are the functions of lipids in the human body?

2.4. Nucleic Acids

Learning Outcome

1. Describe the structure of DNA and RNA;
2. Understand the role of nucleic acids in heredity;
3. Understand the importance of nucleotides in metabolism.

DNA and RNA, which are types of nucleic acids, carry the genetic code that is vital for the growth and proper functioning of every living being. DNA, which is deoxyribonucleic acid, shares and passes on hereditary information by having a special double helix shape made up of four bases: adenine, thymine, cytosine, and guanine. All the genetic data is protected by base pairs, as their specific sequence determines many aspects of our bodies and cells. Unlike DNA, RNA, or ribonucleic acid, mainly supports protein synthesis and helps control genes by translating the genetic code into useful proteins using its single-stranded form. The difference between DNA and RNA proves their importance in biology and makes nucleic acids essential in molecular biology. Many factors in the environment, including metal ions like magnesium and calcium, play a big role in shaping the structure and roles of nucleic acids. They are important for holding nucleic acids together and taking part in biochemical activities such as folding DNA and enzyme actions. It is very important to correctly define these interactions for accurate simulation of biological systems. According to studies, using generic ion parameters may result in wrong predictions about the structure and function of nucleic acids. Studies in this area have tried to improve the ion settings by using experimental results and have helped to better study nucleic acids in various biochemical conditions. By refining these parameters, scientists can improve biomolecular simulations and gain deeper insights into nucleic acid dynamics and interactions (Cruz-León et al., 2021). Nucleic acids have more roles than just holding genetic data; they are also involved in cellular activities including transcription, translation, and regulation. Emerging protein families, such as the La-related proteins (LARPs), exemplify the diverse roles nucleic acids play in regulating gene expression and cellular behavior. They work with RNA at different points during its life, from processing to translation, and this affects both oncogenesis and other important biological processes. It is worth noting that LARP1 is connected to cancer, proving that problems with nucleic acids can lead to illnesses. Seeing how these relationships work provides insight into basic biology and gives chances for treating diseases such as cancer. As research advances, targeting components of nucleic acid complexes may yield promising strategies for novel cancer treatments (Blagden et al., 2015) (Figure 2.13).

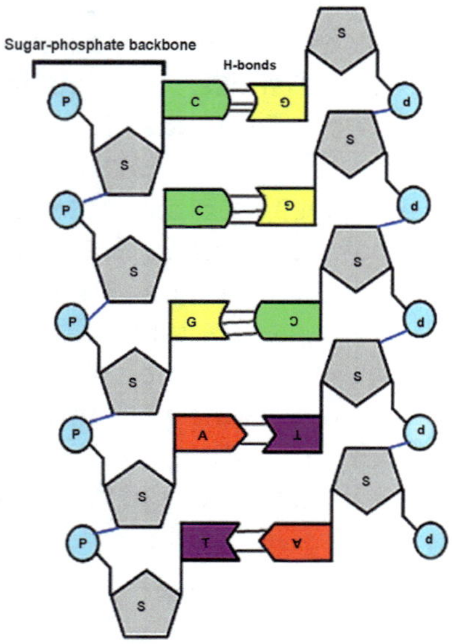

Figure 2.13. Nucleic acids.

Source: https://cdn.entrance360.com/media/uploads/2018/03/04/24.png.

2.4.1. Structure of DNA and RNA

Both DNA and RNA have a basic structure that is important for their roles as biomolecules, and each has its own special traits to carry out its own function in living organisms. DNA is made up of two intertwined strands that are each made up of nucleotide subunits. Nucleotides have a sugar, a phosphate, and a nitrogenous base as their main parts. The order of adenine, thymine, cytosine, and guanine in DNA is what determines how proteins are made and other important cell functions. Unlike DNA, RNA is usually a single-stranded molecule made of ribose sugar and substituting uracil for thymine. This structural difference allows RNA to play diverse roles in the cell, from mRNA carrying genetic information from DNA to ribosomes to transfer RNA (tRNA) facilitating the translation of that information into proteins. Analyses of RNA structure reveal remarkable complexity and adaptability. The arrangement of RNA molecules in three dimensions is determined by their nucleotide sequences and plays a big role in their functions. Research investigating the size and flexibility of RNA molecules have found that these molecules tend to obey the Flory scaling law, where the radius of gyration (R_G) is related to the number of nucleotides (N) in the molecule. Such actions are important since they control the way RNA connects with DNA and proteins. As an example, many RNA structures have unusual shapes, which means they are not like the usual shapes found in other molecules and underline the different functions RNA plays in catalysis and regulation of gene expression through RNA interference. Besides, knowing the persistence length of RNA is necessary to understand its stability and how it interacts with other molecules, since it seems that flexibility increases with the size of the RNA. RNA is important in health and disease, and this is often shown by the actions of ribonucleases such as DIS3. This enzyme in the exosome complex is very well conserved and is important for breaking down and processing

RNA. It has been found lately that genetic changes in DIS3 can result in serious outcomes, such as multiple myeloma, where about 11% of cases have repeated mutations. Studies of DIS3 and its similar proteins have highlighted its part in regulating cell-cycle events and microtubule assembly. As a result, scientists study the structure and function of such RNA-linked enzymes to figure out how they can lead to oncogenesis and highlight the close connection between RNA structure and biological effects (Figure 2.14).

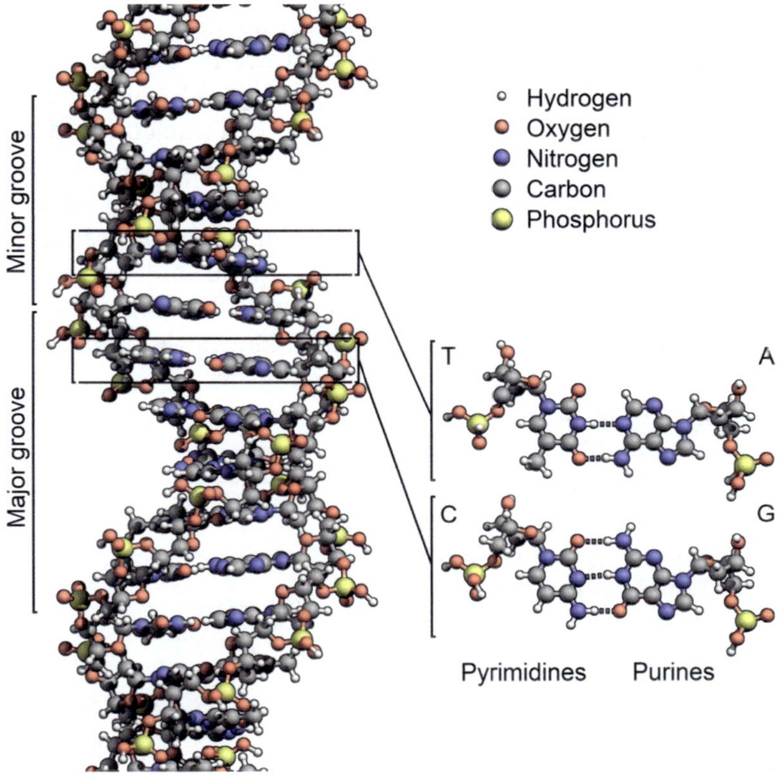

Figure 2.14. Structure of DNA and RNA.

Source: By Zephyris - Own work, CC BY-SA 3.0, https://commons.wikimedia.org/w/index.php?curid=15027555

2.4.2. Role of Nucleic Acids in Heredity

Nucleic acids play a key part in heredity since they carry the main genetic information in living things. All three processes of replication, transcription, and translation, which explain heredity, depend on DNA and RNA. DNA, because of its double-helix shape, carries the genetic code that passes traits from parents to their children. Cells ensure that their children get the same genetic information by replicating the guide. In addition, RNA is involved in making proteins and controls the way genes are regulated and used. This intricate interplay among nucleic acids exemplifies the complexity of biological systems, highlighting how genetic information drives organismal development and trait manifestation, thereby establishing a robust foundation for heredity (Griffiths et al., 2017). Nucleic acids are important for genetics and also affect the way genes are expressed through epigenetic factors that do not change the DNA. Epigenetics adds more details, since environmental factors can induce changes that affect the expression of genes. It shows that heredity covers more than just passing on DNA from one generation to the next. Epigenetic changes, for example methylation and histone modification, can be passed on from one generation to another, allowing organisms to cope with changes in their environment. This knowledge makes us see that heredity involves more than just genes, since epigenetic signals also play a role. The complementary roles of these systems illuminate the intricate network that supports development and evolution, highlighting the sophisticated architecture of life itself (Griffiths et al., 2017). Also, nucleic acids are studied for their possible contribution to the evolution of life, especially in relation to the lipid world hypothesis. It suggests that amphiphilic molecules, which could make compartments, were important in the early stages of life by providing a suitable environment for nucleic acids to develop. It is possible that the first genetic material started in lipid-bound areas, which helped start the processing and copying of information. To understand how nucleic acids developed, one must look at how they changed from simple molecules to the key structures they are today. As scientists keep studying these topics, they might discover new facts about how genetic systems developed and why nucleic acids are so important for heredity and life itself.

2.4.3. Importance of Nucleotides in Metabolism

Nucleotides are important in metabolism because they build nucleic acids and also function as coenzymes and help carry energy for different biochemical reactions. Nucleotides are made of a nitrogenous base, a sugar, and phosphate groups and are needed for cellular signaling, energy transfer, and important metabolic activities in living organisms. Adenosine triphosphate (ATP), the most recognized nucleotide, is crucial as it provides the energy needed for muscle contraction, conduction of nerve impulses, and biosynthesis. Its application emphasizes nucleotides' contribution to maintaining cellular homeostasis as well as promoting processes of life as essential. It also takes part in cellular control and signaling, which shows how important it is for metabolic functions in living organisms. Apart from energy, nucleotides are important in various metabolic reactions, mainly during the production and management of different biomolecules. As an example, 3′-phosphoadenosine-5′-phosphosulfate (PAPS) is a nucleotide that is important in the sulfation reaction needed for detoxification and glycosaminoglycan biosynthesis. The enzymes that produce PAPS have two functions, allowing sulfate to be converted into PAPS through adenosine-5′-phosphosulfate (APS), which shows the importance of nucleotides in metabolism.

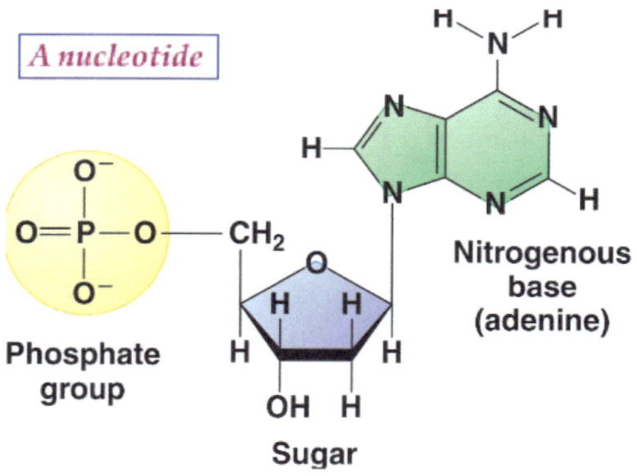

Figure 2.15. Nucleotide.

Source: https://bookdown.org/jcog196013/BS2003/_book/_main_files/figure-html/nucleotide.PNG.

Also, nucleotides are involved in signal transduction chains, which helps to control metabolic processes and guide the cell's reactions to changes in its surroundings. The way nucleotides interact in metabolism highlights how important they are in various physiological situations and shows their key role in life. Balancing nucleotide metabolism is important because any imbalances can cause severe changes in the body. Their effects on fish stress responses show that the nucleotide synthesis and breakdown are carefully managed by the cell to keep homeostasis. The use of nucleotide precursors and other helpful additives in animal feed is being studied to deal with the stress-related changes in metabolism and immunity seen in studies of dietary supplements. Such discoveries highlight the far-reaching significance of nucleotides as mere building blocks for DNA and RNA; they are also key modulators of metabolic wellbeing and welfare in a wide range of biological processes, substantiating their significant role in biomolecule research (Allali-Hassani et al., 2013; Herrera et al., 2019) (Figure 2.15).

Test Your Knowledge

1. What is the role of nucleic acids in heredity?
2. What is the importance of nucleotides in metabolism?

2.5. Metabolism of Biomolecules

Learning Outcome

1. Describe the cellular processes of catabolism and anabolism;
2. Describe the energy production from biomolecules;
3. Understand the regulation of metabolic pathways.

Biochemical reactions that take place in living organisms allow biomolecules to support growth, reproduction, and the normal functioning of cells. Carbohydrates, proteins, lipids, and nucleic acids are important biomolecules in this process, as they each have a special part in sustaining life. They take part in different metabolic processes, for example, catabolism and anabolism. Catabolic pathways break down big molecules to make energy, but anabolic pathways build up complex molecules using energy. It is essential to know these pathways since they explain cellular activities and can also affect health and disease. The fact that organisms have different metabolic abilities shows that life on Earth is strong and able to adjust to many different environments. At first, it was believed that biochemical reactions in metabolism did not need phosphate, a key component in today's metabolic processes. New studies indicate that the main metabolic processes might have formed first without phosphate, showing that simple prebiotic materials could have given rise to them. It brings up interesting questions regarding the early stages of life's development. The identified metabolic system that does not need phosphate supports the generation of vital biomolecules and points out the important role of iron-sulfur clusters in enzymes. By exploring these avenues, researchers provide fresh perspectives on how primitive life forms may have functioned and adapted long before the emergence of more complex biochemical mechanisms, suggesting a profound evolutionary legacy in biomolecular metabolism (Goldford et al., 2017). Those who conduct research and offer funding agree that metabolic processes must be understood in theory and in practice. The help from the Junta de Comunidades de Castilla-La Mancha and the Ministerio de Economía y Competitividad has greatly supported research in biomolecular metabolism. Thanks to such support, scientists can study the details of metabolic pathways and their development, which helps them better understand the molecular aspects of life.

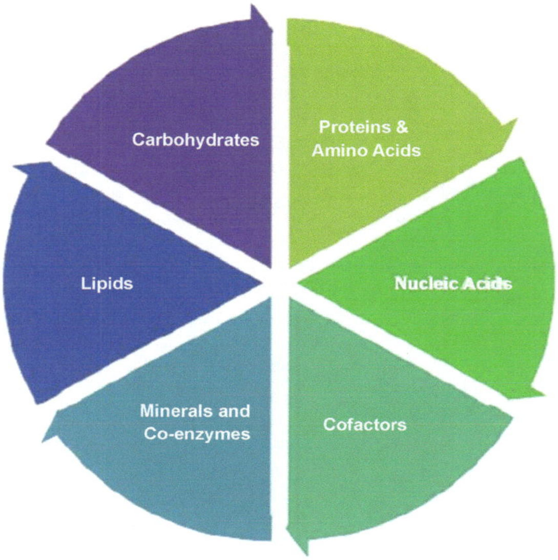

Figure 2.16. Different types of biochemicals that are involved in various metabolic processes of a living cell and organism.

Source: https://cdn-ildfibj.nitrocdn.com/qaWeLntkRcyxNUcEoWbLpZLQkcgLFsiJ/assets/images/optimized/www.biologyonline.com/wp-content/uploads/2019/10/different-biochemicals-for-metabolic-processes-768x723.jpg.

The partnership between those who provide funding and academic institutions encourages new research on biomolecules, which results in major advances in health, biotechnology, and environmental science. This collaborative effort is vital not only for academic advancement but also for the applicable benefits that a better understanding of metabolism can provide in diverse fields, illustrating the significance of ongoing research in biomolecules and their metabolic pathways (Fariñas et al., 2017) (Figure 2.16).

2.5.1. Catabolism and Anabolism

The breakdown of biomolecules through catabolism and their building up through anabolism are important for the metabolism of biomolecules and for creating energy and biosynthesis. Catabolism breaks down complex substances into simpler ones and in doing so, energy is released. This energy is largely trapped in the form of ATP, which also acts as a universal energy currency in living organisms. When catabolic processes occur, carbohydrates, lipids, and proteins are broken down so that important metabolic processes can happen.

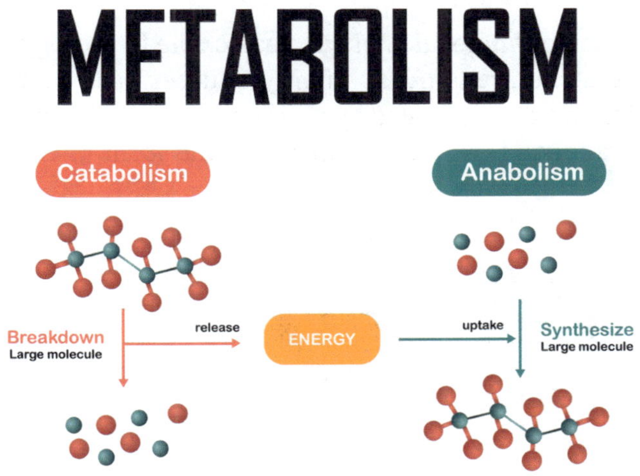

Figure 2.17. Catabolism and anabolism.

Source: https://carbyne.sg/cdn/shop/articles/6475f7bf5406b3331e3104f2c3f65489_7c812714-2079-4c7f-ac89-9c17048c2de4.png?v=1730621044.

Especially, anaerobic organisms use various catabolic ways to break down different substrates and are strong when energy is scarce. These adaptations reflect the essential link between catabolism and energy production, stressing the metabolic adaptability that enables survival under divergent physiological states (Lankiewicz et al., 2025). On the other hand, anabolism is the process of making complex molecules from smaller ones, which generally needs energy. For growth, repair, and maintenance of cells, this phase of metabolism is necessary and forms an important part of homeostasis in the body. ATP from catabolic reactions is used by anabolic pathways to create proteins, nucleic acids, lipids, and polysaccharides for the proper functioning of cells. Besides, the anabolic pathways are controlled by various things such as hormones and the presence of nutrients. For example, nutrient deficiency leads to a switch to catabolic pathways to break down energy reserves, and one will notice that both catabolism and anabolism are finely balanced with each other (Aditya et al., 2024). Exploring the link between catabolism and anabolism will provide insight into metabolic disorders and the treatments that could be used. The way metabolic control and energy homeostasis work in living things depends on the coordination of catabolism and anabolism. When these pathways are coordinated, the use and production of energy are in line with the cell's needs to make the most of its resources. If the glucose level is high, cells tend to use it for making glycogen rather than for other tasks. In case of fasting or greater energy use, the body increases catabolic pathways to access its stored energy. Because of this, organisms can survive in various environments and under different amounts of food. Losing the balance between anabolic and catabolic activities leads to serious problems such as obesity and diabetes. Knowledge about these dynamics is important for the progress of biochemical science and the development of interventions to enhance metabolic well-being (Lankiewicz et al., 2025). As a result, biochemistry gives special attention to the study of catabolism and anabolism in biomolecules since it helps guide both health and disease management (Figure 2.17).

2.5.2. Energy Production from Biomolecules

The production of energy from biomolecules plays a basic role in biology since organic compounds are used both for building structures and as energy sources. The metabolic pathways of living organisms, such as glycolysis and the citric acid cycle, exemplify how biomolecules like carbohydrates, lipids, and proteins are catabolized to release energy in the form of ATP.

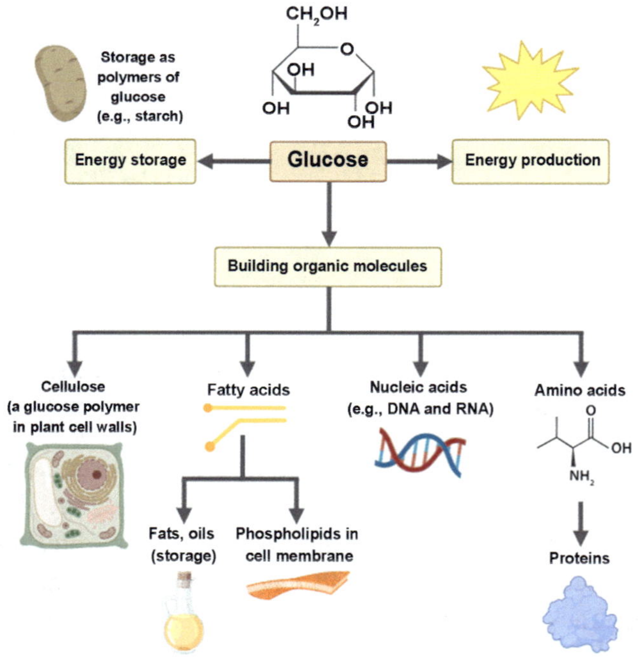

Figure 2.18. Glucose is one of the most abundant carbohydrates. Cells can use glucose for immediate energy or store glucose for later use as a polysaccharide, such as starch. In addition, cells use glucose to build various organic molecules.

Source: https://cdn.kastatic.org/ka-content-images/77938451e8c5c8119a4f8bcacd1037720501 6d67.png.

Because of ATP, cells can perform many tasks, including muscle movement and signaling. Studying these biochemical pathways reveals how living organisms convert energy and also shows possible ways to use them for producing bioenergy that helps meet the world's energy needs. Biomolecules are also studied in exobiology, which looks into the beginnings and possibilities of life in other worlds. Experts in this area research ways to produce biomolecules outside of Earth, to learn about energy production on other planets. In particular, the research agenda includes experiments for the Space Station that try to reproduce the atmosphere of early Earth or other planets. By studying the high-energy chemical processes responsible for biomolecule formation in these simulated environments, scientists can gain valuable knowledge regarding the conditions necessary for life and the possible biogenic pathways that could lead to sustainable energy sources beyond our planet (Devincenzi et al., 2025). Moreover, studying low-energy electron collisions with biomolecules gives important information about how these important molecules react and remain stable.

These studies provide not only foundational knowledge about how biomolecules like DNA, amino acids, and peptides behave under various conditions but also highlight the potential for utilizing these reactions in energy production and storage applications (Allan et al., 2017). Once biomolecules' reactions to energy are understood, researchers can create new strategies to improve bioengineering and biomass digestibility, which is key for making energy through fermentation and similar processes. The area where molecular biology and energy research meet highlights how biomolecules are important for sustainable energy and for learning more about life's biochemistry (Figure 2.18).

2.5.3. Regulation of Metabolic Pathways

A significant part of cellular homeostasis is controlling the pathways of cell metabolism and the interactions between enzymes and feedback loops. Through these pathways, many substances are turned into energy and important molecules that support all cellular activities. Often, enzymatic regulation happens at important points in metabolism by changing the enzyme's structure or by adding or removing groups from the enzyme. In some cases, the presence of metabolic intermediate or end-product can either block or stimulate an enzyme, which allows cells to react to changes in the levels of nutrients and energy. The high level of regulation around enzymes shows they are important targets in the body for new treatments of metabolic diseases. Enzymes play an even bigger role in regulating metabolic pathways when it comes to cancer. Cancer cells tend to have changed metabolism that allows them to reproduce quickly even in places where nutrients are scarce. It is known that changes in metabolic enzymes in cancer cells lead to other pathways being altered to maintain the cells' energy balance. For example, one study illustrated that oral cancer cells with knockdown of transketolase (TKT) via small interfering RNA (siRNA) increased the uptake of glucose and glutamine with enhanced lactate production as a survival mechanism for counteracting metabolic impairments. These findings underscore the adaptive metabolism of cancer and potential multiple metabolic pathways engaging with one another, calling for the need to target intervention based on these complex regulation systems (Brumbaugh et al., 2014). Besides cancer, controlling metabolic pathways is important in both developmental biology and cell differentiation. DIS3, which is an exoribonuclease that helps break down RNA, proves that metabolism and gene expression are always linked. Many types of human cancer are linked to DIS3 disruption, which underlines its role in RNA quality control and in regulating the cell cycle. It is shown by experiments that changes in DIS3 genes can disrupt cellular processes and trigger a series of metabolic problems that help cancer develop. Knowledge of the structure and function of DIS3 not only sheds light on its role in the regulation of metabolic pathways but also provides insights into the development of targeted therapies for cancer treatment (Carazo-Salas et al., 2015). So, controlling metabolic pathways is important in many ways, relating to both health and disease.

Test Your Knowledge

1. What are the cellular processes of catabolism and anabolism?
2. What biomolecules can be used to produce energy?

2.6. Biomolecules in Health and Disease

Learning Outcome

1. Understand the role of biomolecules in nutrition;
2. Know the biomolecules and their link to diseases;
3. Describe the therapeutic applications of biomolecules.

The connection between biomolecules and health is well shown by dental calculus, which is a calcified layer in the mouth where microbes and human biomolecules are stored. Thanks to these biomolecules, scientists can examine earlier microbiome communities and look at how the host responded. Notably, even though oral microbiome studies now mainly examine living dental plaque, dental calculus gives important clues about how oral biofilms have changed over the years. When scientists study microbes in modern dental plaque, modern calculus, and historic samples, they can see differences that show different health conditions. Such examinations reveal that while health-associated communities of plaque and calculus continue to differ, distinct microbial signatures indicative of both health and disease persist through time, emphasizing the relevance of these biomolecules in understanding oral health dynamics (Velsko et al., 2019). The significance of biomolecules extends beyond oral health to encompass broader nutritional influences on disease, particularly evident in conditions such as alcoholic liver disease (ALD). At the symposium, research focused on the impact of nutrition on ALD pointed out significant gains in understanding the disease's development. Experts pointed out that certain fats and carbohydrates in our diet can worsen alcohol-related damage to multiple organs, proving that what we eat can have a big effect on our health. Besides, the study of new nutritional treatments involving betaine and zinc demonstrates the link between nutrition, biomolecules, and treating diseases. Implementing effective nutrition-related interventions has critical implications for treating ALD and emphasizes the pivotal role biomolecules play in both exacerbating and mitigating disease states (Feldstein et al., 2018). Besides looking at biomolecules in certain diseases, one should also consider how they work within the entire biological system, as it adds to the complexity of health outcomes. In particular, the immune system works by using proteins, lipids, and nucleic acids that all work together to defend the body against diseases and help it heal. Problems with these biomolecular interactions may result in chronic inflammatory diseases, autoimmune disorders, and other health problems. That's why it is important to know how these biomolecules act by themselves and together to create new treatments and prevention methods. New studies are showing that working with biomolecules can greatly improve how diseases are managed and a person's overall health, proving that biomolecules play a key role in health and disease (Figure 2.19).

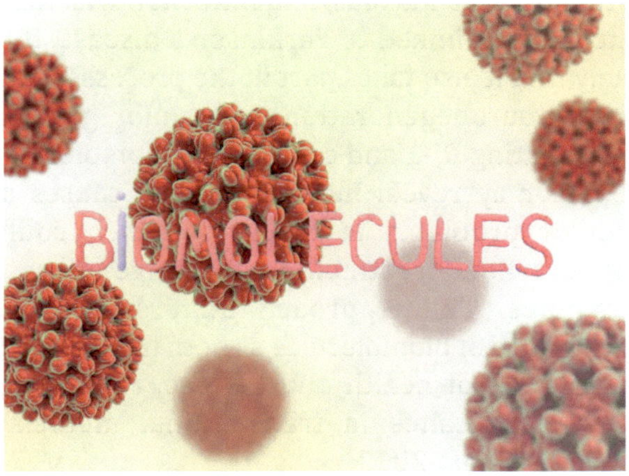

Figure 2.19. Graphic representation of biomolecules surrounded by virus-like particles.

Source: https://cbirt.net/wp-content/uploads/2023/01/Cover-Biomolecules1.webp.

2.6.1. Role of Biomolecules in Nutrition

Biomolecules are very important in nutrition for supporting life and health. Carbohydrates, proteins, lipids, vitamins, and minerals are the basic needs for body processes such as metabolism, energy generation, and repair of cells. Carbohydrates give the body energy, and proteins are important for growing tissues and making enzymes. Lipids are important for keeping cell membranes steady and for creating hormones. Besides, micronutrients, such as vitamins and minerals, help different biochemical reactions and are necessary for maintaining homeostasis. The network of these biomolecules stresses the role they play in nutrition overall, especially when we eat a variety of foods for better health. New findings about biomolecules have increased the roles they play in medical nutrition therapy. For instance, studies presented at the European Society for Biomedical Research on Alcoholism Congress underscored the role of dietary fats and carbohydrates in conditions like ALD. It was found through such research that special diets may help to slow down the progress of ALD and related dietary diseases. The research also points out that the right balance of macronutrients can help tackle malnutrition and help affected people recover. Because nutrition is seen as important for preventing and managing diseases, findings from biomolecule studies will play a key role in designing new nutritional guidelines and treatments. In addition, phenolic compounds are important in biomolecules because they play many roles in nutrition and agriculture. These small compounds that are often in plants have antioxidant properties that might be good for health when eaten.

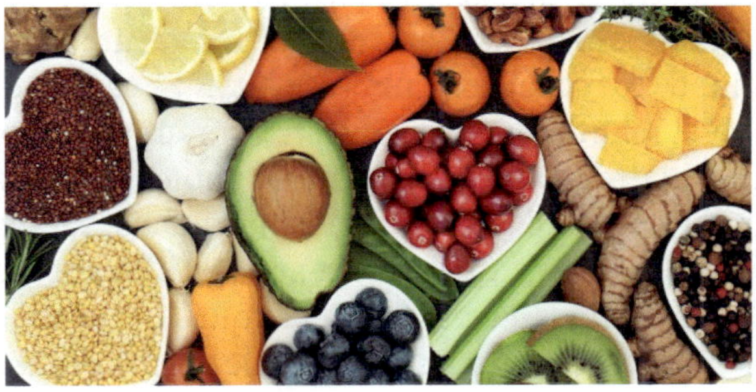

Figure 2.20. Role of biomolecules in nutrition.

Source: https://cdn.labmanager.com/assets/articleNo/28328/aImg/51188/exploring-the-biomolecules-that-will-help-us-get-to-know-our-food-l.jpg.

The presence of these compounds in diets can help other nutrients make essential minerals more available and useful, which is good for mineral element nutrition. In addition, phenolics play a major part in ecological interactions by defending crops against pests and diseases, which helps them grow in a healthier way. Further, the fact that by understanding the bioecological relevance of these compounds, it is possible to inform agricultural practices that enhance the nutritional quality of plant-based foods and therefore promote better public health outcomes, which has been the case in recent studies on their importance in the rhizosphere of legumes and other crops (Makoi et al., 2010) (Figure 2.20).

2.6.2. Biomolecules and Their Link to Diseases

Researchers in biomedicine have paid special attention to the connection between biomolecules and diseases, since they can show the presence of disease and also be treated to help cure it. Within living organisms, proteins, lipids, carbohydrates, and nucleic acids play very important roles. Protein homeostasis is important because, if it is disturbed, proteins may clump and cause harm, as happens in Alzheimer's disease. Also, problems with the metabolism of lipids and carbohydrates are linked to diabetes and obesity. Because of new technologies, scientists can now study the relationships among these molecules and understand their roles in causing and worsening diseases. New developments in biosensors and biochips have improved our knowledge of biomolecules that cause diseases. Because of these advanced technologies, it is possible to keep an eye on disease biomarkers and treat patients with personalized care as soon as needed. As an illustration, devices inserted under the skin can monitor glucose in diabetic people, and this idea can be applied to other metabolites related to additional conditions. Still, there are issues to overcome in developing such technologies, for example, guaranteeing their safety and privacy over time. Working on these issues is important to reach the goal of creating devices that monitor patients with little impact and better results. Initiatives aimed at resolving these challenges may lead to significant advancements in the management of chronic diseases and enhance our comprehension of biomolecular interactions in health and illness (Baj-Rossi et al., 2012). The role of proteins such as DJ-1 in diseases is also shown by their ability to remove sugars from other molecules. It is connected to various cellular processes and might be why the protein appears in the cytoplasm, the nucleus, and mitochondria. Also, since DJ-1 is linked to Parkinson's disease, it is likely that it also takes part in the processes that cause neurodegeneration and tumor growth. Investigating DJ-1 and comparable biomolecules further may reveal more about the causes of cellular problems in diseases, which could support new treatments to change disease outcomes. This approach underscores the importance of biomolecules as both markers and modulators of health and disease, reinforcing their significance in translational medicine (Bisaglia et al., 2017).

2.6.3. Therapeutic Applications of Biomolecules

Biomolecules have a major role in advancing medical science and different forms of treatment. The existence of proteins, nucleic acids, and lipids in the body means that several treatment methods can be developed for different diseases. For example, monoclonal antibodies are a kind of protein biomolecule that is designed to attach to specific antigens and is now very important in treating both cancer and autoimmune diseases. Parallel to this, nucleic acid therapies like small interfering RNAs (siRNAs) and mRNAs offer novel methodologies in gene therapy. With the help of biomolecules, scientists are able to target and stop diseases at the molecular level, which proves their great significance and potential in therapeutics. Extracellular vesicles (EVs) are another notable development within biomolecule-based therapies. They are released by cells of many types and serve as means for cells to communicate, carrying proteins, lipids, and nucleic acids between them and encouraging changes in how the cells act or look. As a result, the sudden release of EVs in abnormal states can trigger communication between cells that may manage or change how the immune system or disease functions. Experts are currently studying the use of EVs as possible tools for diagnosis, prevention, and therapy, mainly in infectious diseases, which could change the way we deal with these diseases. The scientific community can draw significant insights into the role of EVs in disease pathways by studying the differing compositions of EVs across various stressors or disease states, and they can exploit these insights toward innovative therapeutic strategies; such is the therapeutic promise of these biomolecules in clinics, according to Gavinho et al. (2019). Indeed, by highlighting how biological systems are connected, integrative systems biology gives a solid framework to study how biomolecules can be used in medicine. Unlike the old approach that studies only one biomolecule, the systems approach examines the many interactions and loops that happen in biological networks. It is very important to see things this way when considering the effects of therapy in different types of cells and tissues. It supports the development of fair and testable ideas that may reveal new details about diseases and the ways to treat them. By reusing existing data and employing advanced analytic techniques, researchers can overcome the challenges associated with large-scale data integration, ultimately enhancing the efficacy of biomolecule-based therapies in personalized medicine and pharmacological studies (Fernandes et al., 2014). For this reason, systems biology contributes to the use of biomolecules in medicine and also contributes to the progress of medical research.

Test Your Knowledge

1. What is the role of biomolecules in nutrition?
2. What are the therapeutic applications of biomolecules?

Summary

The summation in biomolecules is an important way to bring together the main themes and findings shown in the chapter. We should realize that proteins, nucleic acids, carbohydrates, and lipids are important for the structure and function of all living beings. Interactions between these molecules highlight the fact that many relationships in biology are what allow life to exist. As explained in the section on genes, both the information in genes and epigenetic effects play a big role in development and evolution. This interaction points out that it is important to learn about the different inheritance systems, since biological information is complex and keeps changing. The evolutionary viewpoint is explained here by pointing out that genetic, epigenetic, and exogenetic inheritance play a key role in determining how heredity works. Having these systems in balance explains how organisms can change with time and still keep their growth processes steady. Hence, the idea of proximate and ultimate biology is especially important in this case. Proximate information is responsible for current changes in development, but ultimate information reveals why these changes happened over time. So, it is important to see information as having two aspects to properly handle the challenges of biological inheritance, covering both short-term and long-term effects. Single molecule manipulation techniques are among the innovative ways that help us study the detailed interactions influencing biomolecule stability. When proteins are pulled in different ways, researchers have found out how their structures remain intact. They reveal the reasons behind biomolecule stability and are in line with the main idea of evolutionary adaptation. By running experiments that show phase transitions like those seen in molecules, this research points out how mechanical forces play a key role in biological functions. All in all, the summation highlights how biomolecules are complex, and it calls for an approach that brings together genetics, evolution, and the mechanical details required for life to continue.

Biomolecules are important for life since they form the foundation and work as necessary parts for cellular activities. These molecules are mainly divided into carbohydrates, lipids, proteins, and nucleic acids, and they are very different in both structure and function. Carbohydrates help store energy and keep the body strong, while lipids are needed for building cell membranes and saving energy for a long time. Proteins are important for helping biochemical reactions and performing several cell functions, mainly because of how their three-dimensional structures are built. Nucleic acids, such as DNA and RNA, are needed for storing and moving genetic information, which helps the expression of biomolecular systems by the genetic code. All in all, these different biomolecules highlight how they are related and how important they are in living organisms. When it comes to proteins, their ability to be attached to nanomaterials using physical adsorption or covalent bonds proves their lasting and flexible nature. It has been found through research that proteins can be properly arranged on carbon nanotubes, keeping much of their original structure and function needed for biotechnology and medicine. By using Raman and Fourier transform infrared spectroscopies and enzyme kinetic analyses, scientists can check how well these conjugates work and remain stable under difficult conditions. This discovery indicates that both covalent and noncovalent attachment routes can produce operationally stable and reusable protein conjugates, leading to innovative applications in the fields of sensor technology and drug delivery, ultimately enhancing our understanding of protein behavior in immobilized states (Asuri et al., 2009). Another fascinating class of biomolecules is the antifreeze glycoproteins (AFGPs), which showcase unique functionalities in extreme environmental conditions, specifically in cold habitats. They consist of repeating tripeptides and are not well structured, which makes it hard to determine their structures.

By employing a unique approach that utilizes dimethyl sulfoxide (DMSO), researchers have been able to elucidate the three-dimensional structures of AFGPs from different species. The results suggest that their overall shapes are not the same, yet they are just as compact, which proves that important motifs are kept the same for their function. So, AFGPs can change from being disordered in solution to being ordered on ice, and they function as linkers that stop ice crystals from forming. This characteristic not only underscores the adaptive significance of AFGPs but also enhances our comprehension of protein design and functionality in extreme conditions (Her et al., 2019).

KEY TERMS FROM THIS CHAPTER

- Biological sciences
- Biomolecules
- Disaccharides
- Glycoproteins
- Monosaccharides
- Nucleic acids
- Polysaccharides
- Starch
- Biomolecular science
- Carbohydrates
- Glycolipids
- Lipids
- Nanotechnology
- Polypeptide chains
- Proteins

CRITICAL THINKING QUESTIONS

1. **Which of the following is a carbohydrate?**
   a. Cholesterol
   b. Cellulose
   c. Hemoglobin
   d. DNA
2. **The building blocks of proteins are:**
   a. Fatty acids
   b. Monosaccharides
   c. Amino acids
   d. Nucleotides
3. **Which lipid molecule is a precursor for steroid hormones?**
   a. Triglycerides
   b. Cholesterol
   c. Phospholipids
   d. Glycolipids
4. **What type of bond links amino acids in a protein?**
   a. Glycosidic bond
   b. Hydrogen bond
   c. Peptide bond
   d. Ester bond
5. **Which of the following is a nucleic acid?**
   a. ATP
   b. RNA
   c. Glucose
   d. Hemoglobin

Answers to Critical Thinking Questions

1. (b); 2. (c); 3. (b); 4. (c); 5. (b)

Short Answer Questions

1. What are 4 main biomolecules?
2. Why is biomolecules importance in biological systems?
3. What are carbohydrates?
4. what are the functions of lipids in the body?
5. What is the metabolism of biomolecules?

References

1. Herrera, M., Mancera, J. M., & Costas, B. (2019). The Use of Dietary Additives in Fish Stress Mitigation: Comparative Endocrine and Physiological Responses. *Frontiers in endocrinology, 10*, 447. https://doi.org/10.3389/fendo.2019.00447 (accessed on 11th June 2025).
2. Aditya, G., Chakraborty, A., Chakraborty, S., Ghosh, R., et al. (2024). Growth of *Allopeas gracile* under starvation: Does it comply with von Bertalanffy growth equation? https://core.ac.uk/download/613191930.pdf (accessed on 11th June 2025).
3. Velsko, I. M., Fellows Yates, J. A., Aron, F., Hagan, R. W., Frantz, L. A. F., Loe, L., Martinez, J. B. R., Chaves, E., Gosden, C., Larson, G., & Warinner, C. (2019). Microbial differences between dental plaque and historic dental calculus are related to oral biofilm maturation stage. *Microbiome, 7*(1), 102. https://doi.org/10.1186/s40168-019-0717-3(accessed on 11th June 2025).
4. Canetta, E., Adya, A.K. (2011). Nano-imaging and Its Applications to Biomedicine. In: Maino, G., Foresti, G.L. (eds) Image Analysis and Processing – ICIAP 2011. ICIAP 2011. Lecture Notes in Computer Science, vol 6978. Springer, Berlin, Heidelberg. https://doi.org/10.1007/978-3-642-24085-0_44(accessed on 11th June 2025).
5. Allali-Hassani, A., Bedford, M. T., Benkovic, S. J., Boom, J., Bradley, A., Chen, D., Choe, J., et al. (2013). Adenosine-5′-phosphosulfate–A multifaceted modulator of bifunctional 3′-phospho-adenosine-5′-phosphosulfate synthases and related enzymes. https://core.ac.uk/download/pdf/16279840.pdf (accessed on 11th June 2025).
6. Allan, M., Allan, M., Bouchiha, D., Calegari, F., Caprasecca, S., Colyer, C. J., Colyer, C. J., et al. (2017). Electron scattering from molecules and molecular aggregates of biological relevance. https://core.ac.uk/download/131317000.pdf (accessed on 11th June 2025).
7. Aranda-Caño, L., Valderrama, R., Chaki, M., Begara-Morales, J. C., Melguizo, M., & Barroso, J. B. (2022). Nitrated Fatty-Acids Distribution in Storage Biomolecules during *Arabidopsis thaliana* Development. *Antioxidants, 11*(10), 1869. https://doi.org/10.3390/antiox11101869 (accessed on 11th June 2025).
8. Asuri, P., Bale, S. S., Banerjee, A., Dordick, J. S., et al. (2009). Preparation and characterization of protein-nanotube conjugates. https://core.ac.uk/download/215441831.pdf (accessed on 11th June 2025).
9. Baj-Rossi, C., Burleson, W., Carrara, S., Cavallini, A., et al. (2012). Fully integrated biochip platforms for advanced healthcare. https://core.ac.uk/download/286729684.pdf (accessed on 11th June 2025).
10. Barron, L. D. (2015). The development of biomolecular Raman optical activity spectroscopy. https://core.ac.uk/download/77601498.pdf (accessed on 11th June 2025).
11. Kallepitis, C., Bergholt, M., Mazo, M. *et al.* Quantitative volumetric Raman imaging of three dimensional cell cultures. *Nat Commun* **8**, 14843 (2017). https://doi.org/10.1038/ncomms14843(accessed on 11th June 2025).
12. Bisaglia, M., De Lazzari, F. (2017). DJ-1 as a deglycation enzyme: A unique function to explain a multifaceted protein? https://core.ac.uk/download/154326989.pdf (accessed on 11th June 2025).
13. Blagden, S., & Stavraka, C. (2015). The La-related proteins, a family with connections to

cancer. https://core.ac.uk/download/77019628.pdf (accessed on 11th June 2025).

14. Brumbaugh, J., Chai, Y. D., Feng, S., Hu, M., et al. (2014). Oral cancer cells may rewire alternative metabolic pathways to survive from siRNA silencing of metabolic enzymes. https://core.ac.uk/download/323080101.pdf (accessed on 11th June 2025).

15. Cang, Z., Mu, L., & Wei, G. (2017). Representability of algebraic topology for biomolecules in machine learning based scoring and virtual screening. http://arxiv.org/abs/1708.08135 (accessed on 11th June 2025).

16. Cantor, C. R., Hyeon, C., Thirumalai, D., Dima, R. I., & Zuker, M. (2006). Size, shape, and flexibility of RNA structures. http://arxiv.org/abs/q-bio/0609035 (accessed on 11th June 2025).

17. Carazo-Salas, R. E., Drach, J., Kinoshita, K., Lim, S., Noguchi, T., Ohkura, H., Sazer, S., et al. (2015). The 3' to 5' exoribonuclease DIS3: From structure and mechanisms to biological functions and role in human disease. https://core.ac.uk/download/30613413.pdf (accessed on 11th June 2025).

18. Chen, Z., Hu, F., Min, W., Shen, Y., et al. (2016). Live-cell bioorthogonal chemical imaging: Stimulated Raman scattering microscopy of vibrational probes. https://core.ac.uk/download/211378096.pdf (accessed on 11th June 2025).

19. Cirone, M., Crispini, A., D'Orazi, G., Federici, M., et al. (2020). Interplay between endoplasmic reticulum (ER) stress and autophagy induces mutant p53H273 degradation. https://core.ac.uk/download/296244523.pdf (accessed on 11th June 2025).

20. Cruz-León, S., Grotz, K. K., & Schwierz, N. (2021). Extended magnesium and calcium force field parameters for accurate ion-nucleic acid interactions in biomolecular simulations. *The Journal of chemical physics, 154*(17), 171102. https://doi.org/10.1063/5.0048113(accessed on 11th June 2025).

21. Devincenzi, D. L., & Griffiths, L. D. (2025). *Exobiology experiment concepts for space station.* https://core.ac.uk/download/pdf/42840862.pdf (accessed on 11th June 2025).

22. Lankiewicz TS, Elisabeth NH, Valentine DL, O'Malley MA. An argument for using anaerobes as microbial cell factories to advance synthetic biology and biomanufacturing. *AIChE J.* 2025; 71(6):e18797. doi:10.1002/aic.18797(accessed on 11th June 2025).

23. Fariñas, N. R., Krupp, E., Martín-Doimeadiosa, R. C. R., Matteo, R. A., et al. (2017). Mercury and selenium binding biomolecules in terrestrial mammals (*Cervus elaphus* and *Sus scrofa*) from a mercury exposed area. https://core.ac.uk/download/131023753.pdf (accessed on 11th June 2025).

24. Feldstein, A. E., Kharbanda, K. K., Kirpich, I. A., McClain, C. J., et al. (2018). Role of nutrition in alcoholic liver disease: Summary of the symposium at the ESBRA 2017 Congress. https://core.ac.uk/download/323064796.pdf (accessed on 11th June 2025).

25. Fernandes, M., Husi, H., & Robinson, S. W. (2014). Current advances in systems and integrative biology. https://core.ac.uk/download/42354777.pdf (accessed on 11th June 2025).

26. Gavinho, B., Combes, V., Dlugonska, H., Hart, M., Evans-Osses, I., Rossi, I. V., Inal, J., et al. (2019). A new landscape of host–protozoa interactions involving the extracellular vesicles world. https://core.ac.uk/download/287580982.pdf (accessed on 11th June 2025).

27. Goldford, J. E., Hartman, H., Marsland, R., 3rd, & Segrè, D. (2019). Environmental boundary

conditions for the origin of life converge to an organo-sulfur metabolism. *Nature ecology & evolution, 3*(12), 1715–1724. https://doi.org/10.1038/s41559-019-1018-8(accessed on 11th June 2025).

28. Goldford, J. E., Hartman, H., Smith, T. F., & Segrè, D. (2017). Remnants of an Ancient Metabolism without Phosphate. *Cell, 168*(6), 1126–1134.e9. https://doi.org/10.1016/j.cell.2017.02.001(accessed on 11th June 2025).
29. Griffiths, P. E., & Stotz, K. (2017). Genetic, epigenetic and exogenetic information. https://core.ac.uk/download/131214859.pdf (accessed on 11th June 2025).
30. Harris, S., & Kendon, V. M. (2010). Quantum-assisted biomolecular modelling. http://arxiv.org/abs/1007.1885 (accessed on 11th June 2025).
31. Her, C., Krishnan, V. V., & Yeh, Y. (2019). The ensemble of conformations of antifreeze glycoproteins (AFGP8): A study using nuclear magnetic resonance spectroscopy. https://core.ac.uk/download/323069163.pdf (accessed on 11th June 2025).
32. Ivankin, A., Jaramillo, A., Warshel, A., Camley, A. B., Lee, B., Li, B., Li, Y., et al. (2016). Variational methods for biomolecular modeling. http://arxiv.org/abs/1611.00610 (accessed on 11th June 2025).
33. Kahana, A., Lancet, D., & Segrè, D. (2019). Twenty years of "Lipid World": A fertile partnership with David Deamer. https://core.ac.uk/download/322973325.pdf (accessed on 11th June 2025).
34. Kamleh, A., Malmendal, A., Malmendal, A., Jackson, A. A., Jeulin, C., Watson, D. G., Watson, D. G., et al. (2013). Mapping an atlas of tissue-specific *Drosophila melanogaster* metabolomes by high resolution mass spectrometry. https://core.ac.uk/download/16462998.pdf (accessed on 11th June 2025).
35. Kolb, B., & Thonhauser, T. (2012). Molecular biology at the quantum level: Can modern density functional theory forge the path? http://arxiv.org/abs/1207.1075 Nano LIFE 2012 02:02 (accessed on 11th June 2025).
36. Kumar, A., & Smith, B. (2003). A framework for protein classification. In Anand Kumar & Barry Smith, *Proceedings of the 2003 German Conference on Bioinformatics, Vol. II*. pp. 55-57 (2003) (accessed on 11th June 2025).
37. Macabuhay, A., Arsova, B., Walker, R., Johnson, A., Watt, M., & Roessner, U. (2021). Modulators or facilitators? Roles of lipids in plant root–microbe interactions. *Trends in Plant Science, 27*, 180–190. https://doi.org/10.1016/j.tplants.2021.08.004 (accessed on 11th June 2025).
38. Makoi, J. H. J. R., & Ndakidemi, P. A. (2010). Biological, ecological and agronomic significance of plant phenolic compounds in rhizosphere of the symbiotic legumes. https://core.ac.uk/download/478322475.pdf (accessed on 11th June 2025).
39. Nusz, J. R. (2014). Incorporating engineering in high school biology. https://core.ac.uk/download/211337597.pdf (accessed on 11th June 2025).
40. Ouweneel, A. B., Thomas, M. J., & Sorci-Thomas, M. G. (2019). The ins and outs of lipid rafts: Functions in intracellular cholesterol homeostasis, microparticles, and cell membranes. *Journal of Lipid Research, 61*, 676–686. https://doi.org/10.1194/jlr.tr119000383 (accessed on 11th June 2025).

41. Peveler, W. J., Rotello, V. M., & Yazdani, M. (2016). Selectivity and specificity: Pros and cons in sensing. https://core.ac.uk/download/132211233.pdf (accessed on 11th June 2025).

42. Sargoytchev, S. S. (2017). A new method for analysis of biomolecules using the BSM-SG atomic models. https://core.ac.uk/download/132155325.pdf (accessed on 11th June 2025).

43. Shahul Hameed, M. S. (2012). *Structural Studies of E. coli Thioredoxin and P. falciparum Triosephosphate Isomerase by NMR and Computational Methods*. https://core.ac.uk/download/154851230.pdf (accessed on 11th June 2025).

44. Vanderzande, C., Giri, D., Doi, M., de Gennes, P. G., & Kumar, S. (2007). Does changing the pulling direction give better insight into biomolecules? http://arxiv.org/abs/cond-mat/0701679 (accessed on 11th June 2025).

45. Wei, G. W. (2017). Mathematics at the eve of a historic transition in biology. http://arxiv.org/abs/1711.02001 (accessed on 11th June 2025).

ENZYMES

3

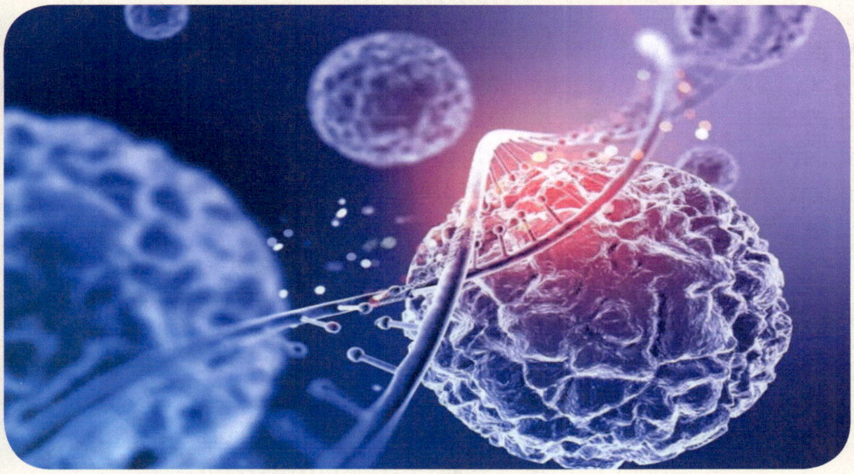

Introduction

Enzymes are important in biochemistry since they speed up chemical reactions in living things. Enzymes are important for various biological functions, such as metabolism, making new DNA, and cell communication. Their three-dimensional shapes as proteins make enzymes able to work in certain ways. The structure of an enzyme and the way it functions are important for knowing how biological systems operate. Enzymes help reactions occur much faster by lowering the energy needed for them, making it possible for life-sustaining processes to happen at the right speed. More research on enzymes shows that temperature, pH, and the amount of substrate affect their activity. So, it is important to learn about enzymes thoroughly to understand their basic functions in biology and also to see their effects in medicine, biotechnology, and environmental science. The significance of glycosylation in enzymatic functions is especially noticeable due to its complexity. The attachment of carbohydrates to proteins and

LEARNING OBJECTIVES

After studying this chapter, you will be able to:

1. Describe the structure of enzymes;
2. Know the mechanism of enzyme action;
3. Describe the types of enzymes;
4. Understand the enzyme kinetics;
5. Describe the role of enzymes in maintaining human health;
6. Know the environmental impact of enzymes.

lipids by glycosylation greatly changes their form and function. A few enzymes are in charge of guiding the process that creates complex glycans. Glycans help with important functions like folding proteins, signaling between cells, and involving the immune system. In addition, the N-linked glycosylation pathways have a modular structure and involve communication between several enzyme modules. They reveal both the complexity of biochemical networks and the way that various cellular molecules and enzymes work together. Exploring these pathways deepens our understanding of how enzymes perform their roles within larger biological systems and lays the groundwork for advancements in therapeutic applications in glycoprotein engineering, as outlined in the findings of research focused on glycan synthesis (Helenius et al., 2009).

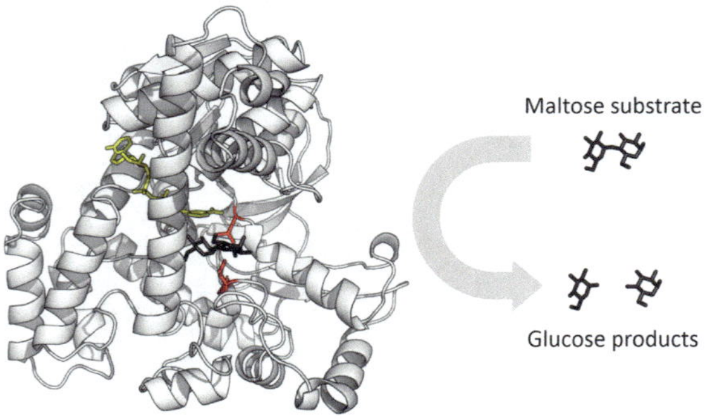

Figure 3.1. Enzymes.

Source: https://en.wikipedia.org/wiki/File:Glucosidase_enzyme.png

Also, genomic data makes it easier to study how enzymes function in both health and disease, especially in cases of infectious diseases such as malaria. Finding possible drug targets starts with mining and organizing genomic information from organisms such as Plasmodium falciparum. Researchers use protein sequences, metabolic pathways, and interactions between molecules to find new targets for enzyme-based treatments. Because of high-throughput tools and bioinformatics, scientists can now rebuild molecular phylogenies and use predictions to see if drug candidates will bind to enzymes. Consequently, this multidisciplinary approach not only enhances our understanding of enzyme activity but also drives innovation in combatting diseases through targeted therapy development (Bastien et al., 2006). As a result, enzymes show their usefulness in biology and in the field of biotechnology (Figure 3.1).

Definition of Enzymes

Enzymes help and speed up chemical reactions that occur in living organisms. They are needed for important biological functions, for example, digestion, metabolism, and DNA replication. Enzymes are usually very specific and only trigger a single reaction or a group of similar reactions. The enzyme's special three-dimensional shape makes it possible for it to connect with its substrate. Enzymes make it easier for reactions in the body to take place at a speed that is necessary for life to continue. Enzymes are important for the metabolic processes that control cellular activity in both single cells and the whole body. The way enzymes work depends on temperature, pH, and the amount of their substrate. Each enzyme has its own best condition, so some work well in alkaline environments, and others do better in acidic ones. When these factors combine, they can greatly change how well enzymes work and the efficiency of metabolism. Presence of inhibitors or activators can either slow down or speed up the activity of enzymes. Because of this, cells can maintain balance and respond to changes in their environment or inside the body. For example, the metabolic shifts observed in organisms like Caenorhabditis elegans demonstrate how enzymatic pathways adjust in response to stressors, showcasing the dynamic nature of enzymatic functions within biological systems (Braeckman et al., 2009). Besides knowing what enzymes are and what they do, it is important to see how they are applied in biotechnology and medicine. Enzymes are used in different industries, such as food and pharmaceuticals, to boost the amount and quality of what is produced. Therapists rely on enzymes for improving drugs, treating illnesses, and carrying out diagnostics. More studies on enzymes and how they interact have resulted in the development of enzyme inhibitors that can treat diseases by stopping certain processes. Meanwhile, the development of enzymatic ontologies can greatly enhance instructional design in educational settings, aiding both instructors and learners in navigating complex biochemical knowledge (Boyce & Pahl, 2007). As a result, enzymes are important in biology and also play a key role in developing technology and healthcare (Figure 3.2).

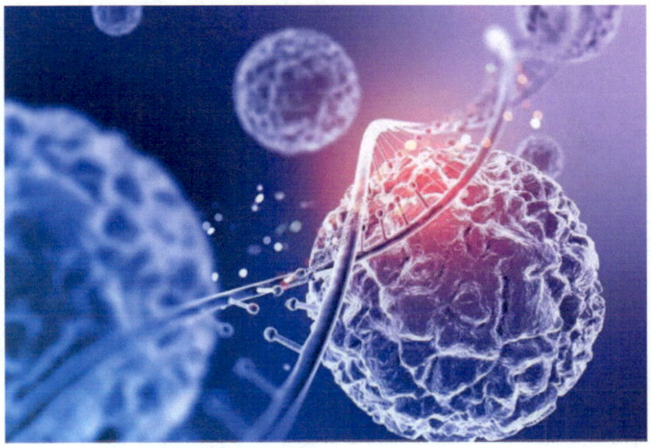

Figure 3.2. Enzymes in body.

Source: https://infinitabiotech.com/wp-content/uploads/2020/08/Enzymes-in-body.webp.

Importance of Enzymes in Biological Processes

Enzymes are important in biological processes mainly because they help speed up and control chemical reactions in living things. Life would not be possible if enzymes did not speed up many biochemical reactions. Thanks to enzymes, the activation energy needed for reactions is reduced, which causes the reactions to happen much faster. As an example, in metabolic pathways, enzymes help change substrates into products so the organism can efficiently produce energy. Thanks to the way they affect the speed and specificity of these reactions, enzymes help the processes of respiration, digestion, and biosynthesis work smoothly and efficiently, which is important for the organism's health. Microbial methane production is a good example of the impressive use of enzymes. Anaerobic archaea called methanogens produce methane using certain enzymes as they metabolize different materials. Studying these enzymes is very important for managing the environment, mainly when it comes to reducing greenhouse gases. Boosting the enzymatic steps in methanogenesis might increase the amount of methane produced and turn it into a reliable source of energy. The genetic manipulation of these archaea via techniques such as the Gibson Kit, while currently challenging, holds promise for improving methane production and thus contributing to biogas solutions for renewable energy (Jennings et al., 2018). Enzymes are important in biology and also play a big role in biotechnology. Using knowledge of enzymes from nature helps create new technologies for making silica-based materials. By creating conditions that mimic natural biosilicifying systems, researchers can develop new materials with a range of applications in sensor technology, drug delivery, and catalysis (Patwardhan et al., 2011). Managing how enzymes work and what they react with increases the usefulness of these materials and makes it possible to produce them on a large scale. The progress of biotechnology makes it clear that enzymes are key to both scientific and industrial activities.

3.1. Structure of Enzymes

Learning Outcome

1. Describe the basic components of enzymes;
2. Understand the role of active sites;
3. Describe the enzyme specificity and substrate interaction.

How amino acids are arranged in the three-dimensional structure of enzymes is what mainly determines their catalytic functions. They mostly take on particular shapes that help them interact with the molecules needed for important reactions in metabolism. Most enzymes have an active site where substrates are bound and several allosteric sites that can change the enzyme's activity. The different ways enzymes are built show their evolutionary backgrounds, as evident when looking at their folds and active sites. This diversity points out that enzymes can react with various substances and also function well in the body. A prime example of structural significance in enzymes can be observed in aldehyde dehydrogenase (ALDH), which plays a critical role in alcohol metabolism. Acetaldehyde is changed into acetate by the enzyme, which stops harmful substances from building up in the body. The special structure of enzymes helps them attach substrates and carry out the changes needed. Besides, the activity and stability of ALDH can be changed through genetic methods, especially by altering the Lys272 amino acid.

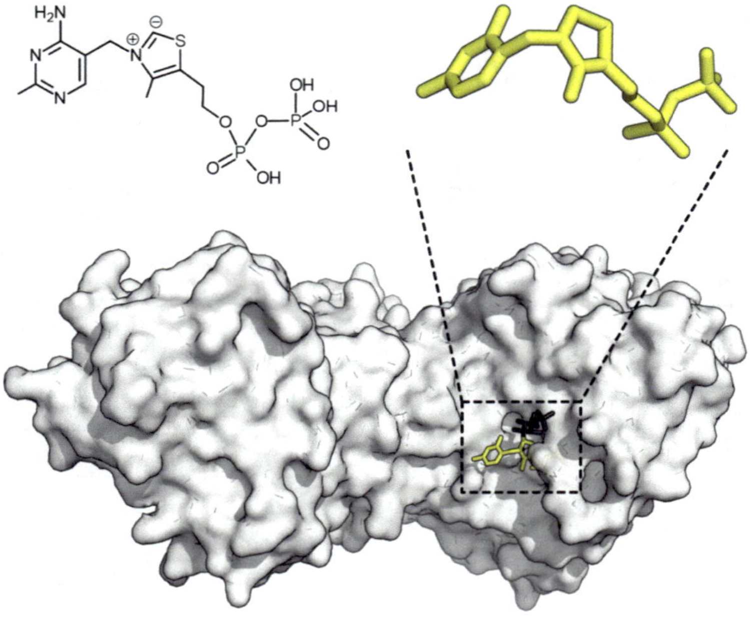

Figure 3.3. Structure of enzymes.

Source: By Thomas Shafee - Own work, CC BY-SA 4.0, https://commons.wikimedia.org/w/index.php?curid=38653926

Such studies enhance understanding of the structural components that are pivotal for enzyme function and overall cellular health, as disturbances in ALDH activity can lead to conditions such as Fetal Alcohol Syndrome, showing the profound implications of enzyme structure on biological processes (Wansbrough, 1998). Also, understanding how enzymes have evolved through their structure is quite fascinating. For instance, the phylogenetic analysis of thiamine pyrophosphate (TPP)-dependent enzymes illustrates the deep evolutionary relationships among this family of enzymes. It is shown in the study that these enzymes developed from a basic homotetramer to more complicated forms, such as $\alpha_2\beta_2$ heterotetramers. The changes in evolution have influenced the domains in these enzymes, for example, the pyrophosphate and pyrimidine binding domains, which are necessary for their functions. According to the findings, although more domains may help enzymes, their main catalytic activity is found in the basic domains. Such evolutionary insights reinforce the idea that enzyme structure is not only vital for function but also signifies the historical development of enzymatic diversity (Costelloe et al., 2008) (Figure 3.3).

3.1.1. Basic Components of Enzymes

Their active sites, substrates, and cofactors are the main parts of enzymes, and all three are important for the reaction to happen. An enzyme's active site is a small part of its surface that is designed to join with substrates and start a chemical reaction. The specificity is necessary since it affects how well and how efficiently the enzyme works.

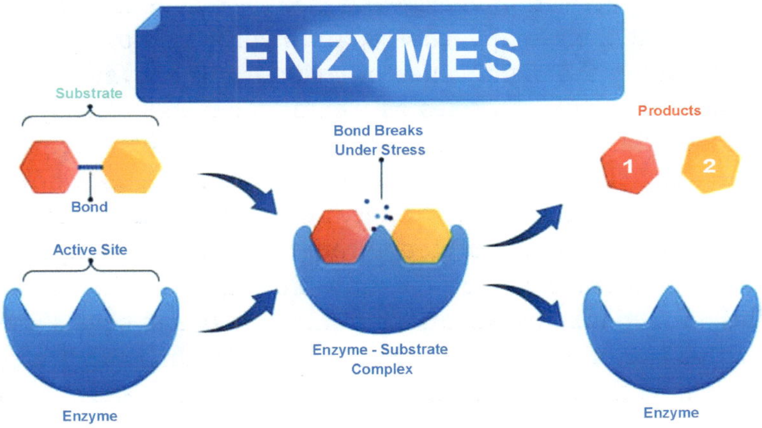

Figure 3.4. Enzymes are proteins.

Source: https://botnam.com/wp-content/uploads/2019/03/Enzymes-are-proteins.jpg.

The interaction between an enzyme and its substrate is often described by the "lock and key" model, which pictures the precise fit needed for the catalysis to be successful. As a result, when the substrate is attached to the active site, it creates an enzyme-substrate (ES) complex that starts a series of reactions that changes the substrate into products. Grasping this relationship forms the base for examining how enzymes work in the body, which is important for understanding many metabolic functions. Some enzymes are grouped depending on whether they depend on cofactors to function. Such additional substances may be metal ions or organic molecules called coenzymes, which help enzymes function as catalysts. In fact, zinc or magnesium can help stabilize enzymes and take part in electron transfers when reactions occur. In metabolism, cofactors are necessary since they usually make enzymes work more effectively and maintain the correct function. A striking example is ALDH, a key enzyme in alcohol metabolism. ALDH needs cofactors to work properly, converts acetaldehyde into less harmful substances and plays a pivotal role in several biochemical pathways (Wansbrough, 1998). If cofactors were not present, enzymatic reactions would not work at all, which clearly shows their vital importance in the enzyme process. Besides, the complexity of their structure can involve a metallocluster that strongly influences how efficiently the enzymes work. Clusters of metal ions and organic ligands are called these, and they play a key role in catalyzing many biochemical reactions, mainly those involving changes in the oxidation state. Enzymes such as nitrogenase and hydrogenase utilize these metalloclusters to process simple molecules like nitrogen and hydrogen, assisting in the generation of energy and basic biological building blocks (Rees et al., 2002). Researchers are still figuring out how these clusters work, since their mechanisms are very hard to uncover. The results of this investigation reveal how metalloclusters are important in biochemical catalysis and show the important relationship between biology and inorganic chemistry in living organisms (Figure 3.4).

3.1.2. The Role of Active Sites

The active site is the main part of an enzyme that helps reactions occur by binding the needed substrates. Because of its special arrangement of amino acids, the region allows ES complexes to form, which helps in lowering activation energy and making reactions occur faster. The reason for active sites' specificity is that their shape, charge, and hydrophilic or hydrophobic nature match the substrate well, underlining the significance of structure in enzyme function. The same level of specificity is important for single enzymes as well as for teams of enzymes working together in metabolic pathways. In this situation, learning about active sites helps us understand how enzymes evolve, because any changes in their composition can influence how well they work and which substances they interact with, thereby affecting the whole metabolism of living beings. It is also significant that active sites are formed through the use of complex adaptive strategies. Enzymes such as TPP-dependent enzymes illustrate how active sites can evolve and diversify while retaining essential functions. Investigations of these enzymes have shown that evolutionary pressures make the active site of enzymes more efficient at binding substrates. Studies show that structural variations, such as the recruitment of the transketolase C-terminal (TKC) domain, bear minimal impact on active site functionality.

Rather, the core components of the active site, including the conserved pyrophosphate (PP) and pyrimidine (Pyr) binding domains, have been fundamental to the role across different species, reinforcing the notion that adaptive evolution sharpens the focus on active site optimization in diverse environments (Costelloe et al., 2008). Biochemical pathways are also influenced by the intricate architecture of active sites found within bacterial microcompartments (BMCs). For instance, the phosphotransacylase (PTAC) enzyme showcases how active sites can adapt to facilitate specific metabolic needs within encapsulated environments. While the Pta enzyme is found everywhere, the PduL variant of PTAC in metabolosomes works differently and still performs the same function. The finding of the dimetal active site in PduLs points out the flexibility of enzymes in various parts of the cell. Such adaptations serve as compelling examples of functional convergence in enzymatic processes, illustrating how active sites can evolve structurally and functionally to optimize metabolism and cofactor recycling in a variety of ecological niches (Erbilgin et al., 2016) (Figure 3.5).

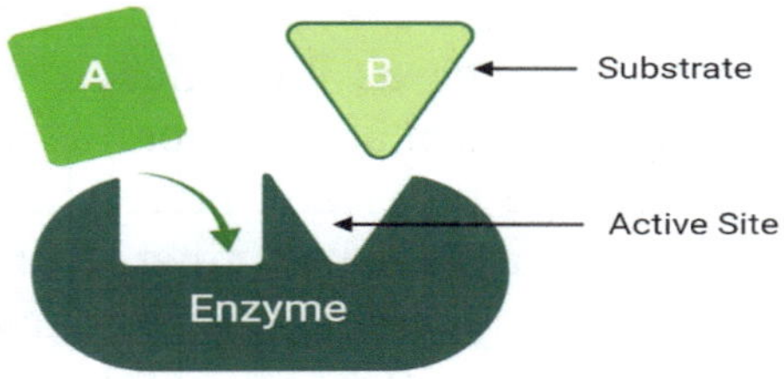

Figure 3.5. Active site of an enzyme.

Source: https://microbenotes.com/wp-content/uploads/2020/12/Active-site-of-enzymes.jpeg.

3.1.3. Enzyme Specificity and Substrate Interaction

Enzymes work well because they are specific, and this is mainly due to the special structure of their active sites. Enzymes are excellent biological agents that help reactions happen by making it easier for them to start. Usually, the active site on the enzyme is shaped in such a way that it fits with the substrate. It makes sure enzymes only catalyze reactions in some substrates and not in others, which is important for the cell's metabolic process. The relationship between enzymes and substrates can be noticed by looking at the active site structure. For instance, in cystathionine γ-lyase from Toxoplasma gondii, specific amino acid residues significantly influence the catalytic function and substrate specificity, illustrating the critical interplay between structure and function in enzymes (Astegno et al., 2018). How enzymes interact with the substances they act on is very significant in determining the final outcome of the reaction. Such forces as hydrogen bonding, hydrophobic interactions, and ionic bonds usually hold the ES complex together. As an illustration, the depolymerases of the bacteriophage Podoviridae demonstrate how specificity happens at the molecular level. The enzyme locates and binds to certain polysaccharides found on the bacterial surface and cuts them very carefully. The design of phage enzymes and their substrates was made to assist in infection and also to carry out a wide range of enzymatic activities. This specificity is at least as important for generating an effective propagation of bacteriophages and novel biotechnological applications (Fieseler et al., 2020). Exploring enzyme specificity includes not only knowing what substrates are but also looking at how the structure of enzymes affects their performance and the ways reactions take place. Small adjustments in the amino acids located in the active site may cause important changes in how the enzyme interacts with its substrate and reacts. As an example, changes in cystathionine γ-lyase show that even tiny alterations in an enzyme can seriously affect its activity and the pathways it influences in the body. This points out that evolution helps enzymes become more efficient and specific at the same time. By understanding how enzymes interact with their substrates, scientists can develop better and more effective biocatalysts for many industrial bioprocesses and advance both research and practical use of biotechnology (Figure 3.6).

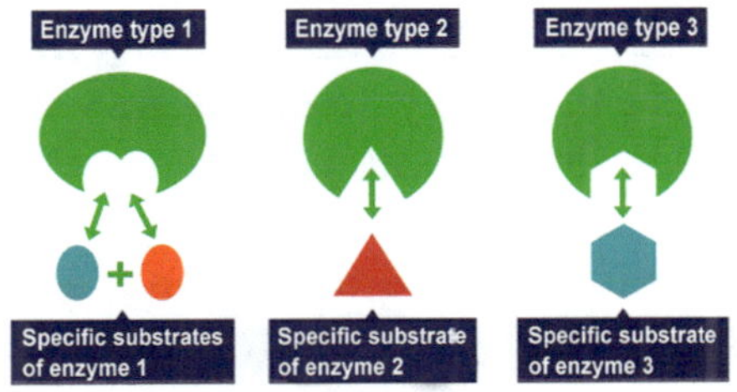

Figure 3.6. Enzyme specificity.

Source: https://bam.files.bbci.co.uk/bam/live/content/zv4gkqt/large.

Test Your Knowledge

1. What is the basic component of an enzyme?
2. What is the role of the active site of an enzyme?

3.2. Mechanism of Enzyme Action

Learning Outcome

1. Describe the lock and key model;
2. Describe the induced fit model;
3. Know the factors affecting enzyme activity.

The way an enzyme functions is complex, as it requires many important molecular interactions to start biochemical reactions. Enzymes mainly help reactions by lowering the energy needed for the change from substrate to product. At the beginning of this process, substrates are attracted to the active site of the enzyme because it is specially designed for them. After bonding, the enzyme weakens the substrates' bonds, which helps the substrates change into the product. Seeing how enzymes interact with their substrates explains why they are specific and points out the importance of the ES complex in carrying out reactions in cells. Apart from binding to their substrates, the actions of enzymes can be changed by things such as temperature, pH, and the presence of either activators or inhibitors. When these variables change the shape of an enzyme, its ability to work is also changed. As an example, some substances called enzyme inhibitors can either be removed or remain attached, both ways preventing the active site from participating in the reaction. On the other hand, activators increase enzyme activity, which makes the processing of substrates faster. Thanks to adaptability, metabolic pathways can manage their tasks well, so enzymes play a key role in keeping biological systems stable, mainly in complex processes like metabolism or signal transduction. In addition, new studies suggest that using ultrasound alongside enzymes can help biotechnology and environmental science advance. Researchers have looked into how ultrasound influences enzyme systems, mainly in bioprocesses such as bioremediation and enzymatic hydrolysis of biopolymers, as it helps these reactions go faster and more efficiently. Even though ultrasound is known to benefit enzymes and bioprocessing, the exact reasons are not yet fully understood, which means this is a major topic for further investigation. Additionally, specific enzymes, such as ALDH, play crucial roles in metabolic processes, including alcohol metabolism and the removal of toxic substances, underscoring the complex interplay between enzyme mechanisms and wider physiological functions (Wansbrough, 1998; Kwiatkowska et al., 2011) (Figure 3.7).

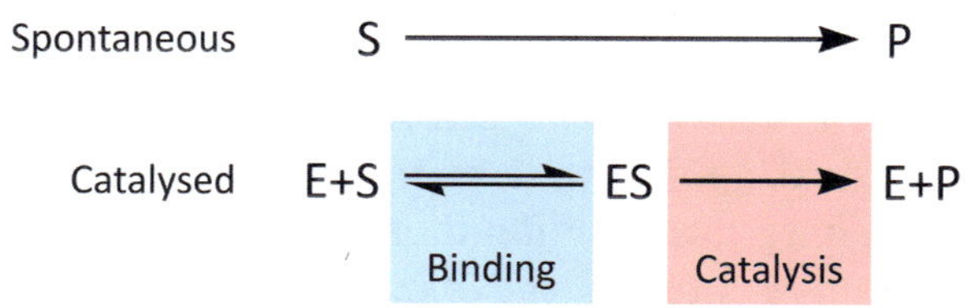

Figure 3.7. Mechanism of enzyme action describes how the substrate reacts with the enzyme, which results in the formation of the enzyme-substrate complex finally, this complex is converted into products and leaves the enzyme without any changes.

Source: By Thomas Shafee - Own work, CC BY 4.0, https://commons.wikimedia.org/w/index.php?curid=38914724

3.2.1. The Lock and Key Model

Emil Fischer's suggestion of the lock and key model at the end of the 19th century was the first step in describing how enzymes work and their specific roles. According to this model, enzymes fit with great precision onto the substrates, much as a key fit into a lock. Therefore, enzymes seem to have particular areas, called active sites, which fit the shape of their substrates. Enzymes take an active part in biochemical reactions by stabilizing the transition states, which helps change substrates into products. The model stresses that for enzymes to work well, they must fit their substrates perfectly, and this is due to the importance of the molecules' structure. Thus, the lock and key model supports the complex relationship between an enzyme's architecture and its functional ability in biological systems. Although the lock and key model helps us understand enzyme action, the induced fit model is used to consider that enzymes are flexible. The induced fit model proposes that the substrate binds to the enzyme, causing the enzyme to change its shape to interact well. Because of this, enzymes are better able to hold the transition states, which improves the speed of their reactions. Rather than the strict lock and key model, the induced fit mechanism takes into account the way enzymes have evolved. Enzyme activity depends on these changes, as the structure of an enzyme can be affected by factors in the environment and the kind of substrate, proving their importance in enzyme evolution. The ideas developed from the lock and key approach are important for biotechnology and pharmaceutical applications. It is important to understand the details of ES interactions to make enzyme inhibitors or drugs aimed at influencing a certain group of enzymes. As an example, inhibitors can be made to look like substrates, so they fit into the active site and prevent the substrates from entering, thereby stopping the unwanted reactions. Furthermore, appreciation of these mechanisms is vital in applications, such as the food industry, where enzymes, for example, pectinase (Srichantra, 2002), are used to change the texture and the achievement of uniformity in the product. Further, enzyme dynamics, how they work, revealed by the help of molecular evolution studies, emphasize that each sequence, structure, and function is in an interdependent relationship (Bhabha et al., 2013). Therefore, the lock and key model is important in explaining enzymes and in other scientific and industrial processes (Figure 3.8).

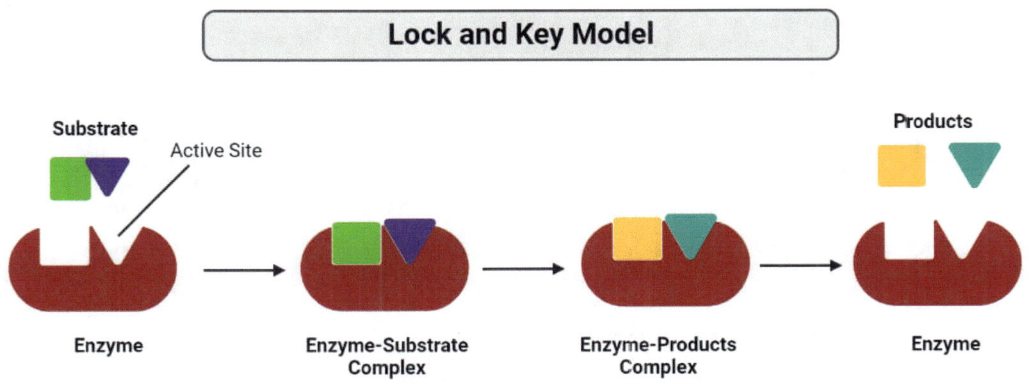

Figure 3.8. Lock and key model.

Source: https://microbenotes.com/wp-content/uploads/2022/09/Lock-and-key-model-of-Enzymes.jpg.

3.2.2. The Induced Fit Model

The induced fit model gives a more detailed explanation of ES specificity than the previous lock-and-key model. Here, the binding of the enzyme to its substrate causes the enzyme's structure to change its shape. The change boosts the efficiency of the enzyme by making sure the active site matches well with the substrate's reactive parts. Because the enzyme can change, it can work with different substances and perform more tasks. Things like pH and temperature in the environment can play a big part in this, affecting how well the enzyme works and how fast the reaction takes place. The ability of the induced fit model to adapt shows how enzymes can work well in different situations and help create a wider range of biochemical reactions. According to the induced fit model, binding of substrate to an enzyme causes changes that can further influence the enzyme's activity. After substrate attaches to the enzyme, the enzyme structure changes to a form that is ready for catalysis, showing the importance of the model for more than just bringing the substrate together with the enzyme. This feature is most common in allosteric enzymes, since binding of an effector molecule at a different site can cause changes in the enzyme's shape, which may boost or reduce its function. The induced fit model points out that enzymes act efficiently because they can adjust to different biochemical signals in the cell. The induced fit model has effects on both medicine and the engineering of enzymes. Seeing how enzymes change their shape when they interact with substrates allows researchers to invent better inhibitors or activators for different diseases. As an example, in pharmaceutical research, affinity-based drug design can rely on the induced fit model to produce molecules that bind and also change the structure of enzymes to achieve better results. This strategic approach is further evidenced by the continuous exploration of regulatory mechanisms within enzymes, as stated in research illustrating the significance of adaptive metabolism in interfacing with environmental changes and pollutant responses (Avilla et al., 2020). Knowing these dynamics is important for progress in biotechnology and medicine since it relates to how enzymes function in their use in science and medicine (Figure 3.9).

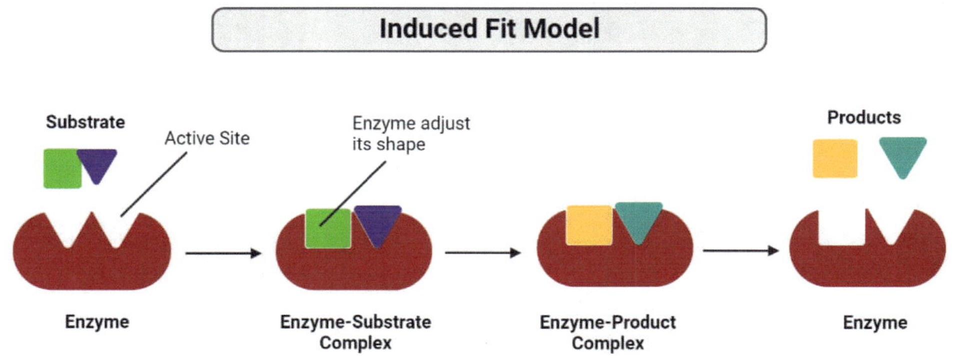

Figure 3.9. Induced fit model of enzymes.

Source: https://microbenotes.com/wp-content/uploads/2022/09/Induced-fit-model-of-Enzymes.jpg.

3.2.3. Factors Affecting Enzyme Activity

Many internal and external factors control how enzymes work, which greatly affects the speed of biochemical reactions. The concentration of the enzyme is a main factor; as it goes up, the rate of reaction tends to rise, as long as the substrate is not changing. Even so, this is not a straight relationship, since having all active sites occupied by substrate can cause the enzyme to reach saturation, which stops the reaction rate from increasing further. Moreover, the structure of the enzyme should be kept intact since changing it decreases its ability to catalyze reactions. Temperature and pH also greatly influence it. Raising the temperature can speed up reactions to the best level, but if it is raised further, denaturation takes place. In addition, enzymes show their best activities within certain pH ranges. So, it is necessary to control these conditions precisely to help enzymes function optimally. Enzymatic activity is greatly affected by inhibitors and activators. Inhibitors are classified as competitive or non-competitive and they affect the enzyme's function in different ways. Competitive inhibitors prevent substrate from attaching to the active site, but non-competitive inhibitors bind in a different place and still change how the enzyme works. Alternatively, activators increase how much an enzyme works, usually by making its shape more active or by helping it hold onto its substrate. It is important to know about these dynamics in areas such as pharmacology, where inhibitors are used as drugs, and in industry, where enzyme efficiency decides the amount of products produced. The fact that enzymes are controlled by both inhibitors and activators proves that it is important to carefully regulate conditions in both natural and artificial systems to get the desired outcomes. Biotechnology and biochemistry have recently made it clear that ultrasound can help boost the activity of enzymes. It has been found that ultrasound can help enzymatic reactions by adjusting the environment, making it easier for the substrate to reach the enzyme, or causing slight changes in the enzyme's shape that boost its activity. For instance, studies have provided insights into the effects of ultrasound on specific enzyme systems, suggesting they might enhance bioprocesses such as enzymatic hydrolysis and bioremediation (Kwiatkowska et al., 2011). Additionally, understanding how certain enzymes function within specific metabolic pathways or contribute to critical biological processes, like those involving the CYP26 subfamily, underscores the intricate balance of factors that govern enzyme activity and the implications of their regulation for developmental and physiological health (Roberts, 2020). Because of these details, it is important to keep studying the variety of enzyme activity and its possible uses in different scientific sectors (Figure 3.10).

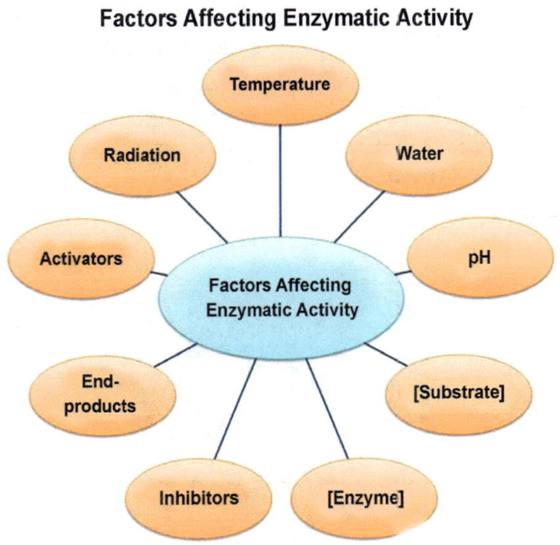

Figure 3.10. Factors affecting enzyme activity.

Source: https://easybiologyclass.com/wp-content/uploads/2019/02/What-are-the-factors-affecting-enzymatic-activity.jpg.

Test Your Knowledge

1. Who proposed the lock and key model?
2. What is the induced fit model?

3.3. Types of Enzymes

Learning Outcome

1. Classify the enzymes based on function;
2. Understand the role of enzymes in facilitating metabolic pathways;
3. Describe the industrial enzymes and their applications.

Enzymes are divided into several groups depending on their functions and the reactions they help with. Many hydrolases are important, as they help break down substrates by adding water, which happens in the digestion process. As an example, amylase helps break starch into sugars, so that the nutrients can be absorbed in the intestines. Ligases are also very important because they help combine two substrates to make new compounds, usually using energy from ATP. Because there are many types of enzymes, we can see that metabolic pathways in living things are very complex and support different processes. Isomerases are another type of enzymes that change a molecule from one type of isomer to another but do not alter its formula. Thanks to this function, organisms can adjust their chemical reactions to cope with different environmental changes. Phosphoglucose isomerase is an example of isomerase because it helps change glucose-6-phosphate into fructose-6-phosphate in glycolysis. Besides, some enzymes, like TKT from the TPP-dependent group, change their structures to match their roles in metabolism. Recent studies have indicated that evolutionary adaptations in these enzyme families demonstrate a remarkable ability to alter functionality, suggesting that gene loss can influence substrate specificity and enzyme efficiency over time (Costelloe et al., 2008; Juárez-Vázquez et al., 2017). Oxidoreductases are enzymes that take part in oxidation-reduction reactions by moving electrons between molecules. In this class, dehydrogenases and oxidases are enzymes that help in cellular respiration and produce energy. Besides, enzymes usually team up with coenzymes, such as NAD+ or FAD, to ensure the proper functioning of their reactions. Since different enzymes are linked, it becomes clear that metabolic networks are complex and that enzymatic activity is necessary to keep cellular balance. Being aware of these enzyme groups improves our knowledge of biochemistry and also highlights how we can treat disorders related to enzymes by studying them further (Figure 3.11).

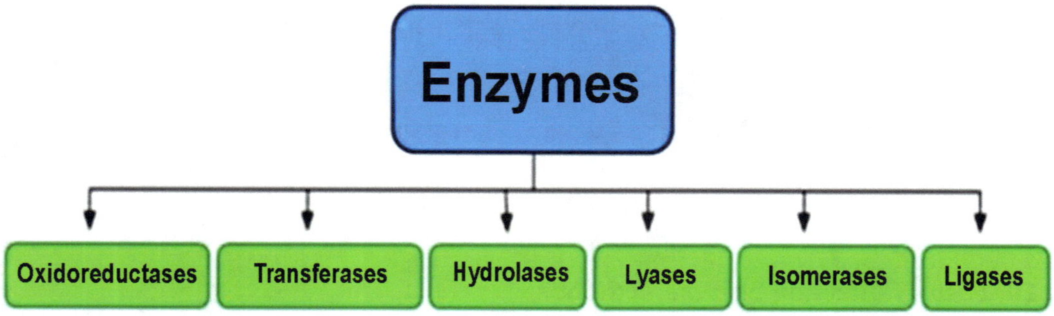

Figure 3.11. Types of enzymes.

Source: https://cdn1.byjus.com/wp-content/uploads/2018/11/chemistry/2016/10/16074509/word-image2.png.

3.3.1. Classification Based on Function

The main way to study enzymes is to first classify them by their functions. Enzymes are sorted into different groups, depending on the type of reaction they help with. As an illustration, oxidoreductases help with redox reactions and make it possible for electrons to move between molecules. The transfer of functional groups is very important in metabolism, and this is mainly done by transferases for substrates that bring a lot of chemical changes. With enzymes sorted by their functions, researchers can better predict their actions in different biological systems and help develop new ideas in biotechnology and medicine. The effectiveness of this classification scheme lies in its ability to correlate enzyme structure with function, offering insights into how alterations at the molecular level can influence biochemical reactions (Johansson et al., 2020). Hydrolases are another important category of enzymes because they help break down substrates by adding water. Enzymes such as proteases and lipases are in this group and help digest proteins and fats. The exact role of these enzymes demonstrates why they are key to maintaining the body's metabolism and absorbing nutrients. Lyases also participate in adding or removing groups to double bonds or cyclic compounds, proving that enzymes are flexible in many biochemical reactions. This functional classification not only simplifies the study of enzymes but also underlines their intricate roles in cellular metabolism, supporting the view that enzymes are indispensable to life (Wansbrough, 1998). Also, ligases are unique since they help create covalent bonds by using energy released during ATP hydrolysis. This group of enzymes is essential for DNA replication and repair, since joining the nucleotide parts is important for the genome's health. It is clear from the function of ligases that various biochemical pathways are linked since substrates usually need several enzymes to interact properly. When research advances, the ways enzymes are grouped will be updated, and new findings about their mechanisms or uses in medicine will be found. To cut it short, the determination of enzyme function is important for the newly emerging fields, such as synthetic biology, wherein the developed enzymes may be utilized for novel purposes in health and industry (Johansson et al., 2020).

3.3.2. Enzymes in Metabolic Pathways

Enzymes are key to helping metabolic pathways, which are necessary for keeping the cell's balance and energy supply. Biochemical processes in the body are made up of a series of reactions that enzymes help to speed up and make easier. Every enzyme works only with its specific substrate, so the metabolic pathways function smoothly without being disturbed by other molecules. Because enzymes are carefully controlled, cells can handle different situations and change their metabolism as needed. During shortages of nutrients or extreme temperatures, enzymes can adjust what they do to support survival, which underlines their role in helping cells adapt. Because of different enzymes, organisms are able to change their metabolic processes depending on the resources they have. The conservation of important enzymes for intermediary metabolism in Caenorhabditis elegans points to the fact that the main metabolic pathways are common to all eukaryotes. There are important changes in metabolism during the development of *C. elegans* and when it encounters stress. Such shifts usually increase resistance to stress from oxygen or make it possible for microaerobic respiration, which can be seen by the use of the malate dismutation and glyoxylate pathways during Dauer diapause. Such metabolic reconfiguration not only promotes survival but also suggests that enzymatic changes can have broader implications for lifespan and health in various organisms (Braeckman et al., 2009). Understanding the role of enzymes in drug metabolism further underscores their significance in metabolic pathways, particularly in pharmacokinetics, the study of drug absorption, distribution, metabolism, and excretion (ADME). Cytochrome P450s and other drug-metabolizing enzymes are important in deciding how a medicine will work and how safe it is. The study of new metabolic pathways and the effects of drugs on unusual enzymes proves that metabolic regulation in the body is very complex. It has been proven that changes in these metabolic processes can cause significant differences in patients' reactions to medicines. Thus, understanding the intricacies of enzyme activity not only offers insights into metabolic processes but also holds the potential for enhancing therapeutic strategies and individualizing medical treatment based on metabolic profiles (Li et al., 2019) (Figure 3.12).

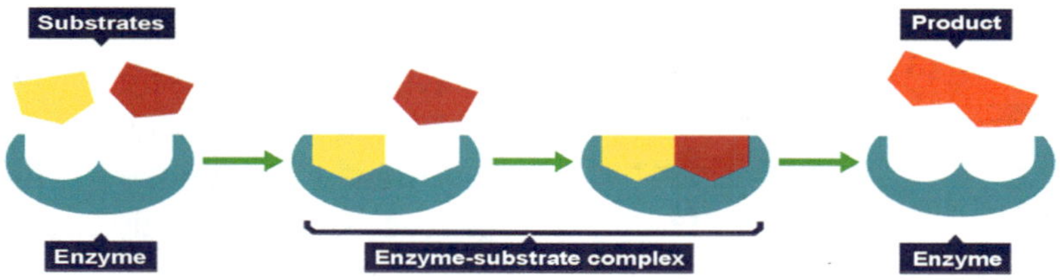

Figure 3.12. Control of metabolic pathways using enzymes.

Source: https://bam.files.bbci.co.uk/bam/live/content/z66rwmn/large.

3.3.3. Industrial Enzymes and Their Applications

The use of industrial enzymes has greatly improved different sectors by making them more efficient and sustainable. For biofuel and biodegradable material production, enzymes such as cellulases are important because they change cellulose into glucose. Because cellulose is the most common biomaterial, it is mainly obtained from plants. Since the use of renewable energy is increasing in industry, it is very important to convert cellulose into glucose monomers. Working together, cellulases made up of endoglucanases, exoglucanases, and β-glucosidases, break down cellulose into glucose, making fermentation reactions possible and producing ethanol and other products. The reliance on fungi to produce cellulases effectively underscores the innovation in biotechnology that seeks to utilize natural processes for industrial advancements (Amer et al., 2018). Apart from being used in biofuel, β-glucosidases are also important in several industries, like food and beverages. Since these enzymes are found everywhere in living organisms, their strong qualities make them useful in industries. They can make food processing faster, improve the taste of drinks, and boost the synthesis of oligosaccharides, which is important in nutritional products. Industries find microbial β-glucosidases especially valuable because they have selective biochemical properties. Hence, industries depend more on these enzymes being stable and effective, so research is mainly aimed at their molecular features and how to produce them. It is crucial to learn about enzymatic attributes and tailor operating conditions for applications in industries, as the demand for enzyme-based technology in food technology continues to increase (Ahmed et al., 2017). Because the biotechnology of enzymes is advancing, it is now more important than ever to optimize their production and use. Fungi are now preferred for making cellulase because they can produce a lot of these enzymes in the culture medium. This feature eases the way enzymes are extracted and saves money in their production. In addition, looking into parameters that influence cellulase yield, such as pH, temperature, and what materials the enzyme can digest, can help increase the efficiency of the process. Using enzymes in industry is a sign of a bigger effort to be sustainable and green, in line with worldwide goals for the environment. As research continues, the ability to leverage industrial enzymes for an array of applications is exciting and a necessity to drive future evolution within biotechnology (Amer et al., 2018).

Test Your Knowledge

1. What is the classification of enzymes on the basis of their functions?
2. What is the role of enzymes in facilitating metabolic pathways?

3.4. Enzyme Kinetics

Learning Outcome

1. Understand the reaction rates;
2. Describe the Michaelis–Menten kinetics;
3. Know the enzyme inhibitors and activators.

Biochemistry pays special attention to enzyme kinetics, which looks into how fast enzymatic reactions take place and what affects their speed. The Michaelis–Menten equation is central in this area because it shows the link between how much product is made and the amount of substrate present. It is assumed in this model that ES complexes can form and break down reversibly, so that the rate of formation and breakdown is equal. Enzyme kinetics helps to explain how enzymes work and what factors affect their performance, as it also lets researchers find out the V_{max} and K_M values for each enzyme. The information about kinetics helps both in understanding enzymes and in making progress in biotechnology and pharmacology. Identifying and understanding different enzymes, especially those that are new, matters a lot in various fields like industry. The enzyme Ppo-Er1 from *Paenibacillus polymyxa* shows how our understanding of enzyme kinetics is progressing. Because of its high specificity and ability to work even at low temperatures, this enzyme could be used for industrial biocatalysis. By studying Ppo-Er1, scientists noticed that it has a high specificity constant for maleimide and also pointed out that enzyme stability is important. Such characteristics contribute to a deeper understanding of how enzymes can be tailored for specific reactions, expanding the biocatalytic toolbox and enhancing the efficiency of synthetic pathways, particularly in the production of valuable chiral compounds (Aregger et al., 2020). In the food industry, controlling enzyme activity is vital for ensuring the best quality products, so efforts to manipulate enzyme kinetics are also used there. As an illustration, tomatoes use pectic enzymes to help maintain the right viscosity during processing. The texture and consistency of the product can be changed by adjusting the temperature and the time the fruit is held in the tank. With mathematical models, researchers are able to see how changes in processing affect enzyme activity and pectin levels, which helps them optimize industrial methods. This understanding not only reinforces the principles of enzyme kinetics but also highlights the practical applications that arise from such knowledge, showcasing the intricate balance between enzyme function and product quality in food processing industries (Srichantra, 2002) (Figure 3.13).

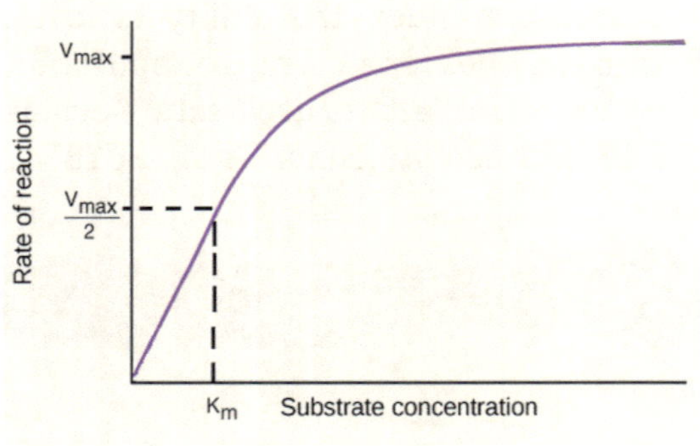

Figure 3.13. Enzyme kinetics.

Source: https://cdn.kastatic.org/ka-perseus-images/3f92b1bf5bc6c5fb4de1d4ca3b8be2aed414f2b8.png.

3.4.1. Understanding Reaction Rates

This concept is the basis of biochemistry because it explains the enzymatic reactions that are important in most metabolic processes. An enzyme works as a catalyst in the body by lowering the energy needed for the reaction to occur, which speeds up the process. The rate of a reaction can be changed by the concentration of the substrate, the temperature, the pH, and the presence of inhibitors or activators. Often, the rate at which enzymes work is highest in a particular temperature range. If the conditions go beyond the optimal range, enzymes may change their shape and become much less active. To understand how enzymes function in all kinds of environments, it is necessary to examine their kinetics. Besides, enzymatic reactions have many aspects and may take a significant amount of time to reach their steady-state rates. Several recent investigations have revealed that enzymatic responses have time delays when the concentration of substrates is changed, proving the complexity of how microbial communities are regulated. A model that relates how enzymes work in the community rather than focusing only on species groups is now better at explaining reaction rates and biogeochemical processes. Here, transcriptional response plays a big role in deciding how enzymes react to changes in their environment. The simulation of models' results prove that the delayed enzymatic reactions could be regulated mainly at the transcriptional level, which sheds light on the relationship between transcript levels and enzymatic activity, as evidenced in different experimental situations (Chen et al., 2017). Their role in nonaqueous media has added a lot to what we know about the speed of reactions. According to research, enzymes work in organic solvents and gaseous systems, meaning that some conditions that are usually considered unsuitable for enzymes can actually help reactions go faster. For example, when mass transfer is less in gas-phase systems, they become more stable and efficient as catalysts. Yet, it is important to maintain the moisture at the right level because it greatly affects how enzymes behave and function. Investigation into gas-phase lipase-catalyzed reactions shows that although an increase in temperature generally augments the reaction rate at low relative humidity, a high humidity leads to a striking loss of enzyme activity (Cameron et al., 1999). Because of this, we can see that temperature and humidity must be optimized together to get the best reaction rates and important knowledge about bioprocessing.

3.4.2. Michaelis–Menten Kinetics

Understanding how enzymes act, mainly by using Michaelis–Menten kinetics, is important for explaining how enzymes and substrates interact. According to the Michaelis–Menten model, from 1913, the rate of enzyme-catalyzed reactions is affected by the concentration of the substrate. Central to this concept is the formation of the ES complex, which is a temporary union that facilitates the conversion of substrates into products. As substrate concentration increases, the rate of reaction escalates until it approaches a maximum velocity (V_{max}) where all enzyme active sites are saturated. Enzymes are clearly efficient, as shown by their ability to catalyze reactions even when the substrate levels change, and they are very important for the cell's metabolic processes. Further investigation into Michaelis–Menten kinetics reveals the importance of two critical parameters: the maximum reaction velocity (V_{max}) and the Michaelis constant (K_M). V_{max} indicates the rate of the reaction when the enzyme is fully saturated with substrate, while K_M reflects the substrate concentration at which the reaction rate is half of V_{max}. This constant serves as an essential metric for enzyme affinity; a low K_M signifies high affinity between the enzyme and substrate, indicating that the enzyme effectively binds to the substrate even at low concentrations. Studies have also found that specific enzymes, like the novel ene reductase Ppo-Er1 derived from *Paenibacillus polymyxa*, exhibit distinct K_M values reflecting their unique interactions with various substrates. Notably, Ppo-Er1 demonstrated the highest specificity constant for maleimide, pointing to the diverse applications of enzymes in biocatalysis (Aregger et al., 2020). Applying Michaelis–Menten kinetics theories, scientists can model complicated biological systems more precisely. Modern computer tools make it possible to study enzyme kinetics and the effects of various factors on reactions inside the cell. They reveal how various biochemical pathways are linked and how the environment can change the activity of enzymes. For example, using stochastic modeling techniques, as shown by research done with the BlenX programming language, increases our knowledge of enzyme kinetics, together with other biochemical reactions. By leveraging these conceptual frameworks, scientists can better predict the outcomes of enzymatic reactions and develop innovative strategies to manipulate metabolic pathways for applications in biotechnology and medicine (Priami et al., 2010) (Figure 3.14).

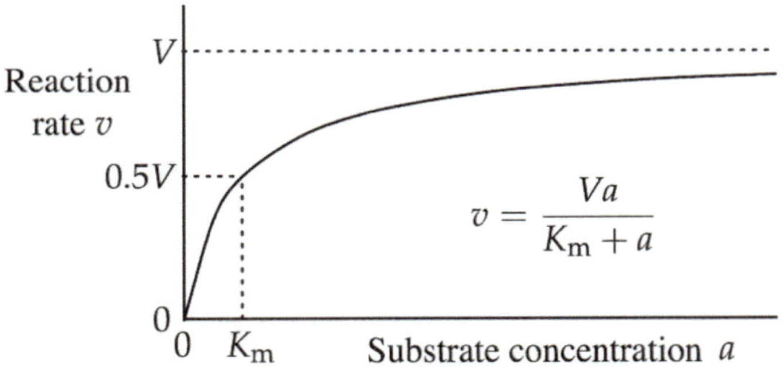

Figure 3.14. Curve of the Michaelis–Menten equation labelled in accordance with IUBMB recommendations.

Source: https://upload.wikimedia.org/wikipedia/commons/2/22/MM-curve.jpg.

3.4.3. Enzyme Inhibitors and Activators

The control of enzyme activity by the use of inhibitors and activators is very important for maintaining balance in the body. They can bind an enzyme either to the active site or allosteric sites and further inhibit an enzyme's catalytic activity. It helps control metabolic processes and also keeps the cell's functions in balance. For example, using allosteric inhibition, the final product of a metabolic pathway prevents an early stage from working too much, so the substrate does not build up too much. It is not easy to understand all these interactions, but learning more about small-molecule regulators is necessary. It has been demonstrated that these small molecules play a critical role in catalytic activity, highlighting the value of combining biochemical investigation with measurements of metabolomics to reveal the subtleties of enzyme regulation in organisms, as illustrated in current research of *Escherichia coli* (Briars et al., 2017). On the other hand, enzyme activators boost the speed and amount of reactions, which influences signal transduction and energy production. Activators can cause enzymes to become active when they get signals, usually because of feedback mechanisms in the cell. For instance, an allosteric activator makes the enzyme work more strongly, meeting the different needs of the cell. Such interactions at the molecular level are significant since drugs that target certain enzymes related to various diseases are being made. In addition, the specificity of these activators may be targeted in drug development, especially under conditions such as diabetes and cancer, where the metabolic pathways are disrupted, representing an exciting therapeutic target for pharmacological intervention (Casas et al., 2015). In the field of drug development, researchers keep searching for enzyme inhibitors and activators, since having effective pharmacologic agents is very important. These regulators need to be balanced carefully, since they are important for using them in medical treatments, mainly for conditions related to oxidative stress. Although a lot of enzymes and isoforms linked to diseases have been identified, it is necessary to test them thoroughly and in preclinical settings to check that they are safe and effective. It is difficult to design such drugs because multitasking enzymes are important in many physiological functions, so it's hard to figure out how to target or affect specific enzyme pathways. At the same time, further research should involve a closer cooperation between academia and clinical research, improving the process of drug discovery before new therapeutic strategies are created, exploiting the potential of enzymatic regulation(Figure 3.15).

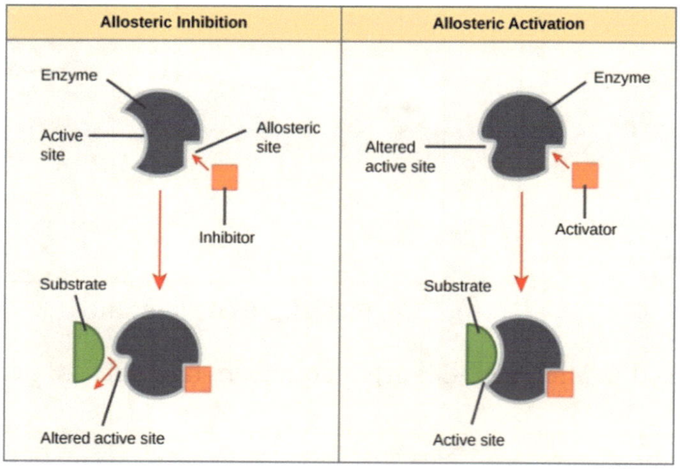

Figure 3.15. Allosteric inhibition works by indirectly inducing a conformational change to the active site such that the substrate no longer fits. In contrast, in allosteric activation, the activator molecule modifies the shape of the active site to allow a better fit of the substrate.

Source: http://biol1113temp.pressbooks.tru.ca/wp-content/uploads/sites/75/2021/10/Figure_04_01_082.jpg.

Test Your Knowledge

1. What is the rate of reaction in biochemistry?
2. Who proposed the Michaelis-Menten equation?

3.5. Enzymes in Human Health

Learning Outcome

1. Understand the role of enzymes in digestion;
2. Describe the role of enzymes in the diagnosis of various diseases;
3. Know the therapeutic enzymes and treatments.

Enzymes are important for human health since they help many biochemical reactions needed for life. The role of enzymes in peroxisomes is especially important since they take part in fatty acid processing and help eliminate harmful oxygen species. This way, peroxisomes can efficiently handle substances that could be dangerous, which highlights their role in keeping metabolism stable. Scientific research has revealed that peroxisomes affect metabolism and are also related to many health problems caused by their dysfunction. For instance, inherited disorders arising from peroxisomal enzyme deficiencies manifest in significant health challenges, emphasizing the need for further exploration of these organelles (Delille et al., 2016). So, knowing how enzymes work in peroxisomes is important for progress in treating metabolic diseases. Besides, the role of enzymes in exercise points to a key part of human health. Redox homeostasis is regulated by enzymes when you are physically active. The combination of superoxide dismutase (SOD) and catalase lessens the oxidative stress caused by exercise and aids in recovery and lowering inflammation. Still, it is difficult to study redox biology because enzymes work differently and oxidative stress varies from one situation to another. It is difficult for investigators to measure enzyme activities correctly, which stresses the need for using suitable methods and biomarkers when analyzing changes caused by exercise. Addressing these issues will enhance our understanding of how exercise impacts health through enzymatic pathways, ultimately advancing public health strategies related to physical fitness (Cobley et al., 2017). It is important to consider how enzymes play a part in health problems such as inflammation and cancer.

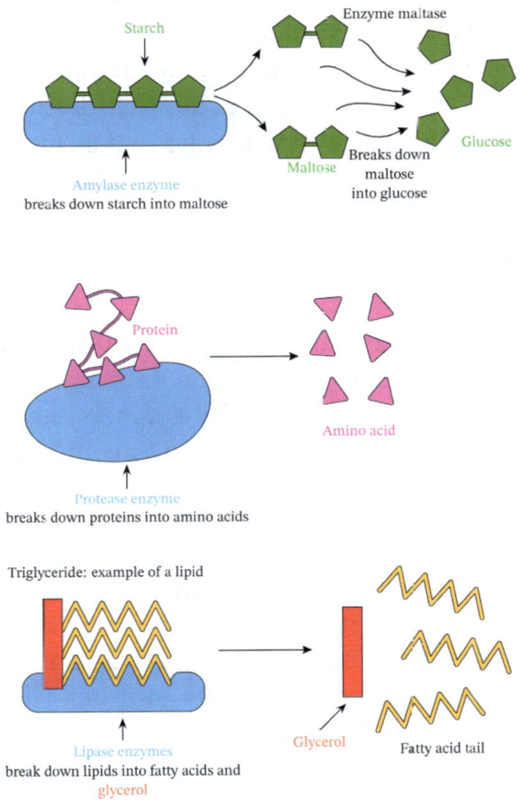

Figure 3.16. A diagram showing the three main enzymes involved in digestion, breaking down three large polymers into their monomer subunits.

Source: https://images.nagwa.com/figures/explainers/480180810123/4.svg.

How inflammation functions are strongly affected by enzyme activity, mainly those that participate in making and breaking down prostaglandins and cytokines. In cancer, there are enzymes that aid the growth of tumors and others that help protect against tumors. It is important to realize these two functions to create effective therapies that make use of enzymes. As an example, inhibiting certain enzymes that encourage cancer could be a helpful approach in oncology. In addition, since many enzymes depend on cofactors and are affected by oxidative stress, exploring their mechanisms might lead to discovering new ways to deal with diseases linked to inflammation or oxidation. Thus, enzymes serve as both key players in biochemical pathways and as targets for therapeutic innovation in human health (Delille et al., 2016) (Figure 3.16).

3.5.1. Role of Enzymes in Digestion

Enzymes are key to the process of digestion because they help break food into units the body can use. Enzymes help speed up the digestion of carbohydrates, proteins, and fats by helping biochemical reactions occur. Saliva contains salivary amylase, which starts to digest carbohydrates in the mouth, and pepsin is one of the gastric enzymes that breaks down proteins into peptides in the stomach. In the small intestine, pancreatic enzymes such as lipase and pancreatic amylase join in to help digest food, so that nutrients are turned into monomers that can be absorbed by the intestinal wall. The important role of enzymes in digestion is clear, as their specificity and effectiveness show that without them, our bodies would not be able to absorb nutrients well. Also, the way enzymes work with food's physical structure is very important for digestion. The digestion of nutrients is affected by the makeup of plant cell walls. Because cell walls have complex polysaccharides, enzymes may find it hard to access the nutrients inside. This is more important in plant-based foods, since cellulose and hemicellulose prevent digestive enzymes from working properly, which may limit the release of nutrients. It is important to know these dynamics to interpret how digestion affects nutrition and health. As highlighted in recent reviews, advancements in characterizing food matrices and cell wall composition illuminate how structural properties influence enzymatic action, further reinforcing the synergistic relationship between enzymes and their substrates in human digestion (Edwards et al., 2020). Besides helping reactions, enzymes also take part in regulating digestive activities. Hormones and nerves make sure that digestive enzymes are released at the proper time and in the right amount. As soon as food goes into the stomach, gastrin is released, which then leads to pepsinogen secretion and increases the movement of the stomach. In addition, the way enzymes and substrates interact can manage the rate of digestion and absorption, indicating a complex system that maintains the digestive tract's stability. As studies continue to analyze the complex processes behind enzyme function and regulation, it is apparent that enzymes are not just facilitators of digestion but play an active role in controlling nutritional outcomes, thereby enhancing overall well-being (Abdulkarim et al., 2019) (Figure 3.17).

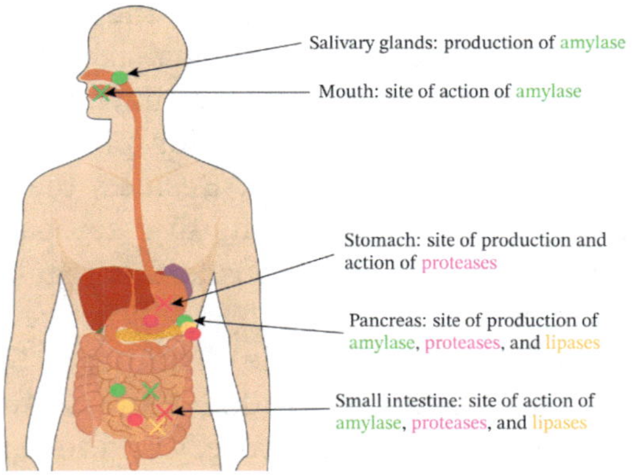

Figure 3.17. A diagram showing the main organs of the human digestive system, with the sites of production (shown by circles) and action (shown by crosses) of amylases in green, those of proteases in pink, and those of lipases in orange.

Source: https://images.nagwa.com/figures/explainers/480180810123/7.svg.

3.5.2. Enzymes in Disease Diagnosis

Enzymes are important for diagnosing different diseases because they help detect and control medical issues at an early stage. Checking the levels of certain enzymes in biological samples can give important details about how organs are working and whether there are any diseases. For instance, elevated serum levels of liver enzymes, such as alanine aminotransferase (ALT) and aspartate aminotransferase (AST), are commonly associated with hepatic injury and diseases like hepatitis. Also, changes in enzyme activities can point to problems in the liver as well as in other organs, showing how important enzymes are in diagnosing diseases. Therefore, using better enzyme assay methods has made it easier and more accurate to diagnose diseases, which benefits patients. Diagnosing genetic disorders is greatly helped by looking at enzyme abnormalities. Conditions such as orotic aciduria, which results from a deficit in the enzyme UMPS, can be detected through elevated urinary orotic acid levels. Some of the symptoms of this disorder are megaloblastic anemia and delays in development. Their importance in pediatric and metabolic medicine is shown by how vital enzymes are in diagnosing rare disorders. Since early detection helps a lot, scientists keep working to improve the methods used for screening. As highlighted by recent findings, timely enzyme assessments can lead to profound shifts in treatment strategies, improving quality of life and reducing morbidity associated with metabolic disorders (Fonteh, 2018). In autoimmune diseases, enzymes are also valuable diagnostic tools, particularly in identifying specific autoantibodies associated with conditions such as systemic sclerosis (SSc) and primary biliary cholangitis (PBC). Research has shown that the presence of anti-mitochondrial antibodies (AMA) in SSc patients can indicate a potential overlap with PBC, even in the absence of elevated alkaline phosphatase or gamma-glutamyl transferase levels (Bonroy et al., 2020). This proves that enzyme-related tests can point out the early stages of autoimmune disorders before any clear symptoms appear. With enzyme assays being used in routine diagnostics, clinicians can assess the risk of disease, predict its advancement, and develop appropriate treatment, proving the key role of enzymes in current medicine (Figure 3.18).

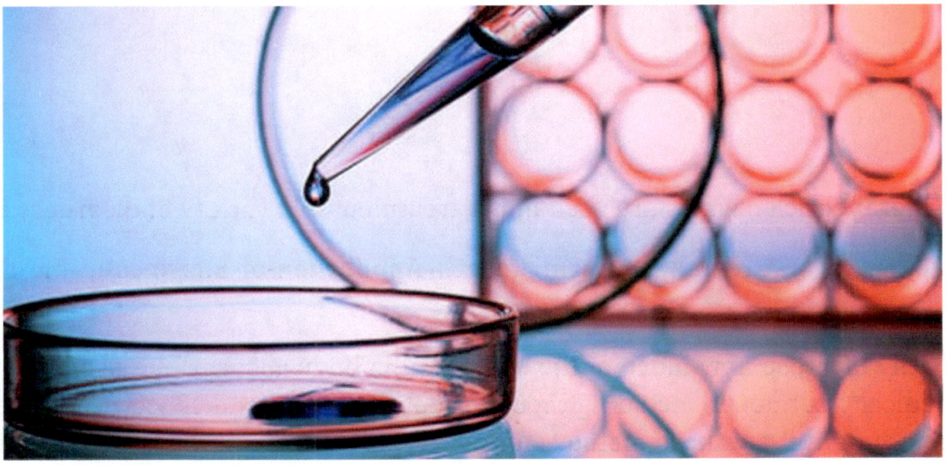

Figure 3.18. Enzymes for disease diagnosis.

Source: https://labinsights.nl/wp-content/uploads/sites/4/2023/05/Nave-Bacillus-licheniformis-Protease.jpg.

3.5.3. Therapeutic Enzymes and Treatments

The use of enzymes in therapy has greatly modified medical care for many metabolic conditions where enzyme shortages stop important biochemical processes. They target specific substances and change them into safe products, which helps improve the body's healthy functions. For example, in enzyme replacement therapy (ERT), the production of therapeutic enzymes replaces the deficiency of natural enzymes, such as in Gaucher disease and Fabry disease. While highly effective, the clinical applicability of enzymes administered parenterally is still plagued by factors like short half-lives within circulatory systems and the risk of immunogenic responses, which reduce therapeutic benefit (Bax et al., 2020). It is very important to address these limitations, as using therapeutic enzymes in medicine depends on solving the issues and making the best use of their benefits. A promising way to improve how enzymes work as therapy is by delivering them through erythrocyte carriers, which makes them stay in the body for longer. If erythrocytes are chosen as carriers, therapeutic enzymes can be released slowly at the right places without being quickly cleared from the bloodstream. This innovative strategy has garnered significant interest over the past five decades and encompasses various applications, including targeted delivery to the monocyte-macrophage system and the engineering of $CD34^+$ hematopoietic precursor cells for enzyme expression (Bax et al., 2020).

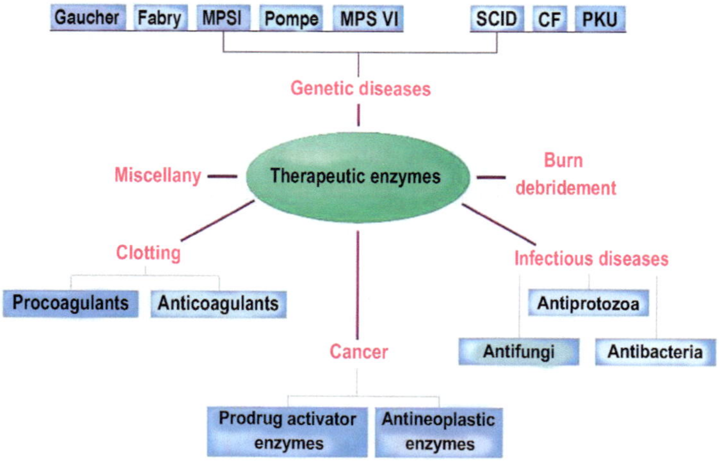

Figure 3.19. Therapeutic enzymes are used in the treatment of a variety of disorders and diseases.

Source: https://www.creative-enzymes.com/images/Application-of-Enzymes-in-the-Treatment-of-Diseases-1.png.

They not only increase how much of the enzymes the body absorbs but also make them useful in more biomedical treatments, including those for detoxification and cancer. With the progress of enzyme therapy, the use of advanced methods for delivering the enzymes will become very important. At the same time, studying phage therapy is an interesting way to handle bacterial infections, especially since antibiotic resistance is on the rise. Using phage therapy, bacteriophages are able to attack and destroy harmful bacteria, making it a good alternative to antibiotics. Thanks to recent progress in biotechnology, phages can be engineered and their lytic proteins isolated, giving them the ability to be used with other treatments or by themselves to fight infections from multidrug-resistant organisms. Although therapeutic enzymes and phage therapy appear to be different, they both aim to give effective and precise treatments for diseases. Clinics should start using enzyme therapy and phage therapy to improve health results as researchers keep uncovering the connections between these biological agents and humans (Figure 3.19).

Test Your Knowledge

1. What is the role of enzymes in digestion?
2. What is the role of enzymes in the diagnosis of various diseases?

3.6. Environmental Impact of Enzymes

Learning Outcome

1. Describe the enzymes in bioremediation;
2. Understand the role of enzymes in agriculture;
3. Understand the role of enzymes in promoting sustainability.

Enzymes contribute greatly to biogeochemical cycles and industrial activities, which have a big effect on the environment. Thanks to their ability to help reactions, they can help break down pollutants, which is very important for cleaning the environment. Some enzymes from microbes can split plastics and petroleum into simpler and safer materials. The enzymatic process makes it possible for waste to decompose naturally, and it also offers eco-friendly options to the harmful and energy-intensive chemical ways of managing waste. Using enzymes in waste treatment, industries may cut down on their negative impact on the environment and support a circular economy. Enzymes are helpful for the environment in waste management and also support positive changes in agriculture. Biofertilizers are made with the help of cellulases and amylases, which increase the amount of nutrients and improve the quality of soil. As a result of this, we need less chemical fertilizer, which is important because it can cause damage to soil and pollute water. Besides, enzymes assist in sustainable agriculture by helping to break down organic substances, which improves the quality and structure of the soil. Because sustainability is now a priority in farming, using enzymes is a good way to address the problems caused by traditional farming and support nature's diversity, ensuring enough food for everyone. Even though enzymes are environmentally friendly, their use and production should be controlled to avoid any negative effects. For instance, introducing genetically modified microorganisms that make certain enzymes into nature may cause concerns about the environment and the variety of living things. Moreover, the methods used in industry to produce enzymes often cause high carbon emissions, so it is necessary to look for greener ways to make them. It is important to carry out research on the environmental impact that enzymes have. Emerging studies suggest that targeting specific pathways, such as those involving ten-eleven translocation 1 (TET1), may help alleviate the negative impacts associated with environmental exposures (Brown et al., 2020). Therefore, understanding the broader implications of enzyme utilization and developing strategies to minimize any adverse effects is essential for maximizing their benefits while protecting the environment (Boyen et al., 2025).

3.6.1. Enzymes in Bioremediation

The process of bioremediation depends a lot on enzymes that are secreted by microorganisms and help remove environmental toxins. Mostly bacteria, fungi, and plants use enzymes to change hazardous organic pollutants into substances that are less harmful. Not only does the process help the environment, but it also uses the natural activities of living organisms to clean up polluted sites. Experts have proven that oxido-reductases and hydrolases are important for biodegradation, since they help to break down pollutants into harmless substances. By advancing our understanding of these bioremediation-related enzymes, the potential for creating efficient and cost-effective strategies to reduce toxic waste significantly increases, ultimately contributing to a more sustainable future for environmental management (Karigar et al., 2011). *Pichia anomala* is a microorganism that is especially strong in bioremediation because of its strong metabolic and physiological abilities. The yeast is adaptable, since it has been found in different places, including food items and wastewater. *P. anomala* can survive in many types of environments, so it is suitable for bioremediation. Because of its different metabolic activities, it can target and remove pollutants from contaminated places. Besides, the antimicrobial abilities of *P. anomala* make it suitable for both biological control and bioremediation. Ongoing research highlights the need for further exploration of its cellular physiology and genetic makeup, which could unlock even more applications in environmental biotechnology, emphasizing its potential significance in tackling pollutant challenges (Walker et al., 2010). Many people in environmental science are excited about enzymatic bioremediation, but there are also several challenges to deal with. Even though enzymes can handle many types of pollutants, their performance and stability may be affected by different environmental factors. To ensure bioremediation works well, it is necessary to keep researching how temperature, pH, and the amount of contaminants influence enzyme activity. Besides, the creation of genetically modified microbes that make specific enzymes allows for better bioremediation. When researchers study enzymes more closely, they may discover ways to remove dangerous toxins and create valuable products at the same time. This line of research represents a significant step in the use of enzymatic remedies for environmental cleanup (Karigar et al., 2011) (Figure 3.20).

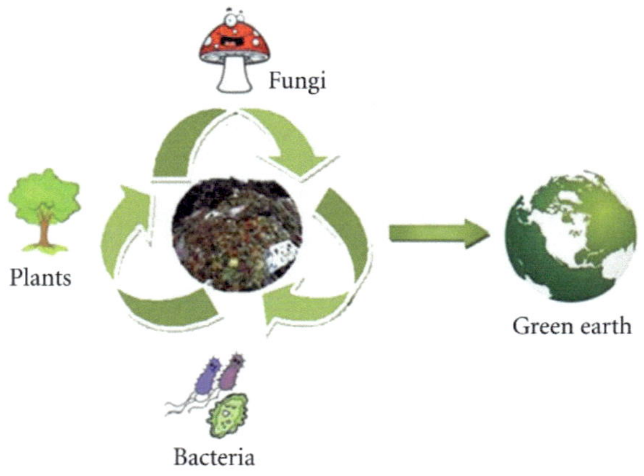

Figure 3.20. Application of enzymes in the bioremediation of solid wastes and soils.

Source: https://www.creative-enzymes.com/images/Application-of-enzymes-in-bioremediation-of-solid-wastes-and-soil.jpg.

3.6.2. Role of Enzymes in Agriculture

Enzymes are very important in agriculture since they support biochemical activities that boost crop yields and improve their health. Enzymes help speed up chemical reactions in soil, so they are important for soil respiration, nutrient recycling, and plant growth. Microorganisms in the soil make enzymes that help in the breakdown of organic matter and release nutrients needed by plants. It increases the quality of the soil and supports sustainable methods in farming. In addition, making these enzymatic reactions more efficient provides nutrients to plants in a timely way, which results in more yields and stronger resistance to both biotic and abiotic stresses. Besides, using enzymes in farming has led to positive results, especially in organic farming. Research points out that using certain enzymes in food processing helps keep organic products intact and of good quality. For example, adding enzymes to the production of organic foods can boost their flavor, texture, and shelf-life, so they are both safe and satisfying to consumers. This is in line with quality of origin, which focuses on both the origin of food and the ways it is prepared. Concept papers have identified critical factors influencing the evaluation of additives and processing methods, aligning with the enzymatic-driven advancements that underscore the overall quality and sustainability of organic food (Beck et al., 2006).

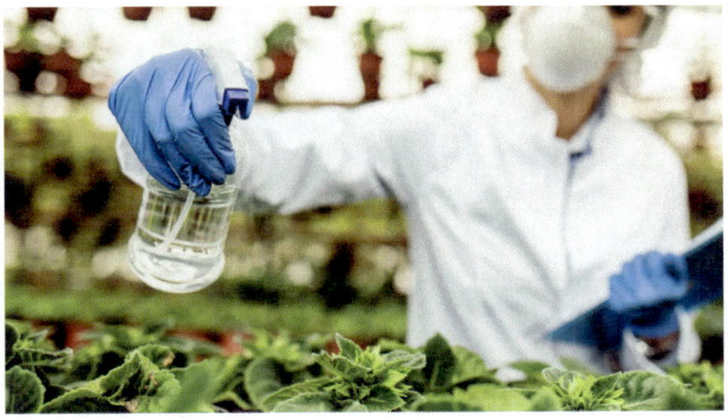

Figure 3.21. Enzymes used in agriculture.

Source: https://infinitabiotech.com/wp-content/uploads/2021/12/Enzymes-Used-in-Agriculture-1.webp.

Besides making soil better and improving the quality of food, enzymes from helpful microorganisms have also been noticed for their positive impact on plant growth. Investigations done lately on endophytic bacteria have found that they can produce indole-3-acetic acid and enzymes that help plants take up phosphate. They help the plant get nutrients and also boost the development of roots, which improves how much water and nutrients the plant can absorb. With more research, it is becoming obvious that beneficial bacteria can be used as biofertilizers, promoting sustainable management of vineyards with the help of microbial enzymes. The multifaceted benefits presented by these microbial communities underscore their critical role in developing agricultural systems that are both productive and environmentally sustainable (Baldan et al., 2015) (Figure 3.21).

3.6.3. Enzymes and Sustainability

Enzymes are recognized as helping sustainability in all areas, including agriculture and waste management. Enzymes help reactions go faster and use very little energy and create little waste. This matters a lot in creating lasting systems, especially in organic farming, where the use of conventional synthetic chemicals is either not allowed or limited. Thanks to enzymes, soil is kept healthy and fertile, which helps crops grow well for a long time and without causing harm to the environment. Besides, applying enzymes in agriculture can boost sustainability by increasing the ability of crops to resist pests and diseases through biology, which helps create stronger and more durable farming environments. Besides being used in farming, enzymes help make waste treatment and industry more sustainable. Using enzymes, industries can change organic wastes into biogas or compost, which helps decrease the amount of waste sent to landfills and the release of greenhouse gases. Enzymes are involved in bioremediation to help break down pollutants in soil and water, which supports renewing the environment. As an example, enzymes can easily break down petroleum products and other harmful substances, showing that they can help deal with pollution and still meet sustainability goals. It is clear from examples that enzymes are important in biology and also help create sustainable practices for everyone. With new biotechnology, the use and production of enzymes are both improved, leading to better, sustainable results. Using enzyme engineering, scientists can make enzymes that work well under specific environmental conditions, making them more useful. For instance, the Marine Board has targeted scientific cooperation with innovation in marine research, which, among other things, presents an opportunity to explore enzymatic processes within marine ecosystems that can substantially impact sustainability on a larger scale (Boyen et al., 2025). Moreover, as organic farming expands to over 24 million hectares worldwide, the emphasis on biological processes, including enzyme activity for nutrient release, illustrates their crucial role in maintaining soil health and promoting a sustainable agricultural future (Araújo et al., 2010). Such developments show that enzyme technology can play a major role in solving important sustainability issues in various sectors.

Test Your Knowledge

1. What is the role of enzymes in agriculture?
2. What is the role of enzymes in promoting sustainability?

SUMMARY

All in all, enzymes are necessary for many biochemical activities and help move science and technology forward. Because they help reactions proceed very quickly in living systems, factories, and hospitals, enzymes are extremely important. It is clear from this chapter that enzymes improve reaction speeds and also allow for more specificity, which helps many biochemical reactions occur. The detrimental effects of oxidative damage, as seen in diseases like Parkinson's, underscore the need for enzymes such as SOD to counteract such harm, further emphasizing their significance in health and disease management (Beltramini et al., 2016). Besides, enzymes are investigated in the fields of biotechnology and renewable energy. Research on fungal enzymes that break down sugarcane bagasse demonstrates their possible use in making biofuels. Learning how *Aspergillus nidulans* uses enzymes to use different substrates gives us ideas for sustainable methods and new biotechnology. The hydrophobins that assist in biofilm formation not only promote enzyme efficiency but also illustrate the intricate interactions between enzymes and their environments, thus presenting avenues for further research and practical implementation (Brown et al., 2016). All in all, the many roles that enzymes can play in different fields, such as medicine and environmental science, prove their major importance. To handle issues such as oxidative stress or good biomass conversion, researchers keep making new discoveries and applying enzymes. If scientists and practitioners keep studying enzyme mechanisms and their effects in living systems, they can discover new approaches for medicine and resource preservation. Studies on enzymes have huge implications; using their abilities will surely contribute to many important advancements outside of research.

Enzymes help to make important reactions in the body that are necessary for life. The presence of these proteins lessens the energy needed for reactions, which makes metabolic pathways go much faster. Inside the cell, enzymes and nucleic acids, mainly DNA and RNA, help manage creating, fixing, and obtaining genetic information. Because of this, it is important to know how enzymes work since this knowledge helps explain important cellular functions and supports the development of genetic engineering. The recent 'Machines on Genes' meeting convened by the Biochemical Society emphasized this point, illustrating how advancements in enzymatic understanding can lead to revolutionary applications in molecular biology, thereby underscoring the ongoing relevance of enzyme research in both basic and applied sciences (Bates et al., 2010). Directed evolution shows how scientists are using deliberate experiments to make enzymes more effective. The process includes repeating cycles of making changes to the enzyme and selecting the ones that work better. The results point out that a small change in just one amino acid can make a big difference in how well an enzyme works. Besides, directed evolution demonstrates that proteins can evolve in the lab under pressure, much like they do in the natural world. As an example, certain mutations can be spotted that improve current functions and also support future changes in enzymes. Such knowledge expands our understanding of the mechanisms governing protein evolution and offers potential pathways for engineering enzymes with novel or improved functionalities (Aharoni et al., 2009). Enzymatic mechanisms have effects that go beyond what happens in laboratories. As scientists learn more about the different roles of enzymes and the rules behind their reactions, the use of biotechnology in many areas increases rapidly. Enzymes are designed for different jobs in pharmaceuticals, agriculture, and biofuels, which helps push forward sustainable technology.

With the help of studies on enzymes, scientists can make enzymes that address urgent problems in society. They demonstrate that more research in enzymology is needed to explain cellular processes and use that knowledge to help people everywhere. The goal of enzyme research is to learn and also to create new innovations that rely on life's basic functions.

KEY TERMS FROM THIS CHAPTER

- Aldehyde dehydrogenase
- Caenorhabditis elegans
- Cell signaling
- Digestion
- DNA replication
- Drug development
- Enzymatic reactions
- Enzymes
- Glycans
- Glycosylation
- Metabolism
- Methanogens
- Plasmodium falciparum
- Renewable energy
- Sensor technology

CRITICAL THINKING QUESTIONS

1. **What is the primary function of an enzyme?**
   a. Provide energy to the reaction
   b. Act as a structural component
   c. Catalyze biochemical reactions
   d. Serve as a source of genetic information
2. **Enzymes are primarily composed of:**
   a. Lipids
   b. Proteins
   c. Carbohydrates
   d. Nucleic acids
3. **Which part of the enzyme binds to the substrate?**
   a. Active site
   b. Allosteric site
   c. Binding groove
   d. Regulatory site
4. **What is the term for the molecule upon which an enzyme acts?**
   a. Product
   b. Substrate
   c. Cofactor
   d. Catalyst
5. **Which of the following acts as a coenzyme?**
   a. Magnesium
   b. ATP
   c. NAD+
   d. Zinc

Answers to Critical Thinking Questions

1. (c); 2. (b); 3. (a); 4. (b); 5. (c)

Short Answer Questions

1. What are enzymes?
2. Describe the role of enzymes in biological processes.
3. What is the basic structure of an enzyme?
4. What are the 3 main types of enzymes?
5. What do you mean by enzyme kinetics?

REFERENCES

1. Li, Y., Meng, Q., Yang, M., Liu, D., Hou, X., Tang, L., Wang, X., Lyu, Y., Chen, X., Liu, K., Yu, A. M., Zuo, Z., & Bi, H. (2019). Current trends in drug metabolism and pharmacokinetics. *Acta pharmaceutica Sinica. B*, *9*(6), 1113–1144. https://doi.org/10.1016/j.apsb.2019.10.001 (accessed on 11th June 2025).
2. Abdulkarim, A. Y., Abdulsalam, S., El-Nafaty, U. A., Muhammad, M., et al. (2019). Bio-fertilizers via co-digestion: A review. https://core.ac.uk/download/220112834.pdf (accessed on 11th June 2025).
3. Aharoni, A., Besenmatter, W., Bloom, J. D., Bloom, J. D., Blundell, T. L., Castle, K., et al. (2009). In the light of directed evolution: Pathways of adaptive protein evolution. https://core.ac.uk/download/4882054.pdf (accessed on 11th June 2025).
4. Ahmed, A., & Bibi, A. (2018). Fungal cellulase; production and applications: Minireview. https://core.ac.uk/download/188826333.pdf (accessed on 11th June 2025).
5. Ahmed, A., Ashraf, M., Aslam, M., Batool, K., et al. (2017). Microbial β-glucosidases: Screening, characterization, cloning and applications. https://core.ac.uk/download/188825641.pdf (accessed on 11th June 2025).
6. Kwiatkowska, B., Bennett, J., Akunna, J., Walker, G. M., & Bremner, D. H. (2011). Stimulation of bioprocesses by ultrasound. *Biotechnology advances*, *29*(6), 768–780. https://doi.org/10.1016/j.biotechadv.2011.06.005(accessed on 11th June 2025).
7. Araújo, A. S. F. de, Melo, W. J. de. (2010). Soil microbial biomass in organic farming system. https://core.ac.uk/download/10933187.pdf (accessed on 11th June 2025).
8. Aregger, D., Buller, R., & Peters, C. (2020). Characterization of the novel ene reductase Ppo-Er1 from *Paenibacillus polymyxa*. https://core.ac.uk/download/289121447.pdf (accessed on 11th June 2025).
9. Astegno, A., Dominici, P., Fruncillo, S., Janson, G., et al. (2018). Functional characterization and structure-guided mutational analysis of the transculturation enzyme cystathionine γ-lyase from *Toxoplasma gondii*. https://core.ac.uk/download/188825581.pdf (accessed on 11th June 2025).
10. Avilla, M. N., Malecki, K. M. C., Hahn, M. E., Wilson, R. H., & Bradfield, C. A. (2020). The Ah Receptor: Adaptive Metabolism, Ligand Diversity, and the Xenokine Model. *Chemical research in toxicology*, *33*(4), 860–879. https://doi.org/10.1021/acs.chemrestox.9b00476(accessed on 11th June 2025).
11. Juárez-Vázquez, A. L., Edirisinghe, J. N., Verduzco-Castro, E. A., Michalska, K., Wu, C., Noda-García, L., Babnigg, G., Endres, M., Medina-Ruíz, S., Santoyo-Flores, J., Carrillo-Tripp, M., Ton-That, H., Joachimiak, A., Henry, C. S., & Barona-Gómez, F. (2017). Evolution of substrate specificity in a retained enzyme driven by gene loss. *eLife*, *6*, e22679. https://doi.org/10.7554/eLife.22679(accessed on 11th June 2025).
12. Cobley, J. N., Close, G. L., Bailey, D. M., & Davison, G. W. (2017). Exercise redox biochemistry: Conceptual, methodological and technical recommendations. *Redox biology*, *12*, 540–548. https://doi.org/10.1016/j.redox.2017.03.022(accessed on 11th June 2025).

13. Baldan, B., Baldan, E., Clocchiatti, A., D'Alessandro, G., et al. (2015). Beneficial bacteria isolated from grapevine inner tissues shape *Arabidopsis thaliana* roots. https://core.ac.uk/download/53521506.pdf (accessed on 11th June 2025).

14. Bastien, O., Birkholtz, L. M., Breton, V., Grando, D., et al. (2006). Integration and mining of malaria molecular, functional and pharmacological data: How far are we from a chemogenomic knowledge space? https://core.ac.uk/download/pdf/4135055.pdf (accessed on 11th June 2025).

15. Bates, S., Belousoff, M., Luisi, B. F., Lilley, D. M. J., Marshall, D., Olorunniji, F. J., Rice, P. A., et al. (2010). Machines on genes: Enzymes that make, break and move DNA and RNA. https://core.ac.uk/download/2776072.pdf (accessed on 11th June 2025).

16. Bax, B. E. (2020). Erythrocytes as carriers of therapeutic enzymes. https://core.ac.uk/download/323114170.pdf (accessed on 11th June 2025).

17. Beck, A., Kretzschmar, U., & Schmid, O. (2006). Concept papers outlining parameters for further development of organic food processing–Crucial topics for the revision of the EU regulation 2092/91. https://core.ac.uk/download/10924657.pdf (accessed on 11th June 2025).

18. Beltramini, M., Bisaglia, M., Bubacco, L., Casella, L., et al. (2016). Superoxide dismutase (SOD)-mimetic M40403 is protective in cell and fly models of paraquat toxicity: Implications for Parkinson disease. https://core.ac.uk/download/53531285.pdf (accessed on 11th June 2025).

19. Bhabha, G., Dyson, H. J., Ekiert, D. C., Godzik, A., et al. (2013). Divergent evolution of protein conformational dynamics in dihydrofolate reductase. https://core.ac.uk/download/323067559.pdf (accessed on 11th June 2025).

20. Delille, H. K., Bonekamp, N. A., & Schrader, M. (2006). Peroxisomes and disease - an overview. *International journal of biomedical science : IJBS, 2*(4), 308–314. (accessed on 11th June 2025).

21. Bonroy, C., De Keyser, F., Devreese, K., Florin, T., et al. (2020). Evaluation of the primary biliary cholangitis-related serologic profile in a large cohort of Belgian systemic sclerosis patients. https://core.ac.uk/download/322829047.pdf (accessed on 11th June 2025).

22. Boyce, S., & Pahl, C. (2007). Developing domain ontologies for course content. Journal of Educational Technology and Society (ETS)., Vol.10(3), pp.275-288(accessed on 11th June 2025).

23. Boyen, C., Børresen, T., Dobson, A., Höfle, M., et al. (2025). *Marine Biotechnology: A New Vision and Strategy for Europe.* https://core.ac.uk/download/pdf/29241634.pdf (accessed on 11th June 2025).

24. Braeckman, B., Houthoofd, K., & Vanfleteren, J. (2009). Intermediary metabolism. https://core.ac.uk/download/84042477.pdf (accessed on 11th June 2025).

25. Briars, E., Christodoulou, D., Goldford, J. E., Noor, E., et al. (2017). Genome-scale architecture of small molecule regulatory networks and the fundamental trade-off between regulation and enzymatic activity. https://core.ac.uk/download/142082717.pdf (accessed on 11th June 2025).

26. Brown, A. P., Ji, H., & Zhu, T. (2020). The emerging role of Ten-Eleven Translocation 1 in epigenetic responses to environmental exposures. https://core.ac.uk/download/323070431.pdf (accessed on 11th June 2025).

27. Brown, N. A., Corrêa Dos Santos, R. A., Goldman, G. H., Rajendran, R., et al. (2016). RNAseq reveals hydrophobins that are involved in the adaptation of *Aspergillus nidulans* to lignocellulose. https://core.ac.uk/download/46165079.pdf (accessed on 11th June 2025).

28. Cameron, P. A. (1999). *Gas Phase Enzyme Catalysis for Esterification and Transesterification Reactions Using Immobilized Lipase*. https://core.ac.uk/download/588288189.pdf (accessed on 11th June 2025).

29. Casas, A. I., Cuadrado, A., Dao, V. T. V., Di Lisa, F., et al. (2015). Pharmacology and clinical drug candidates in redox medicine. https://core.ac.uk/download/30614148.pdf (accessed on 11th June 2025).

30. Chen, X., Fredrickson, J. K., Li, M., Liu, Y., et al. (2017). Regulation-structured dynamic metabolic model provides a potential mechanism for delayed enzyme response in denitrification process. https://core.ac.uk/download/286729904.pdf (accessed on 11th June 2025).

31. Costelloe, S. J., Ward, J. M., & Dalby, P. A. (2008). Evolutionary analysis of the TPP-dependent enzyme family. *Journal of molecular evolution*, *66*(1), 36–49. https://doi.org/10.1007/s00239-007-9056-2(accessed on 11th June 2025).

32. Edwards, C. H., Grundy, M. M. L., Holland, C., Ryden, P., et al. (2020). Plant cell walls: Impact on nutrient bio accessibility and digestibility. https://core.ac.uk/download/287579488.pdf (accessed on 11th June 2025).

33. Erbilgin, O., Kerfeld, C. A., & Sutter, M. (2016). The structural basis of coenzyme A recycling in a bacterial organelle. https://core.ac.uk/download/323063514.pdf (accessed on 11th June 2025).

34. Fieseler, L., Knecht, L. E., & Veljkovic, M. (2020). Diversity and function of phage encoded depolymerases. https://core.ac.uk/download/286703673.pdf (accessed on 11th June 2025).

35. Fonteh, Aliah L. (2018) "Orotic Aciduria," *Fidei et Veritatis: The Liberty University Journal of Graduate Research*: Vol. 2: Iss. 1, Article 1. Available at: https://digitalcommons.liberty.edu/fidei_et_veritatis/vol2/iss1/1 (accessed on 11th June 2025).

36. Helenius, A., Ishii, A., Lal, A., Varki, A., Barabási, A. L., Feist, A. M., Sburlati, A. R., et al. (2009). Centralized modularity of N-linked glycosylation pathways in mammalian cells. https://core.ac.uk/download/pdf/8332683.pdf (accessed on 11th June 2025).

37. Jennings, M. (2018). Optimizing genetic manipulation of methanogens through faster cloning techniques. https://core.ac.uk/download/158200172.pdf (accessed on 11th June 2025).

38. Johansson, F. D., Kriege, N. M., & Morris, C. (2020). A survey on graph kernels. https://core.ac.uk/download/326728403.pdf (accessed on 11th June 2025).

39. Karigar, C. S., & Rao, S. S. (2011). Role of microbial enzymes in the bioremediation of pollutants: A review. https://core.ac.uk/download/pdf/8614112.pdf (accessed on 11th June 2025).

40. Koskella, B., Lin, D., & Lin, H. (2017). Phage therapy: An alternative to antibiotics in the age of multi-drug resistance. https://core.ac.uk/download/323081265.pdf (accessed on 11th June 2025).

41. Patwardhan, S. (2011). *Biomimetic and Bioinspired Silica: Recent Developments and Applications*. https://core.ac.uk/download/9032722.pdf (accessed on 11th June 2025).

42. Powell, J. S., & Raffa, K. F. (2018). Tolerance of plant monoterpenes and diterpene acids by four species of Lymantriid (*Lepidoptera*) exhibiting a range of feeding specificities. https://core.ac.uk/download/216807297.pdf (accessed on 11th June 2025).

43. Priami, C., & Zámborszky, J. (2010). BlenX-based compositional modeling of complex reaction mechanisms. http://arxiv.org/abs/1002.4065 (accessed on 11th June 2025).

44. Rees, D. C. (2002). Great metalloclusters in enzymology. https://core.ac.uk/download/4875844.pdf (accessed on 11th June 2025).

45. Roberts, C. (2020). Regulating retinoic acid availability during development and regeneration: The role of the CYP26 enzymes. https://core.ac.uk/download/pdf/322832230.pdf (accessed on 11th June 2025).

46. Srichantra, A. (2002). *Modeling of the Break Process to Improve Tomato Paste Production Quality: A Thesis Presented in Partial Fulfilment for The Degree of Master of Engineering in Bioprocess at Massey University*. https://core.ac.uk/download/148644111.pdf (accessed on 11th June 2025).

47. Walker, G. M. (2010). *Pichia anomaly: Cell Physiology and Biotechnology Relative to Other Yeasts*. https://core.ac.uk/download/228176756.pdf (accessed on 11th June 2025).

48. Wansbrough, E. M. (1998). *Site Directed Mutagenesis and Purification of The CDNA for Human Class I Aldehyde Dehydrogenase: A Thesis Presented in Partial Fulfilment of The Requirements for The Degree of Master of Science at Massey University*. https://core.ac.uk/download/162616931.pdf (accessed on 11th June 2025).

BIOENERGETICS

4

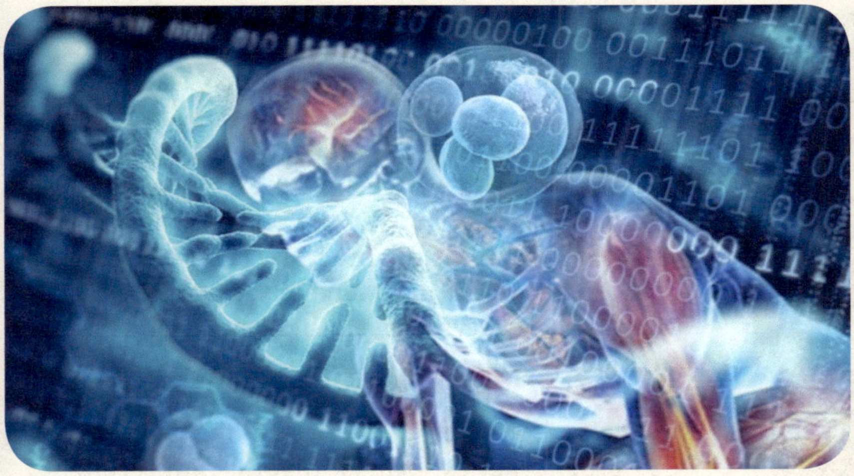

LEARNING OBJECTIVES

After studying this chapter, you will be able to:

1. Understand the fundamental concepts of energy in biology;
2. Describe cellular respiration and photosynthesis;
3. Understand the bioenergetics in muscle function;
4. Understand the relationship between bioenergetics and metabolism;
5. Describe the applications of bioenergetics.

Introduction

Bioenergetics looks at the movement of energy within living organisms, mainly focusing on how cells use and process energy. Since it is an interdisciplinary subject, it uses ideas from biochemistry, physiology, and molecular biology to study how cells gain and use energy. At the core of bioenergetics is the concept of adenosine triphosphate (ATP), the primary energy currency in cells, which is produced through processes such as oxidative phosphorylation and substrate-level phosphorylation. It is essential to understand energy flow both inside and outside the cell, since this explains how metabolic processes respond to the needs of the cell. It is important to note that energy changes happening in the mitochondria are key to cell health, as they affect both metabolism and important signaling pathways that help the cell stay stable and survive. Bioenergetics places a lot of emphasis on how the nuclear and mitochondrial genomes influence each other, demonstrating that energy metabolism is well coordinated. A special trait of mammalian cells is that they have two different genomes that work together. Although mitochondrial DNA makes some proteins needed for energy, more than 98% of the mitochondrial proteins are coded by the nuclear genome. This means that mitochondria and the cell can exchange signals, as new studies indicate that mitochondrial energy production can help coordinate with the cell's need for energy during cell division. Mainly, cyclin B1/CDK1 has been found to coordinate the actions of these genomes to change the energy supply in a cell based on its needs. This way, understanding this sophisticated interaction gives us knowledge about how cells are strong and adaptable in their energy use. Mitochondrial transplantation is an example of how bioenergetics research is being used in practical ways, mainly in the clinical field. Many doctors now use the novel treatment for disorders like cardiac dysfunction since energy deficiency in cells is a main feature of these conditions.

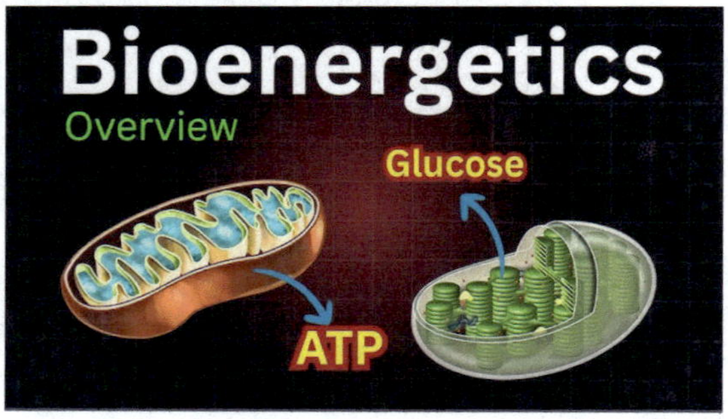

Figure 4.1. Bioenergetics.

Source: https://i.ytimg.com/vi/ORSoZzsiZ7o/hq720.jpg?sqp=-oaymwEhCK4FEIIDSFryq4qpAxMIARUAAAAAGAElAADIQj0AgKJD&rs=AOn4CLAUys3TLsEaiyzULlmNHKhl2Z6bzA.

It has been shown through research that non-autologous mitochondrial transplantation can help boost the energy levels in the heart cells of the recipient for a short time by increasing ATP production and respiration. Still, the fact that these benefits are temporary implies that implanted mitochondria might have a hard time fitting into the cellular environment in the long run. It is important to understand these factors, since the quick enhancement points out the need for creating strategies to maintain bioenergetic improvements, which could open doors to new treatments in urgent situations. They prove that bioenergetics is important for both science and medicine (Figure 4.1).

Definition of Bioenergetics

Bioenergetics is a basic way to understand energy changes and transfers in biological systems. Bioenergetics, in general, looks at how energy moves through living organisms, covering many processes such as respiration and photosynthesis. Bioenergetics at the cellular level looks at the ways cells use energy to keep living. The main benefit of this field is that it explains the energy processes that support metabolism, cell maintenance, and growth. When researchers use physics and chemistry in biology, they can explain how energy is used inside cells and how this is connected to the overall energy balance of living things. So, bioenergetics brings together different scientific fields and explains how evolutionary changes are related to energy efficiency. Energy flow in biology is closely related to major biochemical changes, for example, those that happen in the electron transport chain in mitochondria and thylakoid membranes in chloroplasts. For example, investigations into the Q-cycle mechanism highlight a sophisticated interplay between electron and proton transfer during photosynthesis, which can be modeled using quantum mechanical principles (Tacchino et al., 2019). It increases our knowledge of energy efficiency in these important pathways and also reveals the quantum aspects of biochemical actions. By studying thermodynamics in energy transfer, bioenergetics helps scientists understand how organisms change their metabolism when facing environmental problems and changes in resources. This approach highlights the key role that bioenergetics has in understanding complicated biological processes. In addition, using bioenergetics together with ecohydraulics demonstrates that it is relevant and flexible in different research fields. Ecohydraulics focuses on the interactions between water movement and aquatic ecosystems, melding principles from hydrology with aquatic ecology (Aristotle et al., 2016). Because energy transfer plays a key role in these ecosystems, it is necessary to understand it well when studying different habitats. An example is how organisms move in water depends on their need for energy and the resources they have. When bioenergetics is combined with ecological models, researchers can learn important facts about ecosystems, species, and how to manage the environment. So, bioenergetics is recognized as a key discipline on its own and also for helping us grasp the connections between different ecological and biological systems (Figure 4.2).

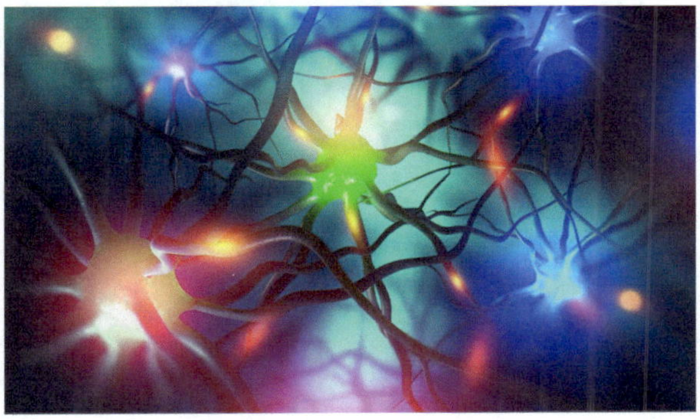

Figure 4.2. Artistic representation of neural activity and bioenergetic signaling in the brain.

Source: https://www.e4l.com/hubfs/what-is-bioenergetics-HUBSPOTSIZE-1.jpg.

4.1. Fundamental Concepts of Energy in Biology

Learning Outcome

1. Describe the types of energy relevant to biological processes;
2. Learn about laws of thermodynamics and their application;
3. Know the energy transformations in living organisms.

Knowing the basic concepts of energy is necessary in bioenergetics, mainly because they affect the many metabolic processes inside an organism. At the center of understanding is ATP, the cell's main energy currency. Energy released by the hydrolysis of ATP allows many biological reactions to occur, so reaction coupling is important in metabolism. To ensure students understand energy and free energy well, it is important to correct any wrong ideas they may have. Active-learning strategies like video modules can further contribute to understanding by summarizing chemistry topics, covering reaction coupling, and setting up for more sophisticated biochemical discussions (Pulukuri & Abrams, 2020). They help students grasp energy processes better and learn bioenergetics as a whole. It reveals how different parts of cells and energy production are connected to the body's balance and cell activity. Mitochondria, usually referred to as the cell's powerhouse, play a central role in energy metabolism, allowing ATP synthesis via cellular respiration.

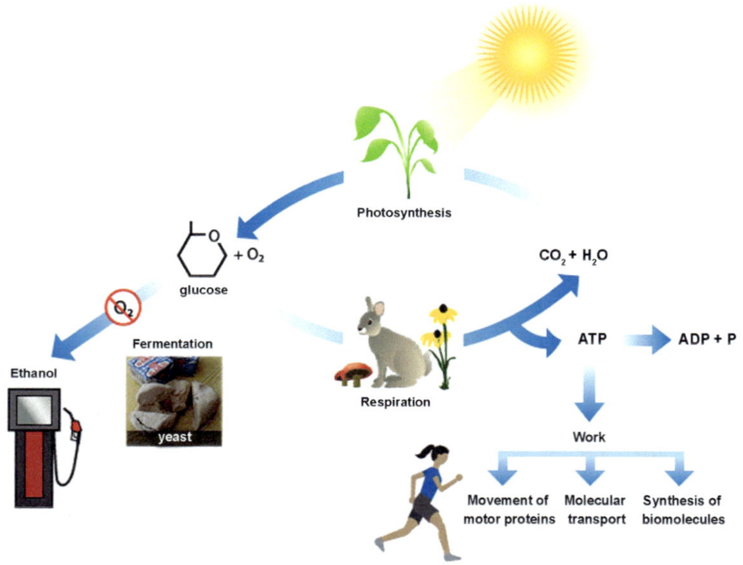

Figure 4.3. Energy and metabolism.

Source: https://s3-us-west-2.amazonaws.com/courses-images-archive-read-only/wp-content/uploads/sites/690/2015/07/23014122/Reactions_whole.png.

The process creates ATP and also joins in with signaling networks that connect mitochondrial activities with the control of nuclear genes. Essentially, the way mitochondrial energy generation links with the cell cycle demonstrates how cells' actions are affected by energy needs. It has been observed that cyclin B1/CDK1 activation helps control mitochondria, so that changes in energy metabolism are linked to the progression of the cell cycle and dealing with stress. Such precise coordination is characteristic of the interface between bioenergetics and cellular processes; it is an excellent example of dynamic regulation of energy transfer in biological systems (Xie et al., 2019). Bioenergetic studies are also very important for learning about both normal and abnormal body functions. As changes in energy metabolism may cause metabolic diseases, it is very important for mitochondria to function well. Therefore, studies have tried to explain how mitochondrial bioenergetics affects a cell's response to various stimuli, such as treatment. Lately, it has been suggested that by adjusting these pathways, adaptive resistance in tumors may be addressed, and mitochondrial metabolism could be a useful approach for cancer treatment. Studies on the connection between energy production and cellular signaling help scientists discover new ways to treat diseases. Therefore, knowing the basic ideas of energy in biology improves discussions in academia and supports progress in medical science, considering how bioenergetics is important in many fields (Figure 4.3).

4.1.1. Types of Energy Relevant to Biological Processes

The main idea of bioenergetics is that biological systems change and use different types of energy. The main part of these processes is chemical energy, which is stored in molecules and can be released by metabolic reactions. Organisms primarily extract chemical energy from food through cellular respiration, a process that converts glucose and other nutrients into ATP, the energy currency of cells. In addition, photosynthetic organisms rely on light energy, as chlorophyll helps change carbon dioxide and water into glucose and oxygen. Because of this connection between chemical and light energy, food webs in ecosystems exist, proving that energy is essential for life on Earth and its survival and growth. Thermal energy is another form of energy important in biology, since it is the heat produced during metabolic processes. Endotherms like mammals and birds control their body temperature to ensure the best conditions for enzymes and their metabolism. Having this thermoregulation is necessary for keeping many body functions going, including digestion and immunity. In addition, losing the right amount of thermal energy can result in problems such as hypothermia or heatstroke, showing the need for proper energy management in living things. Interestingly, recent research has explored bioenergetics in the context of mitochondrial transplantation, revealing short-term bioenergetic enhancements in cardiomyocytes that correspond to improved heat production (Pour et al., 2020).

They show that thermal energy is important for life and that bioenergetics may lead to new medical treatments. Mechanical energy is also important in biological processes, mainly helping with muscle contractions and the movement of cells. Chemical energy is changed into mechanical work by the action of ATP hydrolysis. To facilitate movement in the heart and skeletal muscles, both types of muscles depend on this transformation. How efficiently the body converts energy is very important for the survival of organisms and affects their movement, hunting, and reproduction. Also, motor proteins in cells rely on mechanical energy from ATP to move different components along the cytoskeleton. Understanding these various energy types and their roles in biological processes is essential for grasping the complex bioenergetic dynamics that sustain life, thereby offering insight into future research directions in bioenergetics (Dumas et al., 2008) (Figure 4.4).

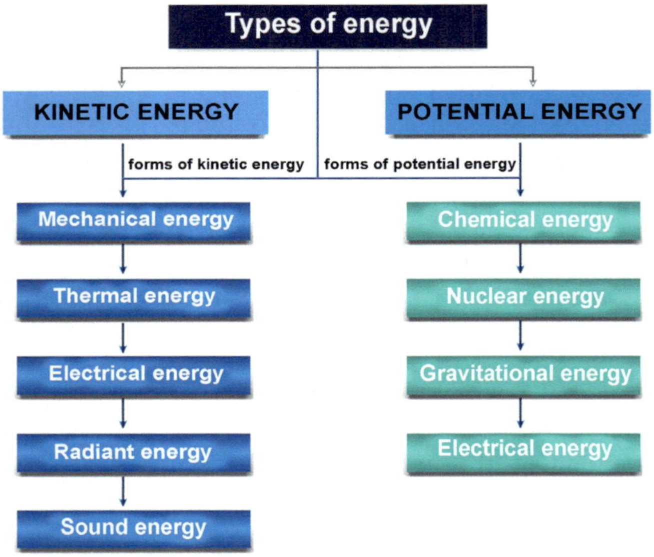

Figure 4.4. Types of energy.

Source: https://www.priyamstudycentre.com/wp-content/uploads/2021/11/different-types-and-forms-of-energy.png.

4.1.2. Laws of Thermodynamics and Their Application

Thermodynamic laws control how energy is used in all living systems and are the basis of bioenergetics. It is known as the first law that energy cannot disappear or appear, but it can be transformed into different types of energy. According to the law, cells use energy from nutrients to do the tasks necessary for survival. For instance, during cellular respiration, glucose molecules are broken down to produce energy, which is stored in the form of ATP. This process exemplifies the transformation of chemical energy into usable cellular energy, representing how the first law of thermodynamics works in living organisms and emphasizing the budget for energy necessary for living organisms to survive (Xie et al., 2019). The second law of thermodynamics points out that energy cannot be used fully and that systems move towards a more disordered state. It is especially important in biology since it points out how metabolic pathways are not perfectly efficient. As an example, the process of getting energy from food does not always result in ATP; some energy is lost as heat, which increases the overall disorder in the system. It is very important for understanding the energy limits that cells must deal with. The ability to maintain order and utilize energy efficiently in the face of these constraints informs our understanding of cellular functions and adaptations in diverse environments (Gerbaud et al., 2020). For this reason, it is important to understand the second law to see how living things handle their energy problems. Besides, using thermodynamics in bioenergetics encourages us to rethink our strategies in energy engineering and metabolic design. Nature-inspired chemical engineering (NICE) exemplifies this intersection, emphasizing the need for frameworks that transcend traditional equilibrium-based assumptions. Using nonequilibrium thermodynamics and nonlinear control, scientists can build better bioengineering processes that match the changing nature of biological systems. Systems such as hierarchical transport networks and dynamic self-organization help to use energy efficiently and stay within thermodynamic rules. Consequently, applying these advanced thermodynamic concepts allows for the innovation of sustainable strategies that optimize energy consumption and resilience in biotechnological applications, further advancing our understanding of the intricate relationship between energy and life (Gerbaud et al., 2020) (Figure 4.5).

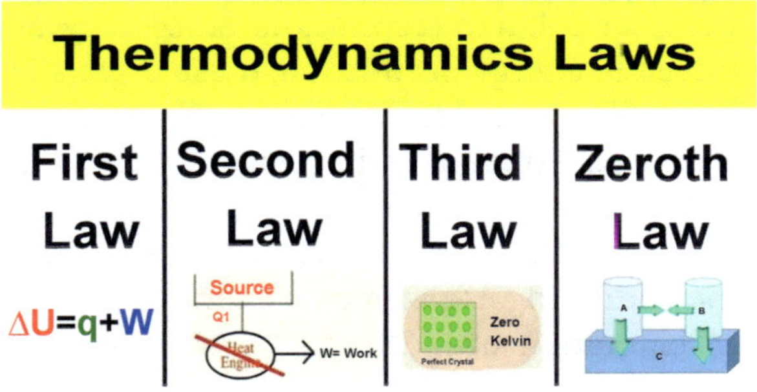

Figure 4.5. Laws of thermodynamics.

Source: https://i.ytimg.com/vi/FGWmzMAFTSY/maxresdefault.jpg.

4.1.3. Energy Transformations in Living Organisms

The conversion of energy is important for all living things, and this happens through complicated biochemical reactions. The main part of these changes is metabolism, which includes both catabolic and anabolic pathways. Catabolism is when organic materials are broken down to give out energy, and anabolism uses that energy to build the components needed for growth and repair. The coupling of these metabolic pathways is vital; energy derived from the degradation of carbohydrates, fats, and proteins is ultimately captured in the form of ATP, the energy currency of the cell. The efficiency of these biochemical processes illustrates the intricate nature of energy flow within biological systems, highlighting how vital energy transformations underpin the life processes essential for survival and adaptation (Goldford et al., 2018). Systems biology methods can give a better view of energy transformations by analyzing metabolic networks in different ways. They show how metabolism changed over time and why it helps life cope with different conditions. Researchers can use computational models to study and examine how metabolic processes work and how efficiently they help organisms use energy. For instance, empirical and theoretical models allow scientists to study energy transformations in specific contexts, such as aquaculture systems, where understanding the metabolism of species like Nile tilapia is crucial for optimizing production and sustainability (Cuenco et al., 2025). Therefore, systems biology helps us better understand bioenergetics and also gives us ways to manage living systems in both ecological and agricultural areas. The link between energy changes and evolutionary biology sheds light on how organisms adapt. The way an organism uses energy can change its place in the environment, its method of reproduction, and how fit it is. All in all, efficient energy use allows an organism to thrive in its environment since energy shortages can affect its growth, reproduction, and chances of survival. The development of photosynthesis and cellular respiration shows how energy is used and stored, giving various ecosystems many benefits. As research advances in understanding these energy transformations, it becomes increasingly apparent that they are not merely biological processes but are also deeply entwined with evolutionary history, highlighting the significance of bioenergetics in shaping life on Earth (Goldford et al., 2018).

Test Your Knowledge

1. What are the types of energy important to biological processes?
2. What are the applications of the laws of thermodynamics?

4.2. Cellular Respiration

Learning Outcome

1. Give an overview of aerobic and anaerobic respiration;
2. Describe the key metabolic pathways involved in bioenergetics;
3. Understand the role of ATP in energy transfer.

Cellular respiration is a basic metabolic process through which living organisms are able to take nutrients and transform them into useful energy, mostly ATP. The process includes several stages, for example, glycolysis, the citric acid cycle, and oxidative phosphorylation. In the cytoplasm, glycolysis changes glucose into pyruvate and produces only a little ATP and NADH. In the mitochondria, the citric acid cycle changes pyruvate into carbon dioxide and makes more NADH and FADH2. Oxidative phosphorylation is the final process, and it happens within the inner mitochondrial membrane, as the electron transport chain uses high-energy electrons to build a proton gradient that helps make ATP. To understand bioenergetics well, you need to understand the details of every stage in cellular respiration because it points out how energy is produced and regulated in both prokaryotic and eukaryotic cells. The role of mitochondria is extremely important in the process of cellular respiration. Since they are involved in energy production, these organelles are commonly called the cell's powerhouses. It has been established in research that when mitochondria do not function properly, it can result in metabolic disorders and diseases that come with aging. Experiments on mitochondrial transplantation over the past few years have supplied useful knowledge about cellular energy systems. Notably, transplanting non-autologous mitochondria into cardiomyocytes resulted in temporarily enhanced ATP production and basal respiration, indicative of a temporarily supercharged bioenergetic state (Pour et al., 2020).

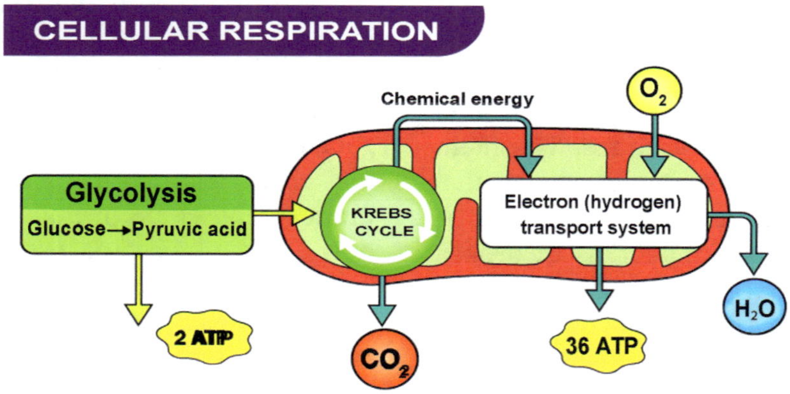

Figure 4.6. Cellular respiration.

Source: https://cdn1.byjus.com/wp-content/uploads/2019/04/Cellular-Respiration-2.png.

Even though these developments are helpful, they point out that cells must maintain a certain balance of energy, which is possible only if mitochondria function consistently. Also, the way mitochondria and cellular signaling interact is key to maintaining the right amount of energy in the cell. The cell's nuclear and mitochondrial genomes interact in many ways to adjust energy use and metabolic activities. The role of cyclin B1/CDK1 in regulating mitochondrial activities is critical, as it integrates energy metabolism with cellular processes like the cell cycle and stress response (Xie et al., 2019). This means that mitochondria can change the amount of energy they produce to fit the needs of the cell, which is very important when the cell grows or faces stress. Furthermore, the way the nucleus and mitochondria interact is a clear sign of the complex control needed for the energy supply in living things, especially during the development of tumors. Exploring these connections further may increase our knowledge of cellular respiration and how to treat metabolic disorders and cancer (Figure 4.6).

4.2.1. Overview of Aerobic and Anaerobic Respiration

Energy in living organisms is mainly produced by aerobic and anaerobic respiration, which is the main concept of bioenergetics. Aerobic respiration occurs in the presence of oxygen and primarily takes place in the mitochondria of cells, where glucose is metabolized into carbon dioxide, water, and ATP, the primary energy currency of the cell. It is a very efficient way, as each glucose molecule can produce up to 36 ATP molecules and involves glycolysis, the citric acid cycle, and oxidative phosphorylation. Because oxygen helps both with energy production and with the survival of cells, aerobic respiration is the main way most eukaryotic organisms generate energy. However, when there is no oxygen, anaerobic respiration takes place by using fermentation to generate energy. Yeast and some bacteria are able to do anaerobic respiration, where they turn sugar into energy and also produce ethanol or lactic acid.

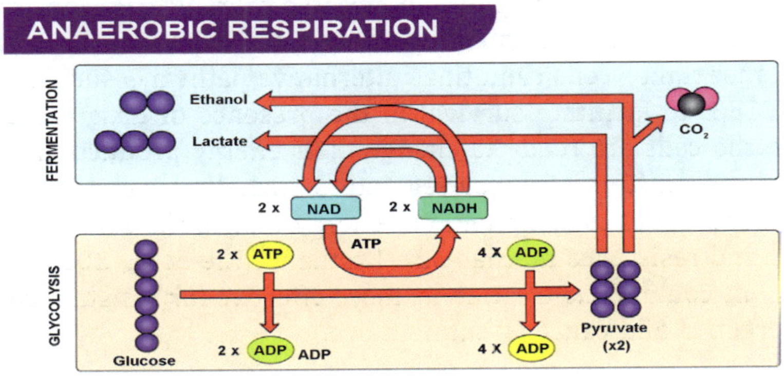

Figure 4.7. Anaerobic respiration.

Source: https://cdn1.byjus.com/wp-content/uploads/2019/04/Aerobic-And-Anaerobic-Respiration-2.png.

The number of ATP molecules produced by anaerobic respiration is lower than what of aerobic respiration. Although anaerobic respiration is necessary in low-oxygen places, the byproducts it forms can be harmful if they reach high levels. Because organisms can use aerobic or anaerobic respiration, they can live and balance their energy levels in different environments. In addition, research on anaerobic processes has become very important in relation to diseases and metabolism. Lactate, which is created during anaerobic respiration, has been suggested to play a role in cancer biology besides just being waste. It has been found that lactate can change the way genes are expressed in cancer cells, affecting cell growth and oncogenic pathways. In this light, understanding the intricate balance between aerobic and anaerobic respiration not only enhances our comprehension of bioenergetics but also opens avenues for exploring therapeutic targets in metabolic disorders and cancer, illustrating the profound implications of these metabolic processes in health and disease (Becker et al., 2017; Brooks et al., 2019) (Figure 4.7).

4.2.2. Key Metabolic Pathways Involved

It is important to understand key metabolic pathways in bioenergetics since they oversee the conversion of nutrients into energy that cells can use. Cellular metabolism is mainly split into catabolic and anabolic parts, and catabolism is the one that breaks down organic molecules to produce energy. The process of glycolysis changes glucose into pyruvate, and while doing so, it produces ATP and NADH. After glycolysis, pyruvate can be carried into the mitochondria and oxidized in the citric acid cycle to play a role in ATP synthesis by forming part of the proton gradient. Because of this interaction, we see how cells use energy, making it necessary to study these pathways for both healthy and diseased states. Bioenergetics is regulated by ATP as well as by the way the nuclear and mitochondrial genomes interact. This relationship plays a critical role in maintaining cellular homeostasis, as the nucleus encodes over 98% of mitochondrial proteins, while mitochondria contribute to gene regulation (Thiagarajan et al., 2016). Such cases show that mitochondrial bioenergetics helps the cell manage its energy use and metabolism, mainly during the cell cycle and when responding to stress. When cells are stressed, special pathways are turned on to help them survive, proving how flexible energy-related processes are. Therefore, these changes may prevent effective treatment of cancer cells and require experts to know in detail how these mechanisms work to help design targeted therapies. Besides showing how cancer cells become resistant to treatment, metabolic pathways are important in cancer biology. Recent studies have revealed that tumor cells can utilize alternative pathways such as autocrine signaling through factors like $TGF\beta_2$ to facilitate survival in the presence of drug therapy (Thiagarajan et al., 2016). As a result, the cells are ready to change their energy production and survive without glutamine. In addition, the function of major regulators, including cyclin B1/CDK1, demonstrates how mitochondrial bioenergetics is symphonic in energy distribution and cell growth, impacting tumor responsiveness and resistance mechanisms firsthand (Xie et al., 2019). So, interfering with these metabolic functions could make treatments more effective for resistant cancers, proving how closely related bioenergetics and cancer treatment are.

4.2.3. Role of ATP in Energy Transfer

ATP is often described as the energy currency of the cell, serving as a pivotal molecule in the transfer and utilization of energy across various biological processes. The structure of ATP, which has ribose sugar, adenine base, and three phosphate groups, makes it possible for ATP to store energy in the bonds between the phosphate groups. When a cell needs energy, ATP is broken down by hydrolysis to provide the energy that is used for muscle contraction, making biochemicals, and active transport. Besides, this system is not limited to one area; it supports major metabolic pathways, proving that ATP is required for both making and using energy in the cell. All in all, ATP plays a key part in explaining how energy is used and controlled in living things. Besides giving energy, ATP is important in many metabolic processes. As an example, anaerobic bacteria use carbon dioxide and molecular hydrogen to make acetate, which demonstrates an old way of producing energy and ATP. Unlike in other bacteria, *Acetobacterium woodii* uses a sodium ion potential instead of cytochromes and quinones to help with ATP synthesis. This unique coupling of ATP production with energy conservation reflects a remarkable adaptation to energetic barriers through electron bifurcation and soluble enzymes, revealing its critical role in sustaining metabolism in diverse environmental contexts (Bertsch et al., 2012). So, when we realize how ATP is involved in many biochemical processes, we can value its role in bioenergetics. New discoveries about mitochondria have pointed out how ATP is produced and regulated, which is vital for keeping cells balanced. Since mitochondria are the energy factories of cells, they make ATP and also regularly communicate with the nucleus to ensure energy is used and produced at the same time. A good example of this connection is the cyclin B1/CDK1 complex, which helps manage mitochondrial energy production based on the cell cycle and stress in the cell. As a result, the cell can use the right amount of ATP for its needs, especially when it comes to tumor growth and reacting to treatment. As more research delineates these complex interactions, the role of ATP in establishing a functional balance between energy metabolism and consumption becomes increasingly clear, emphasizing its centrality in understanding bioenergetics on a cellular and organismal level (Xie et al., 2019) (Figure 4.8).

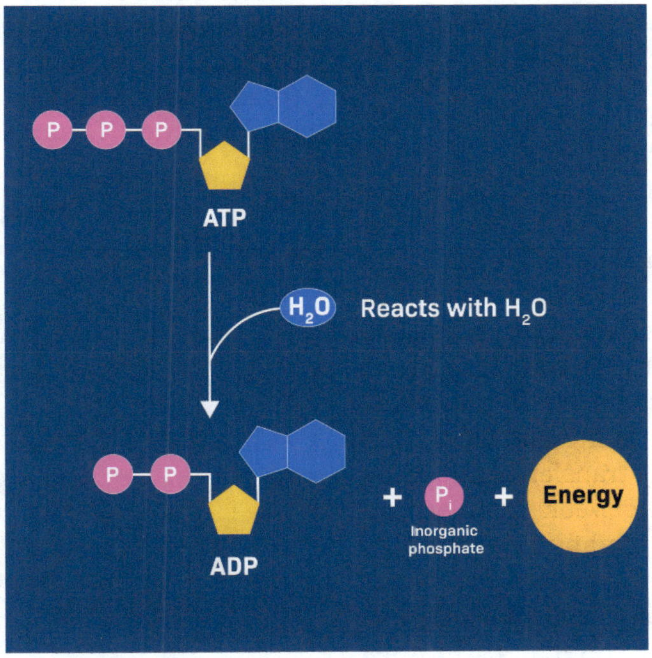

Figure 4.8. ATP hydrolysis. The high-energy bonds of ATP can be broken through the addition of water, which releases high amounts of energy in addition to ADP and an inorganic phosphate.

Source: https://api.www.labxchange.org/api/v1/xblocks/lb:LabXchange:8ef89bac:html:1/storage/copy-of-lxc_ap1_p6_a4_adenosine-triphosphate-atp-and-its-role-in-cellular-energetics_figure-2150x1711463616402-437dcc1ef44c823f3d559eac0e77bdb1.png.

Test Your Knowledge

1. What is aerobic and anaerobic respiration?
2. What is the role of ATP in energy transfer?

4.3. Photosynthesis

Learning Outcome

1. Describe the process of converting light energy into chemical energy;
2. Understand the importance of chlorophyll and light-dependent reactions;
3. Know the Calvin cycle and the synthesis of glucose.

· Photosynthesis is important for life on Earth since it uses light energy to produce the chemical energy that living things need. Mostly, this process happens in chloroplasts, as chlorophyll captures sunlight and helps change carbon dioxide and water into glucose and oxygen. Besides providing energy, photosynthesis is important because it makes the organic compounds that become the basis for food webs in the biosphere. Recent advancements in understanding the bioenergetics of photosynthesis have unveiled its complex mechanisms, including electron transport chains and the role of various protein complexes, such as the cytochrome b_6f complex. This complex operates within a quantum framework that promotes efficient energy transfer, highlighting the delicate interplay between light energy capture and thermodynamic principles (Tacchino et al., 2019). Photosynthesis is not as efficient as thermodynamics would suggest, which means that other elements besides energy are very important. It has been shown by recent studies that the exchange of materials, especially water and carbon dioxide, can affect photosynthesis greatly. Data indicate a median conversion efficiency of approximately 0.78% in terrestrial ecosystems, suggesting that the limiting factors lie not in energy capture but rather in the availability and exchange of essential materials (Kleidon, 2020). It points out that both thermodynamic and ecological aspects are important to study when talking about photosynthesis. Evaporation and precipitation play a major role in forming the environment where photosynthesis needs to function well. To understand photosynthesis from the point of view of bioenergetics, one must combine ecological and biochemical aspects. There is a direct link between how much water evaporates and how efficiently photosynthesis happens. As stated in recent research, the best photosynthesis rates happen when there is enough moisture and sunlight. Therefore, to understand the intricacies of photosynthesis, one has to pay attention not only to the biochemical processes involved but also to the encompassing environmental interactions that determine the thermodynamic effectiveness of the process (Kleidon, 2020). To fully understand photosynthesis and its effect on the environment, you need to consider it from different angles within the context of bioenergetics (Figure 4.9).

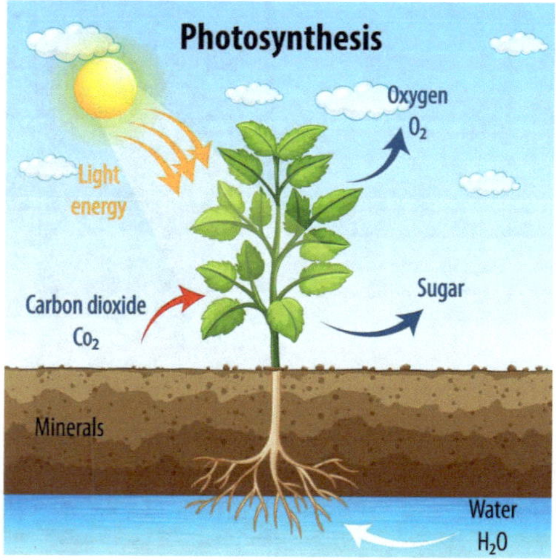

Figure 4.9. Photosynthesis.

Source: https://bartonhillfarms.com/wp-content/uploads/2021/08/photosynthesis-1015x1024.jpg.

4.3.1. Process of Converting Light Energy into Chemical Energy

Bioenergetics relies on the main process of changing light energy into chemical energy, and this mainly happens through photosynthesis in plants, algae, and some bacteria. As a result of this pathway, sunlight is turned into energy by producing glucose from carbon dioxide and water. Chlorophyll in chloroplasts catches the light, which causes electrons to move through a chain of reactions. In the end, photochemical reactions produce ATP and NADPH, which carry energy throughout the cell. The process of light turning into chemical energy supports the organism, and it also helps the whole terrestrial ecosystem by feeding other life and raising oxygen in the air. The process is very efficient, though it does not reach the maximum efficiency possible with thermodynamics. It has been found that photosynthesis is not as efficient as it could be since it only converts light into energy at around 0.78%. It is clear that the main reason for this limit is not energy absorption, but the exchange of important materials such as carbon dioxide and water. The strong link between photosynthetic efficiency and evaporation proves that sunlight helps transfer materials and that the amount of water and air exchange has a big effect on photosynthesis. This research suggests that we should revisit the basic beliefs about how energy is used in living organisms and look further into how the environment and biochemical processes are connected. New discoveries about the cytochrome complex show how energy is transferred during photosynthesis. The Q-cycle mechanism is a good example of how quantum and classical theories can join to help us understand energy transfer in biology. When we study the cytochrome b_6f protein complex and its functions, we find that its electron and proton transport is done most efficiently according to the body's needs. The way quantum mechanics and biochemistry meet in photosynthesis shows how advanced it is and stresses the significance of studying energy movement through cell membranes. The insights gained through these analyses can significantly enhance our grasp of bioenergetics, reinforcing the need for interdisciplinary approaches that unify thermodynamic principles with biological phenomena (Tacchino et al., 2019; Kleidon, 2020) (Figure 4.10).

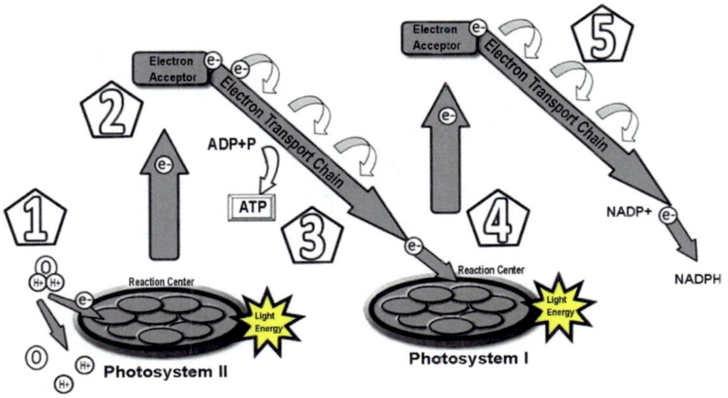

Figure 4.10. Converting light energy to chemical energy.

Source: https://www.biologycorner.com/resources/photosystem_label.jpg.

4.3.2. Importance of Chlorophyll and Light-Dependent Reactions

Chlorophyll is important for photosynthesis, mainly because it absorbs light. It causes a series of light-dependent reactions that are needed to change solar energy into chemical energy. Blue and red light from the electromagnetic spectrum is best absorbed by the chlorophyll molecules in the thylakoid membranes of chloroplasts. When chlorophyll captures photons, it is energized and triggers a series of electron transport processes important for the synthesis of ATP and nicotinamide adenine dinucleotide phosphate (NADPH), which are both essential for the following light-independent reactions. Because of how these reactions are regulated and how chlorophyll uses light, a vital link is formed between light and the energy plants need to live. The light-dependent part of photosynthesis can be explored in more detail to help us understand bioenergetics. Absorption of light by chlorophyll is crucial since it excites the electrons. Through this process, the electrons are pushed along the chain of reactions. Notably, energy-dependent quenching mechanisms, such as excitation dissipation, significantly influence the efficiency of photosystem II (PSII). It has been found that the special way chlorophyll is arranged in the thylakoid membranes can improve the process of excitation transfer. Thanks to these structures, PSII works better, which results in a faster rate of photosynthesis. Thus, the intricate interplay between chlorophylls photochemical properties and its role in facilitating these reactions is paramount for optimizing energy capture and utilization in plant systems (Bennett et al., 2018). Besides the main reactions in the thylakoid membranes, the way in which chlorophylls interact with phycocyanin and other pigments proves its key role in light reactions. Such as, the process of photochemistry in C-phycocyanins is used to explain the complicated ways chlorophyll takes part in energy transfer. The way chlorophyll changes under various conditions, for example, its reversible isomerization, is included in bioenergetics. The fact that chlorophyll and phycocyanin help with energy transfer means that there is an irreversible pathway involved in light absorption and electron movement. Consequently, an in-depth understanding of chlorophylls biochemical properties and interactions is essential for comprehending how plants optimize energy capture and effectively convert it into biochemical forms necessary for growth and metabolism (Bode et al., 1987) (Figure 4.11).

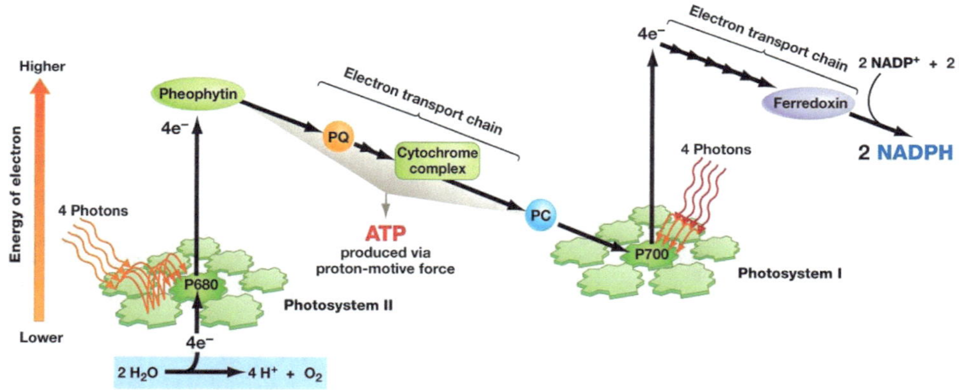

Figure 4.11. The light-dependent reactions.

Source: https://blogger.googleusercontent.com/img/b/R29vZ2xl/AVvXsEihmAa17JvjG3pOSbU9ke3AAbHWT91A54sub4WzwffLguqFIVyN-wjrzoDgqrZyaVjnnL-teUJZ2ufUn3BYpnJ5dk5urB73qu9aIre3LvxASLHEqGx76M2HMpDiZ10pgmN8ASgeXOvEqWM/s1600/lightdependent+reaction.png.

4.3.3. Calvin Cycle and the Synthesis of Glucose

Photosynthesis relies on the Calvin cycle, which helps change carbon dioxide from the air into glucose, which is a main source of energy for many living things. The cycle occurs in the stroma of chloroplasts and is made up of carbon fixation, reduction, and regeneration. During carbon fixation, CO_2 is enzymatically incorporated into ribulose bisphosphate (RuBP) by the enzyme ribulose-1,5-bisphosphate carboxylase/oxygenase (RuBisCO), forming a transient six-carbon compound that swiftly splits into two three-carbon molecules known as 3-phosphoglycerate (3-PGA). The first step is very important because it lays the groundwork for the next process, highlighting how light energy is involved in forming carbohydrates in nature. In the reduction phase of the Calvin cycle, the energy necessary for converting 3-PGA into glyceraldehyde-3-phosphate (G3P) predominantly comes from the ATP and NADPH generated during the light-dependent reactions of photosynthesis. This process changes 3-PGA into G3P by making use of sunlight's energy, so G3P can be used in different biosynthetic pathways. The Calvin cycle shows its biochemical strength by using the energy created from capturing light to synthesize glucose. In addition, G3P can be used by metabolic pathways to create glucose and other carbohydrates, making it an essential point in plant energy processes. The last part of the Calvin cycle regenerates RuBP, so the process of carbon fixation can continue. A set of enzymatic reactions turns G3P back into RuBP, so the cycle can keep happening. It demonstrates that photosynthesis is sustained by a cycle and by maintaining a balance between the things it takes in and the things it gives out. Also, the variety of products made by the Calvin cycle, such as glucose, makes it important for energy as well as for building important biomolecules such as nucleotides, lipids, and amino acids. The interdependencies established in the synthesis of glucose reveal the underlying complexity of metabolic networks in organisms, laying the groundwork for a deeper understanding of metabolic processes (Hakala et al., 2007; Mills et al., 2020) (Figure 4.12).

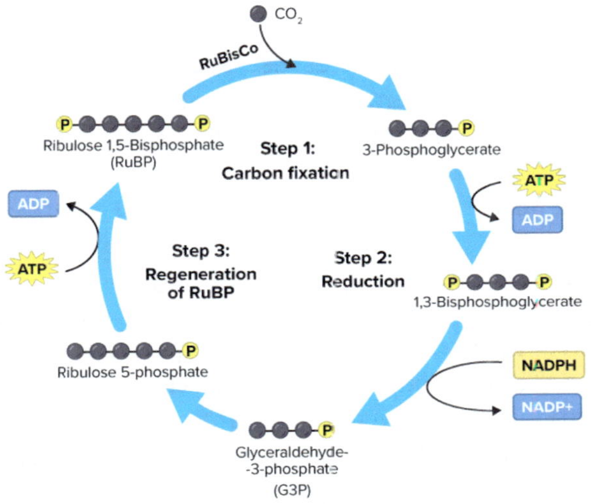

Figure 4.12. Overview of the Calvin cycle pathway.

Source: https://dr282zn36sxxg.cloudfront.net/datastreams/f-d%3A9d587bcc0e6ec7bc11dce4ae9c553eda1048dfadf5a32f973e0296dc%2BIMAGE_TINY%2BIMAGE_TINY.1.

Test Your Knowledge

1. What is the process of converting light energy into chemical energy?
2. What is the importance of chlorophyll and light-dependent reactions?

4.4. Bioenergetics in Muscle Function

Learning Outcome

1. Know the energy requirements during muscle contraction;
2. Understand the role of creatine phosphate (CP) and glycolysis;
3. Describe the impact of aerobic vs. anaerobic metabolism on performance.

To know how muscles use and create energy during movement, the study of bioenergetics is very important. Muscle tissues rely heavily on ATP as the primary energy currency. The first step is for nutrients to be changed into ATP by pathways such as glycolysis and oxidative phosphorylation. Glycolysis gives us quick energy for brief actions, and oxidative phosphorylation in mitochondria is responsible for ATP production when we exercise for a longer time. The combination of energy production ensures muscles function well and are able to adapt to different types of stress in the long run. A careful study of bioenergetics shows that it has important effects on muscle diseases. For instance, research has demonstrated that conditions like Barth syndrome (BTHS) severely impair cardiac and skeletal muscle bioenergetics, leading to diminished exercise tolerance. The phosphocreatine-to-ATP ratio is much lower in affected people than in those without the disease, which shows that the muscle's energy supply is not sufficient. Patients with BTHS also have a significant decrease in the ATP production process called oxidative phosphorylation. These findings elucidate the structural and functional consequences of disrupted bioenergetic processes, showing that not only is energy production compromised, but the overall capacity for muscle recovery post-exercise is also adversely impacted, potentially resulting in exercise intolerance and reduced quality of life for those affected by such disorders (Bashir et al., 2017). Furthermore, the balance of calcium in mitochondria is very important for muscle energy production. If the amount of calcium in mitochondria is not regulated, it can affect ATP production and result in cell death. Studying the molecular processes of mitochondrial calcium uniporters (CUs) explains how signals and metabolism are regulated within cells, which is necessary for muscle function. Appropriate calcium levels in the body, thanks to mitochondria, help produce enough ATP to make muscles contract. A lack of balance in these processes can lead to more muscle fatigue and issues, so focusing on mitochondria is important in medical treatments. This interplay between bioenergetics, calcium signaling, and muscle health is the foundation for current research in maximizing performance and managing muscular disorders, and it has been indicated that developing these advances would see huge increases in athletic training and rehabilitation practice (Quintana et al., 2017) (Figure 4.13).

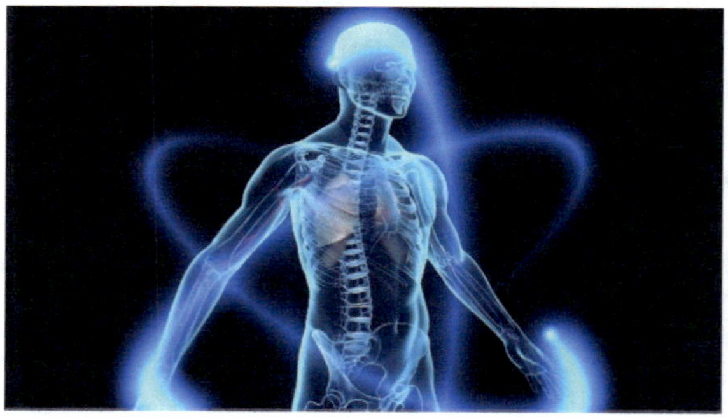

Figure 4.13. Bioenergetics in muscle function.

Source: https://sparkvitalhealth.com/wp-content/uploads/2024/06/maxresdefault.jpg.

4.4.1. Energy Requirements During Muscle Contraction

Effective movement and function of muscles require a lot of energy because the process of contraction is complex. The primary energy molecule utilized during muscle contraction is ATP, which is stored in limited amounts within muscle fibers. As soon as ATP is stimulated, it is quickly broken down by hydrolysis to release energy that helps activate the muscle fibers. Nonetheless, the energy provided by glycolysis is temporary, so it is important to have ways that restore ATP. Specifically, during high-intensity activities, such as sprinting or weightlifting, the body primarily relies on anaerobic pathways, including the phosphagen system and glycolysis, to replenish ATP swiftly, thereby maintaining muscular function during short bursts of strenuous activity, as evidenced in studies examining muscle bioenergetics and their implications for physical performance (Smith, 2016). After the muscles have worked for a longer period, the body relies on other ways to provide the required energy. Within 10 seconds of intense exercise, the glycolytic pathway begins to play a bigger role in making ATP, though it is not as efficient as the phosphagen system. As a result of this process, glucose turns into pyruvate, producing ATP and lactic acid, which may build up and cause tired muscles. Athletes and coaches should understand these metabolic changes to create the best training plans. Further studies show that different activities need different amounts of energy from muscles. For instance, vocalization activities among music and classroom teachers illustrate how laryngeal muscles rely on immediate energy systems due to their brief exertion patterns, emphasizing the specificity of energy demands across diverse forms of muscle contraction (Hill et al., 2013). The ability of an organism to sustain muscle contraction is mostly controlled by the balance between anaerobic and aerobic processes. When exercise lasts longer than the anaerobic threshold, the main source of energy used is aerobic metabolism that takes place in mitochondria. The process takes more time to produce ATP, but it produces much more ATP from every molecule of glucose. Using aerobic metabolism is key for endurance and goes along with how the body adjusts to working out for a long time. For this reason, knowing the energy systems behind muscle contraction helps explain the basics of physical performance and suggests useful ways to improve training. By recognizing how energy demands fluctuate across varying muscle activities, practitioners can tailor interventions to improve muscular efficiency and overall athletic output (Smith, 2016).

4.4.2. Role of Creatine Phosphate and Glycolysis

In the intricate world of bioenergetics, the relationship between CP and glycolysis becomes paramount in ensuring energy homeostasis at the cellular level. CP functions as an instant energy reserve, providing the immediate replenishment of ATP during intense exercise. When the muscles need energy very quickly, the phosphagen system provides it in a short amount of time. Creatine kinase helps convert creatine to CP, which makes sure there is enough ATP for the body at the beginning of exercise. Also, in muscles that use a lot of energy, it becomes clear that CPs play a direct role in glycolysis and metabolism, showing that they are important for better athletic results. Glycolysis is a key way of producing energy without oxygen, especially when someone is working very hard. The mechanism helps change glucose to pyruvate to produce ATP in the absence of oxygen, in addition to the fast ATP formation from CP. Under conditions with low oxygen, such as during high-intensity exercise, the cooperation between glycolysis and CP is very important. Experiments show that, for instance, glycolytic flux can be drastically increased in certain metabolic disorders, such as Huntington's disease, alongside changes in cellular ATP content and phosphocreatine levels (Cunha-Oliveira et al., 2011). These findings suggest that glycolysis can step in for mitochondria when they are not working properly and show the strong connection between these routes in keeping the body's energy and cellular functions stable. Besides, alterations in glycolysis can affect the entire energy system of cells, especially during different diseases. When glioblastoma occurs, major changes in mitochondria can reduce the effectiveness of both glycolysis and CP use.

Research has shown that changes in mitochondrial-associated proteins in such conditions can lead to a reduction in proteins essential for energy metabolism, specifically within respiratory chain complexes (Acharya et al., 2014). It points out that any problem in one area, for example, the mitochondria, can cause changes in glycolysis and CP. This information is necessary for designing treatments that take into account the lack of energy in cells and stresses the importance of CP and glycolysis in meeting the energy needs of the body (Figure 4.14).

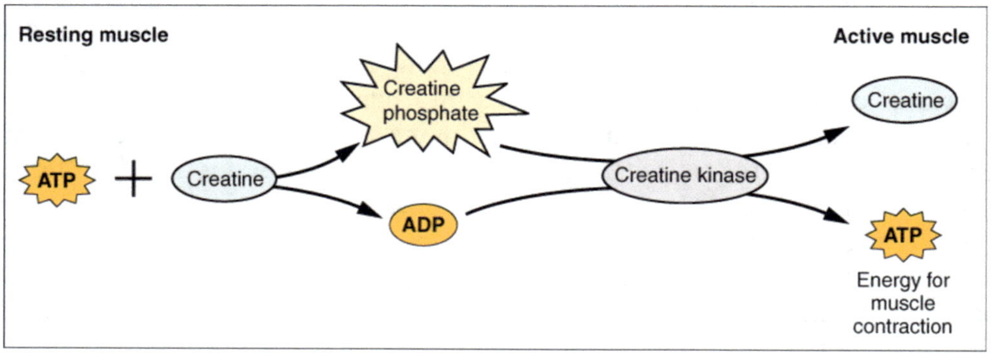

Figure 4.14. A simplified diagram showing the role of creatine phosphate in transporting energy for muscle contraction.

Source: https://upload.wikimedia.org/wikipedia/commons/6/67/1016_Muscle_Metabolism_%28cropped%29.jpg.

4.4.3. Impact of Aerobic vs. Anaerobic Metabolism on Performance

Looking into how aerobic and anaerobic metabolism affect sports performance is important in the field of bioenergetics. When people exercise at a steady low to moderate pace, aerobic metabolism is mainly used to produce energy. It promotes the efficient breakdown of carbohydrates and fats, yielding a high ATP output over an extended period. Thanks to this mechanism, athletes can keep up their performance for a long time, like in marathon running and cycling events. Anaerobic metabolism, on the other hand, is needed for quick, intense workouts because it uses phosphocreatine and glycogen as energy. This route is most important for sprinting or heavy weightlifting, since the body's energy needs are higher than what aerobic energy can provide at that moment. All in all, knowing these metabolic pathways allows for training plans that boost athletic performance. The kind of energy system chosen affects the length of performance as well as the procedures for recovering from intense activity. Taking part in intense exercises without oxygen can cause lactate to build up, which can result in tired and uncomfortable muscles. Hence, after a workout, it is important to use active recovery to remove lactate and restore balance in the body. At the same time, aerobic activities help the body recover faster since they improve blood flow and allow nutrients to reach and remove waste from the muscles more efficiently. By learning about these reactions, athletes and coaches realize why it is important to train periodically for strength and endurance. For instance, training modalities that cleverly integrate both energy systems may yield superior results as athletes not only enhance their anaerobic power but also build a robust aerobic base for sustained performance (Short et al., 2023). Also, the use of both metabolic pathways applies outside sports, such as in voice habilitation, where knowing muscle bioenergetics is very important. Research has shown that vocal performance engages immediate energy systems similar to high-intensity exercises, suggesting that educators, such as music and classroom teachers, rely predominantly on anaerobic metabolism during speaking engagements (Smith, 2016). This point demonstrates that metabolic pathways influence many fields, including those that require vocal endurance. Using strategies that build up both aerobic and anaerobic abilities, people in non-athletic jobs can perform better, proving that bioenergetics is useful everywhere. So, using knowledge from exercise science gives a complete plan for improving performance in various areas (Figure 4.15).

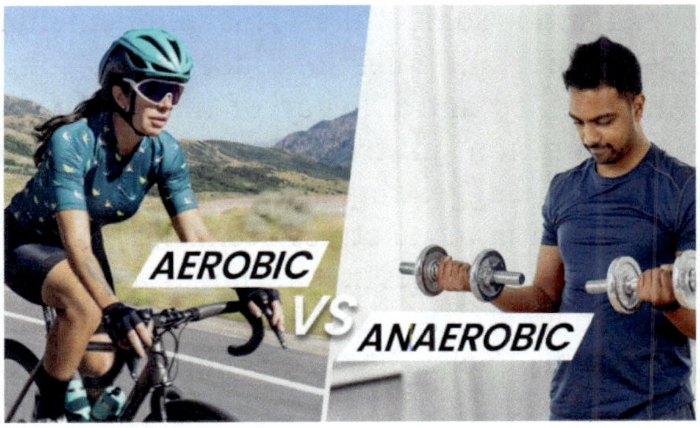

Figure 4.15. Aerobic and anaerobic exercise.

Source: https://www.fitterfly.com/blog/wp-content/uploads/2024/11/Whats-the-Difference-Between-Aerobic-and-Anaerobic-Exercise-1200x720.webp.

Test Your Knowledge

1. What are the energy requirements for muscle contraction?
2. What is the role of creatine phosphate?

4.5. Bioenergetics and Metabolism

Learning Outcome

1. Distinguish between catabolic and anabolic pathways;
2. Understand the regulation of metabolic pathways;
3. Describe the role of enzymes in bioenergetic processes.

To understand how cells work with energy, it is important to look at the link between bioenergetics and metabolism. A center of great importance is the mitochondrion, frequently called the powerhouse of the cell, responsible not only for generating ATP through oxidative phosphorylation but also for playing a critical role in the regulation of many metabolic pathways, promoting cellular function and homeostasis. The connection between mitochondrial and nuclear genomes allows them to work together and manage energy levels in the cell as well as respond to changes in the environment. As emerging research illustrates, the coordination of energy metabolism with cell cycle progression signifies a sophisticated mechanism of control that underscores the dynamic nature of bioenergetics, particularly in tumor biology, where energy demands fluctuate significantly (Xie et al., 2019). The clinical world is interested in mitochondrial bioenergetics because of its potential for treatment. Transplanting mitochondria, either from the patient's own cells or from donors, is a new way to boost cellular energy, especially helping cardiac muscle, which needs a lot of energy to function and heal. According to investigations, ATP production and respiratory capacity in transplanted cardiomyocytes have improved, which is similar to a temporary rise in bioenergetics. Still, these changes usually don't last long and the symptoms return to normal after some time. This phenomenon raises important questions about the long-term viability and efficacy of mitochondrial transplantation in treating energy-deplete conditions, suggesting a potential path for intervention in acute stress scenarios (Pour et al., 2020). The changes in mitochondrial function can also have effects that go further than cellular respiration. Cyclin B1/CDK1 signaling gives important clues about how energy in the cell affects both growth and the body's response to stress. As a result of this regulatory axis, mitochondria can handle different fuel needs, which can change the cell cycle and metabolic processes in cancer. The switch between nuclear and mitochondrial signaling pathways is a key topic, since it shows how tumors use energy to survive treatments. In finding these interactions, the possibility for targeted therapeutics that modulate mitochondrial activity becomes open, creating a profound avenue for improving the treatment of resistant malignancies (Xie et al., 2019) (Figure 4.16).

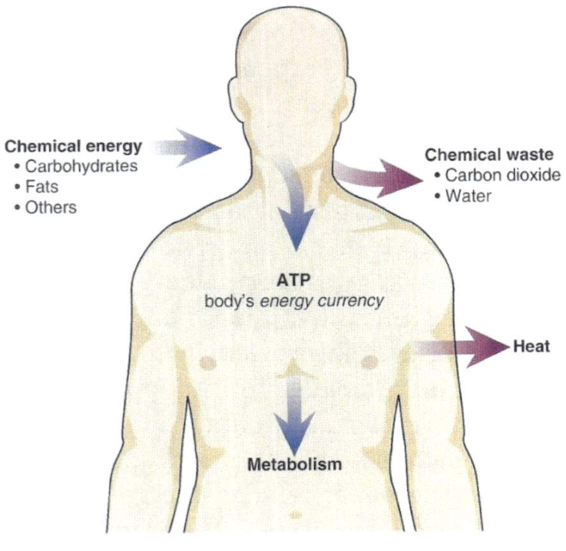

Figure 4.16. Bioenergetics and metabolism.

Source: https://sciencetallis.weebly.com/uploads/9/9/6/6/99666290/scan_orig.jpeg.

4.5.1. Catabolic vs. Anabolic Pathways

Bioenergetics relies on the difference between catabolic and anabolic pathways to show how energy is handled by living things. Catabolic pathways help break down big molecules into smaller ones, and the process also results in ATP energy. Cells need this energy for many functions, and they get it from the oxidation of carbohydrates, fats, and proteins. During catabolism, the Gibbs energy change of the metabolic reaction (ΔG_{met}) reflects the energy available for cellular work, which is intricately linked to ΔG_{cat}, the Gibbs energy change associated with catabolic reactions. The interplay between these energy changes is essential for predicting microbial growth yields and metabolic efficiency, and advances in methods like the Gibbs energy dynamic yield method (GEDYM) enhance our understanding of these catabolic processes under varying environmental conditions, affirming their significance in bioenergetics (Smeaton et al., 2018). Alternatively, anabolic pathways help make complex biomolecules using the energy provided by catabolic reactions. For growth, repair, and maintenance of cells, these processes are very important. To function, anabolic pathways, which are also called biosynthesis, need energy, which is mainly provided by ATP made in catabolic processes. The amount of anabolic and catabolic activities in an organism decides its metabolic condition and energy efficiency. Knowing how ΔG_{an} and ΔG_{cat} work together gives information on the energy needed for various metabolic conditions. The ability to reconcile these two pathways is not only crucial for cellular homeostasis but also for adapting to fluctuating environmental conditions that might impose challenges on energy availability and resource allocation in organisms (Hentscher et al., 2012). The balance between catabolic and anabolic pathways is important for keeping life going. This balance is noticeable in ecosystems because organisms use nutrient cycling to change organic and inorganic materials into energy and to keep their roles in the ecosystem. As an example, in hydrothermal systems, chemosynthesis helps life survive in places without many nutrients by producing energy from catabolic reactions. With the help of advanced thermodynamic models that measure Gibbs energy, we see that these metabolic pathways are very complex and flexible. These insights into metabolic flexibility highlight the importance of both catabolism and anabolism in bioenergetics, reflecting their fundamental roles in sustaining life in diverse habitats (Hentscher et al., 2012; Smeaton et al., 2018) (Figure 4.17).

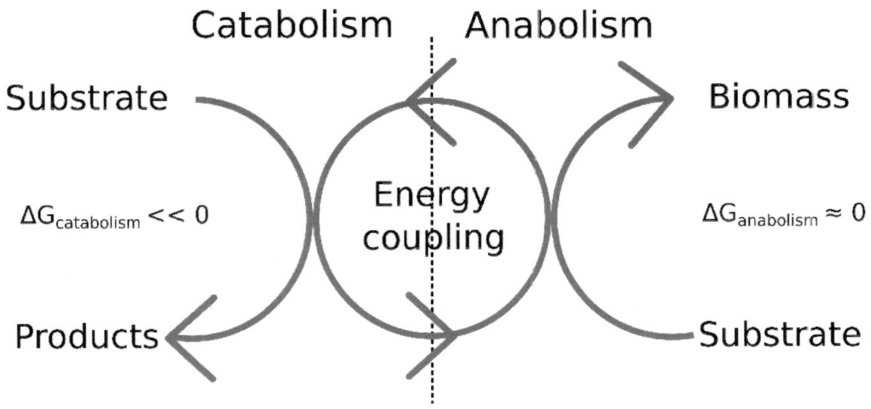

Figure 4.17. The view of microbial metabolism as a thermodynamic energy converter. Catabolic reactions have a large negative free energy gradient, driving anabolic reactions.

Source: Ebenhöh O, Ebeling J, Meyer R, Pohlkotte F, Nies T. Microbial Pathway Thermodynamics: Stoichiometric Models Unveil Anabolic and Catabolic Processes. *Life*. 2024; 14(2):247. https://doi.org/10.3390/life14020247

4.5.2. Regulation of Metabolic Pathways

Proper metabolic control is necessary to keep the cell's balance and supply enough energy. Many mechanisms are involved in tightly regulating metabolic processes, among them are allosteric control, covalent modification, and regulation of gene expression. Because of these mechanisms, cells can react to changes in the body and its energy levels. As an example, when nutrients are scarce, cells could change their metabolic patterns to focus on making ATP, so they can survive. Because of this, tumor cells in cancer metabolism show different metabolic patterns to help them grow rapidly. Understanding these complex regulatory mechanisms is important for developing the therapeutic strategies targeting the metabolic vulnerabilities of cancer cells, thereby ultimately enhancing the treatments' efficacy against resistant tumors. The metabolic process is mainly controlled by the way the mitochondrial and nuclear genomes interact. Besides producing ATP, mitochondria also take part in signaling pathways that tell the nucleus about the cell's energy level. Because of these interactions, metabolic pathways are controlled so that the amount of energy made matches what the cell needs. It has been proven that cyclin B1/CDK1 is the main regulator of the connection between mitochondrial energy and the cell cycle. With these functions in the fine-tuning of metabolic pathways through coordination of the nucleus-mitochondria conversation as cells respond to oscillations in energy demands or environmental stressors, cyclin B1/CDK1 could be crucial for the survival of cancer cells and drug resistance (Xie et al., 2019). Also, the flexibility of tumor cells in dealing with therapies demonstrates how metabolic pathways are regulated. More specifically, research has highlighted the process of early adaptive drug resistance in EGFR-mutant lung cancer cells, where rapid metabolic reprogramming is induced against therapy (Thiagarajan et al., 2016). They are able to become inactive, which helps them survive the harmful effects of targeted therapy. Changes in metabolism are controlled by autocrine signaling that boosts the readiness of mitochondria and lowers the use of glycolysis. So, knowing about these adaptations reveals both the defensive features of cancer cells and the possible approaches for treatment. When clinicians focus on metabolic pathways, they can avoid the development of drug resistance and thus raise the chances of success for bioenergetic cancer therapies.

4.5.3. Role of Enzymes in Bioenergetic Processes

Enzymes help speed up the reactions needed for making energy in cells. With these proteins, reactions can happen more easily, so the products are formed from substrates more efficiently. In cellular respiration, for example, enzymes such as dehydrogenases and kinases play vital roles in pathways like glycolysis and the Krebs cycle, where they facilitate the breakdown of glucose to generate ATP. The ATP made in the cell provides the main source of energy that fuels different biological functions.

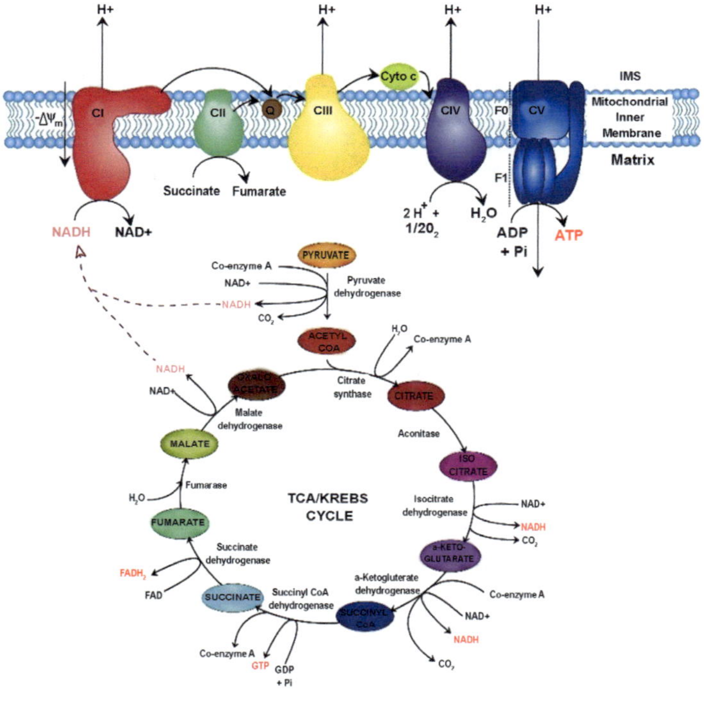

Figure 4.18. Bioenergetics of the electron transport chain and the TCA/Krebs cycle.

Source: https://ars.els-cdn.com/content/image/1-s2.0-S1521690X12000644-gr1_lrg.jpg.

Enzymes that control these metabolic pathways help the cell by increasing energy and making sure energy production is suitable for the cell's needs. Because of this, their function points out how important enzymes are for cellular energy and for supporting life and proper cell activity.

Mitochondria, which are called the powerhouse of the cell, use enzymes greatly in their role in energy production. They have enzymes that make it possible for ATP to be created during oxidative phosphorylation using the energy generated by electron transport chains. Enzymes such as ATP synthase harness the proton gradient generated during electron transport to phosphorylate adenosine diphosphate (ADP), converting it into ATP. Besides, the enzymes in the citric acid cycle are necessary for breaking down metabolites and producing the reducing equivalents that power the electron transport chain. Interactions between mitochondrial and nuclear genomes are important because they affect the enzymes that produce energy in the cell, showing how these interactions are key for regulating metabolism. This shows that enzymes play a key role in both generating energy and managing the cell's reactions to different needs.

New research points out that enzymes play a key role in the way energy metabolism affects cellular functions besides just producing ATP. It has been found recently that enzymes not only take part in metabolism but also play a role in cell cycle and stress signaling. It has been found that the cyclin B1/CDK1 complex is a major link between mitochondrial energy and the cell's progress through the cycle. It illustrates that enzymes are able to change metabolic processes to respond to the cell's changing state, especially in cases of cancer and resistance to drugs. Showing how enzymes work in both metabolism and signaling proves that understanding these mechanisms is very important for designing treatments for diseases. Because of this, enzymes in bioenergetics show more than just their catalytic side, revealing many details of how the body is regulated (Figure 4.18).

Test Your Knowledge

1. What is the regulation of the metabolic pathway?
2. What is the role of enzymes in bioenergetic processes?

4.6. Applications of Bioenergetics

Learning Outcome

1. Describe the role of bioenergetics in medicine and health;
2. Understand the environmental implications of bioenergetics;
3. Describe the future research directions in bioenergetics.

Bioenergetics is useful in different scientific and technological areas, showing how energy changes in living organisms. Bioenergetics is very important in photosynthesis, as plants use sunlight and biochemical reactions to make energy. Q-cycle is a perfect illustration of this process, as it is found in the electron transport chain. Recent studies have modeled the cytochrome b_6f protein complex to analyze energy transport across cellular membranes, revealing optimal thermodynamic efficiency under physiologically relevant conditions. By applying quantum open systems theory, researchers can deepen their understanding of these complex biological systems, providing insights that not only elucidate photosynthetic efficiency but also offer potential applications in enhancing agricultural productivity and biofuel production by optimizing energy conversion processes (Tacchino et al., 2019). Moreover, bioenergetics has far-reaching implications in the development of biological fuel cells, particularly microbial fuel cells (MFCs), which exemplify sustainable energy solutions. As a new technology, MFCs use the reactions of certain bacteria to turn wastewater into electricity. By using this approach, energy is recovered and the environment is treated, which is good for both the energy industry and the environment. The latest developments have shown that enzyme-based fuel cells can be built, and these use immobilized enzymes on electrodes to provide power for portable gadgets. The integration of bioenergetics into these novel fuel cells could revolutionize environmental management and renewable energy sectors by enhancing efficiency, promoting organic matter removal, and supporting onsite applications in remote locations (Duţeanu et al., 2012). The role of bioenergetics in healthcare and biomedical fields shows how important it is to different fields. Bioelectronic devices that use enzymatic biofuel cells can result in new medical technology that lets doctors monitor and treat patients in real time. By turning biochemical changes into electrical signals, these interfaces can regularly give information about metabolism, which helps with personalized medicine. The fact that these devices run on energy from our bodies is a good example of how bioenergetics can help in health care and medical tests. As researchers explore innovative methods for enzyme immobilization and improve energy output, the potential for bioenergetics in clinical settings becomes increasingly promising, reflecting a significant evolution in both energy harvesting and healthcare applications (Duţeanu et al., 2012).

4.6.1. Bioenergetics in Medicine and Health

Bioenergetics is growing as a field, and it has great importance for health and medicine because it explains how cellular energy affects different health conditions. Bioenergetics is important because it can indicate how healthy the body is, mainly in cases of Type 2 diabetes. Recent studies have demonstrated that assessing mitochondrial function in peripheral blood mononuclear cells (PBMCs) can reveal essential insights into systemic bioenergetic capacity. How PBMCs use oxygen in affected people relates to changes in brain structure, showing that mitochondrial efficiency affects both physical and mental health. This dual role of mitochondrial function as both a marker and a mediator vouch for the importance of bioenergetics in decoding disease mechanisms and shaping therapeutic strategies, paving the way for more targeted interventions in chronic diseases (Freedman et al., 2018). As well as being important in metabolic issues, bioenergetics affects many other health areas, including the lungs. Studies on mitochondrial dysfunction have shown that it links to lung injuries and diseases, mainly due to changes in the permeability of the lung's blood vessels. Experiments have found that blocking mitochondrial complexes in cells leads to lower ATP levels, higher ADP:ATP and lactate:pyruvate ratios, and this is seen as a sign of a metabolic crisis in the lungs. Such disturbances can interfere with energy production and also weaken the lungs' blood vessels, which makes it harder to treat both short-term and long-term breathing problems. The insights derived from studying bioenergetics in this context indicate that therapeutic strategies aimed at restoring mitochondrial function could be essential in mitigating lung injuries and improving overall pulmonary health, highlighting the need for a more integrated approach to respiratory care (Audi et al., 2013). Bioenergetics also plays a role in mental health, since it suggests that energy metabolism may be connected to neurological problems. It is believed that changes in how mitochondria work can lead to disorders of the brain and to mental decline. Researchers can use systemic bioenergetic profiles to study how mitochondrial problems affect brain structure, which might help find new ways to discover and track neurodegenerative diseases early on. Because mitochondrial efficiency is linked to cognitive health, metabolic treatments could be helpful in treating diseases. This information proves that bioenergetics is essential for both studying the effects of energy metabolism on various diseases and for finding new ways to improve mental and physical health in many populations (Figure 4.19).

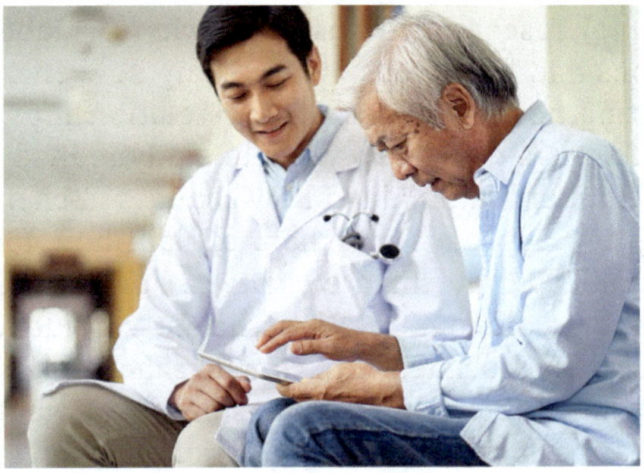

Figure 4.19. Physician consulting with an elderly patient in a clinical setting.

Source: https://www.ifm.org/sites/default/files/styles/alternating_content_image_row_image_desktop_1x/public/2024-07/140806606_lel_1340-x-960-.jpg?h=02c844e9&itok=MUPciXPH.

4.6.2. Environmental Implications and Bioenergetics

It is important to understand how bioenergetics affects the environment to judge the effects of climate change on water ecosystems. Organisms' energy use is closely connected to the environment since temperature can affect their metabolism and the amount of available prey. It has been seen in rainbow trout studies that the amount of energy needed by the fish is affected by changes in the availability of their food. The dominant prey item, the common smelt, plays a significant role in sustaining juvenile and adult trout populations, revealing how energy acquisition strategies can determine population dynamics and ecosystem health, while highlighting the consequences of altered food webs due to environmental changes (Blair et al., 2012). Besides, climate change is a threat to fish adaptations, and it greatly influences bioenergetics at different stages. Higher temperatures change the growth of fish, how they reproduce, and how they use their energy. These changes in the body mean that fish need more food to grow well, mainly in warmer waters. Because of these changes in temperature, some species might do well and others might suffer, which can change the makeup of the community and affect the whole ecosystem. Thus, the intricacies of bioenergetics clearly demonstrate the link between environmental health and species viability, underlining the importance of addressing climate changes in fisheries management and conservation strategies (Vivekanandan, 2013). These adaptations have effects that spread beyond a single species to the whole environment. When predators and prey interact differently, the movement of energy through the food chain may cause big changes in both the types of organisms and the processes in the community. Problems for these animals are made worse by people destroying their habitats and interfering with the environment. It is necessary to use integrated management strategies to strengthen the habitats of fish and ensure the sustainability of fisheries. It is important to have reliable indicators that show changes in ecosystems to help predict them and respond with the right management actions. By understanding the interdependency of environmental health and bioenergetics, we can strive to minimize the harmful impacts of climate change and conserve aquatic biodiversity for generations to come (Vivekanandan, 2013).

4.6.3. Future Research Directions in Bioenergetics

With the development of bioenergetics, scientists need to focus on the major effects of climate change on marine ecosystems. The new and complicated environmental conditions call for a different way of modeling. These models can help us understand how climate change changes the metabolism and actions of marine creatures, which aids our understanding of how ecosystems function. Enhancing how bioenergetics are simulated will make it possible for researchers to predict the individual responses needed to understand the wider effects these changes have on ecosystems. By focusing on the nuances of energy acquisition and utilization, scientists can create more accurate projections concerning marine species' growth, reproduction, and habitat usage under climate pressures, thereby advancing the field significantly through applied research that connects theory with real-world implications (Bednarsek et al., 2024). A further important direction for research is to use what we learn about bioenergetics at the individual level to study populations and food webs. Recognizing how energy is transferred in ecosystems is important for anticipating how species and their relationships in the community will react to environmental problems. Through using new ways to study individual bioenergetics and their effects on the environment, researchers can find out how changes in energy and surroundings affect a population's growth. Using this approach may help explain how food webs remain stable and how trophic relationships are affected by climate changes. Furthermore, enhancing model validation techniques will ensure that predictions retain sufficient confidence, creating a robust framework for assessing the ecological risks associated with climate change (Banha et al., 2024). The way space is used will play an important role in future studies of bioenergetics. The combination of bioenergetics models and spatial data can show how the environment around marine species changes their distribution and numbers. When geographic differences are included in bioenergetics, researchers can spot areas where species are most at risk from climate change and check how they can adapt. This area of research will play a key role in managing fisheries and saving biodiversity as the environment keeps changing. With these models, we can decide how to act in ways that are good for the environment and ensure marine life can survive. Such integrative approaches will ultimately enhance our ability to predict and mitigate the impacts of climate change on marine life (Bednarsek et al., 2024) (Figure 4.20).

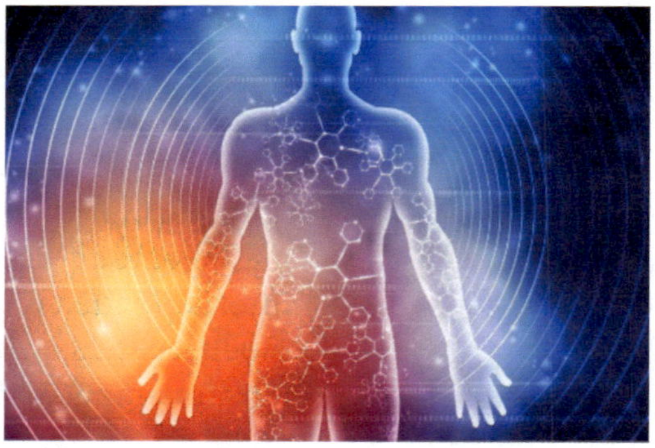

Figure 4.20. Conceptual illustration of human bioenergetics and molecular pathways.

Source: https://neshealthstorage.blob.core.windows.net/articlemedia/123445/images/8d9066ff-e008-480b-a812-029cd02dc98b.jpg.

Test Your Knowledge

1. What is the role of bioenergetics in health and disease?
2. What are the environmental implications of bioenergetics?

Summary

All in all, bioenergetics sheds light on the ways living things turn and make use of energy. This study finds out how cells produce energy and how different living things have adapted to extreme conditions. For instance, organisms thriving in polar regions demonstrate remarkable physiological strategies to maintain metabolic activities despite harsh climate conditions, as highlighted by Arrigo et al. (2014). Because bioenergetics deals with the relationship between metabolism and the environment, it is important in many areas, including biology, biotechnology, and astrobiology. Moreover, how cancer cells use energy shows the wide range of metabolic approaches used by living things. The results on glycolysis and oxidative phosphorylation in breast cancer cells explain that energy production is not the same in normal and malignant tissues. The research documented by Janjic (2012) draws attention to the metabolic variations that exist across different types of tumors, which can inform therapeutic approaches and improve patient outcomes. Thanks to bioenergetics, we can understand cellular health better and it also helps develop new ways to treat cancer. All in all, bioenergetics forms a key basis for understanding energy movements in living systems and how they affect health and disease. With the help of omics technologies, we have learned a lot more about how metabolism changes in extreme conditions and diseases. As shown by research on polar microbes and cancer cell lines, the findings in bioenergetics will keep influencing both research and biotechnology in the future. This way of studying biology helps us understand more about basic life functions and how energy metabolism contributes to a healthy environment and better human health.

Bioenergetics studies the movement of energy in living organisms, which greatly affects cellular metabolism and the body's functions. A major aspect here is how mitochondria are important for energy production. Many people refer to mitochondria as the cell's power source since they produce ATP using oxidative phosphorylation. It is needed for energy generation and also closely linked to signaling in cells and managing metabolism. Besides, problems with mitochondria can cause major changes in energy production, which can harm cells and play a role in many diseases, mainly those related to degenerative changes or cancer, where disrupted energy processes may support tumor growth and new metabolic patterns. Bioenergetics also highlights the important role that calcium and magnesium play as they interact in the cellular environment, mainly in the mitochondria of the heart. Calcium plays a significant role in stimulating mitochondrial energy production through the CU, which facilitates the uptake of calcium ions into the mitochondrial matrix. The process increases the amount of ATP that is produced through NADH oxidation and respiration. On the other hand, when magnesium is present in high amounts outside the cells, it can stop calcium from being taken up by the CU, revealing how the ions influence mitochondrial energy production in a complicated way. For instance, higher extracellular magnesium concentrations have been shown to alter the dynamics of calcium intake, affecting mitochondrial respiration and energy metabolism without altering intracellular magnesium levels, thus suggesting a finely tuned regulatory mechanism at play in bioenergetic processes (Blomeyer et al., 2013). Scientists have recently noticed that EGFR-mutant lung cancer cells can develop adaptive resistance to drugs, and this affects the cell's energy supply. It is found that early changes in cancer cells can cause them to use less energy and change their mitochondria, enabling them to survive treatments. When this happens, the cells become quiet and produce less energy, which changes their cellular communication. It also points out that using EGFR inhibitors together with agents that stop mitochondrial priming could be a good way to overcome resistance. Thus, understanding these intricate bioenergetic adaptations not only aids in therapeutic development but also underscores the importance of targeting metabolic pathways to enhance treatment outcomes in cancer therapy (Thiagarajan et al., 2016).

KEY TERMS FROM THIS CHAPTER

- Adenosine triphosphate
- Carbon dioxide
- Energy conservation
- Glucose
- Mitochondrial genomes
- Nuclear genome
- Photosynthesis
- Thermodynamics
- Bioenergetics
- Cardiac dysfunction
- Energy metabolism
- Medical science
- Mitochondrial transplantation
- Oxidative phosphorylation
- Substrate-level phosphorylation

Critical Thinking Questions

1. What are bioenergetics?
a. The study of genetic material
b. The study of energy flow in living systems
c. The study of protein synthesis
d. The study of cellular respiration only

2. Which of the following is the primary energy currency of the cell?
a. NADH
b. ATP
c. FADH2
d. Glucose

3. The process of breaking down glucose to release energy is called:
a. Glycolysis
b. Photosynthesis
c. Oxidative phosphorylation
d. Gluconeogenesis

4. In which part of the cell does glycolysis occur?
a. Nucleus
b. Cytoplasm
c. Mitochondria
d. Endoplasmic reticulum

5. Which organelle is known as the "powerhouse" of the cell?
a. Nucleus
b. Golgi apparatus
c. Mitochondria
d. Lysosome

Answers to Critical Thinking Questions

1. (b); 2. (b); 3. (a); 4. (b); 5. (c)

Short Answer Questions

1. What do you mean by bioenergetics?
2. What is the fundamental concept of energy?
3. What is meant by cellular respiration?
4. What is photosynthesis?
5. What are the applications of bioenergetics?

References

1. Acharya, A., Herrmann, A., Herrmann, A. G., Gerth, A. M. J., Gallegos, A. M., Venkatesan, B., Ordys, B. B., et al. (2014). Interactions among mitochondrial proteins altered in glioblastoma. https://core.ac.uk/download/20480281.pdf (accessed on 11th June 2025).
2. Ali Pour, P., Kenney, M. C., & Kheradvar, A. (2020). Bioenergetics Consequences of Mitochondrial Transplantation in Cardiomyocytes. *Journal of the American Heart Association*, *9*(7), e014501. https://doi.org/10.1161/JAHA.119.014501(accessed on 11th June 2025).
3. Bashir, A., Bohnert, K. L., Reeds, D. N., Peterson, L. R., Bittel, A. J., de las Fuentes, L., Pacak, C. A., Byrne, B. J., & Cade, W. T. (2017). Impaired cardiac and skeletal muscle bioenergetics in children, adolescents, and young adults with Barth syndrome. *Physiological reports*, *5*(3), e13130. https://doi.org/10.14814/phy2.13130 (accessed on 11th June 2025).
4. Bennett, D. I. G., Fleming, G. R., & Amarnath, K. (2018). Energy-dependent quenching adjusts the excitation diffusion length to regulate photosynthetic light harvesting. *Proceedings of the National Academy of Sciences of the United States of America*, *115*(41), E9523–E9531. https://doi.org/10.1073/pnas.1806597115 (accessed on 11th June 2025).
5. Aristotle, B., Bovee, K., Ginot, V., Gotelli, N. J., Jowett, I. G., Kuhn, T. S., et al. (2016). Eco hydraulics exemplifies the emerging "paradigm of the interdisciplines." https://core.ac.uk/download/82971033.pdf (accessed on 11th June 2025).
6. Arrigo, K. R., Comeau, L. A., Comiso, J. C., Devos, A., DiTullio, G. R., Ferrara, R. M., Gabric, A. J., et al. (2014). Polar microalgae: New approaches towards understanding adaptations to an extreme and changing environment. https://core.ac.uk/download/41989130.pdf (accessed on 11th June 2025).
7. Audi, S. H., Bongard, R. D., Hoffmann, R. G., Lindemer, B. J., et al. (2013). Depleted energy charge and increased pulmonary endothelial permeability induced by mitochondrial complex I inhibition are mitigated by coenzyme Q_1 in the isolated perfused rat lung. https://core.ac.uk/download/213076451.pdf (accessed on 11th June 2025).
8. Thiagarajan, P. S., Wu, X., Zhang, W., Shi, I., Bagai, R., Leahy, P., Feng, Y., Veigl, M., Lindner, D., Danielpour, D., Yin, L., Rosell, R., Bivona, T. G., Zhang, Z., & Ma, P. C. (2016). Transcriptomic-metabolomic reprogramming in EGFR-mutant NSCLC early adaptive drug escape linking TGFβ2-bioenergetics-mitochondrial priming. *Oncotarget*, *7*(50), 82013–82027. https://doi.org/10.18632/oncotarget.13307(accessed on 11th June 2025).
9. Banha, T. N. S., Bednaršek, N., Bueno-Pardo, J., Deslauriers, E., et al. (2024). Advancing bioenergetics-based modeling to improve climate change projections of marine ecosystems. https://core.ac.uk/download/619690506.pdf (accessed on 11th June 2025).
10. Becker, M. (2017). Medium alkalization due to carbon metabolism is largely responsible for inhibition of bacterial growth by *Vibrio cholerae* supernatants. https://core.ac.uk/download/211344058.pdf (accessed on 11th June 2025).
11. Bednaršek, N., Holsman, K. K., Huebert, K. B., Huret, M., et al. (2024). Advancing bioenergetics-based modeling to improve climate change projections of marine ecosystems. https://core.ac.uk/download/654486466.pdf (accessed on 11th June 2025).

12. Bertsch, J., Daniel, R., Goenrich, M., Gottschalk, G., et al. (2012). An ancient pathway combining carbon dioxide fixation with the generation and utilization of a sodium ion gradient for ATP synthesis. https://core.ac.uk/download/14524565.pdf (accessed on 11th June 2025).

13. Blair, J. M., Hicks, B. J., Ling, N., Pitkethley, R., et al. (2012). Diet of rainbow trout in Lake Rotoiti: An energetic perspective. https://core.ac.uk/download/29201346.pdf (accessed on 11th June 2025).

14. Blomeyer, C. A., Boelens, A. D., Camara, A. K. S., Dash, R. K., et al. (2013). Extra-matrix Mg^{2+} limits Ca^{2+} uptake and modulates Ca^{2+} uptake-independent respiration and redox state in cardiac isolated mitochondria. https://core.ac.uk/download/213086441.pdf (accessed on 11th June 2025).

15. Bode, W., Fischer, R., Huber, R., Rüdiger, W., et al. (1987). ZZE-configuration of chromophore ß-153 in C-phycocyanin from *Mastigocladus laminosus*. https://core.ac.uk/download/12163146.pdf (accessed on 11th June 2025).

16. Brooks, G. A., Julian, C. G., Martinez, J., Matarazzo, M., et al. (2019). Is lactate an oncometabolite? Evidence supporting a role for lactate in the regulation of transcriptional activity of cancer-related genes in MCF7 breast cancer cells. https://core.ac.uk/download/305124017.pdf (accessed on 11th June 2025).

17. Cuenco, M. L. (2025). *Aquaculture Systems Modeling: An Introduction with Emphasis on Warmwater Aquaculture*. https://core.ac.uk/download/pdf/6514866.pdf (accessed on 11th June 2025).

18. Cunha-Oliveira, T., Ferreira, I. L., Januário, C., Nascimento, C., et al. (2011). Bioenergetic dysfunction in Huntington's disease human cybrids. https://core.ac.uk/download/61496666.pdf (accessed on 11th June 2025).

19. Gerbaud, V., Shcherbakova, N., & da Cunha, S. (2020). A nonequilibrium thermodynamics perspective on nature-inspired chemical engineering processes. *Chemical Engineering Research & Design*, *154*, 316–330. https://doi.org/10.1016/J.CHERD.2019.10.037(accessed on 11th June 2025).

20. Dumas, A., Armsby, H., Atwater, W., Baldwin, B., Beever, D., Bergman, E., et al. (2008). Mathematical modelling in animal nutrition: A centenary review. https://core.ac.uk/download/pdf/29258963.pdf (accessed on 11th June 2025).

21. Duţeanu, N. M., Erable, B., Ghangrekar, M. M., Scott, K., et al. (2012). Biological and microbial fuel cells. https://core.ac.uk/download/16754572.pdf (accessed on 11th June 2025).

22. Tacchino, F., Succurro, A., Ebenhöh, O. *et al.* Optimal efficiency of the Q-cycle mechanism around physiological temperatures from an open quantum systems approach. *Sci Rep* **9**, 16657 (2019). https://doi.org/10.1038/s41598-019-52842-x (accessed on 11th June 2025).

23. Freedman, B. I., Hughes, T. M., Mahapatra, G., Maldjian, J. A., et al. (2018). Blood-based bioenergetic profiling is related to differences in brain morphology in African Americans with Type 2 diabetes. https://core.ac.uk/download/323066358.pdf (accessed on 11th June 2025).

24. Goldford, J. E., & Segrè, D. (2018). Modern views of ancient metabolic networks. https://core.ac.uk/download/322972862.pdf (accessed on 11th June 2025).

25. Goldford, J. E., Hartman, H., Smith, T. F., & Segrè, D. (2017). Remnants of an Ancient Metabolism without Phosphate. *Cell*, *168*(6), 1126–1134.e9. https://doi.org/10.1016/j.cell.2017.02.001(accessed on 11th June 2025).

26. Hakala, M. (2007). Photodamage to oxygen evolving complex–An initial event in photoinhibition of Photosystem II. https://core.ac.uk/download/197988246.pdf (accessed on 11th June 2025).

27. Hentscher, M. (2012). *Thermodynamic Investigations of Microbial Metabolism and Abiotic Organic Synthesis in Seafloor Hydrothermal Systems*. https://core.ac.uk/download/46919487.pdf (accessed on 11th June 2025).

28. Hill, C. (2013). The acute effect of whole-body vibration on cycling peak power output. https://core.ac.uk/download/13598835.pdf (accessed on 11th June 2025).

29. Janjic, B. M. (2012). Analysis of the level of oxidative phosphorylatin in breast cancer cell types. https://core.ac.uk/download/12210775.pdf (accessed on 11th June 2025).

30. Xie, B., Wang, S., Jiang, N., & Li, J. J. (2019). Cyclin B1/CDK1-regulated mitochondrial bioenergetics in cell cycle progression and tumor resistance. *Cancer letters*, *443*, 56–66. https://doi.org/10.1016/j.canlet.2018.11.019f (accessed on 11th June 2025).

31. Kleidon, A. (2020). What limits photosynthesis? Identifying the thermodynamic constraints of the biosphere within the Earth system. http://arxiv.org/abs/2005.06529 (accessed on 11th June 2025).

32. Mills, L. A., McCormick, A. J., & Lea-Smith, D. J. (2020). Current knowledge and recent advances in understanding metabolism of the model cyanobacterium Synechocystis sp. PCC 6803. *Bioscience reports*, *40*(4), BSR20193325. https://doi.org/10.1042/BSR20193325(accessed on 11th June 2025).

33. Quintana, A., Raffaello, A., Rasola, A., Tosatto, A., Varadi, A., Rowland, A. A., Tarasov, A. I., et al. (2017). The mitochondrial Ca(2+) uniporter: Structure, function, and pharmacology. https://core.ac.uk/download/129191720.pdf (accessed on 11th June 2025).

34. Short, T. (2023). *The Pursuit of Peak Athletic Performance*. https://digitalscholarship.unlv.edu/cgi/viewcontent.cgi?article=1054&context=scholarship_kin (accessed on 11th June 2025).

35. Smeaton, Christina M., & Van Cappellen, Philippe. *Gibbs Energy Dynamic Yield Method (GEDYM): Predicting microbial growth yields under energy-limiting conditions*. United States. https://doi.org/10.1016/j.gca.2018.08.023(accessed on 11th June 2025).

36. Smith, A. (2016). Temporal features of voice in connected speech: Bioenergetic implications. https://holocron.lib.auburn.edu/handle/10415/5164(accessed on 11th June 2025).

37. van Deurs, M., Christensen, A., & Rindorf, A. (2013). Patchy zooplankton grazing and high energy conversion efficiency: Ecological implications of sandeel behavior and strategy. https://core.ac.uk/download/30436810.pdf (accessed on 11th June 2025).

38. Vivekanandan, E. (2013). *Climate Change: Challenging The Sustainability of Marine Fisheries and Ecosystems*. https://core.ac.uk/download/95776376.pdf (accessed on 11th June 2025).

CARBOHYDRATE METABOLISM

5

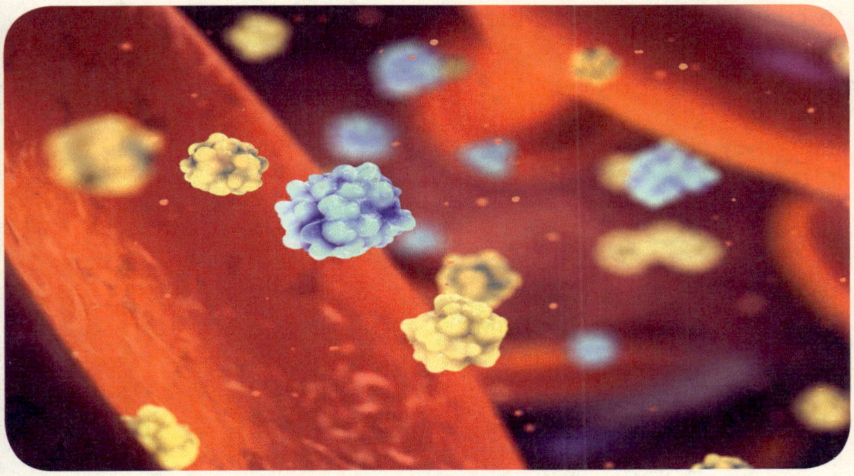

LEARNING OBJECTIVES

After studying this chapter, you will be able to:

1. Describe the types of carbohydrates;
2. Learn about the digestion of carbohydrates;
3. Explain the processes of glycolysis;
4. Summarize the process of gluconeogenesis;
5. Understand the glycogen metabolism;
6. Understand the role of insulin and glucagon.

Introduction

Looking at how carbohydrates are used in the body is important for understanding how living things create energy. Food energy is mainly converted and stored in the body through the use of carbohydrates. There are many biochemical reactions in the pathways that change glucose and other sugars into energy that our bodies use. They show the significance of carbohydrates for nutrition and reveal their key part in cellular activities and maintaining balance in the body. When researchers look at these pathways, they can understand different metabolic disorders such as diabetes and obesity, which highlights the role of carbohydrate metabolism in medical care. Apart from being important in energy production, carbohydrates are also needed for several cellular processes. Breaking down carbohydrates in the body results in the formation of substances that are used to make nucleotides, amino acids, and lipids. Also, the process of regulating carbohydrate metabolism is done by hormones such as insulin and glucagon, which keep blood glucose within a narrow range. Problems with these metabolic controls may cause energy balance to become unbalanced, leading to MS. For this reason, knowing about carbohydrate metabolism improves our understanding of healthy body functions and helps deal with health issues related to metabolic diseases. Studies on carbohydrate metabolism rely on a large body of scientific literature that keeps developing with new technology and techniques. Important biochemical pathways and mechanisms have been explained in scholarly articles and reports, which is crucial for further studies. For instance, metabolomics has been created, which allows scientists to study metabolic profiles and what they mean for health and disease. It is important in this field to relate the detailed aspects of carbohydrate metabolism to larger physiological and medical situations. As outlined in various bibliographies of scientific publications, including those documented by Hess et al. (1992), continual advancements in our understanding of carbohydrate metabolism not only enrich academic inquiry but also inform practical applications in clinical nutrition and metabolic health (Figure 5.1).

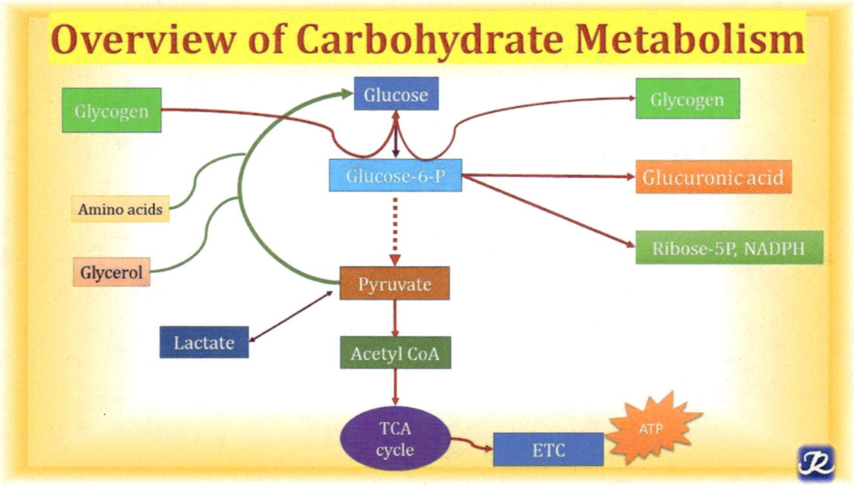

Figure 5.1. Overview of carbohydrate metabolism.

Source: https://i.ytimg.com/vi/a3hy-i8Usj4/maxresdefault.jpg.

Definition of Carbohydrate Metabolism

Carbohydrate metabolism includes the steps by which carbohydrates are broken up and changed into energy that the body can use. This intricate web of reactions primarily entails glycolysis, the citric acid cycle, and oxidative phosphorylation, all of which facilitate the conversion of carbohydrates into usable energy in the form of ATP. In the cytoplasm, glycolysis takes place and converts glucose to pyruvate, resulting in a little ATP and reducing equivalents. As pyruvate enters the mitochondria, it goes through the citric acid cycle to help obtain more energy from carbohydrates and release carbon dioxide. All in all, these processes reveal the importance of carbohydrate metabolism for maintaining cellular activities and energy balance in organisms. In addition, proper control of carbohydrate metabolism is needed to maintain safe glucose levels in the body for good health. The process is mainly controlled by hormones such as insulin and glucagon. Insulin makes it possible for tissues to absorb glucose and creates glycogen, while glucagon causes glycogen to break down into glucose when required. These hormones make sure that there is enough glucose as fuel without causing either high or low blood sugar levels. The metabolic flexibility in utilizing carbohydrates is particularly evident in different dietary scenarios, as individuals may experience variable nutrient digestibility and energy excretion based on their carbohydrate intake and macronutrient composition, demonstrating the complexity of the body's adaptive mechanisms in carbohydrate metabolism (Zou, 2007). To create good diet and exercise plans for fitness and health, you need to know about carbohydrate metabolism. Carbohydrates are the main source of energy and also affect the changes in metabolism that happen during exercise. For instance, the right amount and kind of carbohydrates eaten after exercise can help enhance performance by speeding up glycogen restoration. Apart from energy production, recent studies indicate that carbohydrate metabolism is linked to weight control and diseases of the metabolism. If carbohydrate metabolism is not normal, for example, insulin resistance, it may result in type 2 diabetes. Exploring the underlying mechanisms, including the role of gut microbiota and metabolic pathways, provides further insights into how carbohydrate metabolism can be manipulated for health benefits (Cho et al., 2017). Because of this, learning about carbohydrate metabolism is important for dealing with overall public health issues connected to diet and lifestyle.

Importance of Carbohydrates in Human Nutrition

Carbohydrates are important in our nutrition because they mainly provide energy for our bodies. Since carbohydrates are easy to find, they are important for brain activity, muscle movements, and metabolism. When carbohydrates are broken down, glucose is formed and the brain and central nervous system prefer it as their main fuel. A lack of carbohydrates in the diet could result in tiredness, a drop in mental performance, and weaker physical abilities. Besides, choosing complex carbohydrates is important since they give you long-lasting energy and important nutrients. On the other hand, simple carbohydrates in processed foods make blood sugar levels rise quickly and then fall quickly, which could cause people to feel tired and hungry. For this reason, it is important to know how much and what type of carbohydrates you eat for your health. The way carbohydrates affect your metabolism is important for controlling weight and avoiding chronic diseases. According to several studies, a diet that contains complex carbohydrates and fiber may help reduce the chances of getting obesity, heart disease, and type 2 diabetes. Fiber helps your digestion and also controls your blood sugar levels and makes you feel full longer. Especially, researchers are looking at how changing the amount of carbohydrates in the diet may help manage insulin resistance, which is important in the development of type 2 diabetes. Having too many high-glycemic carbohydrates in your diet can make insulin resistance worse, but eating low-glycemic foods can have a better effect on your metabolism. Consequently, a careful consideration of carbohydrate quality and composition is vital for mitigating health risks associated with poor dietary habits (Weickert, 2012). In addition, the ease with which carbohydrates are digested plays a big role in their usefulness for nutrition and metabolism. New studies have shown that the digestibility of nutrients in feces is not the same for all carbohydrate-rich diets, which proves that the composition of the diet impacts how nutrients are absorbed and used for energy. For instance, refined carbohydrates tend to have higher digestibility compared to high-fiber diets, which may lead to significant disparities in metabolizable energy (ME) availability. It appears that the Atwater factors do not always accurately show the energy from all carbohydrate foods. As such, the implications of carbohydrate choices on human nutrition extend beyond mere caloric intake; they encompass the potential for various health outcomes influenced by how carbohydrates are metabolized by the body (Zou, 2007). Awareness of these factors can guide nutrition advice and help improve health programs meant for the public (Figure 5.2).

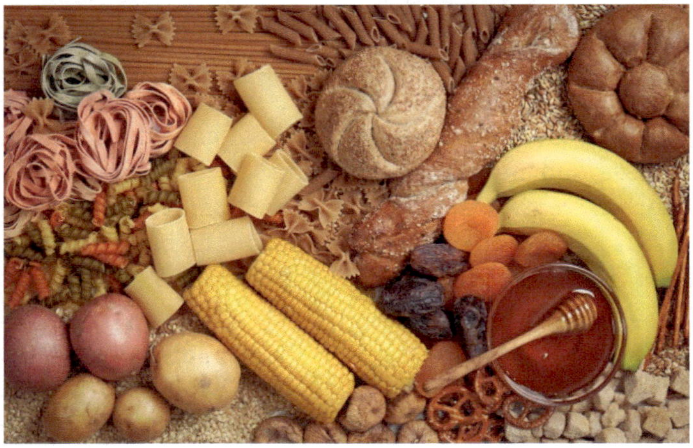

Figure 5.2. Importance of carbohydrates in human nutrition.

Source: https://cdn.britannica.com/16/203316-050-822EE04E/food-carbohydrates.jpg.

5.1. Types of Carbohydrates

Learning Outcome

1. Describe the category of simple carbohydrates;
2. Understand the complex carbohydrates;
3. Describe the dietary fiber.

The main types of carbohydrates in human nutrition are called monosaccharides, disaccharides, and polysaccharides. Glucose and fructose, which are monosaccharides, are important for quick energy and for the body's metabolism. Most importantly, cells depend on glucose for energy, especially when it comes to brain activity. Disaccharides, formed by the linkage of two monosaccharides, include sucrose (table sugar) and lactose (milk sugar), each providing energy through hydrolysis into their constituent monosaccharides in the digestive system. These carbohydrates vary in their glycemic indices, influencing how quickly they raise blood glucose levels, which can have implications for metabolic health, particularly in individuals with insulin resistance, as discussed in relation to dietary management strategies for conditions like PCOS (Ghazeeri et al., 2021). On the other side, polysaccharides are made up of many monosaccharides linked together and are called storage or structural carbohydrates. Storing energy is mainly done by glycogen and starch, which are called storage polysaccharides.

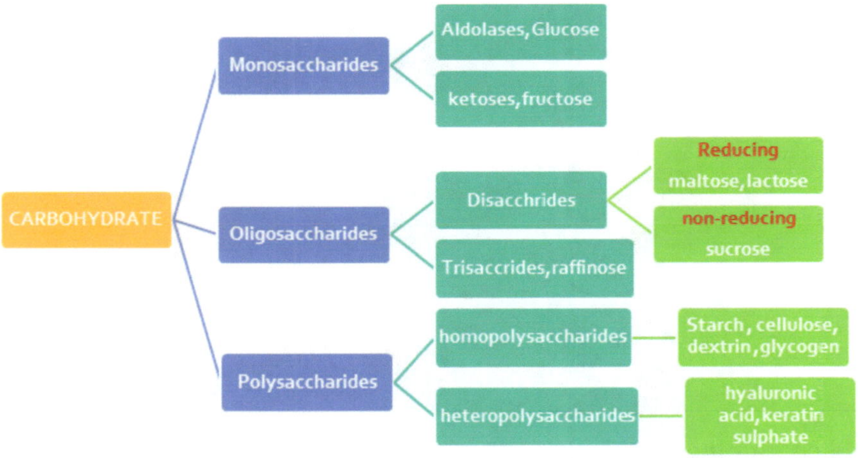

Figure 5.3. Types of carbohydrates.

Source: https://thefuturedentistry.com/wp-content/uploads/2021/05/carbo-meta-1.jpg.

The liver and muscles mainly keep glycogen, which can be quickly released for energy use, while starch is the main energy store in plants and is turned into glucose by humans after digestion. Cellulose and similar structural polysaccharides are important for the fiber in our diet that keeps the gut healthy. Even though humans cannot digest cellulose, it helps manage digestion and makes people feel full. Understanding the diverse functions of these carbohydrate types is critical for appreciating their roles in carbohydrate metabolism and their impact on health (Zou, 2007). The glycemic index (GI) of carbohydrates, which measures how quickly a carbohydrate-containing food raises blood glucose levels, is essential for managing energy intake and metabolic responses. Eating foods with a high GI, for example, white bread and sugary snacks, results in quick rises in insulin and could eventually cause problems with insulin sensitivity and raise the risk of type 2 diabetes. On the other hand, foods with a low GI usually have lots of fiber, which helps blood glucose rise slowly, giving a steady supply of energy and making you feel less hungry. Consuming different types of carbohydrates can greatly affect metabolism, which is especially important for people with PCOS, who should eat a balanced amount of all macronutrients to improve their insulin sensitivity and health. Therefore, selecting the appropriate types of carbohydrates is crucial for effective carbohydrate metabolism and long-term health (Ghazeeri et al., 2021) (Figure 5.3).

5.1.1. Simple Carbohydrates

Monosaccharides and disaccharides, which are part of the simple carbohydrates group, are important in carbohydrate metabolism since they are quickly used as energy. Glucose and fructose, which are monosaccharides, are easily absorbed by the body, which causes blood sugar levels to rise fast. Disaccharides, for example sucrose and lactose, are built from two monosaccharide units and need to be split by enzymes before the body can use them. Since simple carbohydrates are used quickly, they provide fast energy that is helpful during intense exercises.

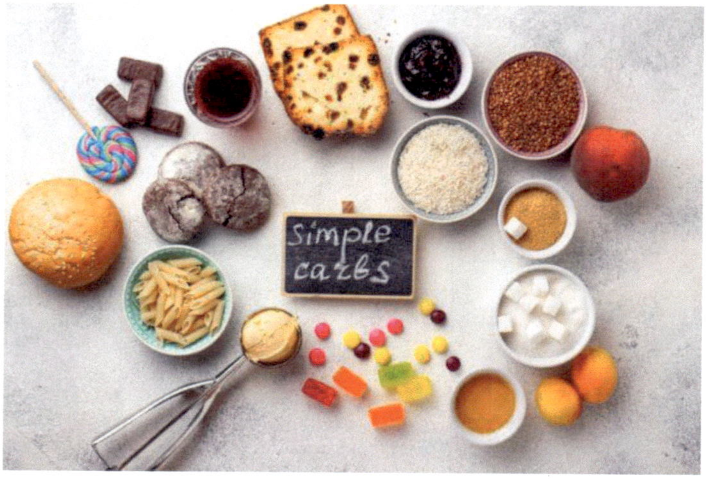

Figure 5.4. Foods containing simple sugars.

Source: https://biologydictionary.net/wp-content/uploads/2021/01/Simple-carbs.jpg.

At the same time, fast absorption of sugars can result in extra insulin being released, which might disturb metabolism and create energy imbalances when people consume too much. That's why it is important to know how simple carbohydrates are metabolized to make sure energy is used efficiently and health is maintained. Besides giving you immediate energy, eating simple carbohydrates also impacts your body's metabolism as you exercise. It has been demonstrated that eating simple carbohydrates like sucrose before exercise can affect the way our bodies use energy during activity. An experiment was carried out to see how different amounts of sucrose before exercise changed blood glucose and fat burning while cycling at a moderate intensity. It was observed that even small doses of sucrose could result in a decline in blood glucose concentration during exercise, accompanied by a stepwise reduction in fat oxidation as the duration progressed (Montzingo et al., 2016). This points out that carbohydrate metabolism is easily influenced by food choices and shows why it is important to know how to consume simple carbs for better performance and metabolism. In addition, simple carbohydrates affect not only humans but also other species, as shown by studies done on farmed animals. When gilthead seabream larvae were provided with extra glucose during key developmental phases, their metabolic systems changed a lot. The study found that recurrent glucose exposure influenced metabolic gene expression and nutrient utilization, indicating enhanced glucose oxidation pathways and improved catabolism in responding larvae (Dias et al., 2016). This proves that simple carbohydrates are important for the efficient functioning of various biological systems. As a result, it is now clear that carbohydrate nutrition influences metabolic programming, which may have wider effects on growth and performance in humans, aquaculture, and livestock management (Figure 5.4).

5.1.2. Complex Carbohydrates

Most of the complex carbohydrates in our diet come from whole grains, legumes, vegetables, and some fruits, and they are very important for human nutrition and energy use. While simple carbohydrates are digested and absorbed fast, complex carbohydrates take more time because they have long chains of glucose molecules. Carbohydrate breakdown starts in the mouth with salivary amylase and finishes in the small intestine, where pancreatic amylase changes them into maltose and glucose. As a result, the body is provided with energy and the digestive system benefits, as it helps avoid high blood sugar after meals and increases the feeling of fullness, which may stop obesity and other metabolic problems. Because complex carbohydrates take longer to digest, they help keep energy and metabolism stable during the whole day. Besides giving energy, complex carbohydrates are a great source of dietary fiber. Having fiber in your diet encourages regular bowel movements and stops constipation. This carbohydrate can also help control the body's insulin levels, which improves how carbohydrates are processed. Besides, oats and legumes contain soluble fibers that are helpful in lowering cholesterol and may protect you from heart problems. Emerging research points to the significant variability in digestibility and ME of complex carbohydrates depending on their source and preparation methods, as indicated in studies assessing different diets.

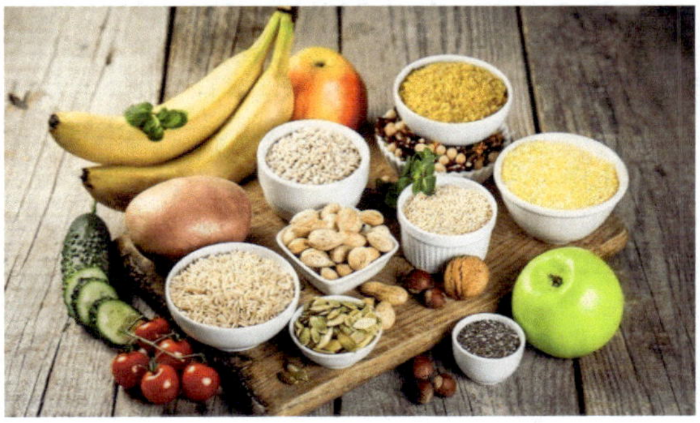

Figure 5.5. Complex carbohydrates.

Source: https://aloha.com/cdn/shop/articles/What_Are_Complex_Carbs-257664.png?v=1732030941.

The differences in nutrient digestibility highlight how fiber-rich diets can vary in their metabolic impact, which is vital for proper dietary planning and weight management (Zou, 2007). Besides other functions, complex carbohydrates take part in several biochemical pathways that help the body store and use energy. In bumble bees, having enough sugars from carbohydrates helps them save glycogen that is necessary for living through times when food is scarce. Research has shown that inadequate sugar intake can significantly impair glycogen accumulation, leading to weight loss and reduced energy reserves, which may jeopardize overall fitness during winter months (Doan et al., 2014). It demonstrates that the right balance between carbohydrate intake and storing energy is important not only for people but also for the environment. So, knowing about complex carbohydrates and their effects on the body helps in designing healthy dietary plans for people and the environment (Figure 5.5).

5.1.3. Dietary Fiber

Optimal digestion and the right use of carbohydrates depend greatly on dietary fiber, which is a type of carbohydrate. Unlike carbs that give immediate energy, dietary fiber is made up of non-starch polysaccharides (NSPs) and resistant starches, which the small intestine does not digest. These fibers travel to the large intestine, where they undergo microbial fermentation, leading to the production of short-chain fatty acids (SCFAs) that significantly influence colonic health. The intricate relationship between dietary fiber and gut microbiota underscores its importance; as fiber ferments, it alters bacterial populations and their metabolite profiles, potentially enhancing overall metabolic health (Bosch et al., 2012). Besides, diets rich in dietary fiber are linked to better blood sugar management and increased feelings of fullness, so they are essential in nutritional advice. How fiber is made and what type it is can change the way it is fermented and the amount of SCFA it produces, which is good for our bodies. Intact fibers in the diet lead to better fermentation than those that are broken. It is important because the characteristics of fiber-rich foods can determine both the kinds of SCFAs and their effects on the body's metabolism. For instance, acetate, one of the most prevalent SCFAs, aids in peripheral metabolism and can serve as a primary energy source for colonocytes, influencing both energy homeostasis and inflammatory responses (Bosch et al., 2012). For this reason, it is important to know the differences between fiber types when trying to enhance carbohydrate metabolism and gut health. Evidence points to the idea that fiber helps digestion and also controls the body's reaction to glucose. Eating fibrous foods in clinical studies usually helps the body regulate blood glucose levels more effectively. Besides, fermentation in the large intestine has been found to increase the levels of hormones that help control appetite and blood sugar. As such, fibers can be considered critical players in the broader context of carbohydrate metabolism, influencing hormonal responses and metabolic pathways that govern energy distribution and utilization in the body (Flint et al., 2019). So, exploring the details of different types of dietary fiber may help experts create better dietary guidelines for improving health and well-being (Figure 5.6).

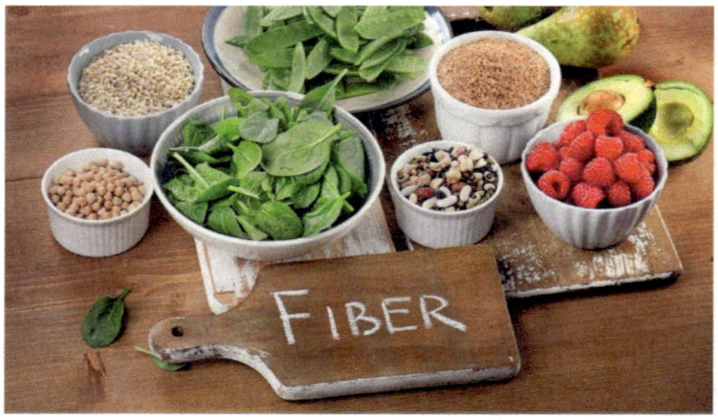

Figure 5.6. Variety of fiber-rich foods including fruits, vegetables, legumes, and grains.

Source: https://steelfitusa.com/cdn/shop/articles/Is-Fiber-a-Carb-Blog-Post.jpg?v=1728672000.

Test Your Knowledge

1. What are simple carbohydrates also called?
2. Which are complex carbohydrates?

5.2. Digestion of Carbohydrates

Learning Outcome

1. Understand the role of salivary amylase in carbohydrate metabolism;
2. Describe the enzymatic breakdown in the small intestine;
3. Know the absorption process of monosaccharides.

Carbohydrates begin to be digested in the mouth and end up being processed in the small intestine. Salivary amylase is an enzyme that the salivary glands produce to start changing starches into maltose. When food is in the small intestine, pancreatic amylase helps to break down the starches that are still present. The enzyme is needed because complex carbohydrates are changed into simple sugars, like glucose, to allow them to enter the bloodstream. It is important for energy and also for the body's metabolism to function properly. Proper digestion of carbohydrates helps nutrients be absorbed and then used by cells for respiration. After enzymes in the small intestine break down carbohydrates, absorption becomes very important in the digestion process. Sodium-glucose co-transporters and similar proteins help cells in the intestines absorb monosaccharides fast. Glucose and galactose enter the cells by active transport, but fructose moves in by facilitated diffusion. This method points out that digestion and absorption interact, and that hormones help control these actions. After getting into epithelial cells, monosaccharides are carried by the bloodstream to the liver, which is in charge of metabolic control. How well the body absorbs nutrients affects both energy levels and health; in case of poor absorption, malabsorption disorders and other health problems may arise. Carbohydrate digestion has effects on energy as well as gut health and the types of microbes living there. If digestion is disrupted, the amount of indigestible carbohydrates can be changed, which is important for the health of the gut microbiota and metabolic health. For instance, unabsorbed carbohydrates can be fermented by colonic bacteria, leading to the production of SCFAs that provide numerous health benefits, including maintaining intestinal integrity and modulating immune responses. According to recent findings, eating certain foods can influence the availability of carbohydrates and positively change the expression of intestinal genes, which helps the gut and reduces related problems. Understanding these interactions helps elucidate the broader implications of carbohydrate metabolism and offers potential therapeutic avenues for targeting digestive health through dietary strategies (Bauer et al., 2011; Arabyan et al., 2016) (Figure 5.7).

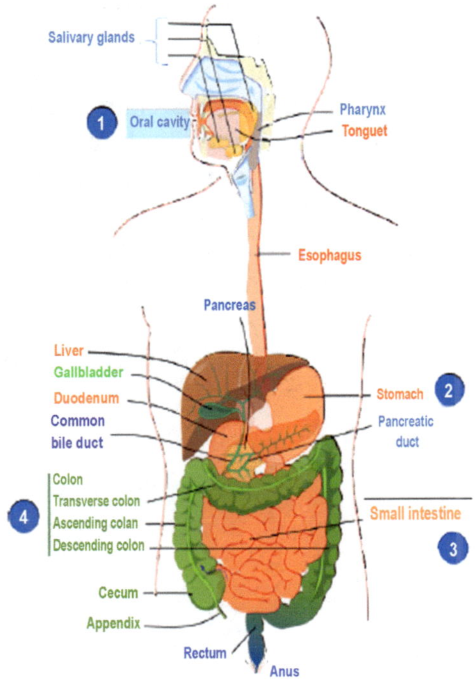

Figure 5.7. The digestive system.

Source: https://openoregon.pressbooks.pub/app/uploads/sites/98/2019/09/image6.png.

5.2.1. Role of Salivary Amylase

Salivary amylase helps in breaking down starches into sugars as soon as food is put in the mouth. Even before food goes to the stomach, salivary amylase helps increase the amount of nutrients that are absorbed. Salivary amylase is especially important for human evolution since eating more starch led to important changes in metabolism. Researchers propose that the development of cooking, which enhances the digestibility of starch, along with variations in the salivary amylase gene (AMY1), were crucial for accommodating the growing metabolic demands of humans, particularly their brains (Brand-Miller et al., 2015). Therefore, the first enzymatic step is important for changing carbohydrates into energy that the body needs for its functions. Besides, the fact that salivary amylase is genetically different in humans adds another challenge to how it affects carbohydrate metabolism. Individuals possess different copy numbers of the AMY1, which correlate with dietary starch consumption. Those who have more copies of this gene tend to make more salivary amylase, which is an evolutionary reaction to eating a lot of carbohydrates. This heightened capacity for starch digestion may contribute to improved glucose tolerance through the cephalic phase insulin release, suggesting a nuanced relationship between salivary amylase levels and metabolic health (Barber et al., 2018). Notably, individuals with lower AMY1 copy numbers may display different metabolic responses, affecting their body mass index (BMI) and overall energy efficiency. So, by knowing about this variability, we can learn how genes affect people's diet and metabolism. In addition to digesting carbohydrates, salivary amylase affects the wellbeing of the gut and the microbiome. The breakdown of starch by enzymes helps to manage the number of undigested carbohydrates in the intestine, which affects SCFAs and the bacteria in the gut. It is important because dietary fibers and resistant starches change the gut environment and affect a person's metabolic health. Studies suggest that the metabolic consequences linked to varying amylase activity may include alterations in appetite regulation and energy expenditure, crucial factors in managing obesity and MS (Barber et al., 2018). Overall, salivary amylase is crucial for digestion and also plays a big role in wider metabolic functions, proving its importance in learning about carbohydrate metabolism and the evolution of human eating habits (Figure 5.8).

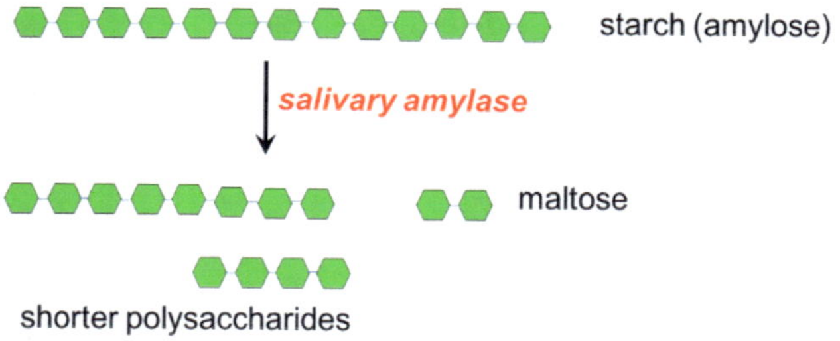

Figure 5.8. The enzyme salivary amylase breaks starch into smaller polysaccharides and maltose.

Source: https://openoregon.pressbooks.pub/app/uploads/sites/98/2019/09/image2-1.png.

5.2.2. Enzymatic Breakdown in the Small Intestine

The main function of the small intestine is to change complex carbohydrates into simple sugars by using enzymes. At the start, salivary amylase in the mouth breaks down the first part of carbohydrates. Most of the important enzyme activities happen in the small intestine, where pancreatic amylase keeps breaking down starches. Together with maltase, isomaltase, and lactase, these enzymes help change disaccharides and oligosaccharides into glucose, fructose, and galactose. The body is able to absorb nutrients from carbohydrates well, because only monosaccharides can cross the intestinal wall and enter the bloodstream, which shows how enzymes are important for this process. Besides, the makeup of carbohydrates in the diet has a strong effect on how well enzymes break down food in the small intestine. Research highlights that NSPs within various cereal-based diets can substantially alter digestive processes. It was discovered in studies that raising the amount of NSPs in feed decreases how well organic matter is digested in the small intestine of pigs. Both soluble and insoluble NSPs were found to have an impact on digestion as well as on the whole gut environment, including pH and the number of microbes. This emphasizes the potential for dietary manipulation to optimize enzymatic activity, thus enhancing carbohydrate metabolism and overall gut health in livestock and potentially other species, including humans (Högberg, 2003). As well as the enzymes in the small intestine, enzyme supplements in diets help to digest carbohydrates more effectively. When exogenous enzymes, for example, those for NSPs, are included, the digestion of parts of the diet that are not normally digested can be enhanced. They help supply more fermentable carbohydrates, which allows the body's digestive enzymes to work less. During controlled studies, it was noted that enzyme supplementation changed the amount of organic acids in the small intestine and encouraged the growth of beneficial microbes in the gut. The proactive use of dietary enzymes holds promise not only for enhancing unabsorbed carbohydrate degradation but also for optimizing the overall metabolic pathways of carbohydrates in agricultural species, paving the way for advancements in sustainable animal nutrition (Jensen et al., 2012) (Figure 5.9).

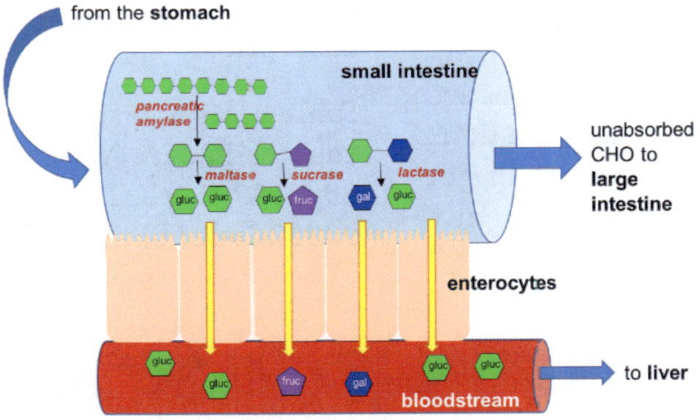

Figure 5.9. Digestion and absorption of carbohydrates in the small intestine.

Source: https://openoregon.pressbooks.pub/app/uploads/sites/98/2019/09/image7-1.png.

5.2.3. Absorption of Monosaccharides

Monosaccharides are absorbed in the body to ensure that simple sugars can be carried into the blood after digestion. During digestion, glucose, fructose, and galactose are set free and then transferred through the intestinal wall. The sodium-dependent transporter SGLT1 helps move glucose and galactose into enterocytes using the sodium gradient made by the sodium-potassium pump. Alternatively, fructose moves into cells by means of facilitated diffusion with the help of the GLUT5 transporter. How efficiently these mechanisms work is crucial since it influences the body's response to carbohydrates and has an impact on metabolism and energy balance. So, the process of monosaccharide absorption provides useful information about the changes in the body when carbohydrates are consumed and used. When inside the enterocytes, monosaccharides are usually sent into the portal circulation by the GLUT2 transporter and then go to the liver for metabolism or storage. The liver is important for controlling blood sugar by using gluconeogenesis, glycogenesis, and glycolysis, so it is essential for monosaccharides to be absorbed efficiently. Hormones such as insulin and glucagon prompt the liver to handle the monosaccharides it receives. It is especially important to follow this regulation since high blood glucose for a long time can result in diabetes and insulin resistance. Thus, knowing how monosaccharides are absorbed and used in the body helps find ways to prevent metabolic disorders caused by eating carbohydrates. Apart from direct ways of absorption, what you eat and how healthy your digestive system is can strongly affect how monosaccharides are taken up. A diet high in NSPs and soluble fibers can change the environment in the gut, which can impact absorption as well as the whole digestive process. Research has indicated that variations in fiber content can lead to alterations in gut microbiota composition, which subsequently affects nutrient absorption and energy extraction from carbohydrates (Högberg, 2003). Moreover, the presence of competing sugars can influence absorption rates, as observed with disaccharides like maltose and trehalose in certain crustacean species, which suggests shared transport pathways for disaccharides and monosaccharides (Scheffler et al., 2016). It is important to understand how these interactions work to design better diets for carbohydrate metabolism and better health (Figure 5.10).

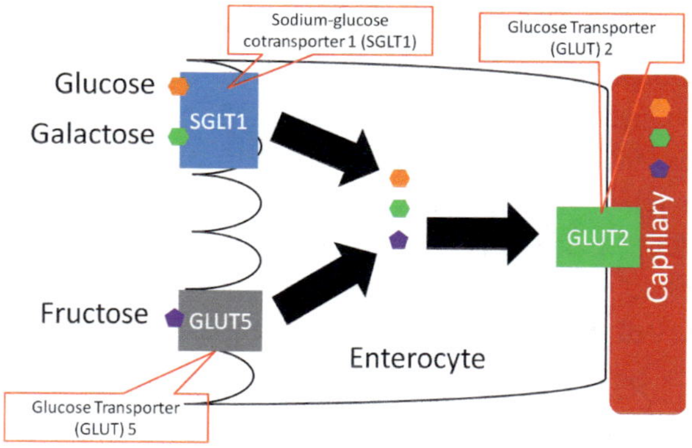

Figure 5.10. Carbohydrate uptake and absorption.

Source: https://s3-us-west-2.amazonaws.com/courses-images/wp-content/uploads/sites/2569/2017/10/23201337/100000000000045F000002C98EA9D4DE.png.

Test Your Knowledge

1. What is the role of salivary amylase in carbohydrate metabolism?
2. What is the absorption process of monosaccharides?

5.3. Glycolysis

Learning Outcome

1. Give an overview of the glycolytic pathway;
2. Describe the energy yield from glycolysis;
3. Understand the regulation of glycolysis.

Glycolysis is important because it helps metabolize carbohydrates, especially by breaking down glucose to give energy. The steps in this process happen in the cytoplasm of cells and are anaerobic, so glucose is changed into pyruvate and ATP and NADH are produced as well. Besides making energy, glycolysis is important for linking different metabolic pathways. As an example, glycolysis links with the pentose phosphate pathways, which produce nucleotides, and with the citric acid cycle, where more oxidation of pyruvate takes place. Since glycolysis supports both breaking down and building up of carbohydrates, it helps organisms respond to changes in their energy needs and the substances they can use. The process of glycolysis is regulated based on the cell's energy level and is affected by things such as the presence of needed substrates and the cell's energy demands. Throughout the glycolytic pathway, important checkpoints are formed by the enzyme's hexokinase, phosphofructokinase, and pyruvate kinase. Hexokinase changes glucose into glucose-6-phosphate, which is trapped within the cell, and phosphofructokinase is a key point that adjusts to the cell's energy levels. High levels of ATP prevent this enzyme from working properly, which slows down glycolysis. On the other hand, more ADP in the cell speeds up this enzyme's activity. Because of this elegant regulation, glycolysis responds to the needs of the cell and supports the balance of energy, showing why it is important in carbohydrate metabolism. The connection between glycolysis and other metabolic reactions helps multicellular organisms adjust and function efficiently. As an example, during times of high energy use, such as when exercising hard, glycolysis speeds up to supply the body with more ATP.

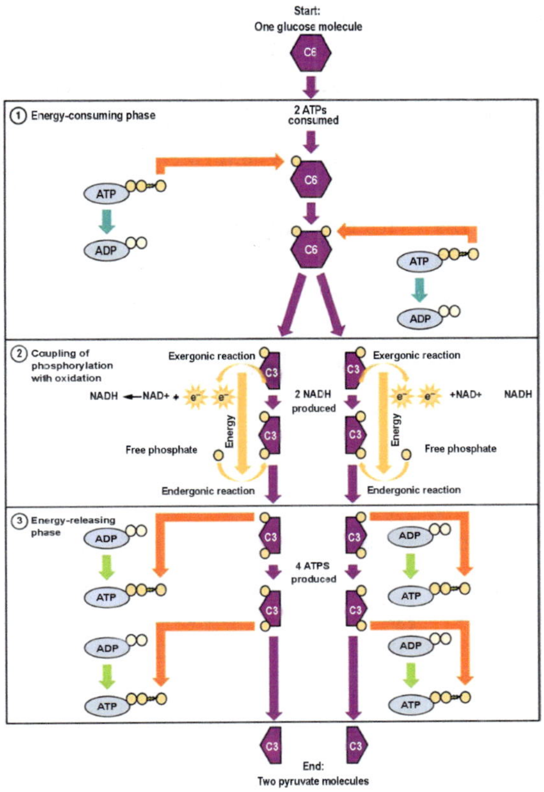

Figure 5.11. During the energy-consuming phase of glycolysis, two ATPs are consumed, transferring two phosphates to the glucose molecule. The glucose molecule then splits into two three-carbon compounds, each containing a phosphate. During the second phase, an additional phosphate is added to each of the three-carbon compounds. The energy for this endergonic reaction is provided by the removal (oxidation) of two electrons from each three-carbon compound. During the energy-releasing phase, the phosphates are removed from both three-carbon compounds and used to produce four ATP molecules.

Source: https://s3-us-west-2.amazonaws.com/courses-images-archive-read-only/wp-content/uploads/sites/403/2015/05/21032118/Screen-Shot-2015-05-21-at-1.39.34-PM.png.

Lactate, which is one of the products of glycolysis, can also be used in various other metabolic reactions, showing that the pathways are connected. In some organisms, modifications in glycolysis can be observed under various developmental and environmental conditions, such as in the model organism Caenorhabditis elegans, where metabolic pathways adapt in response to external stressors (Braeckman et al., 2009). Moreover, the role of key enzymes involved in carbohydrate sensing, like hexokinases, sheds light on how organisms manage energy resources (Olsson et al., 2005). They demonstrate that glycolysis is very versatile and essential for carbohydrate metabolism (Figure 5.11).

5.3.1. Overview of the Glycolytic Pathway

The glycolytic pathway is important because it changes glucose into pyruvate, while making ATP and NADH in the process. The process takes place in the cytoplasm and involves 10 steps, each one guided by a certain enzyme. You can divide glycolysis into an energy investment phase and an energy payoff phase. At the start, glucose is phosphorylated and altered into fructose-1,6-bisphosphate by using ATP. In this part, the cell produces ATP and NADH, which means more energy is available. Glycolysis is very important because it helps produce energy and gives the necessary substances for other processes, including the citric acid cycle, which links carbohydrate metabolism to the entire cellular respiration process. The glycolytic pathway is under strict control and relies on major enzymes that act as key steps. It is the enzymes hexokinase, phosphofructokinase, and pyruvate kinase that decide how glucose moves through the glycolytic pathway. For example, phosphofructokinase is usually thought of as the main regulatory enzyme, which responds to changes in the cell's energy supply. When energy is required, glycolysis increases thanks to the presence of ATP and other important metabolites. Thanks to this mechanism, cells are able to deal with different conditions and keep their metabolism balanced. Because glycolysis can respond to changes in the body, it is important in both healthy and sick states. Also, new developments in metabolomics, especially in analyzing glycolytic intermediates, have given a clearer picture of the pathways involved. Researchers can use liquid chromatography mass spectrometry to measure the changes in metabolites that occur because of nutrients and hormones. These studies show that changes in glycolytic flux are associated with certain physiological reactions, for example, the activation of stress response pathways. For instance, extensive reorganization of intermediary metabolism observed in certain models indicates a coordinated response to environmental changes, suggesting that glycolysis plays a pivotal role not only in energy production but also in the integration of cellular responses to diverse metabolic challenges (Braeckman et al., 2014). Moreover, this increasing understanding contributes to potential therapeutic approaches for metabolic disorders, emphasizing the importance of glycolytic regulation in systemic health (Barbara et al., 2010).

5.3.2. Energy Yield from Glycolysis

In the process of carbohydrate metabolism, glycolysis is important for producing energy by turning glucose into pyruvate. This anaerobic process occurs in the cytoplasm of cells and consists of 10 enzymatic steps, all of which contribute to the breakdown of glucose and the subsequent generation of ATP. During both aerobic and anaerobic situations, glycolysis gives the body two ATP molecules for each glucose molecule it breaks down. After producing pyruvate, glycolysis makes it possible for other metabolic processes, such as the citric acid cycle and fermentation, to occur, depending on whether there is oxygen. Glycolysis is central to energy metabolism since it allows cells to function under different conditions, whether they have oxygen or not, which proves its key role in cellular respiration. The usefulness of glycolysis in making energy is most important when we consider what is left over from the process. The buildup of acetate in *Escherichia coli* can have a negative effect on cell growth and protein synthesis during aerobic fermentation, which usually means altering metabolic pathways to boost yield.

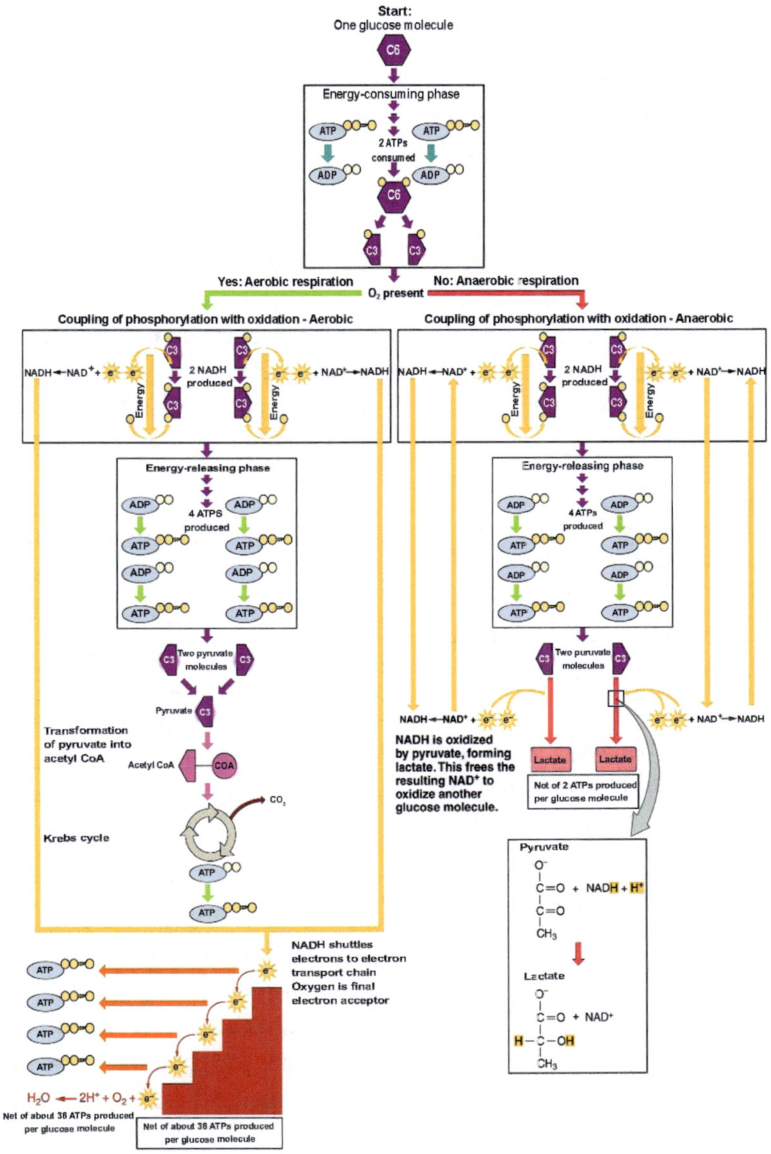

Figure 5.12. The process of anaerobic respiration converts glucose into two lactate molecules in the absence of oxygen or within erythrocytes that lack mitochondria. During aerobic respiration, glucose is oxidized into two pyruvate molecules.

Source: https://s3-us-west-2.amazonaws.com/courses-images/wp-content/uploads/sites/217/2016/10/07181032/2505_Aerobic_Versus_Anaerobic_Respiration.jpg.

This research on *E. coli* to decrease acetate accumulation is an example of how metabolic engineering often works to improve the flow of glycolysis. They show that how a substrate is used and the resulting by-products can greatly influence how efficiently the metabolic process works. By understanding and manipulating the glycolytic pathway, researchers can improve energy yields, addressing both energy demands and by-product management, ultimately leading to advancements in industrial biotechnology and metabolic engineering practices (Maeseneire et al., 2007). Further insights into glycolysis can be drawn from the study of lactic acid bacteria (LAB), particularly those belonging to the Streptococcaceae family, including Lactococcus lactis. The main by-product of these organisms is lactate, which helps make fermented foods acidic and keeps them preserved. Glycolysis in LAB is useful for industry and also helps explain how microbes adapt to different levels of nutrients. Recent advancements in genomic and proteomic technologies have enhanced our understanding of the metabolic pathways in these bacteria, promoting insights into how they optimize energy yield in diverse environments (Kok et al., 2012). As we go deeper into glycolysis, it is clear that the relationship between producing energy and making metabolic waste is important and demonstrates how carbohydrate metabolism varies among different organisms (Figure 5.12).

5.3.3. Regulation of Glycolysis

The biochemical pathway glycolysis is key to the breakdown of glucose into pyruvate without oxygen, which is important in carbohydrate metabolism. The way glycolysis is regulated is important for the cell because it ensures that energy levels are kept constant and the body can meet its energy needs under many different conditions. Hexokinase, phosphofructokinase, and pyruvate kinase are important enzymes that monitor and control the flow of glucose in the glycolytic pathway. Enzymes react to certain signals, so the cell can focus on glycolysis when it needs energy fast and lower the pathway's activity when there is plenty of energy. Moreover, the interplay between glycolysis and other metabolic pathways highlights the importance of coordination in central carbon metabolism, thereby integrating cellular responses and maintaining metabolic balance across various tissue types and developmental stages, such as observed during grape berry development (Dai et al., 2013). When the cell is growing or reacting to the environment, the level of glycolysis can be adjusted over time. As an example, when a cell switches from a low-energy state to a high-energy state, the activity of glycolytic enzymes may be changed by metabolites and hormones that show the cell's energy level, such as ATP, ADP, and AMP.

They shape energy production as well as the supply of intermediates that are important in nucleotide synthesis and lipid metabolism. The way glycolysis is used in both catabolic and anabolic pathways highlights its key role in making sure cells respond properly to changes in energy levels. Dysregulation of glycolysis can lead to metabolic disorders, illustrating the pathways significance in the broader context of carbohydrate metabolism and its impact across various biological functions (Berkers et al., 2013). Researchers have recently found out more about how transcription factors and signaling molecules control glycolysis. In addition to its usual part in cellular responses to stress, p53 has been found to play a major role in regulating metabolism. By affecting genes that control glycolysis, p53 can influence the pathway when metabolic stress occurs and, as a result, affects both cell cycle and metabolism. The fact that glycolysis affects cell fate decisions shows that it is significant in energy production and in the development of diseases such as cancer and diabetes. The ongoing exploration of these regulatory networks may unveil potential therapeutic targets for managing metabolic disorders and improve our understanding of the intricate relationships between carbohydrate metabolism and overall cellular function (Berkers et al., 2013).

Test Your Knowledge

1. What is the glycolytic pathway?
2. What is the regulation of glycolysis?

5.4. Gluconeogenesis

Learning Outcome

1. Define the gluconeogenesis;
2. Describe the key enzymes involved in carbohydrate metabolism;
3. Differentiate between glycolysis and gluconeogenesis.

During prolonged fasting or intense exercise, the pathway of gluconeogenesis is very important because it helps the body make glucose from other substances. The anabolic process happens mainly in the liver, but under some circumstances, the kidneys also play a role. It is responsible for keeping glucose available, since this is a main energy source for the brain and red blood cells. The route helps the body make glucose from lactate, glycerol, and amino acids when there are not many dietary carbohydrates. Gluconeogenesis is controlled by hormones, mainly insulin and glucagon, to help maintain a constant level of blood glucose. Lactate is one of the main materials used in gluconeogenesis and it is produced when glycolysis happens without oxygen. The importance of lactate in gluconeogenesis is highlighted by studies demonstrating its utilization in post-injury recovery protocols, particularly following traumatic brain injury (TBI). In these situations, lactate gives energy and is also broken down to help in the production of glucose. It has also been found that about 70% of the carbohydrates needed by an injured brain come from lactate produced by other parts of the body. This interplay between lactate levels and gluconeogenesis showcases the dynamic adaptability of metabolic processes to meet the energy demands of stressed tissues, emphasizing the critical role of this pathway in overall carbohydrate metabolism in specialized scenarios like TBI recovery (Glenn et al., 2015). Besides, the amount of carbohydrates in the diet can strongly affect gluconeogenesis and carbohydrate metabolism in several situations, including during exercise. Taking carbohydrates before exercise has been found to change the body's metabolism by affecting blood glucose levels and the use of different fuels. For example, when people eat sucrose before exercising, it changes the ratio of carbohydrate and fat burned, which can affect both their performance and recovery. It has been found that the amount of carbohydrates you eat before exercise can change your body's blood sugar and how your body uses energy. Such insights are crucial for athletes and those engaged in rigorous physical activity as they navigate the delicate balance of glycogen stores, blood glucose levels, and overall energy homeostasis necessary for optimal performance (Montzingo et al., 2016). So, it is very important to understand gluconeogenesis as part of carbohydrate metabolism to create useful nutritional plans and improve how the body responds to various metabolic situations (Figure 5.13).

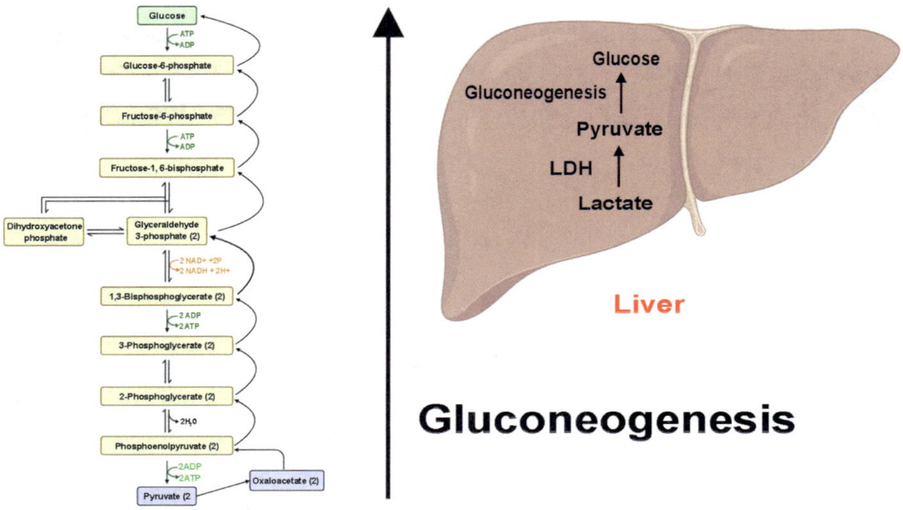

Figure 5.13. Gluconeogenesis.

Source: https://microbenotes.com/wp-content/uploads/2023/10/Gluconeogenesis.jpeg.

5.4.1. Definition and Purpose of Gluconeogenesis

Most of the gluconeogenesis process happens in the liver, and a little bit also happens in the kidneys. It means making glucose from non-carbohydrate substances such as lactate, glycerol, and some amino acids. When a person fasts, exercises for a long time, or does not consume enough carbohydrates, this process matters a lot. Gluconeogenesis makes sure that cells always have enough glucose for their vital activities, mainly in the brain and red blood cells. This adaptation is important for keeping blood glucose within a small range, thus preventing hypoglycemia, which can cause problems with both mental and physical performance. Besides making glucose, gluconeogenesis is important for regulating the level of glucose in the body. If the body does not get enough glucose in the diet, such as during a fast or low-carb meal plan, it makes glucose from gluconeogenesis. As a result, the body's important organs get the glucose they need to function normally and avoid the risks of hypoglycemia. Moreover, gluconeogenesis helps the body switch from using carbohydrates to using fats as an energy source, depending on what is available. It is important to know about this pathway, as problems with gluconeogenesis may result in metabolic diseases such as diabetes mellitus and hypoglycemia. Studies done recently have revealed that gluconeogenesis is regulated by a mix of hormonal and nutritional factors. Glucagon and cortisol cause the pathway to be activated, while insulin slows it down. In addition, recent studies indicate that substances that influence gluconeogenesis might also change energy metabolism as a whole. For instance, the acute effects of propionate, a short-chain fatty acid derived from gut bacterial fermentation, have been shown to modify energy metabolism by influencing substrate oxidation and appetite regulation (Sukkar et al., 2021). They highlight the main role of gluconeogenesis in making glucose and in managing energy levels in the body. So, understanding gluconeogenesis well is necessary to learn about carbohydrate metabolism and the effects on health and disease, especially since metabolic disorders are on the rise globally (Figure 5.14).

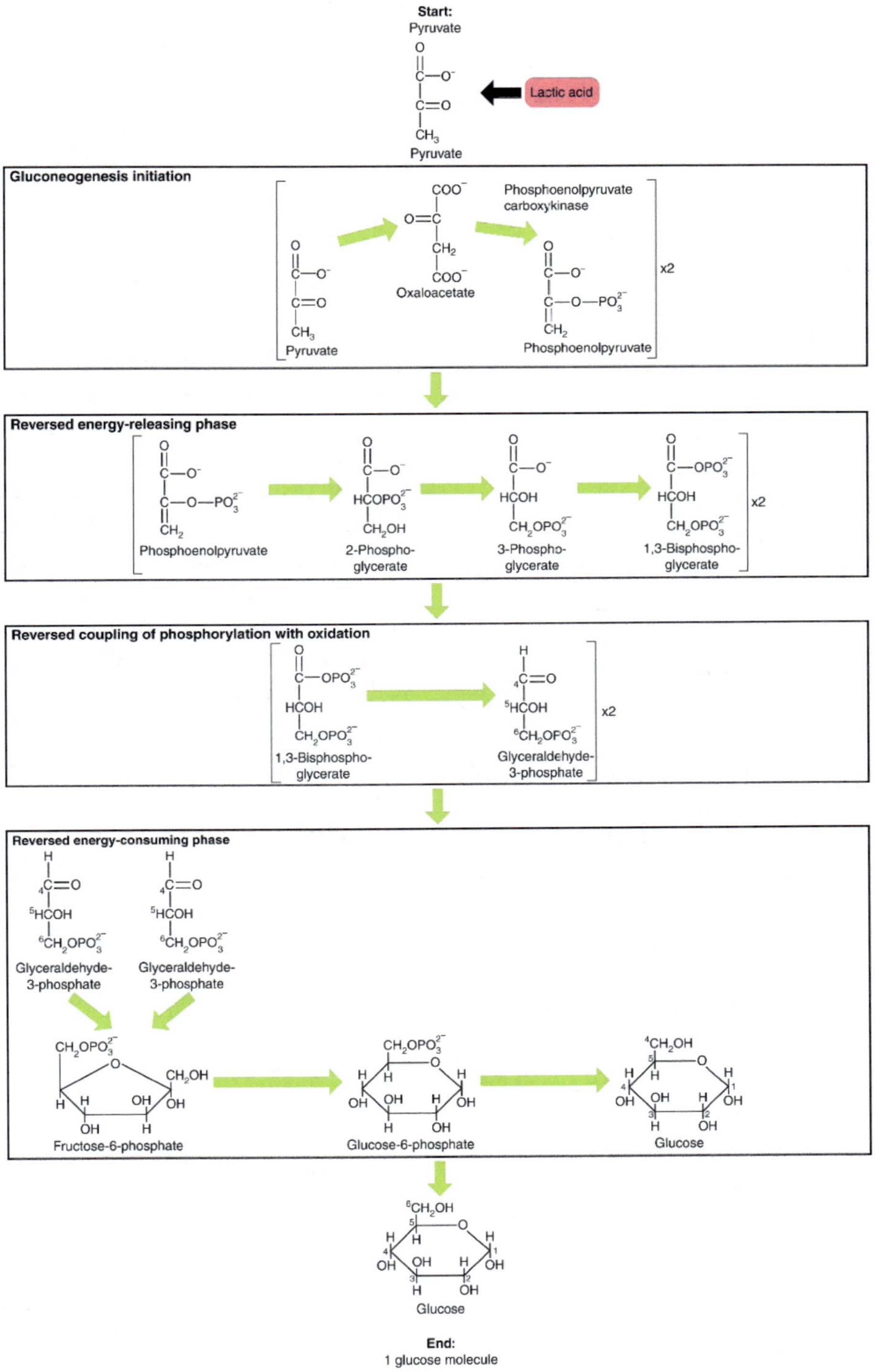

Figure 5.14. Gluconeogenesis is the synthesis of glucose from pyruvate, lactate, glycerol, alanine, or glutamate.

Source: https://s3-us-west-2.amazonaws.com/courses-images/wp-content/uploads/sites/217/2016/10/07181923/2510_Gluconeogenesis.jpg.

5.4.2. Key Enzymes Involved

Breaking down, making, and modifying carbohydrates is guided by different key enzymes in the process of carbohydrate metabolism. At different stages of carbohydrate processing, these enzymes, such as glycoside hydrolases, glycosyltransferases, and isomerases, are very important. As an example, glycoside hydrolases help in breaking down glycosidic bonds, allowing polysaccharides to be changed into simpler sugars. For organisms like *Lactobacillus pentosus*, such enzymes are necessary because they can change oligo- and polysaccharides and live well in the human gut. Understanding these enzymes provides insight into how microorganisms adapt to their surroundings by efficiently utilizing available carbohydrates for energy and growth, which is critical for their survival and functioning in diverse ecosystems (Abriouel et al., 2017). Besides, the actions and levels of these important metabolic enzymes are controlled by different physiological and environmental factors that increase their activity in particular situations. For example, when plants such as cucumber are put under saline stress, studies show that enzymes involved in carbohydrate metabolism are increased. In particular, the use of putrescine from the outside showed a strong effect on the activity of enzymes in this metabolic pathway, proving that external nutrients can regulate enzyme functions. This modulation reflects the dynamic nature of carbohydrate metabolism, which must adjust to both nutrient availability and abiotic stressors, underscoring the adaptability of organisms (Sun et al., 2016). All in all, looking at the main enzymes involved in carbohydrate metabolism shows how enzymes and the environment interact in many ways. Since many factors adjust metabolic pathways, the study of these enzymes is important for understanding how organisms efficiently break down carbohydrates. These enzymes play a key role in evolution since they help determine the energy levels of an organism and also affect the relationships between microbes. This comprehensive approach to analyzing enzymatic roles contributes to a broader understanding of carbohydrate metabolism, with implications for agriculture, industry, and health (Abriouel et al., 2017; Sun et al., 2016).

5.4.3. Differences Between Glycolysis and Gluconeogenesis

The pathways of glycolysis and gluconeogenesis show how complex carbohydrate metabolism is. When oxygen is scarce, glycolysis is important for creating energy by changing glucose into pyruvate. In this pathway, glucose is transformed into pyruvate by 10 enzymatic reactions, which also make ATP and NADH, important energy providers for the cell. On the other hand, gluconeogenesis means making glucose out of other substances, mainly when there is not enough carbohydrate in your diet or when you exercise a lot. This pathway is almost the opposite of glycolysis, involving several reactions that help produce glucose, mostly in the liver and kidneys, to keep supplying glucose to the brain and red blood cells. The way these two processes are regulated is a major difference between them. Glycolysis is turned on when glucose and insulin are high, and it is turned off when ATP and citrate are high, showing there is enough energy and materials. Gluconeogenesis is turned on by fasting and by stress hormones such as glucagon and cortisol, but it is switched off by insulin. The way these two pathways work together shows how active the body's metabolism is and how much energy it requires. As an example, after eating, glycolysis is used to break down extra glucose and produce energy in the form of ATP. In contrast, during periods of low blood glucose, such as after prolonged fasting, gluconeogenesis is prioritized to synthesize glucose from stored substrates, such as lactate and amino acids, thereby maintaining blood glucose homeostasis, as noted in research on lactate in cerebral metabolism following TBI (Glenn et al., 2015). At the enzymatic stage, it is noticeable that certain parts of gluconeogenesis skip the irreversible steps in glycolysis, showing how these pathways are carefully designed for what they do. In other words, while glycolysis has pyruvate kinase, gluconeogenesis uses pyruvate carboxylase and phosphoenolpyruvate carboxykinase to change pyruvate into glucose. Also, important regulatory proteins, for example, Shc proteins, play a role in these metabolic pathways. Studies indicate that Shc proteins may shift metabolism from glycolysis to gluconeogenesis, particularly under fasting conditions, showcasing their regulatory role in fuel selection (Cortopassi et al., 2016). All these aspects highlight how glycolysis and gluconeogenesis are different but still connected in the body's use of carbohydrates (Figure 5.15).

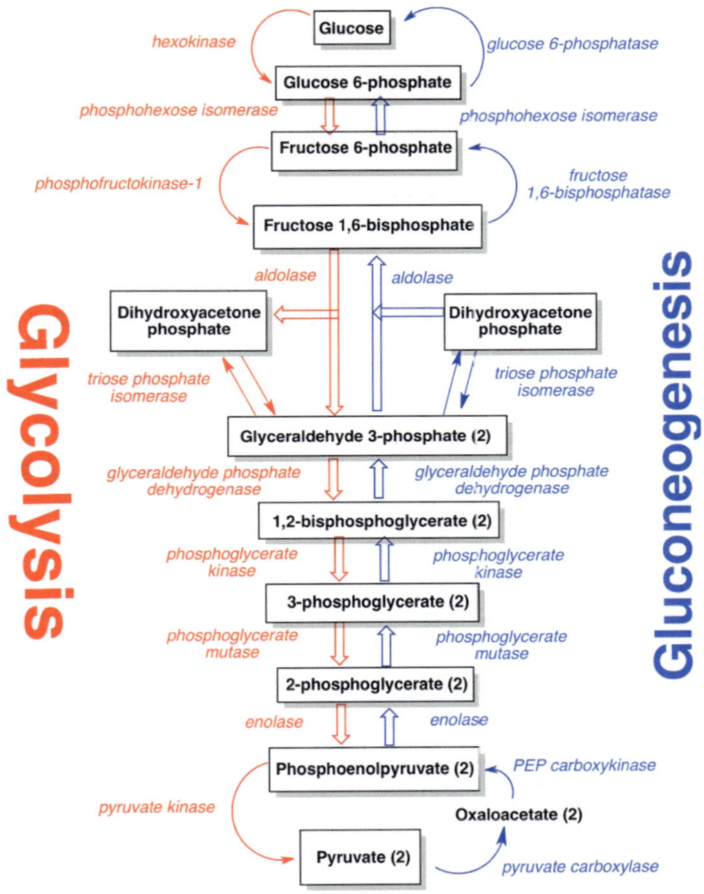

Figure 5.15. Glycolysis vs. gluconeogenesis.

Source: https://upload.wikimedia.org/wikipedia/commons/5/51/Glycolytic_and_gluconeogenic_pathways.jpg.

Test Your Knowledge

1. What is the purpose of gluconeogenesis?
2. What are the key enzymes in carbohydrate metabolism?

5.5. Glycogen Metabolism

Learning Outcome

1. Describe the biochemical process responsible for the formation of glycogen from glucose;
2. Know the biochemical process of glycogenolysis;
3. Understand the hormonal regulation of glycogen metabolism.

Glycogen metabolism is very important for understanding the overall process of carbohydrate metabolism. Glycogen, a polysaccharide that stores glucose in the liver and muscles, is very important for giving us energy when we exercise. When carbohydrates are consumed, insulin prompts the body to change glucose into glycogen. The process helps store energy and also controls blood glucose, which supports the body's metabolic balance. In comparison, glycogenolysis is controlled by hormones such as glucagon and epinephrine, especially when a person is fasting or doing strenuous exercise. Looking at these pathways makes it clear that glycogen is needed to keep up energy levels and is involved in using carbohydrates, showing how the body's energy balance is connected. Glycogen metabolism is greatly influenced by when and how many carbohydrates are consumed, mainly in athletes. It has been found through research that consuming carbohydrates before exercise can affect both blood sugar and what the body uses for energy during exercise. For instance, studies suggest that varying amounts of sucrose taken before exercise can lead to distinct responses in blood glucose and fat oxidation dynamics (Montzingo et al., 2016). This means that glycogen allows the body to quickly get energy when it is needed. On top of this, when carbohydrates are consumed at specific times, they can help restore glycogen and improve both athletic performance and stamina. Athletes who eat certain foods can control their glycogen levels and, as a result, improve their performance. The way glycogen is used and how central fatigue affects each other makes it harder to understand carbohydrate metabolism during and after exercise. While peripheral fatigue has long been a focus, emerging research emphasizes the significance of central nervous system interactions during recovery processes (Argus et al., 2015). Refilling glycogen is good for your physical recovery and may also contribute to better mental recovery and performance. If athletes follow proper post-exercise nutrition to restore glycogen, they may feel more mentally sharp and less tired, which is necessary for excellent performance later. So, recognizing that glycogens help both the body and the mind increases the discussion about carbohydrate metabolism. It points out that nutrition should address both a person's short-term health and their mental development in the future (Figure 5.16).

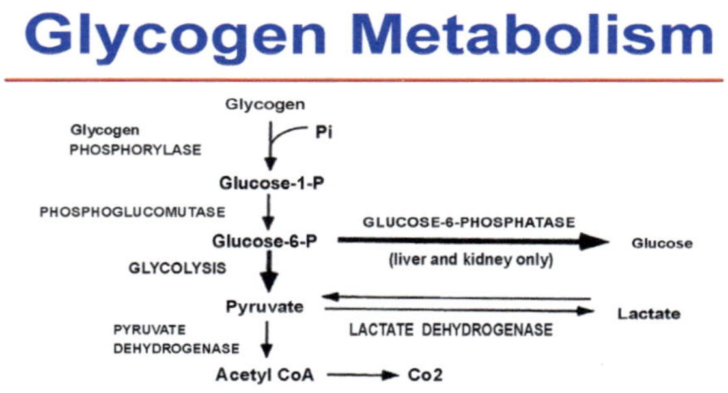

Figure 5.16. Glycogen metabolism.

Source: https://i.ytimg.com/vi/myDJJ_EGM2U/hq720.jpg?sqp=-oaymwEhCK4FEIIDSFryq4qpAxMIARUAAAAAGAElAADIQj0AgKJD&rs=AOn4CLBd9KPfUqvdMxLc_kLssQWv8_HK2w.

5.5.1. Glycogenesis: Formation of Glycogen

Maintaining the right amount of energy in the body depends on glycogenesis, which creates glycogen out of glucose. Excess glucose is mainly turned into glycogen in the liver and muscles for storage and use at a later time. The process of glycogenesis starts by phosphorylating glucose to make glucose-6-phosphate, which is then changed to glucose-1-phosphate. The glycogen polymer gets its characteristic highly branched shape when the enzymes glycogen synthase and branching enzyme add glucose units to it. As a result of branching, glycogen can be broken down more easily and used quickly when more energy is needed, proving the careful balance in glycogenesis. The process of glycogenesis is carefully regulated by hormones and how much of energy is in the cell. Insulin is important because it boosts glycogenesis by turning on glycogen synthase and turning off glycogen phosphorylase.

The hormones show how the body responds to a rise in blood glucose, which happens after consuming food. Besides, metabolic factors such as having enough glucose-6-phosphate and energy charge affect this process. During periods of starvation or low carbohydrate intake, glycogenesis is downregulated to conserve glucose and allow for its utilization in vital physiological processes (Awai et al., 1957). As a result, it is important to understand how glycogenesis is regulated to see how carbohydrates keep the body's energy levels stable in different situations. New studies are helping to reveal the details of glycogenesis and what they mean for health and disease. As an example, sulfonylurea drugs, given for diabetes, have shown how insulin-sensitive tissues are stimulated to produce glycogen. Studies indicate that these drugs enhance glucose utilization and the activity of metabolic enzymes, thereby indirectly promoting glycogen synthesis (Altan et al., 1994). This research points out that glycogenesis matters for energy storage and also for treating diabetic patients by controlling their glucose levels. In short, glycogenesis is a key part of carbohydrate metabolism and explains the importance of linking different biological pathways and their regulation.

5.5.2. Glycogenolysis: Breakdown of Glycogen

Glycogenolysis is important for carbohydrate metabolism since it quickly releases glucose when the body needs extra energy. Glycogen is a polysaccharide kept in the liver and muscles and is used as the body's quick energy source. When a person is active or fasting, glycogenolysis is started to break down glycogen into glucose. Glycogen phosphorylase enzyme helps by breaking down glycogen into glucose-1-phosphate by removing glucose units one by one. After that, glucose-1-phosphate can be turned into glucose-6-phosphate and is set to be used in glycolysis or gluconeogenesis. Glycogenolysis is controlled by hormones such as glucagon and epinephrine, which help the process continue, so glucose is always available when the body needs it. Glycogenolysis helps maintain the balance of blood glucose as well as providing energy. When energy intake is less or energy is used more, glycogenolysis helps to keep blood glucose levels steady, which is important for the body's balance. If there is not enough glucose due to fasting or tough exercise, glucagon from the pancreas makes the liver release glucose into the bloodstream. The brain needs this mechanism a lot since it depends on glucose for most of its energy. Besides, the ability of muscle cells to break down glycogen helps maintain muscle activity and performance, since energy is released as needed during exercise. New research has pointed out the details of glycogenolysis and its role in processes such as lactate use and the way substrates are handled during exercise. It is clear that glycogenolysis and lactate metabolism are connected, meaning that glycogen breakdown provides energy and also works together with other metabolic processes for recovery and better performance. Research has demonstrated that in TBI, the metabolic demands may shift, affecting glucose and lactate metabolism, where glycogenolysis could either directly or indirectly support enhanced cerebral energy requirements through lactate utilization (Glenn et al., 2015). Additionally, carbohydrate ingestion before exercise can significantly influence glycogenolysis, illustrating the adaptability of metabolic pathways in response to varying physiological conditions (Montzingo et al., 2016). Therefore, understanding glycogenolysis increases our knowledge of how carbohydrates are used in the body and affects our health and exercise abilities (Figure 5.17).

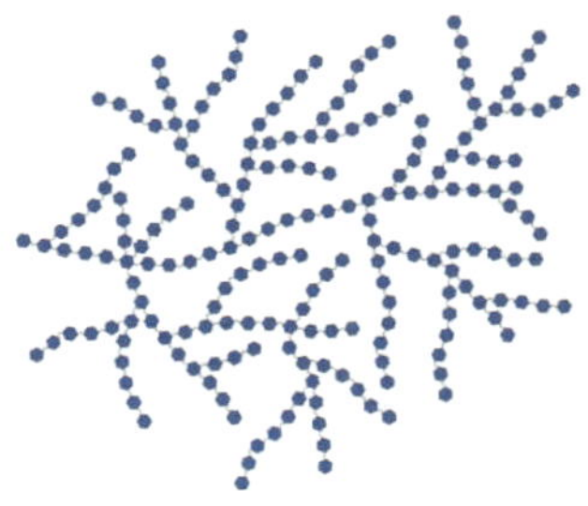

Figure 5.17. Glycogen.

Source: https://microbenotes.com/wp-content/uploads/2023/10/Glycogen.jpeg.

5.5.3. Hormonal Regulation of Glycogen Metabolism

The body uses hormonal control of glycogen metabolism to make sure energy is supplied and used in balance. When fasting or using a lot of energy, glucagon, and epinephrine hormones prompt glycogen to be converted into glucose for instant use. When hormones bind to certain receptors on liver and muscle cells, it starts a series of reactions that turn glycogen into glucose-1-phosphate and then into glucose-6-phosphate for use as energy. Due to the interaction of these hormones, there is always an adequate supply of glucose in the blood. Alternatively, insulin is important for glycogenesis because it helps glucose become stored as glycogen. Keeping this balance is necessary for the body to work well, as any disturbance can result in metabolic disorders, proving that hormones are vital for carbohydrate metabolism. Hormones play a bigger role than simply turning on or off the body's metabolic processes. How the nervous system and humoral factors interact is very important for the regulation of glycogen metabolism. For instance, when people are starving, the body turns more to glycogen, so it is important for the body's regulation to adapt accordingly. Studies have proven that the autonomic nervous system plays an important role in controlling the enzymes involved in storing and releasing glycogen. In particular, tissues without nerves have more fat and different glycogen levels, proving that hormones and nerves are both involved in keeping metabolism stable. This dual regulatory mechanism adapts to various physiological states, such as stress and fasting, ensuring a balance between energy substrates to meet the body's changing demands in different circumstances, reflecting the intricate networks governing carbohydrate metabolism in living organisms (Awai et al., 1957). New studies have suggested ways to study how glycogen metabolism is controlled in different parts of tissues. For instance, the metabolic patterning on a chip (MPOC) platform allows for in vitro examination of metabolic heterogeneity, particularly in liver tissues where zonation affects metabolic capacities. Gradients of metabolic modulators allow researchers to imitate the roles of hormones such as insulin and glucagon on glycogen metabolism. With this approach, we can learn how the efficiency and reaction of glycogen storage and breakdown differ in different tissue areas. Knowing about these differences in the brain is important for both studying normal brain functions and finding out what goes wrong in diseases such as diabetes. As research continues to explore the hormonal and spatial dimensions of glycogen metabolism, it holds promise for developing targeted therapies for metabolic disorders (Eo et al., 2018).

Test Your Knowledge

1. What is the biochemical process of glycogenolysis?
2. What is the hormonal regulation of glycogen metabolism?

5.6. Role of Insulin and Glucagon

Learning Outcome

1. Know the insulin's effect on carbohydrate metabolism;
2. Understand the glucagon's role in energy mobilization;
3. Describe the interaction between insulin and glucagon.

Maintaining the right amount of energy in the body is possible because of how carbohydrate metabolism is controlled by insulin and glucagon. Insulin produced by the pancreas is necessary for bringing down blood glucose levels when we eat carbohydrates. When insulin is present, it allows glucose to enter muscle and adipose cells so that the extra glucose can be changed into glycogen for storage. Insulin also prevents the body from making glucose and breaking down fat, so there is enough glucose for cellular respiration. If carbohydrates are consumed in larger amounts, insulin helps the body use energy and prevents high blood sugar, which is linked to different metabolic problems. Meanwhile, glucagon, made by the alpha cells in the pancreas, raises blood glucose levels when there is not enough carbohydrate or food. When blood glucose is low, glucagon prompts the liver to break down glycogen and make new glucose to be released into the blood for the brain and other vital organs. The body's need to respond to changes in energy is made possible by the interaction between insulin and glucagon. Recent studies have revealed that variations in carbohydrate intake, such as pre-exercise consumption, significantly affect insulin and glucagon dynamics, influencing substrate utilization during physical activity (Montzingo et al., 2016). It shows that carbohydrate metabolism is controlled by many hormones and responds to both the body's need for energy and the energy it receives. Metabolic actions of insulin and glucagon in the body depend greatly on the liver, which demonstrates significant metabolic diversity and zoning required for handling carbohydrates.

Hepatocytes in the periportal area react more to insulin, thus boosting glycolysis and glycogen synthesis, while perivenous hepatocytes are more sensitive to glucagon, helping to produce more glucose and use glycogen. Since the brain and muscles are different in structure, it is important for hormones to be regulated precisely to ensure the best use of carbohydrates. Emerging research using advanced technologies, such as the MPOC platform, further elucidates how gradients of metabolic modulators can mimic and study these zonal responses in vitro (Eo et al., 2018). Scientists studying these hormones and cells will help find new ways to handle diseases such as diabetes and MS (Figure 5.18).

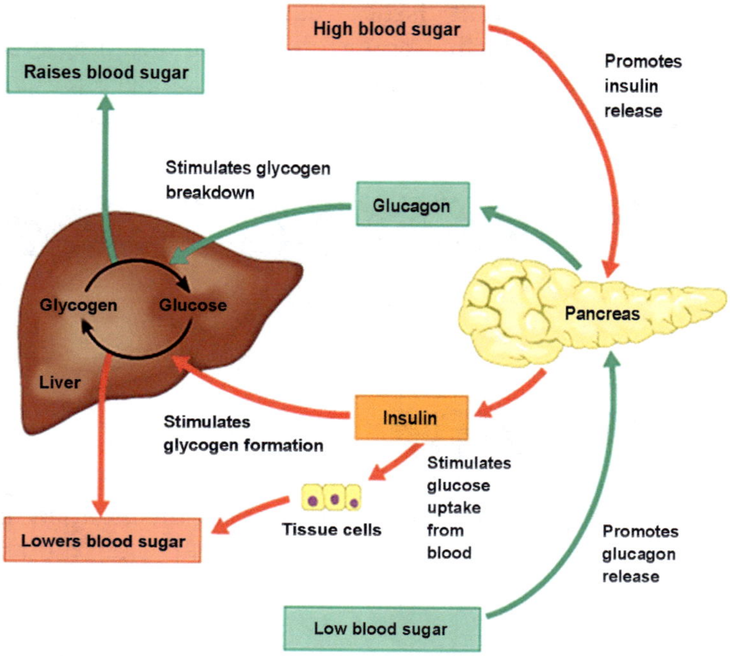

Figure 5.18. Complementary roles of insulin and glucagon.

Source: https://www.atrainceu.com/sites/default/files/diabetes-role-of-insulin-and-glucagon.png.

5.6.1. Insulin's Effect on Carbohydrate Metabolism

Insulin is key in managing the process of using and storing glucose from carbohydrates. When carbohydrates are eaten, glucose in the blood increases, which makes pancreatic beta cells release insulin. It makes it possible for glucose to enter muscle and fat cells, where it may be used right away or saved as glycogen. Insulin helps glucose enter cells and also stimulates the liver and muscle to make glycogen, a step important for managing energy levels in the body. Because insulin is missing in type 1 diabetes, blood glucose levels rise and this causes harmful changes in metabolism, pointing out the important role hormones play in controlling carbohydrate metabolism. In addition, insulins play a role in preventing the metabolic process that creates glucose from things other than carbohydrates. When we fast or eat very few carbohydrates, gluconeogenesis rises to keep blood glucose within a safe range. Insulin causes the body to change its energy source from fat to carbohydrates. It is very important for energy balance and the flexibility of the metabolic system. Besides, insulin helps control other hormones that play a role in glucose metabolism, making sure there is a balanced system in the body. In individuals with type 1 diabetes, improper insulin administration can lead to extreme fluctuations in glucose levels, which underscores the need for careful management of insulin therapy to stabilize carbohydrate metabolism in this population (Heller et al., 2008). When people with type 1 diabetes exercise, it is very important to manage insulin therapy since their glucose levels can change quickly. Exercise may cause the body to experience both low and high blood sugar levels because people do not always understand how insulin and activity are connected. Notably, peri-exercise bolus insulin dose adjustments are essential to mitigate these risks, as studies suggest that without proper management, individuals with type

1 diabetes can suffer from post-exercise and nocturnal hypoglycemia (McCarthy et al., 2021). Such incidents prove that it is necessary to understand each individual's response to insulin and to use personalized treatments that control how the body handles carbohydrates. Therefore, it is very important to manage insulin therapy with exercise to avoid bad outcomes and keep blood sugar under control (Figure 5.19).

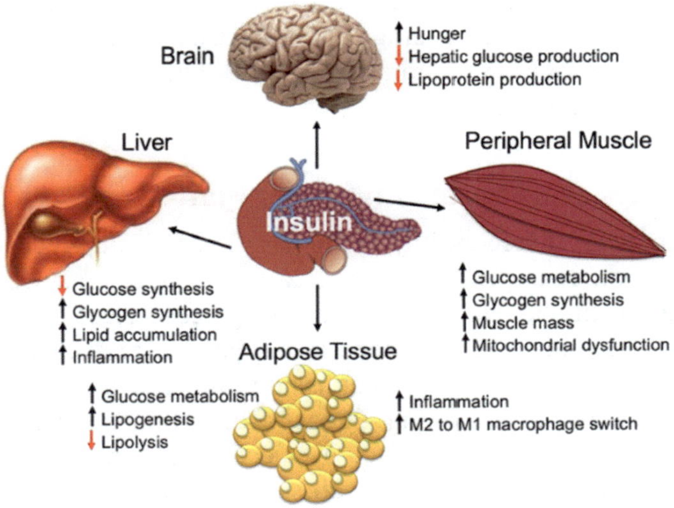

Figure 5.19. Insulin is a major regulator of metabolism and organ function.

Source: Yee LD, Mortimer JE, Natarajan R, Dietze EC and Seewaldt VL (2020) Metabolic Health, Insulin, and Breast Cancer: Why Oncologists Should Care About Insulin. Front. Endocrinol. 11:58. doi: 10.3389/fendo.2020.00058

5.6.2. Glucagon's Role in Energy Mobilization

When there is not enough food or when we exercise a lot, glucagon helps our body use stored energy. Glucagon is produced by the alpha cells in the pancreas and it works against insulin to keep blood glucose levels balanced. When the body runs out of glucose, as during long exercise, glucagon causes glycogen in the liver and muscles to be broken down, letting glucose into the blood. It is necessary to maintain enough energy and for the brain and other organs to keep functioning as usual. The intricate interplay between glucagon and glycogen stores illustrates how the body employs hormonal regulation to adapt to fluctuating energy demands, highlighting its significance in the broader framework of carbohydrate metabolism, particularly under stress conditions or physical exertion (Montzingo et al., 2016). In addition, glucagon is important for gluconeogenesis since it prompts the liver to produce glucose from non-carbohydrate materials. Since this pathway keeps releasing glucose, it is very important when food is not available for a long time. After trauma or hard physical exercise, the body uses lactate and amino acids to help maintain energy balance by producing glucose. Glenn et al. (2015) elaborate on how elevated lactate levels can prompt gluconeogenic activity, demonstrating the interdependence of various metabolic pathways in energy regulation. Therefore, glucagon helps the body use its stored glycogen and also makes new glucose, which is key to dealing with different body challenges. Besides giving energy, glucagon also controls how carbohydrates and fats are used in the body's metabolism.

As a result of promoting lipolysis, glucagon allows adipocytes to break down triglycerides (TGs) and release free fatty acids (FFAs) for energy use, mainly during fasting or exercise. As a result of this hormone's action, the body can easily switch from using carbohydrates to using fat as its main energy source when glucose levels fall. It is very important for athletes to balance the use of carbohydrates and lipids to perform well and maintain balance in the body. Studies illustrate that variations in glucagon levels can influence substrate utilization types, revealing the hormones' essential role in metabolic flexibility (Montzingo et al., 2016). So, knowing how glucagons help with energy mobilization improves our understanding of carbohydrate metabolism and also explains the effects on metabolic health and sport.

5.6.3. Interaction Between Insulin and Glucagon

Carbohydrate metabolism is regulated mainly by the way insulin and glucagon interact to maintain balance in the body. The pancreas produces these two hormones that work in opposite ways to control the level of glucose in the blood. When blood glucose rises, insulin is released to take glucose into tissues and help turn extra glucose into glycogen and fat for storage. On the other hand, glucagon mainly works when blood sugar is low and during fasting; it leads to breaking down glycogen into glucose and also making glucose from other sources. Having enough energy in the body at all times depends on the balance between insulin and glucagon. Diet and exercise are some of the factors that affect the role of insulin and glucagon in maintaining energy balance. If you regularly eat too many energy-dense foods, it can cause insulin resistance and stop insulin from working properly in glucose metabolism. If the body's cells do not react to insulin as they should, the balance between insulin and glucagon is disrupted, which usually leads to high blood sugar and more stored fat. This condition points out the important impact of dietary macronutrients on how sensitive the body is to insulin. While reducing overall caloric intake may improve insulin sensitivity, it is equally important to consider the types of macronutrients consumed because their metabolic pathways directly affect the interaction between these two hormones, impacting health outcomes associated with type 2 diabetes (Weickert, 2012). In addition, insulin and glucagon control glucose and also influence the relationship between adipose tissue and lipid metabolism. Adipose tissue serves as a vital reservoir for energy storage, primarily in the form of TGs, which influence the metabolic response to insulin and glucagon. Insulin stops lipolysis when it is present, which means fat is stored, but glucagon helps release fat from adipose tissue when there is little or no food. This finding shows that adipose tissue is important for metabolism and helps regulate energy use with the help of insulin and glucagon. The complexity of these interactions emphasizes the need for targeted dietary frameworks that can optimize metabolic responses, as evidenced in recent research that explores how different diets can affect insulin sensitivity and lipid metabolism, thus supporting insulin dysfunction associated with obesity and diabetes (Wilson, 1983).

Test Your Knowledge

1. What is the effect of insulin on carbohydrate metabolism?
2. What is the interaction between insulin and glucagon?

SUMMARY

To sum up, studying carbohydrate metabolism has shown how important it is for human health and body functions. The process of digesting and absorbing carbohydrates points out the importance of different carbohydrate types, especially that complex carbohydrates are handled differently than simple sugars. Having complex carbohydrates is better for your energy and health, but eating a lot of added sugars might have negative effects on your metabolism. This knowledge stresses the role of choosing a healthy diet in controlling carbohydrate intake for better health, mainly for those at risk for metabolic conditions. Furthermore, recent studies have indicated a growing concern regarding the relationship between carbohydrate intake and cardiometabolic health, particularly in children with high BMI. According to the data, having too much sugar, mainly from processed foods, can result in higher TGs and more insulin resistance, which may lead to health problems in the future. It is clear from the evidence that some carbohydrates affect the body differently, so we should be careful when giving diet advice. Reducing sugar in youth meals could help stop obesity and its related health problems, since carbohydrate metabolism is a vital part of public health efforts. Lastly, making changes to the amount of carbohydrates in the diet can have a big impact on metabolism-related health issues, as shown by recent studies on lowering skatole production in pigs. Even though it is about livestock, the main ideas about dietary fiber and resistant starch teach us about how carbohydrates can change metabolism and health. With the progress of carbohydrate metabolism, bringing together results from different research areas is necessary for making complete dietary guidelines and interventions. Consequently, ongoing research should focus on optimizing carbohydrate sources in diets to mitigate health risks and enhance metabolic efficiency, reinforcing the critical connection between carbohydrate management and overall health, as evidenced by investigations on the dietary impacts related to pathways of carbohydrate metabolism (Fleming et al., 2010; Jensen et al., 2012).

Carbohydrate metabolism is studied to identify the main steps and processes involved in energy production and how cells work. It is very important to know how these metabolic pathways function and how they are controlled during different times or conditions in the body. How organisms respond to their energy needs is shown by the way enzymatic reactions and energy substrates work together. Moreover, when carbohydrate metabolism links with other metabolic processes, it becomes easier to understand how cells react to their surroundings. All metabolic pathways are linked, so they collaborate to control the production and breakdown of carbohydrates for normal metabolism. Researchers also study how carbohydrate metabolism is regulated during the development of fruit-bearing plants, for example, grapes. Metabolite analyses reveal that there are major changes in grape berries at every stage, especially during veraison. At this point, there is a fast rise in sugar and a drop in organic acids, which indicates important changes in the fruit's metabolism for maturation. Comprehensive studies, including those that assess enzymatic activities and metabolite profiles, illustrate how each developmental phase is marked by distinctive metabolic signatures, enhancing our understanding of how carbohydrates are orchestrated during this critical growth period (Dai et al., 2013). Also, recent findings about how carbohydrate metabolism affects microbial communities give us a better understanding of wider ecological situations. Current studies point out that heterotrophic bacteria are very active in the metabolic processes happening in anammox granules. It appears from the findings that Chlorobi-affiliated bacteria are involved in breaking down proteins and recycling nutrients, which shows how they are connected to other organisms in the process of carbohydrate metabolism. Such interactions illustrate the interconnectedness of microbial metabolism within larger ecological frameworks, whereby carbohydrate pathways not only support individual growth but also contribute to nutrient cycling and ecosystem function (Bhattacharjee et al., 2017).

KEY TERMS FROM THIS CHAPTER

- Carbohydrate metabolism
- Chronic diseases
- Dietary fiber
- Heart disease
- Hypoglycemia
- Lactase
- Pyruvate
- Sucrose
- Carbohydrate nutrition
- Complex carbohydrates
- Gut microbiota
- Hyperglycemia
- Isomaltase
- Maltase
- Salivary amylase

CRITICAL THINKING QUESTIONS

1. **Which process describes the breakdown of glucose to pyruvate?**
   a. Glycogenesis
   b. Glycolysis
   c. Gluconeogenesis
   d. Glycogenolysis
2. **The primary site of gluconeogenesis in the body is:**
   a. Muscle
   b. Brain
   c. Liver
   d. Adipose tissue
3. **What is the end product of anaerobic glycolysis in humans?**
   a. Ethanol
   b. Lactate
   c. Acetyl-CoA
   d. Oxaloacetate
4. **Which process converts glycogen to glucose-1-phosphate?**
   a. Glycogenesis
   b. Glycogenolysis
   c. Glycolysis
   d. Gluconeogenesis
5. **The TCA cycle is fueled by:**
   a. Pyruvate
   b. Acetyl-CoA
   c. Glucose
   d. Glycogen

Answers to Critical Thinking Questions

1. (b); 2. (c); 3. (b); 4. (b); 5. (b)

Short Answer Questions

1. What is carbohydrate metabolism
2. Why are carbohydrates important?
3. Name the 3 types of carbohydrates.
4. What is glycolysis?
5. What is gluconeogenesis?

References

1. Abriouel, H., Pérez Montoro, B., Casimiro-Soriguer, C. S., Pérez Pulido, A. J., Knapp, C. W., Caballero Gómez, N., Castillo-Gutiérrez, S., Estudillo-Martínez, M. D., Gálvez, A., & Benomar, N. (2017). Insight into Potential Probiotic Markers Predicted in *Lactobacillus pentosus* MP-10 Genome Sequence. *Frontiers in microbiology*, *8*, 891. https://doi.org/10.3389/fmicb.2017.00891(accessed on 11th June 2025).

2. McCarthy, O., Deere, R., Churm, R., Dunseath, G. J., Jones, C., Eckstein, M. L., Williams, D. M., Hayes, J., Pitt, J., Bain, S. C., Moser, O., & Bracken, R. M. (2021). Extent and prevalence of post-exercise and nocturnal hypoglycemia following peri-exercise bolus insulin adjustments in individuals with type 1 diabetes. *Nutrition, metabolism, and cardiovascular diseases : NMCD*, *31*(1), 227–236. https://doi.org/10.1016/j.numecd.2020.07.043 (accessed on 11th June 2025).

3. Altan, V. M., Aoki, M., Avruch, J., Bak, M., Begum, M., Brown, S., Caren, D., et al. (1994). Stimulation of glucose utilization in 3T3 adipocytes and rat diaphragm *in vitro* by the sulphonylureas, glimepiride and glipalamide, is correlated with modulations of the cAMP regulatory cascade. https://core.ac.uk/download/12169475.pdf (accessed on 11th June 2025).

4. Andrews, E. (2016). *Design and Basic Verification of A Discrete Event Simulator for Glucose Metabolism in Human Beings*. https://core.ac.uk/download/217190920.pdf (accessed on 11th June 2025).

5. Arabyan, N., Desai, P., Foutouhi, S., Huang, Y., et al. (2016). *Salmonella* degrades the host glycocalyx leading to altered infection and glycan remodeling. https://core.ac.uk/download/323070778.pdf (accessed on 11th June 2025).

6. Argus, C. K., Driller, M. W., Martin, K., Northey, J., et al. (2015). Is it time to turn our attention toward central mechanisms for post-exertional recovery strategies and performance? https://core.ac.uk/download/29202901.pdf (accessed on 11th June 2025).

7. Awai, M., Oda, T., Ohtani, K., Sakai, T., et al. (1957). Histochemical studies on the nervous and humoral regulation of lipids and carbohydrate metabolism. https://core.ac.uk/download/12548410.pdf (accessed on 11th June 2025).

8. Bakker, B. M., Cubbon, A., Barrett, M. P., Breitling, R., & Shim, H. (2010). Metabolomic systems biology of trypanosomes. https://core.ac.uk/download/81325.pdf (accessed on 11th June 2025).

9. Barber, T., Burnett, D., Elder, P. J. D., Ramsden, D. B., et al. (2018). Human amylase gene copy number variation as a determinant of metabolic state. https://core.ac.uk/download/161512004.pdf (accessed on 11th June 2025).

10. Bauer, E., Metzler-Zebeli, B. U., Mosenthin, R., Verstegen, M. W. A., et al. (2011). Intestinal gene expression in pigs: Effects of reduced feed intake during weaning and potential impact of dietary components. https://core.ac.uk/download/pdf/29230036.pdf (accessed on 11th June 2025).

11. Berkers, C. R., Cheung, E. C., Maddocks, O. D. K., Mor, I., et al. (2013). Metabolic regulation by p53 family members. https://core.ac.uk/download/46559680.pdf (accessed on 11th June 2025).

12. Bhattacharjee, A. S., Goel, R., Hamilton, J. J., Lawson, C. E., et al. (2017). Metabolic network analysis reveals microbial community interactions in anammox granules. https://core.ac.uk/download/323308677.pdf (accessed on 11th June 2025).

13. Bosch, G., Depauw, S., Hendriks, W. H., Hesta, M., et al. (2012). Fermentation of animal components in strict carnivores: A comparative study with cheetah fecal inoculum. https://core.ac.uk/download/30640688.pdf (accessed on 11th June 2025).

14. Braeckman, B., Brewer, H. M., Camp, D. G. II., et al. (2014). LC-MS proteomics analysis of the insulin/IGF-1-deficient *Caenorhabditis elegans* daf-2(e1370) mutant reveals extensive restructuring of intermediary metabolism. https://core.ac.uk/download/55799360.pdf (accessed on 11th June 2025).

15. Braeckman, B., Houthoofd, K., & Vanfleteren, J. (2009). Intermediary metabolism. https://core.ac.uk/download/84042477.pdf (accessed on 11th June 2025).

16. Brand-Miller, J., Brown, K. D., Copeland, L., Dykhuizen, D. E., et al. (2015). The importance of dietary carbohydrate in human evolution. https://core.ac.uk/download/79495995.pdf (accessed on 11th June 2025).

17. Glenn, T. C., Martin, N. A., Horning, M. A., McArthur, D. L., Hovda, D. A., Vespa, P., & Brooks, G. A. (2015). Lactate: brain fuel in human traumatic brain injury: a comparison with normal healthy control subjects. *Journal of neurotrauma*, *32*(11), 820–832. https://doi.org/10.1089/neu.2014.3483(accessed on 11th June 2025).

18. Cho, S. K., Ijaz, U. Z., Jung, K. W., Kim, T., et al. (2017). Bacterial community analysis in upflow multilayer anaerobic reactor (UMAR) treating high-solids organic wastes. https://core.ac.uk/download/96882968.pdf (accessed on 11th June 2025).

19. Cortopassi, G. A., Hagopian, K., Kim, K., López-Dominguez, J. A., et al. (2016). Mice with low levels of Shc proteins display reduced glycolytic and increased gluconeogenic activities in liver. https://core.ac.uk/download/323069006.pdf (accessed on 11th June 2025).

20. Dai, Z., Delrot, S., Feil, R., Gomes, E., et al. (2013). Metabolic profiling reveals coordinated switches in primary carbohydrate metabolism in grape berry (*Vitis vinifera* L.), a non-climacteric fleshy fruit. https://core.ac.uk/download/210621820.pdf (accessed on 11th June 2025).

21. De Maeseneire, S., De Mey, M., Soetaert, W., Vandamme, E., et al. (2007). Minimizing acetate formation in *E. coli* fermentations. https://core.ac.uk/download/55794506.pdf (accessed on 11th June 2025).

22. Dias, J., Dinis, M. T., Engrola, S., Geurden, I., et al. (2016). High-glucose feeding of gilthead seabream (*Sparus aurata*) larvae: Effects on molecular and metabolic pathways. https://core.ac.uk/download/186632050.pdf (accessed on 11th June 2025).

23. Elizabeth L. Hess, Janice Wallace-Robinson, Katherine J. Dickson, and Janet V. Powers The George Washington University Washington, D.C (1992). *Publications of the Space Physiology and Countermeasures Program, Regulatory Physiology Discipline: 1980–1990.* Prepared for NASA Office of Space Science and Applications. https://core.ac.uk/download/pdf/42811395.pdf (accessed on 11th June 2025).

24. Doan, A. H. (2014). *Manipulation of Carbohydrate Diet and Ensuing Changes in Weight and Glycogen Storage in Bumble Bee (Bombus impatiens) queens.* https://core.ac.uk/download/211344433.pdf (accessed on 11th June 2025).

25. Eo, J., & Kang, Y. B. (Abraham), Mert, S., Usta, B., et al. (2018). Metabolic patterning on a chip: Towards *in vitro* liver zonation of primary rat and human hepatocytes. https://digitalcommons.georgefox.edu/cgi/viewcontent.cgi?article=1056&context=mece_fac (accessed on 11th June 2025).

26. Fleming, S. E., Lustig, R. H., Roberts, L. S., Sharma, A., et al. (2010). Carbohydrate intake and cardiometabolic risk factors in high BMI African American children. https://core.ac.uk/download/323073095.pdf (accessed on 11th June 2025).

27. Flint, A., Peeters, A., Butland, B., Challis, B., Abbott, C., Byrne, C., Byrne, D., et al. (2019). A study protocol for a randomized crossover study evaluating the effect of diets differing in carbohydrate quality on ileal content and appetite regulation in healthy humans. https://core.ac.uk/download/286269689.pdf (accessed on 11th June 2025).

28. Ghazeeri, G., Ghazeeri, G., Hmedeh, C., Hmedeh, S., et al. (2021). Nutritional management in polycystic ovary syndrome: Challenges and opportunities. https://core.ac.uk/download/161103740.pdf (accessed on 11th June 2025).

29. Heller, S. (2008). Minimizing hypoglycemia while maintaining glycemic control in diabetes. https://core.ac.uk/download/50935.pdf (accessed on 11th June 2025).

30. Högberg, A. (2003). *Cereal Non-Starch Polysaccharides in Pig Diets.* Acta Universitatis Agriculturae Sueciae. Agraria 2003, number: 413 Publisher: Department of Animal Nutrition and Management, Swedish University of Agricultural Sciences https://core.ac.uk/download/11694626.pdf (accessed on 11th June 2025).

31. Jensen, R. L. (2012). *Feed Interventions and Skatole Deposition.* https://core.ac.uk/download/10932999.pdf (accessed on 11th June 2025).

32. Jin, S., Zhong, M., Du, N., Shu, S., Guo, S., & Yuan, Y. (2016). Proteomic and physiological analyses reveal putrescine responses in roots of cucumber stressed by NaCl. https://core.ac.uk/download/pdf/82882950.pdf (accessed on 11th June 2025).

33. Kok, J., Kuipers, O. P., & Price, R. (2012). From meadows to milk to mucosa–adaptation of *Streptococcus* and *Lactococcus* species to their nutritional environments. https://core.ac.uk/download/pdf/12960006.pdf (accessed on 11th June 2025).

34. Montzingo, L. J. (2016). *Effects of Pre-Exercise Carbohydrate Consumption on Metabolism During Exercise.* https://core.ac.uk/download/211339673.pdf (accessed on 11th June 2025).

35. Olsson, T. (2005). *Functional Characterization of Hexokinases in the Moss Physcomitrella Patens.* https://core.ac.uk/download/11694926.pdf (accessed on 11th June 2025).

36. Scheffler, O. (2016). *Functional Characterization of A Novel Disaccharide Membrane Transporter in The Digestive Tract of the American Lobster, Homarus Americanus.* https://core.ac.uk/download/71999260.pdf (accessed on 11th June 2025).

37. Sukkar, A. (2021). The impact of acute oral sodium propionate supplementation on energy metabolism. https://core.ac.uk/download/479016909.pdf (accessed on 11th June 2025).

38. Weickert, M. O. (2012). Nutritional modulation of insulin resistance. https://core.ac.uk/download/18328007.pdf (accessed on 11th June 2025).

39. Wilson, R. D. (1983). *Triacylglycerol Synthesis in Rat Adipose Tissue: A Thesis Presented in Partial Fulfilment of The Requirements for The Degree of Master of Science in Biochemistry at Massey University.* https://core.ac.uk/download/185642042.pdf (accessed on 11th June 2025).

40. Zou, M. L. (2007). *Variation in the Apparent Fecal Digestibility Of Macronutrients and Urinary Energy Excretion for Three Diets Varying in Fat and Fiber Content–Assessment of The Atwater Factors and Related Energy Conversion Factors: A Thesis Presented in Partial Fulfillment of The Requirements for The Degree of Master of Science in Nutritional Science at Massey University, Palmerston North, New Zealand.* https://core.ac.uk/download/162617248.pdf (accessed on 11th June 2025).

LIPID METABOLISM

6

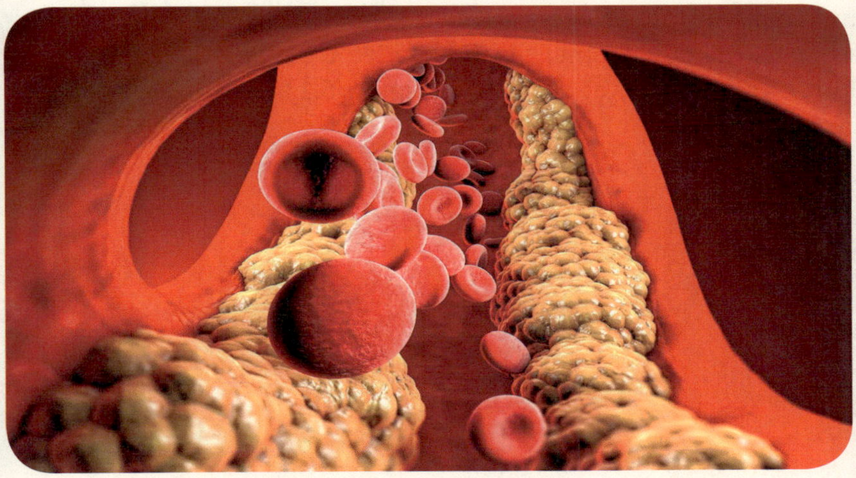

LEARNING OBJECTIVES

After studying this chapter, you will be able to:

1. Describe the types of lipids;
2. Understand the process of lipid digestion and absorption;
3. Describe the transport of lipids in the body;
4. Understand the beta-oxidation of fatty acids;
5. Know lipogenesis;
6. Describe the disorders related to lipid metabolism.

Introduction

Lipid metabolism plays an important role in explaining both healthy and unhealthy processes in cells. Lipids serve many purposes in the body, storing energy and also forming parts of cell membranes. Lipid metabolism involves the biochemical steps for lipids to be formed, altered, and broken down, which shows their role in different body functions. Since lipids come in many different forms and have specific functions, advanced techniques are required to examine them all. As scientists delve deeper into the nuances of lipidomics, their explorations illuminate the critical implications of altered lipid metabolism in diseases such as MS and cancer, emphasizing the importance of this field in both research and therapeutic contexts (Kamphorst et al., 2017). The progress in technology has greatly helped scientists understand how lipids are involved in health and disease. New developments in mass spectrometry and liquid chromatography have greatly helped researchers to learn more about the lipids in biological samples. With new analytical methods, scientists can better study lipid pathways and find out how disturbances in lipid metabolism may result in diseases. It is important to mention that the wide range of lipid structures can make it difficult to identify them, which shows why careful and advanced methods are needed for lipidomics. Efforts to increase the comprehensiveness of lipid analyses not only expand our knowledge base but also provide potential biomarkers for disease, thereby bridging the gap between basic research and clinical application (Kamphorst et al., 2017). Besides being important in science, understanding lipid metabolism may help develop treatments for several diseases. Since lifestyle-related disorders are becoming more common, understanding lipid metabolism in the body can lead to new treatments. Changing lipid metabolism by diet or drugs could greatly help in preventing and treating different diseases. In addition, lipids act as signals, making the process more complex since they can control inflammation and important cell processes. Consequently, ongoing research into lipid metabolism is not merely an academic exercise but a fundamental pursuit with the potential for real-world impact, aiding in the development of innovative treatment strategies for conditions linked to lipid dysregulation (Kamphorst et al., 2017) (Figure 6.1).

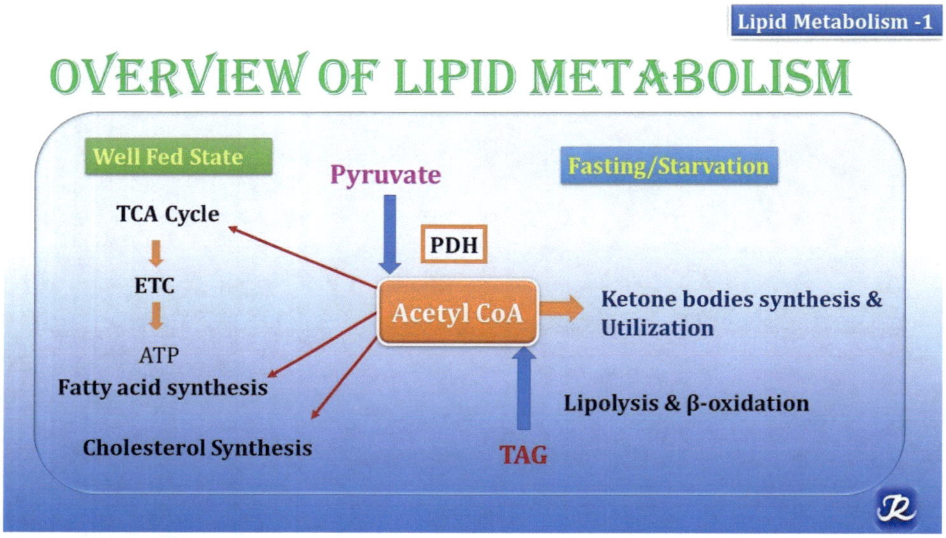

Figure 6.1. Overview of lipid metabolism.

Source: https://i.ytimg.com/vi/CBiP2ptNbUg/maxresdefault.jpg.

Definition of Lipid Metabolism

Lipid metabolism is made up of two main biochemical pathways called lipogenesis and lipolysis. Lipogenesis means making fatty acids and then transforming them into triglycerides (TGs), which store energy in the body. Most of the time, the liver and fatty tissues take excess carbohydrates and proteins and turn them into fats for future use. Lipolysis is the opposite, where TGs are broken down into free fatty acids (FFAs) and glycerol and these are used to produce energy. It is important when you are fasting or exercising heavily, since the body needs an alternative to glucose. It becomes clear from the rules that govern these pathways that lipid metabolism is not simple and is very important for maintaining energy balance and good metabolic health. In addition, the process of cholesterol metabolism plays a key role in lipid metabolism and mostly happens in the liver. A sterol, cholesterol, is needed for cellular membranes and is also used to make steroid hormones and bile acids. Its synthesis is intricately controlled by a feedback mechanism involving low-density lipoprotein (LDL) receptors and various enzymes. Most cholesterol inside the cell is formed by the synthesis pathway, and if this pathway is not regulated well, it can cause diseases such as Familial Hypercholesterolemia. In this way, mathematical models have been made to show how alterations in receptors and diet can change the level of cholesterol in the body. This integrated modeling approach enhances our understanding of lipid metabolism and sets the stage for potential therapeutic interventions, particularly concerning statin therapy, which aims to lower cholesterol levels effectively (Pool et al., 2018). In addition, how lipid metabolism affects health outcomes shows that it is not only about energy balance. Disorders in lipid metabolism are associated with MS, obesity, and cardiovascular diseases (CVDs), so it is important to study the reasons behind them. New studies are focusing on using different omics techniques to find biomarkers linked to cardiometabolic diseases. Looking at lipid metabolism this way helps identify the many processes involved, because each omics data source alone does not give a complete picture. In addition, paying attention to gender differences benefits this field, because metabolism can be affected by both biological and social factors. Therefore, elucidating the definition and implications of lipid metabolism is crucial for developing tailored strategies in the prevention and management of metabolic disorders, thus enhancing public health outcomes (Argano et al., 2019) (Figure 6.2).

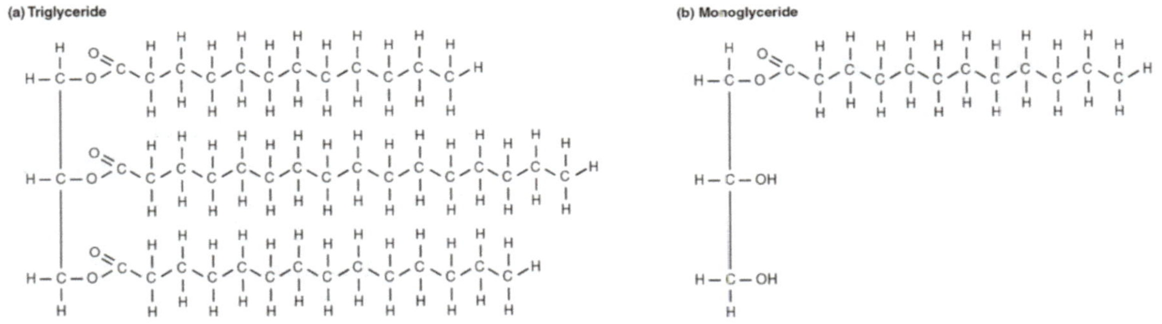

Figure 6.2. A triglyceride molecule (a) breaks down into a monoglyceride (b).

Source: https://s3-us-west-2.amazonaws.com/courses-images/wp-content/uploads/sites/217/2016/10/07182803/2511_A_Triglyceride_Molecule-1024x304.jpg.

Importance of Lipid Metabolism in Human Health

Lipid metabolism is very important for human health since it controls many functions and metabolic routes in the body. It is important to break down and build up lipids to produce energy, build cellular membranes, and produce hormones. A well-balanced way of using lipids is important for the body's energy balance. Disorders in lipid metabolism can cause obesity, type 2 diabetes, and different heart diseases. Many cases of this disease come from accumulating too many lipids, which can harm several tissues and organs, so it is important to study lipid metabolism to prevent health risks. Additionally, researchers have underscored the need for further exploration of how factors such as diet, sleep patterns, and circadian rhythms influence lipid metabolism, thus facilitating preventive health measures and interventions aimed at improving metabolic health in the population (Arble et al., 2015). In addition, the connection between obesity and lipid metabolism has drawn a lot of interest from public health experts. Because obesity is on the rise all over the world, it is now clear that too much body fat can lead to disrupted lipid metabolism. Having obesity can cause different metabolic issues that harm the organs and help diseases develop further. Lipid metabolism and obesity are connected through many factors, for example, inflammation and hormonal changes. When obesity leads to chronic inflammation, it can upset the balance of fats in the body, which may result in a higher chance of getting MS and heart disease. It is important to know these mechanisms to create therapies that treat both obesity and its related metabolic issues. Research efforts are now focusing on identifying specific lipidomic profiles that could serve as biomarkers for evaluating metabolic health and guiding therapeutic strategies for obesity-related disorders (Keller et al., 2019). The use of lipid metabolism research in healthcare is important for encouraging healthy living and better patient outcomes. Studies have revealed that unsaturated fats are good for metabolic health, but eating too many saturated fats can cause problems with lipid balance and health. Studies that are just coming out are stressing the need for better sleep routines and more physical activity, as they are being recognized as important for improving lipid metabolism. For instance, interventions aimed at addressing sleep quality and circadian disruptions have been shown to positively affect metabolic health, further underscoring the multifaceted nature of lipid metabolism (Arble et al., 2015). When we know more about these connections, public health measures can be introduced to help people maintain a healthy lipid profile and enjoy better health.

6.1. Types of Lipids

Learning Outcome

1. Describe the role of fatty acids in lipid metabolism;
2. Describe the role of triglycerides in lipid metabolism;
3 Understand the phospholipids.

It is important to classify lipids to understand their many roles in the body, mainly in the process of lipid metabolism. Lipids are usually divided into TGs, phospholipids, and sterols, and each type has its own function. Adipose tissue mostly stores energy in the form of TGs, which are made of glycerol and three fatty acids. The process of hydrolysis in their metabolism results in FFAs that are then used in β-oxidation for creating energy. Phospholipids are important for cell membranes because their hydrophilic head helps the membrane function, while the two hydrophobic tails make the membrane flexible. Lipids and proteins, especially phospholipids, play an important role in controlling the body's metabolism and keeping cells intact. Another major group of lipids is sterols, and cholesterol, one of them, helps keep cell membranes strong and functional. It is not only a part of cell structures; it also helps form steroid hormones and bile acids. Cholesterol is metabolized using various pathways, like making it from scratch and absorbing it from food, and this process is strictly controlled to avoid hyperlipidemia. It is interesting that lipids can alter the clumping of proteins, and this is especially true for α-synuclein, which has a unique link with lipids that impacts both lipid processing and signaling in cells. Because of this relationship, we see that sterols and other lipids have a key role in keeping metabolism steady and signaling in cells. It is important to know about lipids when dealing with metabolic diseases and their treatments. In particular, lipids are important for energy, movement of cells, and communication, not just for their structure. It seems that lipids and their complexes may have been key in the beginning of life, as new research shows their structure helped form important functions needed for biological evolution. The article states that amphiphiles can explain how lipid assemblies could have helped early life organisms form compartments and process information. Continued exploration of lipid types and their functions will advance our understanding of metabolic pathways and their implications for health and disease, potentially revealing novel avenues for intervention in metabolic disorders (Alza et al., 2019; Kahana et al., 2019) (Figure 6.3).

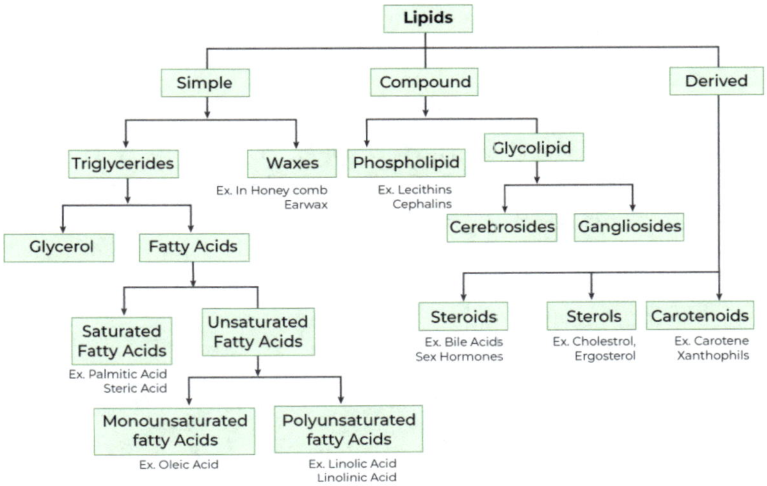

Figure 6.3. Classification of lipids.

Source: https://media.geeksforgeeks.org/wp-content/uploads/20230328093528/Classification-of-Lipids.png.

6.1.1. Fatty Acids

Fatty acids are important in lipid metabolism because they give energy and also affect metabolic pathways. There are saturated and unsaturated fatty acids, and each one has a unique role in the body. Monounsaturated and polyunsaturated fatty acids are helpful for the heart and for the way the body uses insulin. Too many saturated fatty acids can also result in insulin resistance and metabolic problems, showing that lipid metabolism needs to be well-balanced. This balance is further demonstrated by the interplay between fatty acids and glucose metabolism, where elevated fatty acids inhibit glucose oxidation, potentially leading to metabolic disorders when homeostasis is disrupted, as proposed by the glucose-fatty acid cycle introduced by Randle in 1963 (Dulloo et al., 2005). Emerging research highlights the dynamic relationship between FFAs and hormonal mediators like fibroblast growth factor 21 (FGF-21), which significantly influence metabolic outcomes. FGF-21 is now a key subject in exploring how lipids are handled by the body, especially when people are fasting or obese. It is shown that certain FFAs promote the secretion of FGF-21 in a peroxisome proliferator-activated receptor (PPAR)-dependent manner, effectively linking fatty acid levels to enhanced metabolic regulation. For instance, oleate and linoleate seem to boost FGF-21 levels, suggesting that some fatty acids are involved in regulating metabolism, but palmitate does not have the same outcome. This signaling mechanism affirms the importance of fatty acids in not just energy provision but also metabolic regulation, which could further elucidate strategies for managing insulin sensitivity and obesity (Pfeiffer et al., 2009). Fatty acid metabolism is important in clinical practice, mainly for treating metabolic diseases. Exploring the way fatty acids affect different metabolic pathways can give us ideas for treating type 2 diabetes and insulin resistance. Since FGF-21 levels increase when insulin is high, it shows that targeting lipid metabolism could be effective in treating diseases. Moreover, thanks to drugs that influence PPAR activity, it is now possible to use this knowledge to improve cholesterol and boost metabolic health. Therefore, more research on fatty acid metabolism is helping us understand lipids and their effects on health and disease (Figure 6.4).

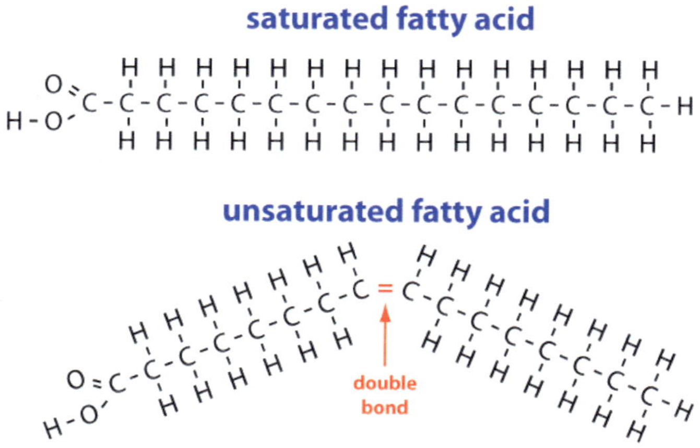

Figure 6.4. Fatty acids.

Source: https://www.creative-proteomics.com/blog/wp-content/uploads/2018/10/fatty-acids-0.png.

6.1.2. Triglycerides (TGs)

Triglycerides (TGs), which are the main type of fat in our bodies, help supply the body with energy and play a significant part in lipid metabolism. Made of glycerol and three fatty acids, TGs are kept in adipose tissue and sent into the bloodstream when required for energy. With the help of lipases, they are hydrolyzed into FFAs and glycerol that can be used by different tissues. A high or low level of TGs is often linked to metabolic disorders, especially when people eat a lot of fat and do not exercise. The consequences of elevated triglyceride levels can be severe, leading to conditions like CVD and Type 2 Diabetes Mellitus (T2DM), highlighting the importance of maintaining healthy triglyceride levels as part of overall metabolic health. Insulin and glucagon, two hormones, are responsible for making sure the body balances the processes of creating and breaking down TGs. High insulin levels cause TGs to be formed, while glucagon breaks them down to supply energy. In insulin resistance, high levels of insulin do not work properly to reduce lipolysis, which causes too much triglyceride to build up. An excess of TGs leads to lipotoxicity, which causes insulin resistance and adds to other metabolic problems, so it is a serious concern for public health. Certain pathways, such as the mTORC1 signaling pathway, have been identified as critical in understanding how triglyceride metabolism becomes dysregulated in the context of obesity and diabetes, offering potential targets for therapeutic intervention (Thimmiah et al., 2016). Other than hormones, external factors such as glucocorticoids have a big impact on triglyceride metabolism. Long-term use of glucocorticoids such as dexamethasone causes hypertriglyceridemia and hepatic steatosis, both resulting from too many TGs in the liver. Angptl4 is responsible for helping lipids be made and stored when glucocorticoids are involved. It has been found that blocking some enzymes can affect the influence of glucocorticoids on TGs, which might help in finding treatments for MS. Understanding the pathways involved in triglyceride regulation, particularly those linked to glucocorticoid signaling, is essential for developing strategies to combat lipid disorders and their associated health risks (Cheang et al., 2019) (Figure 6.5).

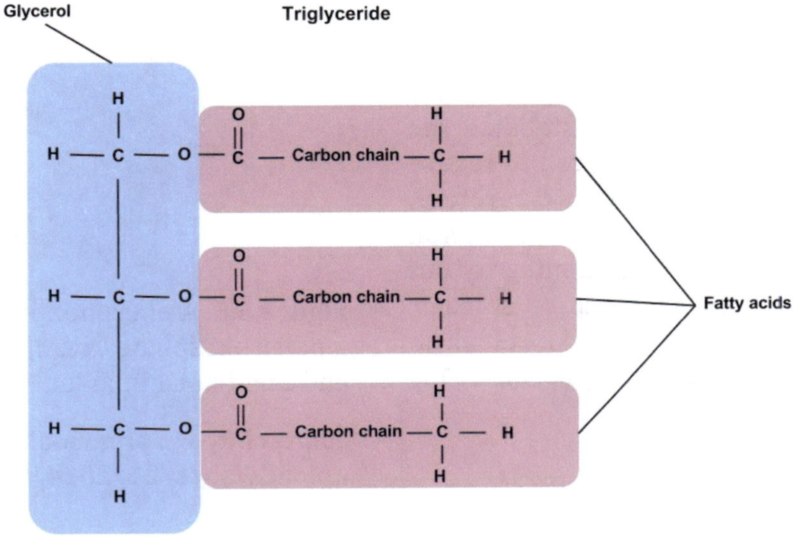

Figure 6.5. The chemical structure of a triglyceride, showing the glycerol backbone and three attached fatty acids.

Source: https://pressbooks.library.vcu.edu/app/uploads/sites/21/2024/07/image4-3.jpg.

6.1.3. Phospholipids

Phospholipids are important for cell structure and function since they are major parts of cell membranes. The way they are built, having a water-loving head and water-repelling tails, helps them form bilayers that stop ions and polar molecules from entering the cell, maintaining its structure. As well as being important for structure, phospholipids affect the flexibility of the membrane and how other molecules and proteins interact there. Because bilayers are dynamic, they help cells carry out important processes such as responding to changes in the environment. As phospholipids are involved in many biochemical reactions, they also help produce signaling molecules, proving their role in both supporting a cell's structure and sending messages to other cells. The pathways involving phospholipids are important and play a key role in many biological activities. The process of making phospholipids begins by adding fatty acids to glycerol or sphingosine, after which more reactions occur. Because of metabolic flexibility, cells can respond to different needs in the body, for example, during stress or when receiving signaling molecules. Besides, phospholipids can be used to make bioactive molecules, such as eicosanoids, which are important for controlling inflammation and immune reactions. How phospholipids are arranged in cell membranes affects the cell's responses and the overall health of the organism, which shows why their metabolism needs to be studied for more than just their structure. Besides, phospholipids' involvement in oxidative stress demonstrates their significant role in keeping cells healthy. As lipid components, phospholipids are susceptible to oxidative damage by reactive oxygen species (ROS), which can lead to alterations in membrane integrity and function. Because phospholipids have polyunsaturated fatty acids, they are easily affected by oxidative changes. Oxidative stress is connected to many neurodegenerative conditions, showing that proper phospholipid levels are important for cell health. Phospholipids help stabilize the membrane and signal inside the cell to reduce the effects of oxidative stress. Therefore, phospholipid metabolism and its regulation are pivotal not only for structural integrity but also for the prevention of oxidative damage, reinforcing their significance in lipid metabolism as a whole (Carla et al., 2018; Singh et al., 2019) (Figure 6.6).

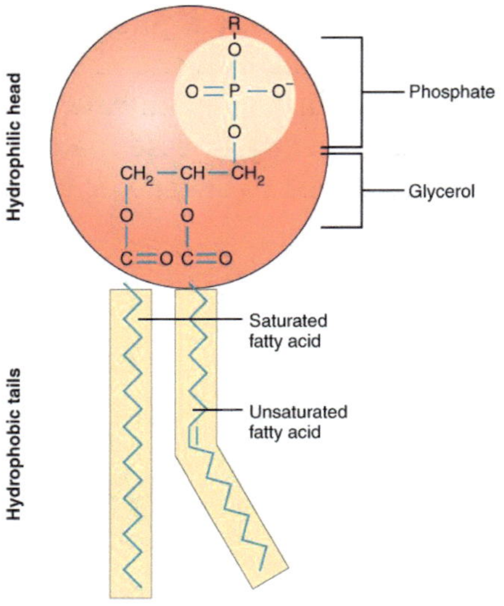

Figure 6.6. A phospholipid molecule consists of a polar phosphate "head," which is hydrophilic, and a non-polar lipid "tail," which is hydrophobic.

Source: https://pressbooks.library.vcu.edu/app/uploads/sites/21/2024/07/image7.jpg.

Test Your Knowledge

1. What is the role of fatty acids in lipid metabolism?
2. What are the phospholipids?

6.2. Digestion and Absorption of Lipids

Learning Outcome

1. Understand the role of bile salts;
2. Describe the enzymatic breakdown of lipids;
3. Know the process of absorption in the intestinal mucosa.

The process starts in the mouth and is mostly finished in the small intestine. In the beginning, bile salts help to break down dietary fats, which allows pancreatic lipases to break TGs into FFAs and monoglycerides. The process happens in the intestine, where emulsification increases the amount of lipid surface, allowing enzymes to reach it more easily. Once hydrolysis is finished, the fatty acids and monoglycerides combine with bile salts to form micelles that help carry them across the watery interior of the intestine to the intestinal lining. This important process helps prepare lipids for absorption, which is important for maintaining energy balance and getting needed fatty acids. At the point of enterocytes, absorption works by allowing lipid components to diffuse and also by using specific proteins that move fatty acids. Within the enterocytes, fatty acids and monoglycerides are reformed into TGs and then wrapped up in chylomicrons so they can be carried by the lymphatic system into the bloodstream. The cell's condition and proper functioning play a major role in how fats are reassembled inside the cell. The dependency on efficient lipoprotein synthesis highlights the metabolic interplay between lipid absorption and overall metabolic health, as disruptions can lead to impaired lipid transport, which is especially detrimental in conditions like cystic fibrosis, where fat malabsorption is a common complication that affects nutritional status and quality of life (Drouin et al., 2005). In addition, when you eat, lipids may be important for their metabolism, according to studies that point to the effects of circadian rhythms on lipid processing. Studies have shown that optimal timing of lipid consumption, particularly during the biological morning or around noon, aligns with metabolic peaks for insulin sensitivity and glucose tolerance (Jamshed et al., 2018). Interrupting the normal circadian rhythms can result in more risk factors for metabolic disorders, so it is important to study how both timing and the body's processes affect lipid absorption and metabolism. As a result, paying attention to both the biochemical steps and the timing of eating lipids can guide dietary advice that helps improve metabolism and avoid different metabolic diseases (Figure 6.7).

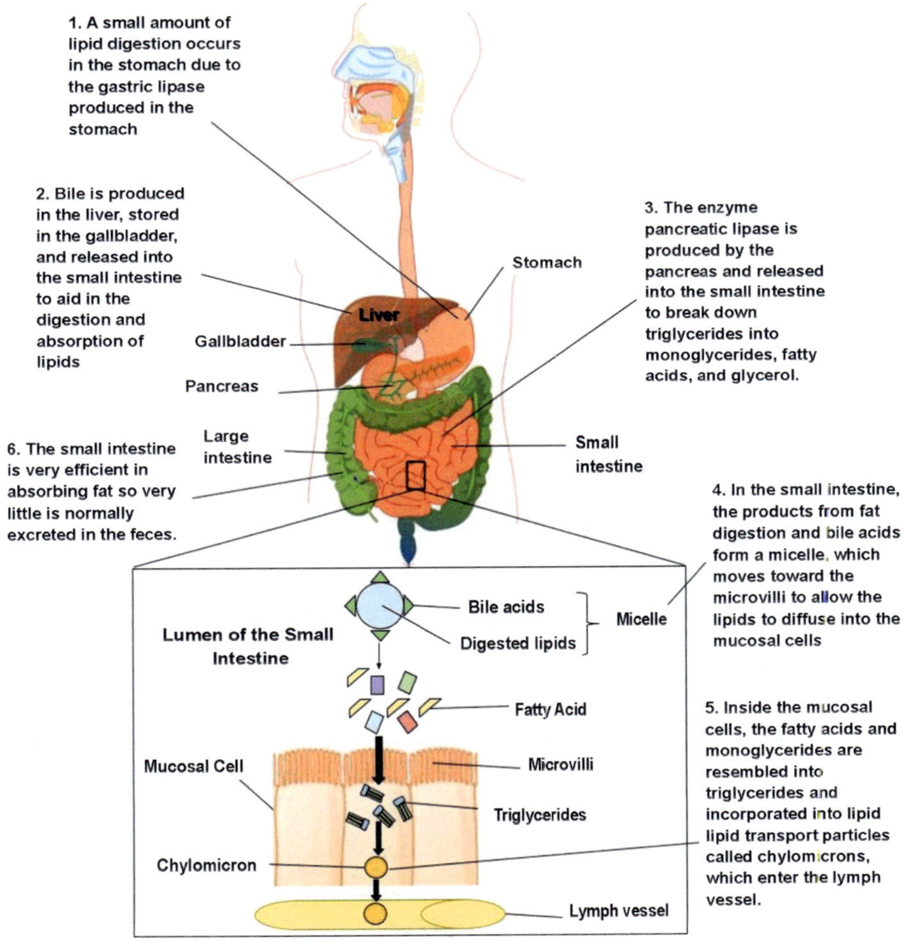

Figure 6.7. Lipid digestion and absorption.

Source: https://pressbooks-dev.oer.hawaii.edu/humannutrition/wp-content/uploads/sites/10/2017/12/Lipid-Digestion-and-absorption-1024x1014.jpg.

6.2.1. Role of Bile Salts

Bile salts are very important in helping the body digest and absorb fats from food. After being produced from cholesterol in the liver, these amphipathic molecules are stored in the gallbladder and take part in breaking up fats in the small intestine. As soon as you eat food with lipids, bile salts are sent into the intestine to break up the fat globules into micelles, making it easier for lipase enzymes to work on them. This process is crucial not only for the absorption of fatty acids and monoglycerides but also for the uptake of fat-soluble vitamins (A, D, E, and K). The close connection between bile salts and dietary lipids proves how important they are for lipid metabolism and general nutrition. Besides, bile salts help to signal and regulate different metabolic pathways that are needed for homeostasis.

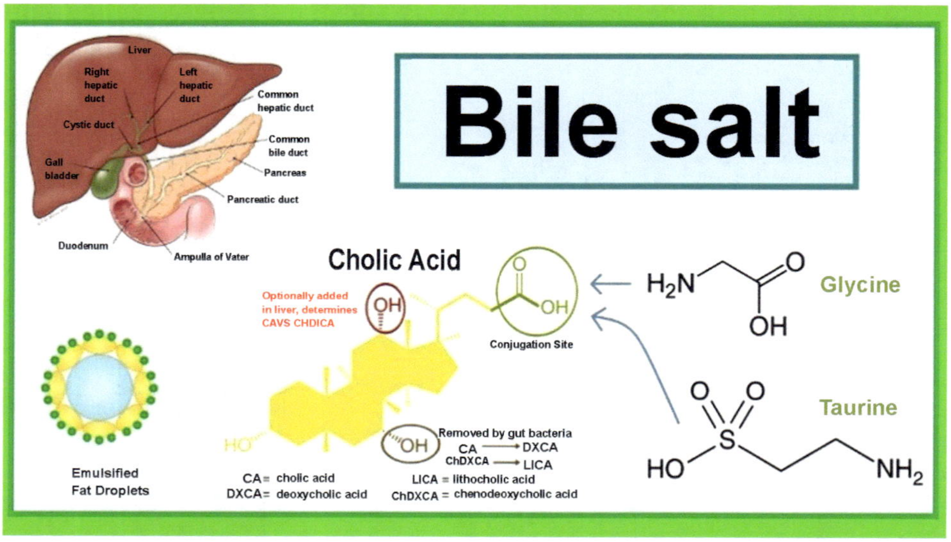

Figure 6.8. Bile salt.

Source: https://i.ytimg.com/vi/87oc75uQ-U4/maxresdefault.jpg.

They exert their effects primarily through activation of specialized receptors such as the farnesoid X receptor (FXR) and Takeda G protein-coupled receptor 5 (TGR5), which are critically involved in lipid and glucose metabolism. When these receptors bind with ligands, it starts a series of events that make the body more sensitive to insulin, burn more energy, and lessen inflammation, which all benefit metabolic health. It has been found that problems in bile salt signaling are involved in the development of obesity and type 2 diabetes. This emerging understanding highlights the complexity of bile salts as multifaceted agents beyond mere digestive facilitators, revealing their extensive influence on metabolic pathways that govern lipid homeostasis in the body (Choucair et al., 2019). Bile salts also play a part in lipid metabolism because they interact with the gut microbiota. Studies done recently prove that gut bacteria can transform primary bile acids into a range of secondary metabolites that can change how metabolic processes work. Such changes in bile salts can influence how well they signal and affect the body's lipid metabolism. Some bacteria may increase or decrease the production of bile acid metabolites, which can change or influence how the body handles obesity and similar diseases, showing that the gut microbiota and host metabolism are related. With more research, the relationship between bile salts, gut bacteria, and lipid metabolism creates new possibilities for treating metabolic diseases. Understanding this relationship may be key to leveraging bile salts in clinical settings for improved metabolic health and disease management (Willem et al., 2022) (Figure 6.8).

6.2.2. Enzymatic Breakdown by Lipases

Most of the breakdown of lipids in the body is carried out by lipases, which is very important for lipid metabolism. Lipases help to break down ester bonds in TGs, phospholipids, and cholesterol esters, which causes fatty acids and glycerol to be released. This is important since FFAs provide energy to different tissues, mainly during fasting or when doing strenuous exercise. In the digestive process, pancreatic lipases are sent to the intestine, where they work on dietary fats. Bile acids help the enzymes by emulsifying lipids, which increases their surface area and makes it easier for lipases to work well. Because of this, the substances produced by lipolysis are taken up by enterocytes and packaged in chylomicrons for transportation through the lymphatic system to different tissues. Lipase activity is controlled in a complicated manner by hormones and different body states. For example, insulin is important for stopping lipolysis in adipose tissue, which is vital for energy balance. During states of energy deprivation, hormones like glucagon and epinephrine stimulate the activity of hormone-sensitive lipase (HSL), promoting the release of fatty acids into the bloodstream. Also, lipases are flexible in the way they function; each isoform is expressed and controlled differently in different tissues. Because of this, lipid metabolism can be carefully managed depending on how much energy the body needs. In pathological conditions, such as Type 2 Diabetes Mellitus, abnormalities in lipid metabolism can occur due to impaired lipase function, leading to dysregulated fatty acid release and consequent metabolic disturbances (Galicia-Garc et al., 2020). There is also evidence that lipase activity and immune cells, mainly macrophages, play a role in dealing with inflammation and metabolic diseases. Macrophages can change their metabolism depending on their surroundings, showing that they can be M1 or M2. While responding to inflammation, M1 macrophages use glycolysis and change their lipid metabolism to help promote inflammation. Conversely, M2 macrophages, which are involved in tissue repair and resolution of inflammation, exhibit a greater dependence on oxidative phosphorylation and possess intact tricarboxylic acid (TCA) cycles for efficient ATP production (Viola et al., 2019). It demonstrates that lipases affect both energy use and immune responses, so they might be useful targets for treating diseases with inflammation and problems in lipid metabolism.

6.2.3. Absorption in the Intestinal Mucosa

For lipid metabolism to work well, dietary fats, their breakdown by-products, and other important nutrients must be absorbed in the intestinal mucosa. The specialized cells of the mucosa help with the movement of fatty acids and monoglycerides from the digestive process. Bile salts first mix these lipids in the small intestine, which makes it possible for more digestive enzymes to act on them. When hydrolysis is finished, FFAs move into the enterocytes by either diffusion or the action of transport proteins. The nutrients in the diet can impact the process of absorption and the metabolic reactions that take place in the mucosal cells, showing that what we eat can control lipid metabolism. In addition, intestinal epithelial cells are not just present in the process; they actively react to different nutrients. Factors such as the presence of SCFAs and other metabolic byproducts significantly influence gene expression in the intestinal mucosa. In particular, the diet can change the activity of genes that control important proteins for digestion and absorption, which enhances how the body deals with lipids. According to research, when feed intake goes down after weaning, it can negatively influence the expression of these genes and result in problems with absorption and metabolism. These observations underscore the possibility that appropriate dietary interventions could enhance mucosal function, thereby improving lipid metabolism and overall gut health, especially in developmental phases like weaning and adaptation to solid diets (Bauer et al., 2011). In addition, the makeup of gut microbiota supports the body's processes for absorbing and metabolizing lipids. A well-balanced microbiota helps break down lipids and release more fatty acids into the body, which are then taken up by the intestine. Thanks to this relationship, the gut ecosystem is healthy because good bacteria outnumber the harmful ones. When microbes ferment what has not been absorbed from the diet, they make SCFAs that positively affect the health of the digestive system and metabolism. The gut barrier is kept intact by the action of microbes, but if there is dysbiosis, it can cause problems with absorption and increase inflammation in the body. Consequently, understanding the interplay between mucosal absorption, dietary composition, and gut microbiota becomes essential in formulating dietary strategies aimed at enhancing lipid metabolism and preventing related disorders (Meheust et al., 2010) (Figure 6.9).

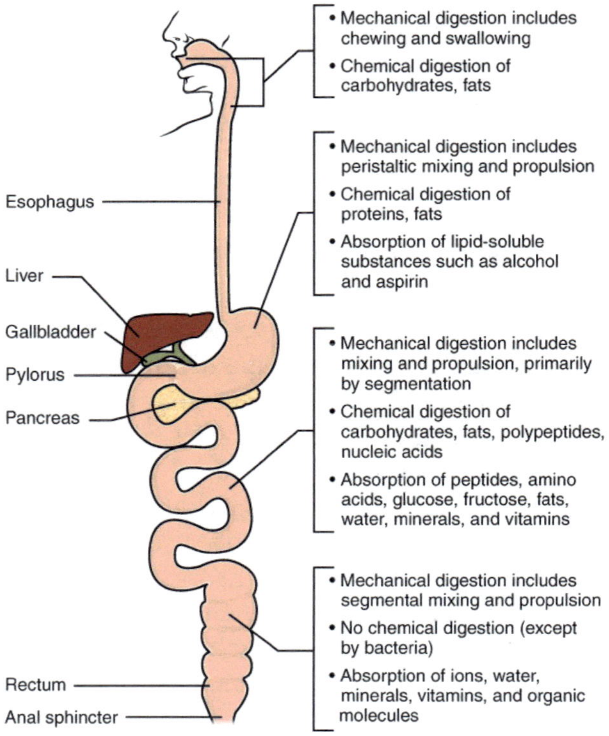

Figure 6.9. Digestion begins in the mouth and continues as food travels through the small intestine. Most absorption occurs in the small intestine.

Source: https://s3-us-west-2.amazonaws.com/courses-images-archive-read-only/wp-content/uploads/sites/403/2015/04/21031749/2426_Mechanical_and_Chemical_DigestionN.jpg.

Test Your Knowledge

1. What is the role of bile salts?
2. What is the process of absorption in the intestinal mucosa?

6.3. Transport of Lipids in the Body

Learning Outcome

1. Learn about chylomicrons and lipoproteins;
2. Describe the role of the lymphatic system in lipid metabolism;
3. Understand the transport of lipids in the bloodstream.

The movement of lipids in the body is important for lipid metabolism since it helps distribute important fatty acids and cholesterol to different tissues. TGs and phospholipids, which are types of lipids, are put into lipoproteins for delivery through the blood. First, the intestine absorbs dietary fats and mixes them with bile salts. Then, enterocytes take in the fats. In the enterocytes, TGs are put back together and team up with proteins to create chylomicrons, which are the biggest lipoproteins. First, chylomicrons go into the lymphatic system and then enter the bloodstream to bring lipids to the tissues around the body. It makes sure that the important energy and building materials are sent in the right amounts to the organs and cells. Once lipids are released into the bloodstream, their transport is further regulated by various lipoproteins, including very low-density lipoproteins (VLDL), LDL, and high-density lipoproteins (HDL). They all have a special function in managing and transporting lipids in the body.

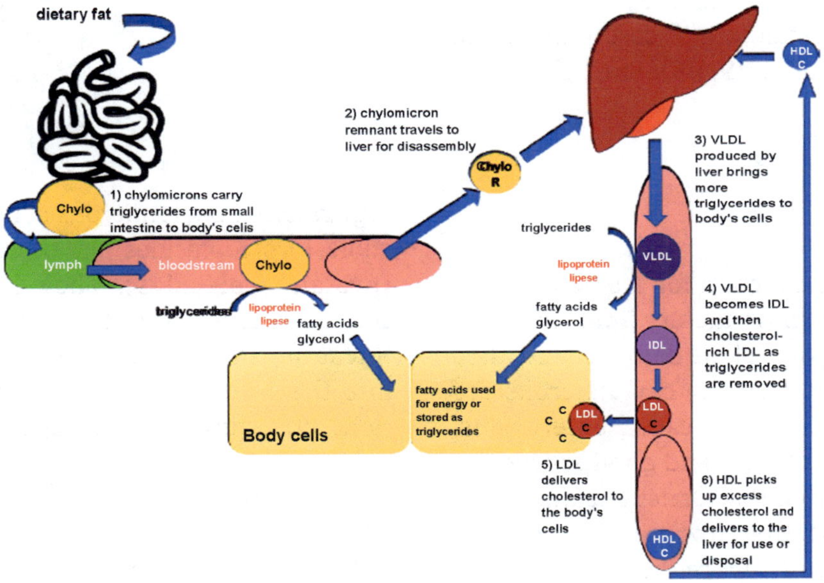

Figure 6.10. Overview of lipoprotein functions in the body.

Source: https://openoregon.pressbooks.pub/app/uploads/sites/98/2019/10/image2-3.png.

As an example, VLDLs carry TGs from the liver to adipose and muscle tissues, which may either make use of them for energy or keep them for later storage. While LDLs are known as bad cholesterol since they transport cholesterol to cells, an excess of LDLs may result in atherosclerosis and CVD. HDLs are referred to as good cholesterol since they carry cholesterol from the body's tissues to the liver for elimination or reuse. Having the right balance of lipoproteins is necessary to keep homeostasis and prevent diseases related to lipids. Peroxisomes are important in lipid transport as they take part in oxidizing fatty acids and making new lipids. It has been found by recent research that peroxisomes take part in lipid metabolism in adipocytes, which are important for energy storage and controlling metabolic processes. Peroxisomes not only facilitate the breakdown of very long-chain fatty acids but also play a significant role in managing oxidative stress by producing and detoxifying ROS and reactive nitrogen species (RNS). The maintenance of redox balance by peroxisomes is key to proper fat cell metabolism and fat cell development, which affects the whole process of lipid transport in the body. Understanding these mechanisms can inform potential therapeutic approaches for metabolic diseases linked to dysfunctions in lipid transport and peroxisomal activity, thereby contributing to a broader understanding of cardiometabolic health (Argano et al., 2019; Klein et al., 2019) (Figure 6.10).

6.3.1. Chylomicrons and Lipoproteins

Chylomicrons are important for the body's lipid metabolism as they move dietary lipids from the intestines to other parts of the body. Because they are the biggest lipoproteins, chylomicrons are produced in intestinal cells called enterocytes, where TGs, phospholipids, and apolipoproteins are combined in the endoplasmic reticulum (ER). After being put together, lipoproteins are sent to the Golgi apparatus, where they are prepared and discharged into the lymphatic system, later reaching the bloodstream. Chylomicrons are essential since they distribute lipids well and help with both energy storage and the delivery of vitamins that need fat to be absorbed. Once chylomicrons are in circulation, they interact with various enzymes, specifically lipoprotein lipase (LPL), which plays a pivotal role in hydrolyzing TGs into FFAs. It is necessary for tissues such as muscle and adipose tissue to use fats, as fatty acids are either burned for energy or stored again. The way chylomicrons and LPL interact points out that lipoprotein metabolism should be regulated, as unbalanced lipids can cause hyperlipidemia. Furthermore, genetic mutations affecting proteins involved in chylomicron metabolism can lead to inherited disorders, emphasizing the complexity of lipid transport and the consequences of its dysregulation in human health (AlSulaiman et al., 2017).

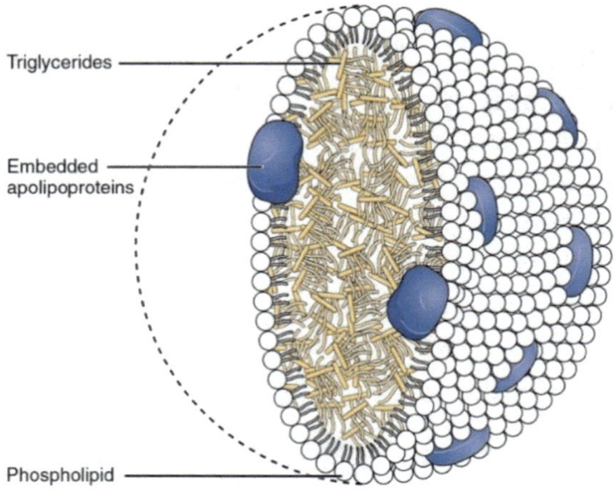

Figure 6.11. Chylomicrons contain triglycerides, cholesterol molecules, and other apolipoproteins (protein molecules). They function to carry these water-insoluble molecules from the intestine, through the lymphatic system, and into the bloodstream, which carries the lipids to adipose tissue for storage.

Source: https://s3-us-west-2.amazonaws.com/courses-images-archive-read-only/wp-content/uploads/sites/403/2015/04/21031804/2512_Chylomicrons_Contain_Triglycerides_Cholesterol_Molecules_and_Other_Lipids.jpg.

The broader family of lipoproteins, which includes VLDL and LDL, is intricately linked to the action and fate of chylomicrons. Even though both chylomicrons and VLDL are involved in moving TGs, they are produced differently and follow different routes in the body. While chylomicrons bring dietary fats to the body,

VLDL carries lipids made in the liver to other parts of the body. For lipid homeostasis to be maintained, the different lipoprotein classes have to interact in the body. Research also suggests that statins help lower cholesterol and may also help prevent ischemic events in patients with high cholesterol. Such findings underscore the intricacy of lipid metabolism and the implications of lipoproteins in cardiovascular health (AlSulaiman et al., 2017) (Figure 6.11).

6.3.2. Role of the Lymphatic System

The lymphatic system is very important for lipid metabolism since it helps absorb and transport the lipids found in foods. Because of the detailed design of lymphatic vessels, especially the lacteals in the intestinal villi, chylomicrons can move lipids from the intestine into the blood. As chylomicrons move into the lymphatic system, they go through several transformations before entering the bloodstream, so that lipids are used properly by the body. Recent advances in understanding the molecular mediators that regulate lymphatic endothelial cell function have highlighted the importance of the lymphatic system in maintaining lipid homeostasis and its implications in metabolic disorders, thus emphasizing its role as a critical player in lipid metabolism overall (Cifarelli & Eichmann, 2019).

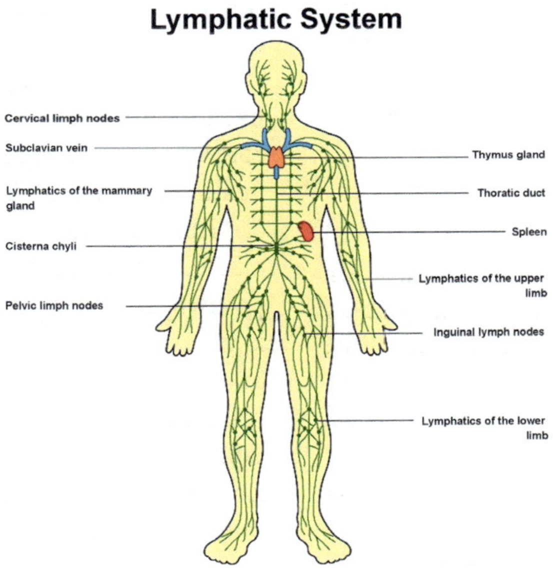

Figure 6.12. Lymphatic system.

Source: https://images.squarespace-cdn.com/content/v1/57853f211b631b3aa7b0053d/43407423-2d0c-4f7a-a2e4-9820000c8992/Acupuncture+Rochester+NY+Lymphatic+2-min.jpeg.

Besides, the lymphatic system helps with immune responses and fluid balance, both of which are important in lipid metabolism. The lymphatic vessels and the immune system communicate, so that immune cells can react to dietary lipids by adjusting their functions. In addition, the lymphatic system helps get rid of interstitial fluid, which stops the buildup of too many lipids and prevents lipotoxicity, which is related to obesity and MS. By ensuring that dietary lipids are efficiently transported and removing excess interstitial fluid, the lymphatic system supports not only metabolic health but also overall physiological balance (Custodis et al., 2019). Moreover, research into the regulatory mechanisms of the lymphatic system has revealed the critical role of vascular endothelial growth factors (VEGFs) in promoting lymphatic vessel growth and function. They take part in controlling the movement of chylomicrons into lymphatic vessels and also affect the organization and efficiency of the lymphatic system. Understanding these pathways provides a chance to develop treatments that help the lymphatic system in people with metabolic disorders. Since the lymphatic system is now seen to play a key part in lipid metabolism, it is important to study its effects on health and disease. This body of knowledge not only broadens our understanding of lipid metabolism but also identifies potential targets for enhancing metabolic health and managing related diseases (Cifarelli & Eichmann, 2019) (Figure 6.12).

6.3.3. Lipid Transport in the Bloodstream

Moving lipids in the blood is necessary for lipid metabolism, since it distributes fatty acids and other lipids to different parts of the body. Since lipids are not water-soluble, they need particular methods to be transported in blood plasma. Lipids are mainly carried in the body by lipoproteins, which are made from both lipids and proteins. The particles are not all the same; they differ in density and size and each one has a special purpose in lipid delivery. For instance, chylomicrons are responsible for transporting dietary TGs from the intestines to peripheral tissues, while LDL facilitate the delivery of cholesterol. The dynamic interplay of these lipoprotein classes is essential for maintaining lipid homeostasis, with disruptions leading to conditions such as hyperlipidemia, insulin resistance, and metabolic disorders noted in contemporary populations (Beard et al., 2018).

When someone eats a high-fat diet, the increased FFAs in their blood worsen the problem of lipid transport and metabolism. When these fatty acids are present in high amounts, they may disrupt the functions of cells in muscles and fat, which causes insulin resistance and increases the risk of type 2 diabetes and similar metabolic problems. How much fat the body takes in is very important for its metabolic functions. It has been found that the way fatty acids are used in the body depends on their transport, which may be changed by the lipid composition and the levels of lipids in the blood. Understanding these dynamics offers insight into how chronic overconsumption of fats disturbs energy regulation and promotes pathological states, highlighting the critical role of lipid transport in sustaining metabolic health (Beard et al., 2018). The liver is important for lipid metabolism since it keeps lipids and also controls their movement through different pathways. Dealing with excess lipids in the liver is greatly helped by the cellular process known as autophagy. It affects the buildup of fat, the breakdown of fats, and the production of bile, which supports the body's metabolic stability. According to research, hepatic autophagy plays a protective role in MS by controlling the body's lipid levels and making sure lipids are transported properly in the bloodstream. In addition, hepatic autophagy is important for lipid transport and metabolism because it affects not only the liver but also other tissues, like skeletal muscle.

Test Your Knowledge

1. What is the role of the lymphatic system in lipid metabolism?
2. What transports lipids in the bloodstream?

6.4. Beta-Oxidation of Fatty Acids

Learning Outcome

1. Know the process of fatty acid activation;
2. Describe the mitochondrial transport of fatty acids;
3. Understand the energy production from beta-oxidation.

The process of beta-oxidation of fatty acids is pivotal in lipid metabolism, serving as the primary mechanism through which fatty acids are catabolized to generate ATP. The process happens inside mitochondria, where fatty acids are split into acetyl-CoA, each having two carbon atoms. Every cycle of beta-oxidation includes four steps, and each step shortens the acyl-CoA chain and creates reduced cofactors, FADH2 and NADH. After that, the cofactors are used in the electron transport chain to boost the production of ATP by oxidative phosphorylation. In addition, beta-oxidation is regulated by the presence of substrates and the cell's energy demands, which demonstrates its key role in keeping the cell balanced and providing enough energy. Apart from helping with energy production, beta-oxidation is involved in different metabolic problems and issues. For example, having too many fatty acids in the body can result in lipotoxicity, which means the extra compounds harm the function of cells, especially those in the pancreatic beta cells. Exposure to fatty acids for a long time can lead to insulin problems and promote cell death, emphasizing the strong link between beta-oxidation and the body's metabolism. Enhanced activity of peroxisome proliferator-activated receptor alpha (PPARα) has been proposed to mitigate these adverse effects by promoting fatty acid oxidation and maintaining glucose homeostasis.

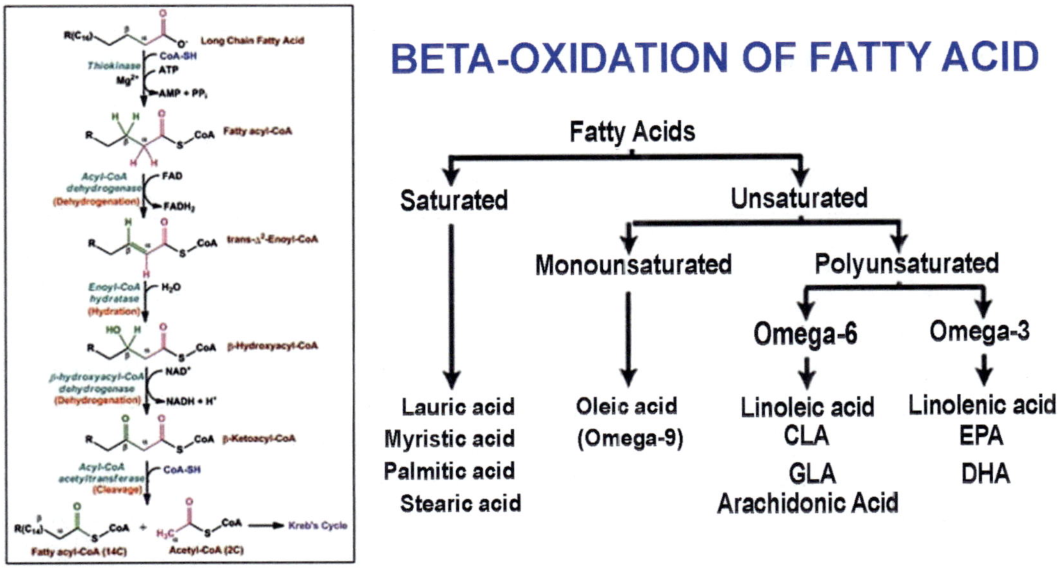

Figure 6.13. Beta-oxidation of fatty acid.

Source: https://microbenotes.com/wp-content/uploads/2018/08/Beta-oxidation-of-Fatty-Acid.jpg.

By regulating critical metabolic pathways, PPARα acts as a guardian against the detrimental outcomes associated with lipid accumulation, thereby highlighting the importance of effective beta-oxidation in preventing metabolic diseases like type 2 diabetes (Bartley et al., 2018). The relationship between beta-oxidation and various liver conditions, particularly nonalcoholic fatty liver disease (NAFLD), further underscores the significance of this metabolic pathway in overall health. Because obesity is becoming more common around the world, the number of people with NAFLD is also increasing, as this condition can lead to cirrhosis or hepatocellular carcinoma. As a result, when beta-oxidation is impaired and there is more triglyceride in the liver, insulin resistance appears, which then causes more lipid to build up and harm the liver. When there is too much fat in the liver and oxidative stress, it becomes clear that good fatty acid metabolism is necessary to avoid liver-related diseases. Addressing these imbalances through targeted metabolic interventions may offer therapeutic avenues to combat the metabolic consequences of obesity and associated liver diseases, thereby emphasizing the importance of beta-oxidation in lipid metabolism (Perla et al., 2017) (Figure 6.13).

6.4.1. Process of Fatty Acid Activation

Activating fatty acids is necessary for their use as energy or as parts of cell membranes. Cytoplasm is the main location where FFAs are changed into acyl-CoA derivatives by acyl-CoA synthetases. To do this, ATP is consumed and is converted into AMP and pyrophosphate, which helps coenzyme A attach to the fatty acid. Fatty acids must first be converted to acyl-CoA to be able to get into the mitochondria for β-oxidation.

Besides, acyl-CoA helps to control and coordinate many metabolic and cellular processes, which shows its role in both energy production and in managing cells. The following major step after activating fatty acids is to move acyl-CoA into mitochondria, where fatty acids are broken down by β-oxidation. The carnitine shuttle system makes sure that the mitochondrial matrix receives long-chain fatty acids from the cytoplasm.

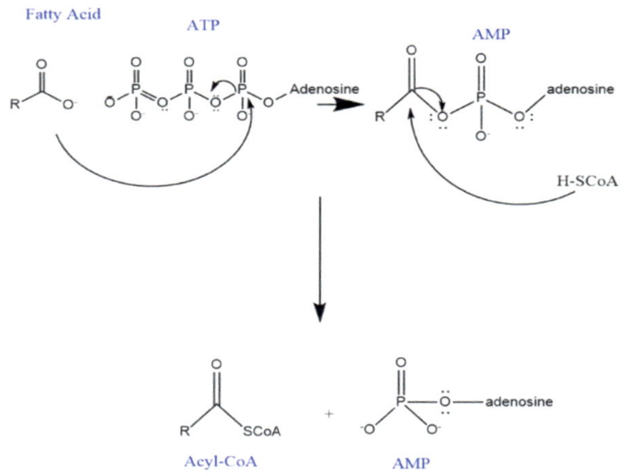

Figure 6.14. Activation of fatty acids through coenzyme A.

Source: https://chemistrytalk.org/wp-content/uploads/2023/10/image-5.png.

The enzyme carnitine palmitoyl transferase I (CPT I) is responsible for converting acyl-CoA to acylcarnitine, allowing it to pass through the mitochondrial membrane. Once inside the matrix, acylcarnitine is reconverted back to acyl-CoA by carnitine palmitoyl transferase II (CPT II). This mechanism is crucial, especially considering that impaired transport can lead to an accumulation of fatty acids, subsequently contributing to metabolic disorders such as NAFLD, where hepatic lipid accumulation plays a pivotal role in disease progression. For metabolic homeostasis to occur, fatty acids need to be activated and transported properly. Besides, it is essential to regulate fatty acid activation to maintain a proper balance of lipids, especially when people eat a high-fat diet. It has been highlighted by recent studies that the liver's management of fatty acids depends closely on the cytochrome P450 system. When P450 activity is compromised, there's an increased accumulation of unsaturated fatty acids, which can influence metabolic pathways by activating nuclear receptors such as CAR (constitutive androstane receptor) and PXR (pregnane X receptor). As a result, dysfunction in fatty acid activation might lead to hepatic steatosis and help cause other metabolic problems linked to obesity and insulin resistance. Understanding the nuances of this regulatory framework aids in elucidating how altered lipid metabolism can lead to chronic conditions, including NAFLD (Perla et al., 2017) and its subsequent complications (Finn et al., 2008) (Figure 6.14).

6.4.2. Mitochondrial Transport of Fatty Acids

Mitochondrial transport of fatty acids plays an important role in lipid metabolism by affecting energy production and the creation of biomolecules. Fatty acids, used for energy, have to enter the mitochondrial matrix through the membrane to go through β-oxidation. The carnitine shuttle mechanism and other carrier proteins help transport fatty acyl groups into mitochondria so they can be further processed. It has been proven that the way mitochondria change their shape by fusing and dividing plays a key role in fatty acid metabolism. These morphological changes can alter the capacity of mitochondria to accommodate varying levels of lipid substrates, as studies have shown that metabolic cues can regulate mitochondrial dynamics, ultimately affecting the efficiency of substrate transport and utilization (Pearce et al., 2018).

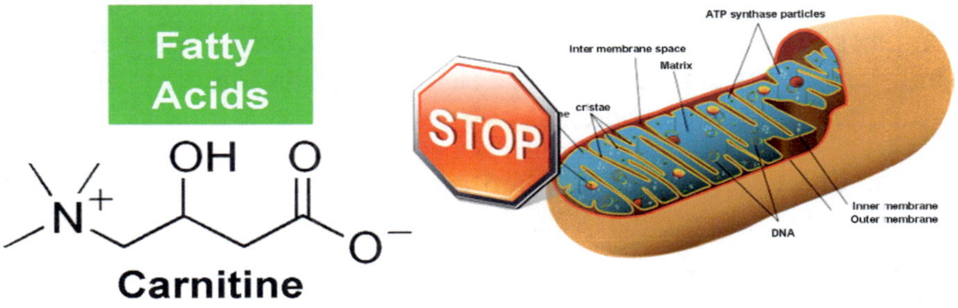

Figure 6.15. Carnitine shuttles fatty acids into the mitochondria.

Source: https://s3-us-west-2.amazonaws.com/courses-images/wp-content/uploads/sites/2569/2017/10/26142746/10000000000000044C000001875F0B71EC.png.

To know how lipids are broken down and how energy-rich molecules are made, we must understand these relationships. As well as physical methods, signaling pathways that control lipid metabolism are important in changing the expression of genes responsible for mitochondrial fatty acid transport. Researchers have found that transcription factors and lipid metabolism genes interact in a complicated way when mice are treated with fenofibrate. This treatment has been observed to upregulate several genes associated with fatty acid transport and β-oxidation, while not significantly altering those involved in fatty acid biosynthesis or the Krebs cycle (Sanoudou et al., 2009). The results point out the detailed systems that oversee mitochondrial actions and underline the importance of fatty acid transport in metabolism. Any problems with this process may result in metabolic disorders, which highlights the need to learn about these pathways in lipid metabolism. Mitochondrial transport of fatty acids is important for keeping the normal functions of the cell. If mitochondrial fatty acid transport is affected, it may lead to problems with energy metabolism, and this can result in obesity, type 2 diabetes, and heart disease. Working on the mechanisms involved in transporting molecules to mitochondria could be a way to improve their function and metabolic health. It is necessary to keep studying the molecular activities in mitochondria, such as the ways different fatty acid types affect their shape and function. By advancing our understanding of the mitochondrial transport of fatty acids, scientists can uncover new strategies for managing lipid metabolism-related diseases and promoting overall metabolic health within diverse populations (Sanoudou et al., 2009; Pearce et al., 2018) (Figure 6.15).

6.4.3. Energy Production from Beta-Oxidation

Among the many processes in lipid metabolism, beta-oxidation is an important way to produce energy. This catabolic pathway facilitates the breakdown of fatty acids into acetyl-CoA units, which subsequently enter the TCA cycle for further energy extraction. The first stage happens in mitochondria, where fatty acids are changed into fatty acyl-CoA with the help of energy. After transport into the mitochondrial matrix through carnitine, beta-oxidation happens in four steps: first, oxidation, then hydration, another oxidation, and finally thiolysis. Beta-oxidation releases a lot of energy mainly as NADH and FADH2, which are important in the electron transport chain and improve the efficiency of lipid energy production. The relationship between energy production from beta-oxidation and metabolic health is increasingly recognized, particularly in the context of diseases such as NAFLD. Accumulation of hepatic TGs, a hallmark of NAFLD, is linked to compromised lipid metabolism that impairs the body's ability to efficiently oxidize fatty acids (Perla et al., 2017). When there is obesity and insulin resistance, the disrupted beta-oxidation may result in more oxidative stress and cause further metabolic problems.

A buildup of FFAs due to less beta-oxidation can both disrupt the body's energy balance and cause liver cells to suffer from lipotoxicity. The relationship between lipid metabolism and energy production calls for more research on how better beta-oxidation could help treat NAFLD and related diseases. Beta-oxidation is also important for cellular reactions to changes in metabolism. Studies in recent times have examined how neurons react to shortages of energy by changing their lipid metabolism. For instance, upon exposure to oxygen glucose deprivation (OGD), a model of metabolic stress, alterations in mitochondrial function and lipid-related proteins were observed, indicating the interconnectedness of energy production and cellular health (Deighton et al., 2013). Beta-oxidation is important in neurodegenerative diseases because poor energy production in neurons is linked to Alzheimer's disease. When energy is needed, efficient beta-oxidation gives neurons the necessary substances, showing its importance for the body and brain. Therefore, knowing about energy production through beta-oxidation is key to dealing with various metabolic and neurological problems in our society.

Test Your Knowledge

1. What is the process of fatty acid activation?
2. What is the energy production of beta-oxidation?

6.5. Lipogenesis

Learning Outcome

1. Know the process of conversion of excess carbohydrates to fat;
2. Describe the role of Acetyl-CoA in lipogenesis;
3. Understand the hormonal regulation of lipogenesis.

Lipogenesis is important for lipid metabolism since it helps the body save energy as fat by converting carbohydrates. Liver and adipose tissues are the main areas where this pathway is active and it is controlled by things like diet and hormones. Insulin, in particular, serves as a powerful initiator of lipogenesis, promoting the expression of enzymes like fatty acid synthase (FASN). It is important to understand lipogenesis to understand normal metabolism and to deal with issues such as obesity and diabetes. With more people consuming high-carbohydrate diets, it becomes clear that lipogenesis is more important, which has led researchers to look for new methods to manage these processes. Recent research reveals that the regulation of *de novo* lipogenesis (DNL) is very complex, and its activity is influenced by the body's nutritional state. It has been noted that there is a lot of interaction between lipid production and the regulation of the sympathetic nervous system in fat cells.

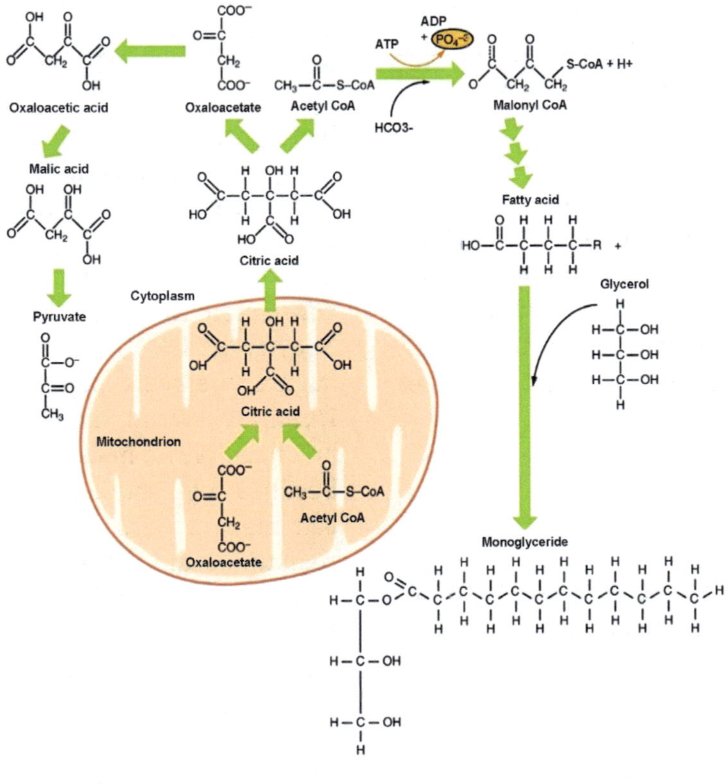

Figure 6.16. Lipids may follow one of several pathways during metabolism. Glycerol and fatty acids follow different pathways.

Source: https://s3-us-west-2.amazonaws.com/courses-images-archive-read-only/wp-content/uploads/sites/403/2015/04/21031811/2516_Lipid_Metabolism.jpg.

In one study, removing FASN from adipocytes boosted glucose tolerance and brought about more beige adipocytes, which are known to have a greater ability to burn energy. The research points out that lipogenesis in white adipose tissue is involved in glucose balance in the body. Particularly, the activation of markers such as uncoupling protein 1 (UCP1) in beige adipocytes reveals a deeper connection between lipid metabolism and the body's ability to maintain energy balance under varying metabolic states (Czech et al., 2017). Looking into how we can manage lipogenesis could result in fresh treatments for metabolic diseases. With the identification of exercise mimetics, the field of metabolic therapy is changing. Resveratrol and AICAR are able to activate the AMPK and SIRT1 pathways, which are usually triggered by physical exercise. Therefore, medicines could be designed to mimic exercise on fat metabolism and help the body use and store fats healthily. As the global prevalence of obesity and related diseases rises, exploiting the mechanisms underlying lipogenesis not only advances our understanding of energy metabolism but also holds promise for innovative treatment strategies to combat these growing health challenges (Handschin et al., 2014) (Figure 6.16).

6.5.1. Conversion of Excess Carbohydrates to Fat

The conversion of excess carbohydrates to fat, known as DNL, is a pivotal metabolic process that underscores the interconnectedness of carbohydrate and lipid metabolism. If carbohydrates are eaten in larger amounts than the body needs for energy, insulin is released to help glucose be stored as glycogen. When glycogen is full, extra glucose is changed into fatty acids that are combined with glycerol to make TGs and stored in adipose tissue. It supports energy balance and points out the effect of food choices on lipid storage in the body. The rate of DNL is affected by diet, hormones, and how fast a person's body metabolizes, which makes the process of lipid metabolism more complex and has important clinical effects. The role of gut microbiota in the conversion of excess carbohydrates to fat is becoming increasingly recognized, particularly through the production of SCFAs during the fermentation of dietary fibers. SCFAs can play a major role in the host's metabolism by serving as signals that may affect appetite, insulin's effects, and where fat is stored. If some carbohydrates are not fully digested, the gut bacteria ferment them and produce SCFAs that can be used by the host's intestinal cells and enter the bloodstream. According to studies, these SCFAs might increase the body's ability to save fat in the periphery and affect metabolism and energy use. However, as noted, there remains a need for further exploration of the molecular mechanisms by which SCFAs affect metabolic pathways, highlighting an area ripe for future investigation in lipid metabolism, especially in the context of obesity and metabolic disorders (Gijs et al., 2013). Besides, changing extra carbohydrates into fat is not a simple process; it is also connected to public health issues, especially obesity and MS. When you eat many simple sugars, the body may put on more fat because it cannot store all the glycogen. It stresses that a balanced diet is necessary to avoid too much fat, because regularly eating a lot of carbohydrates can make a person more likely to get insulin resistance and related problems. Within the clinical approach, healthcare providers should focus on both the balance of macronutrients and the quality of carbohydrates in people's meals. This multifaceted view aligns well with the recommendations outlined in the ESC/EAS Guidelines, which stress the importance of comprehensive assessment and management strategies for maintaining metabolic health (François et al., 2019). For this reason, it is important to understand how carbohydrates are turned into fat for the purpose of dietary advice and maintaining good health.

6.5.2. Role of Acetyl-CoA in Lipogenesis

Acetyl-CoA plays a key part in making fatty acids, which is very important for lipid metabolism. Acetyl-CoA is the main source of carbon in the process that makes fatty acids longer. Enzymatic reactions catalyzed by acetyl-CoA carboxylase (ACC) lead to the conversion of acetyl-CoA into malonyl-CoA, which then enters the FAS complex for further processing. It is regulated by different signals, some of which come from the amount of nutrients and from hormones. It is clear from research that problems with lipogenesis may result in obesity and various related diseases. So, knowing how acetyl-CoA works in lipogenesis may lead to better ways to treat conditions related to lipid metabolism. Acetyl-CoA also helps regulate how much energy and fat your body has by affecting storage. More acetyl-CoA being available, mainly after eating carbohydrates, can result in more lipogenesis and the storage of extra energy as TGs in the body's fat cells. Besides, studies indicate that changes in acetyl-CoA metabolism may contribute to the growth of insulin resistance. For instance, the action of fructose has been implicated as a fat-promoting agent that influences acetyl-CoA availability, consequently altering lipogenic pathways and contributing to obesity-related diseases (Beane et al., 2018). For this reason, controlling acetyl-CoA levels is very important, as it shapes energy storage and is necessary for the health of metabolic processes. New studies have pointed out that acetyl-CoA is important for more than energy metabolism, especially in the development and survival of tumor cells. For example, the connection between acetyl-CoA synthetase 2 (ACSS2) and cancer metabolism reveals how acetyl-CoA derived from acetate can sustain lipid biosynthesis under nutrient-depletion conditions, promoting tumor growth (Schug et al., 2015). In places where nutrients are scarce, cancer cells rely on acetyl-CoA to keep their ability to divide. This means that acetyl-CoA is important for lipogenesis and also helps make lipids in energetically active situations like cancer, thus showing how it is involved in many metabolic functions. Knowing about these relationships points to the value of targeting acetyl-CoA pathways in treating diseases such as metabolic and oncological disorders (Figure 6.17).

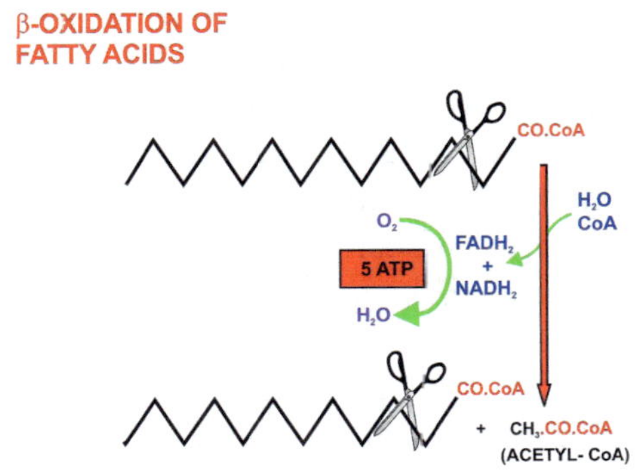

Figure 6.17. Schematic of key steps in lipogenesis: acetyl-CoA is carboxylated by acetyl-CoA carboxylase (ACC) to form malonyl-CoA. In the rate-limiting step, malonyl-CoA is synthesized into palmitic acid and various other fatty acids via fatty acid synthase (FASN). These fatty acids are accumulated and stored as lipid droplets, which can be used as a fuel source in proliferating tumor cells.

Source:By Cruithne9 - Own work, CC BY-SA 4.0, https://commons.wikimedia.org/w/index.php?curid=45500332

6.5.3. Regulation of Lipogenesis by Hormones

Hormones play an important role in controlling the body's production and storage of fats. In response to high blood glucose, insulin released by the pancreas is the major controller of lipogenesis. It encourages the body to turn extra glucose into fatty acids and then store them as TGs in the adipose tissue. Moreover, insulin turns on the production of important enzymes for fatty acid synthesis, such as ACC and FAS. This process reveals the strong relationship between carbohydrate and lipid metabolism, as hormones can control how energy is used and stored. Conversely, in states of insulin resistance, such as obesity, this regulatory pathway can become dysregulated, leading to increased lipogenesis and contributing to metabolic disorders, underscoring the importance of hormonal balance in maintaining metabolic health (Titus et al., 2025). Thyroid hormones (THs) also play a prominent role in regulating lipogenesis, alongside their influence on lipolysis. Because these hormones promote the formation and breakdown of fats, they play a more complicated role in metabolism. Research demonstrates that THs regulate numerous genes associated with lipid metabolism, including the stearoyl-CoA desaturase 1 (SCD1), an enzyme crucial for the production of monounsaturated fatty acids. Having SCD1 deficiency is connected to better lipid storage in tissues, which can prevent obesity. In hypothyroid conditions, however, an increase in triglyceride accumulation within the heart occurs due to unopposed lipogenesis, indicating how hormonal shifts can profoundly affect lipid homeostasis (Olichwier et al., 2020). It is important for the thyroid hormone and lipid balance to avoid obesity and its related health issues. Glucagon also plays a part in controlling lipogenesis by working oppositely to insulin. If blood glucose levels fall, glucagon is released by the pancreas to support the breakdown of fats and stop fat formation. Because of this hormone, stored TGs are transformed into FFAs and glycerol, which can be used to create energy. It also facilitates the activation of AMP-activated protein kinase (AMPK), a critical regulator of energy balance that inhibits lipid synthesis while promoting fatty acid oxidation. The way glucagon and insulin work against each other is an example of the body's wide network of hormones that helps maintain energy balance. Disruptions in these delicate relationships between hormones can lead to metabolic disorders such as type 2 diabetes, emphasizing the necessity of understanding hormonal regulation in the broader context of lipid metabolism (Titus et al., 2025).

Test Your Knowledge

1. What is the process of conversion of excess of carbohydrates into fat?
2. What is the role of Acetyl-CoA in lipogenesis?

6.6. Disorders Related to Lipid Metabolism

Learning Outcome

1. Learn about hyperlipidemia;
2. Describe the fatty liver disease;
3. Understand the metabolic syndrome.

Lipid metabolism disorders refer to many conditions that happen when the body's lipid homeostasis is disturbed. Such disorders usually become lipid storage diseases, where lipids build up in the body because of missing or defective enzymes. Some examples are Tay-Sachs disease and Gaucher disease, which develop because of certain genetic mutations that affect lipid processing. These disorders can be very serious since they may result in several organ failures and severe health problems if not treated. Also, since lipid metabolism is very complex, it is difficult to diagnose these disorders, so doctors need to use detailed metabolic tests to distinguish apart similar symptoms and metabolic problems. Because new technologies in diagnosis are emerging, there is a higher need to identify lipid-related disorders and the genes that play a role in their development. It is important to know how biomarkers can help identify and track lipid metabolism disorders. The presence of biomarkers related to lipid metabolism can explain the causes of certain disorders and help choose the right treatment. Recent studies incorporating multi-omics strategies highlight the potential of integrating genomics, proteomics, and metabolomics to yield a comprehensive view of disease mechanisms (Argano et al., 2019). Using this approach on lipid-related data could help us learn a lot about these disorders and create accurate biomarkers for early detection and individualized treatment. It is also important to consider gender in biomarker research, since there are differences in lipid metabolism that can change the way diseases develop and should be treated. Adding gender medicine to the study of lipidology points out that lipid metabolic disorders are not simple and can vary greatly among people. The field of lipid metabolism is further complicated by the emergence of inborn errors of metabolism (IEMs), which represent a significant class of genetic disorders characterized by enzymatic deficiencies that disrupt lipid pathways (Ismail et al., 2019). Since these disorders may result in both sudden and long-term health problems, it is crucial to detect them early and correctly. Traditional screening for newborns looks at only a few metabolites, which makes it hard to identify many other IEMs. New developments in untargeted metabolomics could lead to better diagnostics, since many metabolites can be identified at once and this increases the chances of spotting significant changes in metabolism. Researchers can find new details about the problems in lipid metabolism by increasing the analysis of lipid profiles. This change in diagnostic methods may help patients recover better and help experts understand the relationship between lipid metabolism and various diseases (Figure 6.18).

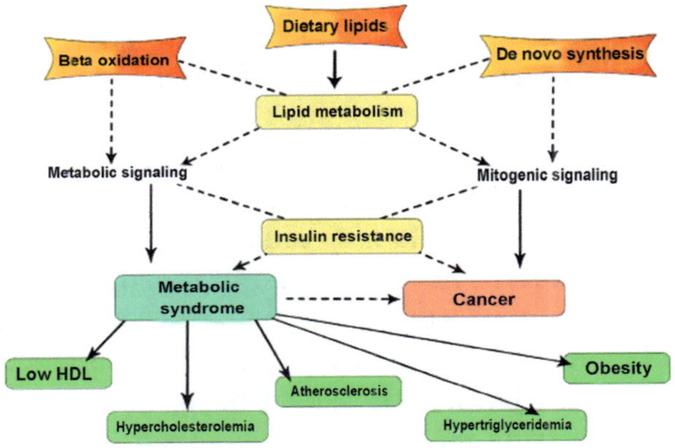

Figure 6.18. Dysregulation of lipid metabolism can confer metabolic disorders and trigger cancer.

Source: https://ars.els-cdn.com/content/image/3-s2.0-B9780128243565000102-f07-01-9780128243565.jpg.

6.6.1. Hyperlipidemia

Hyperlipidemia describes a situation where the blood contains too much triglyceride and cholesterol. Since these imbalances disrupt the usual lipid metabolism, they can cause health issues such as CVDs and pancreatitis. Hyperlipidemia is usually divided into primary and secondary forms, depending on whether it is caused by genes or lifestyle habits and other medical conditions. Understanding how hyperlipidemia develops is very important, since it helps doctors find the best treatments. To control lipid levels, it is important to make changes to your diet and exercise more. Using statins and other drugs is another way modern medicine helps prevent the negative effects of hyperlipidemias on health. Problems in lipid metabolism from hyperlipidemia can influence different body processes and interactions, leading to higher lipid levels. Transporting and metabolizing fatty acids is very important in this condition. It has been found that problems with fatty acid transport can have a big impact on the body's metabolism, especially during pregnancy. In preeclampsia, a condition marked by elevated blood pressure in pregnant women, alterations in fatty acid binding protein (FABP4) levels have been observed, demonstrating how lipid metabolism can be adversely affected during this critical physiological state (Han et al., 2010). This proves that lipid metabolism is complicated and can be linked to many diseases, suggesting that hyperlipidemia may cause and result from other metabolic problems. Hyperlipidemia affects people from different backgrounds, so it is necessary to carefully study how common it is and what health risks it brings. Exploring the effects of obesity in adolescents has shown how the location of fat in the body is linked to metabolic problems. Specifically, visceral fat accumulation is a significant risk factor for developing diabetes and CVDs, further complicating the hyperlipidemic landscape (Akbaezadeh et al., 2017). Because obesity and hyperlipidemia are usually linked, controlling weight may help a lot in managing lipids. All in all, a strategy that takes into account genetics, environment, and behavior is necessary for managing hyperlipidemia well, and stresses the need for more research to understand its different aspects (Figure 6.19).

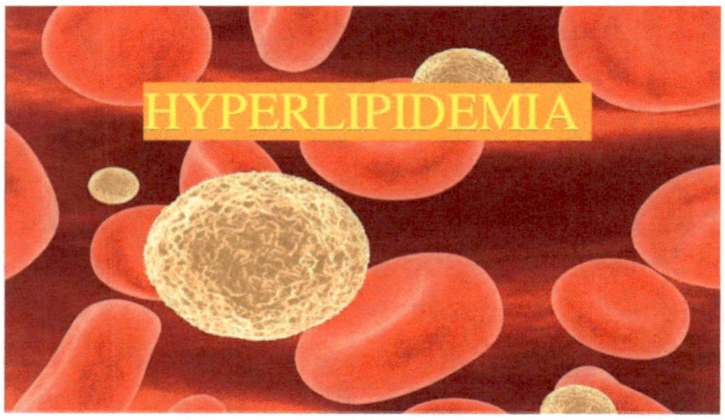

Figure 6.19. Hyperlipidemia.

Source: https://almurshidimed.com/wp-content/uploads/2020/07/team-8-hyperlipidemia-ukraine-1-638.jpg.

6.6.2. Fatty Liver Disease

Fatty liver disease, particularly non-alcoholic fatty liver disease (NAFLD), has emerged as a significant concern due to its association with MS and various chronic health conditions. It happens when too much fat builds up in the liver cells, and this may lead to steatohepatitis, fibrosis, and cirrhosis if left untreated. More and more, this condition is found in people who are obese, insulin-resistant, and have dyslipidemia, which shows how diet and lifestyle are affecting people. NAFLD is a complicated condition, and it is mainly caused by changes in lipid metabolism. Given that the number of people with obesity is rising, it is now very important to learn about the metabolic pathways related to fatty liver disease, as it affects general health and places more demands on healthcare services. Understanding NAFLD relies on the role autophagy plays in breaking down fats. Autophagy helps cells remove and recycle their parts, which supports the balance of lipids in the body under all circumstances. NAFLD has been linked to autophagy that is not working properly, since it does not remove enough lipids from the liver, leading to its disease state. Autophagy and lipid metabolism are not always clear; studies indicate that autophagy can have effects that increase or decrease lipid levels. Therefore, it is important to look closely at how autophagy affects liver lipid regulation, mainly in situations where there is a metabolic disorder and fatty liver disease. The interplay between autophagy and other cellular processes underscores the complexities involved in managing and understanding NAFLD (Francque et al., 2016). Another important feature of fatty liver disease is the problem with how the body handles glucose and lipids. Recent studies have indicated that genetic factors, such as reduced-function polymorphisms in the organic cation transporter 1 (OCT1), critically influence lipid profiles and the risk of associated metabolic disorders, including type 2 diabetes.

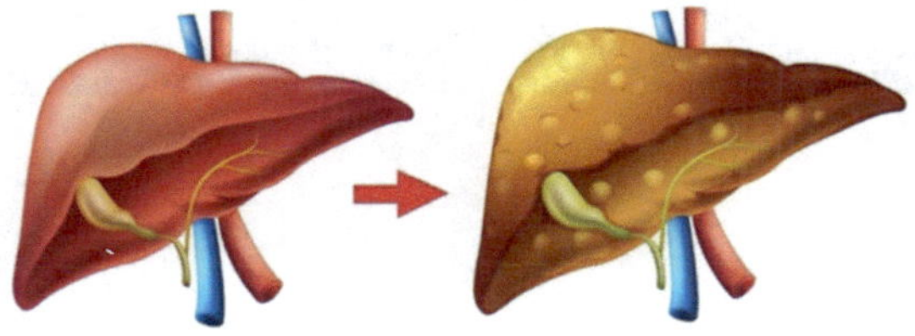

Figure 6.20. Fatty liver disease.

Source: https://www.hindustantimes.com/ht-img/img/2024/04/29/550x309/MixCollage-29-Apr-2024-06-10-PM-6538_1714394014728_1714394044577.jpg.

AUG1 is responsible for bringing thiamine into the liver, which is necessary for different enzymes that handle glucose and lipid metabolism. When OCT1 is lacking, these processes are affected, causing too much fat to build up and making it harder for the body to use glucose, which keeps metabolic inflexibility going. Understanding the genetic underpinnings and the biochemical mechanisms connecting OCT1 to lipid metabolism enhances our insight into the pathogenesis of NAFLD and its complications, revealing potential therapeutic targets aimed at combating this growing public health issue (Liang et al., 2018) (Figure 6.20).

6.6.3. Metabolic Syndrome (MS)

The interrelationship between lipid metabolism and metabolic syndrome (MS) has garnered significant attention in recent years, particularly due to its implications for cardiovascular health. A group of factors, such as insulin resistance, abdominal obesity, dyslipidemia, and hypertension, make up MS and increase the risk of CVDs. Changes in lipid profiles among these biochemical abnormalities indicate how much lipid metabolism affects our general health. For instance, as individuals develop insulin resistance—a core feature of MS—lipid metabolism becomes increasingly impaired, leading to elevated levels of TGs and reduced levels of HDL cholesterol, which are strong predictors of cardiovascular risk. Understanding this nexus allows for the identification of therapeutic targets that could mitigate the onset of related complications associated with MS and thus highlights the need for continued exploration within lipid metabolism research (Ali et al., 2015). The part that adipocytokines play in MS points to the complexity of regulating lipid metabolism, especially with the help of new hormones such as asprosin. Studies carried out recently have found that asprosin, a type of adipokine, is present in much higher amounts in women with MS than in those without. This increase is connected with typical signs of metabolic issues, for example, BMI and insulin levels. Asprosin is important because it indicates that changes in adipose tissues may worsen the symptoms of MS. The relationship between asprosin and lipid profiles further elucidates the intricate dance of metabolic pathways and emphasizes the necessity of elucidating this relationship to inform clinical strategies for managing MS (Sulaiman et al., 2021). Moreover, since MS and dyslipidemia are closely connected, it is important to use combined methods for prevention and treatment. Since MS affects several risk factors, making healthy changes in diet and exercise can improve the way lipids are processed and the overall metabolic health of a person. It is crucial to use management strategies that rely on understanding biochemical mechanisms in lipid metabolism to cut the cardiovascular risks linked to MS. Consequently, elucidating the pathways involved in lipid metabolism provides an avenue for targeted interventions, reinforcing the importance of interdisciplinary approaches in both research and clinical practice within the context of metabolic health (Ali et al., 2015) (Figure 6.21).

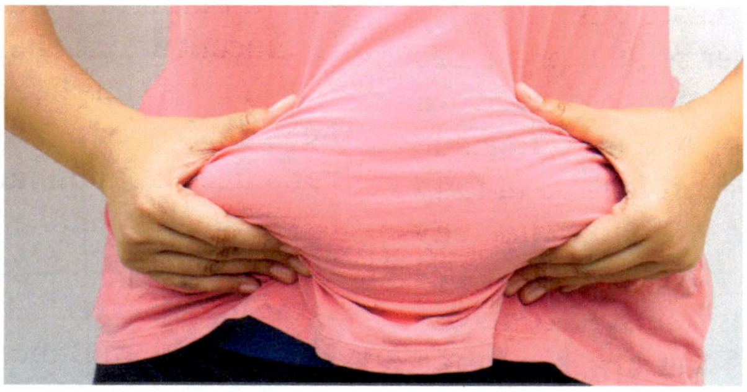

Figure 6.21. Metabolic syndrome.

Source: https://draxe.com/wp-content/uploads/2016/01/DAMetabolicSyndrome_FB.jpg.

Test Your Knowledge

1. What is hyperlipidemia?
2. What is fatty liver disease?

SUMMARY

In short, looking into lipid metabolism shows that it plays a key role in both healthy and diseased states of the body. If the body's lipid homeostasis is disturbed by any problem in its pathways, it can result in metabolic disorders and liver injuries. The results on the hepatotoxicity of Saikosaponins, especially in lipid metabolism, show the need to understand how different lipids are kept in balance. The identification of differentially expressed proteins in response to these bioactive compounds underscores the necessity for caution when utilizing herbal remedies, as their effects can extend beyond intended benefits to detrimentally impact liver function and lipid homeostasis, as demonstrated in recent research (Li et al., 2017). Furthermore, when we look at age, gender, and genetic backgrounds, the details of lipid metabolism become easier to notice, especially in cases of Alzheimer's and similar diseases. A study on lipid profiles linked to these risk factors proves that lipid metabolism is not fixed but can be affected by many different factors. Specifically, the associations discovered between lipid species and age or gender emphasize the potential for tailored therapeutic strategies that consider individual patient profiles, which may enhance treatment efficacy and minimize the risk of lipid-related pathologies, an assertion supported by the comprehensive findings on the lipidomes relationship with Alzheimer's disease (Ames et al., 2020). To sum up, knowing about lipid metabolism is essential for progress in clinical practice and therapy. Research on how lipid homeostasis works improves our knowledge and supports the creation of effective targeted treatments. Because lipid metabolism is involved in liver injury and neurodegeneration, it is necessary to manage health using lifestyle changes, dietary adjustments, and possible drugs. By looking at lipid metabolism as a whole, we can design better ways to prevent and treat metabolic and neurodegenerative diseases for the health of many groups.

To know about metabolic disorders and liver diseases, it is important to understand how lipid metabolism works. One major part of lipid metabolism is controlling fatty acids and their effects on the liver. It has been found that microRNAs, especially miR-155, are very important in this regulatory system. Mice that did not have miR-155 showed more hepatic steatosis when they were fed a high-fat diet. This finding was related to higher weight of the liver and increased levels of cholesterol and alanine transaminase in the blood, proving miR-155's importance in lipid regulation. Also, the expression of genes involved in lipid uptake and metabolism in the liver, for example, Cd36 and Fasn, was greatly affected. These findings emphasize the importance of miR-155 in lipid metabolic processes and its potential implications for conditions like type 2 diabetes and fatty liver disease (Grefhorst et al., 2013). Choline and methionine are important for cell function and metabolism, so their relationship also plays a key role in lipid metabolism. Wilson disease (WD), a genetic disorder marked by copper accumulation, showcases how disrupted lipid metabolism can lead to severe clinical symptoms. Researchers found that the serum levels of WD patients were high in choline and methionine and were also altered in phospholipids. In particular, these disturbances were related to hepatic steatosis, which highlights the connections between several metabolic pathways. Researchers believe that high choline and methionine levels may lead to the disease's progression, suggesting them as possible biomarkers for WD. This underscores the relevance of understanding lipid metabolism in the context of genetic disorders and highlights the need for further research into the metabolic implications of such dysregulations (Czlonkowska et al., 2019). Moreover, when lipid metabolism is not regulated well, it can influence the brain and the whole body's balance. Cholines involvement in making neurotransmitters and its increased presence in WD suggest that lipid processing affects brain function in many ways. If lipid metabolism is altered, it can result in less acetylcholine and might be a reason for cognitive and behavioral problems in people with WD. Also, the connection between elevated aromatic amino acids and lipid problems in these patients calls for further study of their possible effects on the brain and mind. With further research, it will be important to understand how these connections work so that doctors can design better treatments for patients with lipid metabolism disorders. When we mix knowledge from different fields, we can handle the many aspects of these health concerns.

KEY TERMS FROM THIS CHAPTER

- Cardiovascular diseases
- Chronic inflammation
- Farnesoid X receptor
- Free fatty acids
- Hepatic steatosis
- Hypertriglyceridemia
- Lipid metabolism
- Triglycerides
- Cholesterol
- Dexamethasone
- Fatty acids
- Gallbladder
- Hormone-sensitive lipase
- Lipases
- Phospholipids

Critical Thinking Questions

1. **Which of the following is the primary storage form of lipids in the body?**
   a. Phospholipids
   b. Cholesterol
   c. Triglycerides
   d. Free fatty acids
2. **The process of breaking down triglycerides into glycerol and free fatty acids is called:**
   a. Lipogenesis
   b. Lipolysis
   c. Beta-oxidation
   d. Ketogenesis
3. **Which organ is the primary site of fatty acid oxidation?**
   a. Liver
   b. Kidney
   c. Muscle
   d. Adipose tissue
4. **Which enzyme catalyzes the hydrolysis of triglycerides in adipose tissue?**
   a. Hormone-sensitive lipase
   b. Lipoprotein lipase
   c. Acetyl-CoA carboxylase
   d. HMG-CoA reductase
5. **Which process converts acetyl-CoA into ketone bodies?**
   a. Lipolysis
   b. Ketogenesis
   c. Beta-oxidation
   d. Lipogenesis

Answers to Critical Thinking Questions

1. (c); 2. (b); 3. (a); 4. (a); 5. (b)

Short Answer Questions

1. What are the two pathways of lipid metabolism?
2. What is the importance of lipid metabolism to the human body?
3. Name the 3 types of lipids.
4. What is the process of lipid digestion and absorption?
5. What does lipogenesis mean?

REFERENCES

1. Liang, X., Yee, S. W., Chien, H. C., Chen, E. C., Luo, Q., Zou, L., Piao, M., Mifune, A., Chen, L., Calvert, M. E., King, S., Norheim, F., Abad, J., Krauss, R. M., & Giacomini, K. M. (2018). Organic cation transporter 1 (OCT1) modulates multiple cardiometabolic traits through effects on hepatic thiamine content. *PLoS biology*, *16*(4), e2002907. https://doi.org/10.1371/journal.pbio.2002907 (accessed on 11th June 2025).

2. Schug, Z. T., Peck, B., Jones, D. T., Zhang, Q., Grosskurth, S., Alam, I. S., Goodwin, L. M., Smethurst, E., Mason, S., Blyth, K., McGarry, L., James, D., Shanks, E., Kalna, G., Saunders, R. E., Jiang, M., Howell, M., Lassailly, F., Thin, M. Z., Spencer-Dene, B., ... Gottlieb, E. (2015). Acetyl-CoA synthetase 2 promotes acetate utilization and maintains cancer cell growth under metabolic stress. *Cancer cell*, *27*(1), 57–71. https://doi.org/10.1016/j.ccell.2014.12.002 (accessed on 11th June 2025).

3. Akbaezadeh, M. (M.), & Behbahani, B. M. (2017). Central obesity and BMI associated with different phenotypes of polycystic ovary syndrome in adolescents. https://core.ac.uk/download/480549992.pdf (accessed on 11th June 2025).

4. Ali, H., Bushra, S., Ashoor, L., Jasim, Z. J., & Rasha, R. (2015). Prolactin is a novel biochemical marker in sera of Iraqi type-2 diabetic women with metabolic syndrome in Baghdad. https://core.ac.uk/download/234656078.pdf (accessed on 11th June 2025).

5. AlSulaiman, W. (2017). *Assessing the Effect of Statins in Lowering the Risk of Stroke and Preventing Cerebral Ischemia in Patients with Hypercholesterolemia*. https://open.bu.edu/bitstream/2144/23752/5/AlSulaiman_bu_0017N_12798.pdf (accessed on 11th June 2025).

6. Alza, N. P., Conde, M. A., Iglesias González, P. A., Salvador, G. A., et al. (2019). Lipids at the crossroad of α-synuclein function and dysfunction: Biological and pathological implications. https://core.ac.uk/download/287883350.pdf (accessed on 11th June 2025).

7. Ames, D., Australian Imaging, Biomarker & Lifestyle Research Group, Bush, A. I., Chatterjee, P., et al. (2020). Relationships between plasma lipid species, gender, risk factors and Alzheimer's disease. https://core.ac.uk/download/333540058.pdf (accessed on 11th June 2025).

8. Perla, F. M., Prelati, M., Lavorato, M., Visicchio, D., & Anania, C. (2017). The Role of Lipid and Lipoprotein Metabolism in Non-Alcoholic Fatty Liver Disease. *Children (Basel, Switzerland)*, *4*(6), 46. https://doi.org/10.3390/children4060046(accessed on 11th June 2025).

9. Arble, D. M., Bass, J., Behn, C. D., Butler, M. P., Challet, E., Czeisler, C., Depner, C. M., Elmquist, J., Franken, P., Grandner, M. A., Hanlon, E. C., Keene, A. C., Joyner, M. J., Karatsoreos, I., Kern, P. A., Klein, S., Morris, C. J., Pack, A. I., Panda, S., Ptacek, L. J., ... Wright, K. P. (2015). Impact of Sleep and Circadian Disruption on Energy Balance and Diabetes: A Summary of Workshop Discussions. *Sleep*, *38*(12), 1849–1860. https://doi.org/10.5665/sleep.5226(accessed on 11th June 2025).

10. Argano, V., Balistreri, C. R., Giarratana, R. M., Lio, D., et al. (2019). On the road to accurate biomarkers for cardiometabolic diseases by integrating precision and gender medicine approaches. https://core.ac.uk/download/268910274.pdf (accessed on 11th June 2025).

11. Dulloo, A. G., Gubler, M., Montani, J. P., Seydoux, J., & Solinas, G. (2004). Substrate cycling between de novo lipogenesis and lipid oxidation: a thermogenic mechanism against skeletal

muscle lipotoxicity and glucolipotoxicity. *International journal of obesity and related metabolic disorders : journal of the International Association for the Study of Obesity, 28 Suppl 4,* S29–S37. https://doi.org/10.1038/sj.ijo.0802861 (accessed on 11th June 2025).

12. Averna, M., Cefalù, A. B., Giammanco, A., Noto, D., et al. (2015). The pathophysiology of intestinal lipoprotein production. https://core.ac.uk/download/53300204.pdf (accessed on 11th June 2025).

13. Bartley, C., Bosco, D., Brun, T., Frigerio, F., et al. (2018). Peroxisome proliferator-activated receptor α (PPARα) protects against oleate-induced INS-1E beta cell dysfunction by preserving carbohydrate metabolism. https://core.ac.uk/download/159144359.pdf (accessed on 11th June 2025).

14. Bauer, E., Metzler-Zebeli, B. U., Mosenthin, R., Verstegen, M. W. A., et al. (2011). Intestinal gene expression in pigs: Effects of reduced feed intake during weaning and potential impact of dietary components. https://core.ac.uk/download/pdf/29230036.pdf (accessed on 11th June 2025).

15. Beane, K. E., & Montalbano, A. M. (2018). Effects of mitochondrial NADP+-dependent isocitrate dehydrogenase deficiency on fructose-induced obesity in mice. https://core.ac.uk/download/158199987.pdf (accessed on 11th June 2025).

16. Beard, J. K., Mulliniks, T., & Yates, D. T. (2018). Function and dysfunction of fatty acid mobilization: A review. https://core.ac.uk/download/286364498.pdf (accessed on 11th June 2025).

17. Han, V., Lajoie, G., Ballard, J. *et al.* Early onset preeclampsia is characterized by altered placental lipid metabolism and a premature increase in circulating FABP4. *Nat Prec* (2010). https://doi.org/10.1038/npre.2010.4885.1 (accessed on 11th June 2025).

18. Cheang, R. T., Chen, T. C., Fitch, M. D., Gray, S., et al. (2019). An ANGPTL4-ceramide-protein kinase Cζ axis mediates chronic glucocorticoid exposure-induced hepatic steatosis and hypertriglyceridemia in mice. https://core.ac.uk/download/323311253.pdf (accessed on 11th June 2025).

19. Choucair, I., Nemet, I., Li, L., Cole, M. A., Skye, S. M., Kirsop, J. D., Fischbach, M. A., et al. (2019). Quantification of bile acids: A mass spectrometry platform for studying gut microbe connection to metabolic diseases. *Journal of Lipid Research, 61,* 159–177. https://doi.org/10.1194/jlr.ra119000311 (accessed on 11th June 2025).

20. Sanoudou, D., Duka, A., Drosatos, K., Hayes, K. C., & Zannis, V. I. (2010). Role of Esrrg in the fibrate-mediated regulation of lipid metabolism genes in human ApoA-I transgenic mice. *The pharmacogenomics journal, 10*(3), 165–179. https://doi.org/10.1038/tpj.2009.51(accessed on 11th June 2025).

21. Cifarelli, V., & Eichmann, A. (2019). The Intestinal Lymphatic System: Functions and Metabolic Implications. *Cellular and molecular gastroenterology and hepatology, 7*(3), 503–513. https://doi.org/10.1016/j.jcmgh.2018.12.002(accessed on 11th June 2025).

22. Custodis, P., Gemeinhardt, O., Hafez, H. M., Hirschberg, R., et al. (2019). Structure and age-dependent development of the turkey liver: A comparative study of a highly selected meat-type and a wild-type turkey line. https://core.ac.uk/download/288114303.pdf (accessed on 11th June 2025).

23. Czech, M. P., Danai, L. V., Guilherme, A., Henchey, L., et al. (2017). Adipocyte lipid

synthesis coupled to neuronal control of thermogenic programming. https://core.ac.uk/download/84911330.pdf (accessed on 11th June 2025).

24. Czlonkowska, A., Kim, K., Litwin, T., Mazi, J., et al. (2019). Dysregulated choline, methionine, and aromatic amino acid metabolism in patients with Wilson disease: Exploratory metabolomic profiling and implications for hepatic and neurologic phenotypes. https://core.ac.uk/download/323068668.pdf (accessed on 11th June 2025).

25. de Carvalho, C. C. C. R., & Caramujo, M. J. (2018). The various roles of fatty acids. *Molecules, 23*, 2583–2583. https://doi.org/10.3390/molecules23102583 (accessed on 11th June 2025).

26. de Vos, W. M., Tilg, H., Van Hul, M., & Cani, P. D. (2022). Gut microbiome and health: Mechanistic insights. *Gut, 71*, 1020–1032. https://doi.org/10.1136/gutjnl-2021-326789 (accessed on 11th June 2025).

27. Deighton, R. F., Herrmann, A. G., Kerr, L. E., Le Bihan, T., et al. (2013). Adaptive changes in the neuronal proteome: Mitochondrial energy production, endoplasmic reticulum stress, and ribosomal dysfunction in the cellular response to metabolic stress. https://core.ac.uk/download/16459694.pdf (accessed on 11th June 2025).

28. den Besten, G., van Eunen, K., Groen, A. K., Venema, K., Reijngoud, D. J., & Bakker, B. M. (2013). The role of short-chain fatty acids in the interplay between diet, gut microbiota, and host energy metabolism. *Journal of Lipid Research, 54*, 2325–2340. https://doi.org/10.1194/jlr.r036012 (accessed on 11th June 2025).

29. Drouin, É., Levy, E., Marcil, V., Peretti, N., et al. (2005). Mechanisms of lipid malabsorption in cystic fibrosis: The impact of essential fatty acids deficiency. https://core.ac.uk/download/55643433.pdf (accessed on 11th June 2025).

30. Facchiano, A., Gaudio, E., Giampietri, C., Giulitti, F., et al. (2019). The role of autophagy in liver epithelial cells and its impact on systemic homeostasis. https://core.ac.uk/download/196295456.pdf (accessed on 11th June 2025).

31. Ismail, I. T., Showalter, M. R., & Fiehn, O. (2019). Inborn Errors of Metabolism in the Era of Untargeted Metabolomics and Lipidomics. *Metabolites, 9*(10), 242. https://doi.org/10.3390/metabo9100242 (accessed on 11th June 2025).

32. Finn, R., Henderson, C., Scott, C., Wolf, C. R., et al. (2008). Unsaturated fatty acid regulation of cytochrome P450 expression via a CAR-dependent pathway. https://core.ac.uk/download/4148336.pdf (accessed on 11th June 2025).

33. Francque, S. M., Kwanten, W. J., & Martinet, W. (2016). Autophagy in non-alcoholic fatty liver disease (NAFLD). https://core.ac.uk/download/322427771.pdf (accessed on 11th June 2025).

34. Galicia-García, U., Benito-Vicente, A., Jebari, S., Larrea-Sebal, A., Siddiqi, H., Uribe, K. B., Ostolaza, H., et al. (2020). Pathophysiology of type 2 diabetes mellitus. *International Journal of Molecular Sciences, 21*, 6275–6275. https://doi.org/10.3390/ijms21176275 (accessed on 11th June 2025).

35. Grefhorst, A., Kauffmann, A., Calkin, A. C., Lakner, A. M., Miller, A. M., Wang, B., Carvalho, B. S., et al. (2013). MiR-155 has a protective role in the development of non-alcoholic hepatosteatosis in mice. https://core.ac.uk/download/16460549.pdf (accessed on 11th June 2025).

36. Handschin, C., & Svensson, K. (2014). Modulation of PGC-1α activity as a treatment for metabolic and muscle-related diseases. https://core.ac.uk/download/33298388.pdf (accessed on 11th June 2025).

37. Li, X., Li, X., Lu, J., Huang, Y., Lv, L., Luan, Y., Liu, R., & Sun, R. (2017). Saikosaponins induced hepatotoxicity in mice via lipid metabolism dysregulation and oxidative stress: a proteomic study. *BMC complementary and alternative medicine, 17*(1), 219. https://doi.org/10.1186/s12906-017-1733-0 (accessed on 11th June 2025).

38. Jamshed, H., Peterson, C. M., & Poggiogalle, E. (2018). Circadian regulation of glucose, lipid, and energy metabolism in humans. https://core.ac.uk/download/188827386.pdf (accessed on 11th June 2025).

39. Kahana, A., Lancet, D., & Segrè, D. (2019). Twenty years of "Lipid World": A fertile partnership with David Deamer. https://core.ac.uk/download/322973325.pdf (accessed on 11th June 2025).

40. Kamphorst, J. J., & Lewis, I. A. (2017). Editorial overview: Recent innovations in the metabolomics revolution. https://core.ac.uk/download/80696822.pdf (accessed on 11th June 2025).

41. Kamphorst, J. J., & Tumanov, S. (2017). Recent advances in expanding the coverage of the lipidome. https://core.ac.uk/download/74231961.pdf (accessed on 11th June 2025).

42. Keller, J. N., & Uranga, R. M. (2019). The complex interactions between obesity, metabolism and the brain. https://core.ac.uk/download/287882287.pdf (accessed on 11th June 2025).

43. Klein, S., Liu, J., Lu, W., Shi, Y., et al. (2019). Peroxisomal regulation of redox homeostasis and adipocyte metabolism. https://core.ac.uk/download/231816688.pdf (accessed on 11th June 2025).

44. Mach, F., Baigent, C., Catapano, A. L., Koskinas, K. C., Casula, M., Badimón, L., Chapman, M. J., et al. (2019). 2019 ESC/EAS guidelines for the management of dyslipidemias: Lipid modification to reduce cardiovascular risk. *European Heart Journal, 41*, 111–188. https://doi.org/10.1093/eurheartj/ehz455 (accessed on 11th June 2025).

45. Meheust, A., McCartney, A. L., Neyrinck, A. M., Balsari, B., Stahl, B., Watzl, B., et al. (2010). Prebiotic effects: Metabolic and health benefits. https://core.ac.uk/download/9368.pdf (accessed on 11th June 2025).

46. Olichwier, A., Balatskyi, V. V., Wolosiewicz, M., Ntambi, J., & Dobrzyn, P. (2020). Interplay between thyroid hormones and stearoyl-CoA desaturase 1 in the regulation of lipid metabolism in the heart. *International Journal of Molecular Sciences, 22*. https://www.semanticscholar.org/paper/68dacd8869428c8d07a7870203cf88ff59a668db (accessed on 11th June 2025).

47. Pearce, E., & Rambold, A. (2018). Mitochondrial dynamics at the interface of immune cell metabolism and function.

48. Pfeiffer, A. F. H., Arner, P., Carpentier, A., Chen, Y., Reinecke, F., Ferrannini, E., Galman, C., et al. (2009). Free fatty acids link metabolism and regulation of the insulin-sensitizing fibroblast growth factor-21. https://core.ac.uk/download/46323.pdf (accessed on 11th June 2025).

49. Pool, F., Sweby, P. K., & Tindall, M. J. (2018). An integrated mathematical model of cellular cholesterol biosynthesis and lipoprotein metabolism. https://core.ac.uk/download/160748845.pdf (accessed on 11th June 2025).

50. Singh, A., Kukreti, R., Saso, L., & Kukreti, S. (2019). Oxidative stress: A key modulator in neurodegenerative diseases. *Molecules, 24*, 1583–1583. https://doi.org/10.3390/molecules24081583 (accessed on 11th June 2025).

51. Sulaiman, D. M. (2021). Evaluation of serum asprosin levels in women with metabolic syndrome in Duhok City-Kurdistan Region/Iraq. https://core.ac.uk/download/552655014.pdf (accessed on 11th June 2025).

52. Thimmiah, H. (2016). *Developing a Mouse Model to Study the Metabolic Role of The Mammalian Target of Rapamycin Complex 1 in adipose tissue.* https://open.bu.edu/bitstream/2144/14674/9/Thimmiah_bu_0017N_10506.pdf (accessed on 11th June 2025).

53. Titus, S. D., Emmanuel, A., Stephen, E. C., Tatah, S. V., & Arowora, K. A. (2025). Recent advances in lipid metabolism and regulations: A review. *Journal of Multidisciplinary Science: MIKAILALSYS.* https://www.semanticscholar.org/paper/495680ea5a77ceed5f93f27e1362666f4a60d085 (accessed on 11th June 2025).

54. Viola, A., Munari, F., Sánchez-Rodríguez, R., Scolaro, T., & Castegna, A. (2019). The metabolic signature of macrophage responses. *Frontiers in Immunology, 10.* https://doi.org/10.3389/fimmu.2019.01462 (accessed on 11th June 2025).

PROTEIN AND AMINO ACID METABOLISM

7

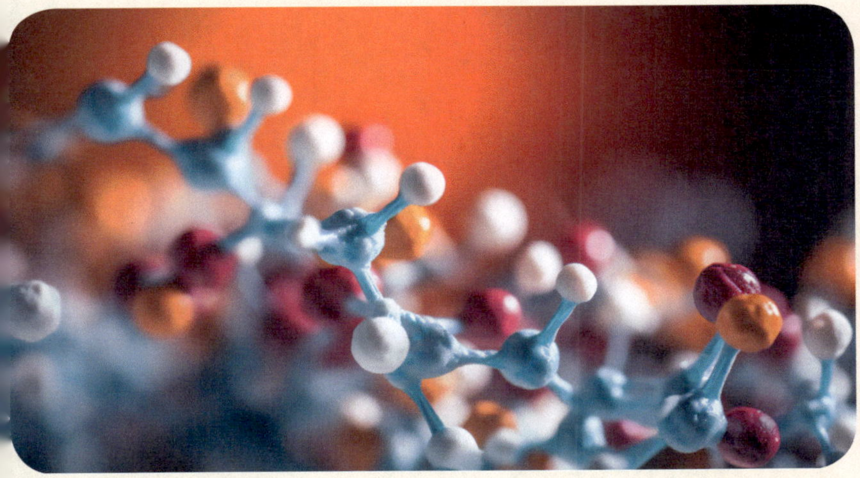

LEARNING OBJECTIVES

After studying this chapter, you will be able to:

1. Describe the structure of proteins;
2. Know the process of protein digestion;
3. Understand the amino acid metabolism;
4. Describe the protein synthesis;
5. Understand the regulation of protein metabolism;
6. Describe the disorders related to protein metabolism.

Introduction

Protein and amino acid metabolism is an important subject in nutritional biochemistry. Proteins are important for life because they provide structure and also take part in metabolic activities. During protein metabolism, dietary proteins are broken down into amino acids that are needed for tissue repair, hormone production, and making energy. Learning about this metabolic pathway is necessary since it helps in developing healthy and nutritious strategies for people in different populations. The main part of protein metabolism is played by amino acids, which are the final products of protein breakdown. Some amino acids are called essential because the body cannot make them and therefore, they must be provided by food. Because of this, diet and nutritional supplements should be planned differently. Scientific studies have pointed out that how well amino acids are digested depends on both the food and the person's metabolism. For instance, studies have shown that the apparent fecal nutrient digestibility can fluctuate based on the composition of the diet, which in turn affects the assessment of dietary ME (Zou, 2007). This points out why we need to know how dietary proteins and amino acids are metabolized, especially when it comes to different food sources. In addition, protein metabolism is important not only for human nutrition, but also for different industries, mainly in dairy manufacturing with strains of Lactococcus lactis. They have learned to move and use peptides well, which helps them survive in places like milk. Recent findings suggest significant variations in peptide metabolism and utilization among different Lactococcus lactis strains, thus enhancing our understanding of microbial protein metabolism (Moore et al., 1994). It is important for both improving the quality of dairy products and enhancing methods that help amino acids and proteins be used better in different parts of the body. By studying how amino acids are metabolized by humans and microbes, we realize how complicated amino acid assimilation is and what this means for our health and industry (Figure 7.1).

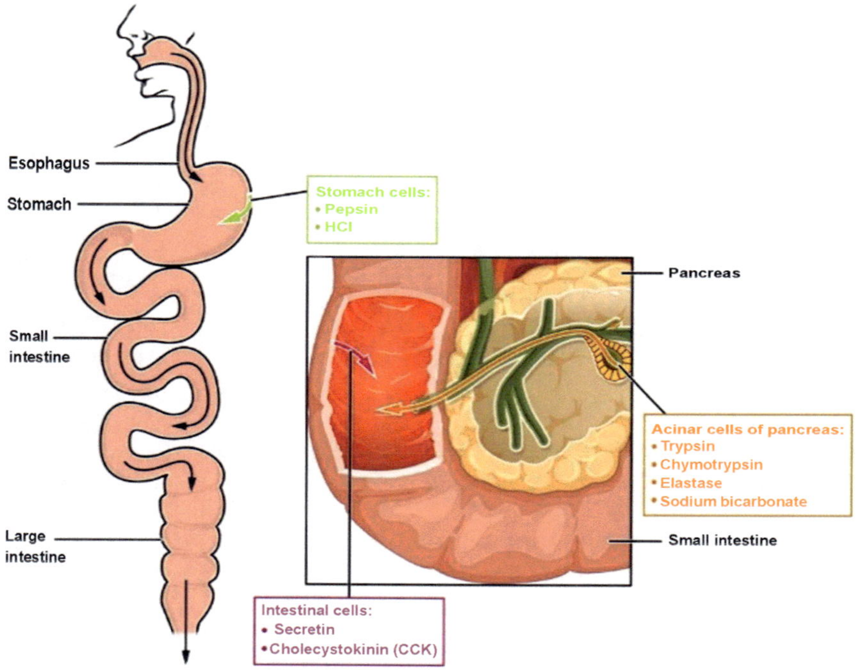

Figure 7.1. Enzymes in the stomach and small intestine break down proteins into amino acids. HCl in the stomach aids in proteolysis, and hormones secreted by intestinal cells direct the digestive processes.

Source: https://s3-us-west-2.amazonaws.com/courses-images-archive-read-only/wp-content/uploads/sites/403/2015/04/21031813/2517_Protein-Digesting_EnzymesN.jpg.

Definition of Proteins and Amino Acids

Long chains of amino acids, which are organic substances, make up proteins, which are the main macromolecules. Since amino acids are made of carbon, hydrogen, oxygen, nitrogen, and sometimes sulfur, they are grouped as essential or non-essential. Since the body does not make essential amino acids, they need to be included in the diet, but non-essential amino acids are produced inside the body. The way these amino acids are put together in a protein gives it its own structure and function, so it can act as a catalyst, support the body's structure, and control gene activity. Proteins are complex because their functions and stability can change a lot when their amino acid sequences are changed. The processes of amino acids and proteins in the body are complicated and are closely controlled to meet the needs of the organism. Proteins eaten in food are broken down into amino acids by the digestive system. After absorption in the blood, these amino acids go to tissues to be used for making proteins, producing energy, or being changed into other active compounds. This connection points out that proteins are necessary for keeping cells stable and carrying out vital metabolic tasks. Besides, the enzymes that work on amino acids are very specific, which means they can adjust the body's metabolic rate as needed. In this situation, proteins are important for structure and function and also control metabolic activities and signaling. The way proteins function is further affected by things in the environment and by genes. It has been found that changes in metabolic pathways may result in health problems such as cardiometabolic diseases, which shows why it is important to study protein and amino acid functions at a molecular level. Multi-omics approaches, which integrate genomics, proteomics, and metabolomics, enhance our understanding of how proteins function in interconnected metabolic networks (Argano et al., 2019). This information is necessary to design specially targeted actions and nutrition plans for each person's metabolic needs. The exploration of interactions between proteins and other biomolecules holds promise for elucidating the complexities of metabolic diseases and can inform future research directions for therapeutic innovations (Avilla et al., 2020) (Figure 7.2).

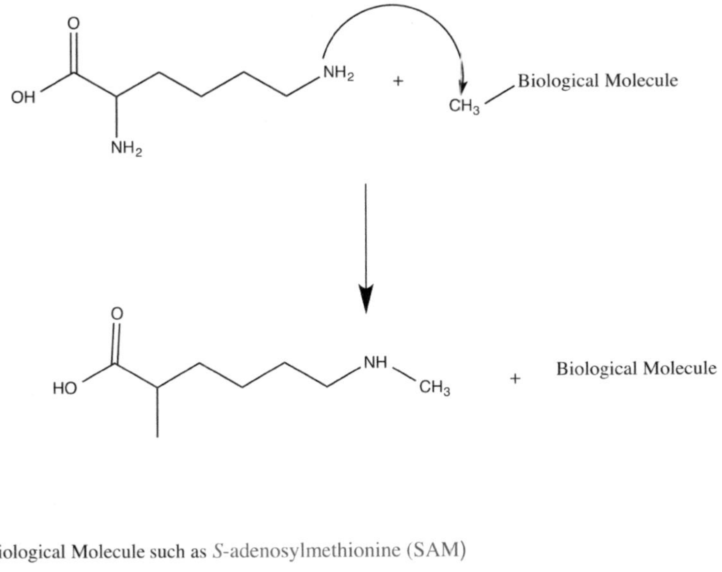

Figure 7.2. Amino acid metabolism.

Source: By Olaneli - Own work, Public Domain, https://commons.wikimedia.org/w/index.php?curid=57016003

Importance of Protein Metabolism in the Body

Protein metabolism is necessary for the body to maintain its shape and how it functions. As well as helping the body grow and heal, proteins are important for creating enzymes and hormones that control different body functions. Proteins are broken down in catabolism to provide amino acids that can be used to make new proteins or changed into energy by gluconeogenesis. Also, knowing how proteins are used in the body is important to decide on the right diet, as eating balanced amounts of protein helps your body work well. It has been observed that discrepancies in protein absorption can lead to various health issues, emphasizing the significance of this metabolic pathway in overall well-being (Zou, 2007). So, protein metabolism helps maintain muscles and also supports the proper functioning of many other biological systems. Besides, protein metabolism plays a key role in managing weight and the composition of the body. Since proteins increase satiety and control appetite, they are especially important in diets meant for weight loss or control. According to studies, consuming foods rich in protein increases the body's energy use. It highlights the fact that proteins are more efficient in boosting metabolism than carbohydrates and fats. Additionally, the permissive nature of amino acids in metabolic pathways suggests that they are indispensable not only as building blocks for proteins but also as regulators of metabolic processes, influencing everything from muscle growth to fatty acid oxidation (Ayuso et al., 2015). That is why protein metabolism is important in the relationship between nutrition, energy use, and body composition. Lastly, disturbances in protein metabolism may cause health problems such as muscle loss and a weakened immune system. A person with chronic illness or starvation may lose muscle mass because the body uses it for energy, which stresses the need for enough protein in the diet. Certain amino acids are important for the immune system because they are used to create neurotransmitters or take part in cell signaling. For instance, branched-chain amino acids (BCAAs) are not only fundamental for muscle recovery but also play roles in immune responses and resistance to stress (Zou, 2007). That's why it is necessary to thoroughly understand protein and amino acid metabolism to create better dietary guidelines and treatments that help improve health and reduce diseases. If people eat a balanced amount of protein, they may improve their health and wellness.

7.1. Structure of Proteins

Learning Outcome

1. Describe the amino acid composition and structure;
2. Describe the levels of protein structure;
3. Understand the role of protein folding in function.

Proteins consist of chains of amino acids and are built in different ways to support many functions in the body. Proteins are usually described in terms of four main structures called primary, secondary, tertiary, and quaternary. A protein's overall shape is determined by the particular sequence of amino acids joined by peptide bonds in the primary structure. When a protein folds, it could develop structures called alpha helices and beta sheets, which are held together by hydrogen bonds. At the tertiary level, the three-dimensional shape is formed through different interactions, for example, hydrophobic interactions, ionic bonds, and disulfide bridges. The way the amino acids are arranged is very important for the protein's job, so any change in the sequence could disrupt its function and influence metabolic processes. Proteins also have a quaternary structure, which happens when different polypeptide chains join to work together. Because of this assembly, proteins can be regulated, bind with others, and have different structures, which are all required in biology. As an example, hemoglobin is a protein made of four subunits and has cooperative binding abilities necessary for carrying oxygen in the blood. It is especially important to understand these structures, especially when proteins are involved in metabolic processes.

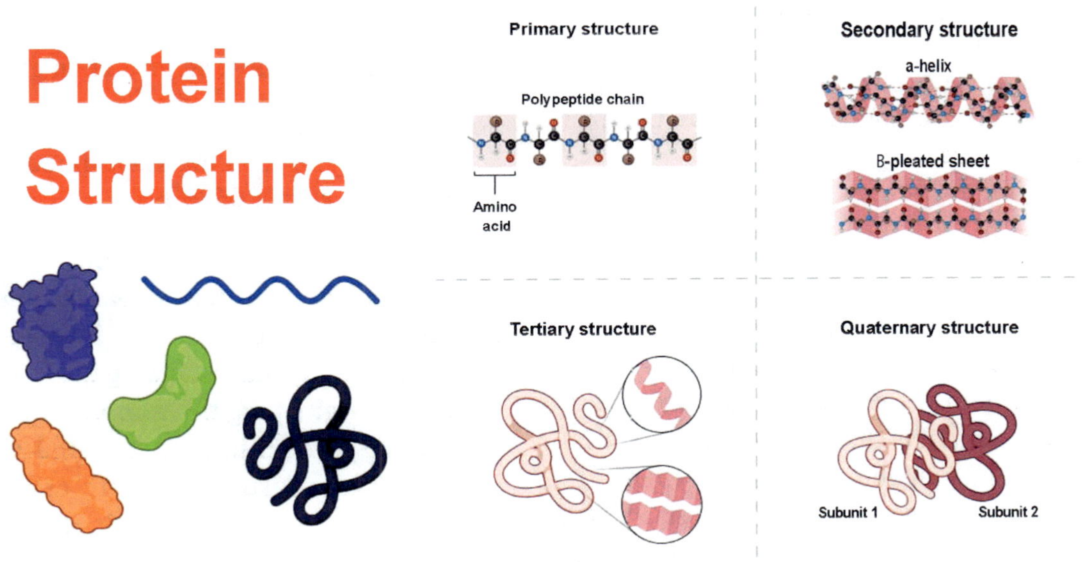

Figure 7.3. Types of protein structure.

Source: https://microbenotes.com/wp-content/uploads/2023/10/Types-of-Protein-Structure.jpeg.

Problems in the structure of proteins can result in different disorders, some of which are neurodegenerative diseases and other forms of pathology. For this reason, it is necessary to understand the structure of proteins to explain their functions in metabolism and what happens when they do not function properly. It is important to look at cases where changes in the structure of proteins affect how metabolism is regulated. For instance, apolipoprotein E (ApoE) exists in three isoforms, ApoE2, ApoE3, and ApoE4, each differing by a mere amino acid substitution yet imparting significant variations in function and disease associations. The way these isoforms are built determines their interaction with lipoprotein receptors, which in turn influences cholesterol levels and the chance of getting Alzheimer's. Researchers believe that the way ApoE4's domains interact causes harmful changes in its structure, which increases the chance of neurodegenerative diseases. Understanding these structural dynamics is key in the realm of protein and amino acid metabolism, as it paves the way for therapeutic innovations targeting these critical biological molecules, as seen in ongoing research focused on structure correctors that address ApoE4-associated pathology (Mahley et al., 2016). Furthermore, enabling a deeper understanding of how structural intricacies relate to functionality can inform targeted interventions to mitigate protein-related metabolic disorders (Chen et al., 2017) (Figure 7.3)

7.1.1. Amino Acid Composition and Structure

How a protein works and is metabolized greatly depends on its amino acid composition and structure. Proteins consist of 20 standard amino acids, and their side chains make each amino acid unique and give the resulting polypeptides special functions. The way amino acids are put together in a protein's sequence determines its three-dimensional shape, which is necessary for its biological function. Proteins fold differently and interact with other molecules because of the presence of hydrophobic or hydrophilic side chains. A thorough understanding of amino acid composition not only elucidates protein structure but also informs research in various applications, such as the use of specific proteins in therapeutic contexts or the development of food sources enriched with beneficial amino acids, as evidenced by studies like those focusing on *M. esculenta* proteins and their metabolic benefits (Gao et al., 2025). The roles of amino acids in proteins are mainly determined by their structure, including chirality and functional groups. Every amino acid has a main carbon atom linked to an amino group, a carboxyl group, a hydrogen atom, and a side chain called the R-group. Because of their ability to form different bonds, amino acids can take part in many biochemical interactions that direct the structure and stability of proteins.

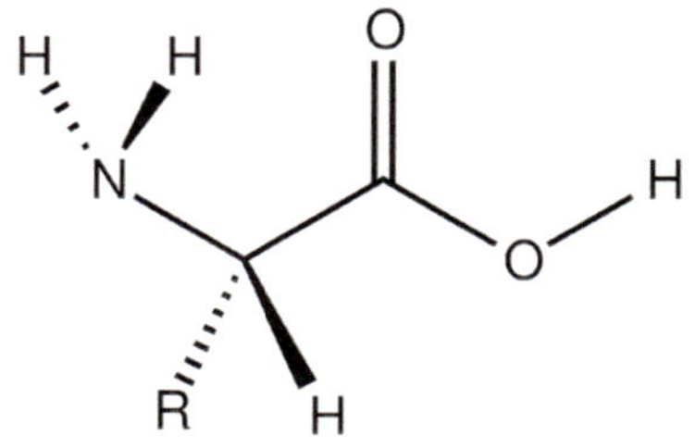

Figure 7.4. General structure of an amino acid.

Source: By Smokefoot - Own work, Public Domain, https://commons.wikimedia.org/w/index.php?curid=106539890

Besides, attaching phosphate or sugar groups to amino acids can increase the number of functions that proteins have and where they are found in the cell. Understanding these nuances is essential for grasping the complex mechanisms underlying protein interactions and metabolic pathways that sustain life (Niu et al., 2025). Looking into how amino acids affect protein structure has significant effects on nutrition and biotechnology. For instance, studies of silk fibroins, as seen in the diamondback moth, highlight how specific amino acid sequences are integral to silk production by affecting the mechanical properties and compatibility of the silk proteins (Niu et al., 2025). It highlights the role of amino acids in setting up a protein's structure as well as in giving it functions that keep the organism alive. Such knowledge can help find new ways to improve protein engineering, ensure proper nutrition, and make new biomaterials, linking the essential science of amino acids to practical uses in health and industry (Figure 7.4).

7.1.2. Levels of Protein Structure: Primary, Secondary, Tertiary, and Quaternary

The main structure of proteins comes from the order of amino acids attached by peptide bonds to create a polypeptide chain. The different side chains of amino acids play a role in the formation and functioning of proteins. The genetic code tells which amino acids go in which order during the translation of mRNA.

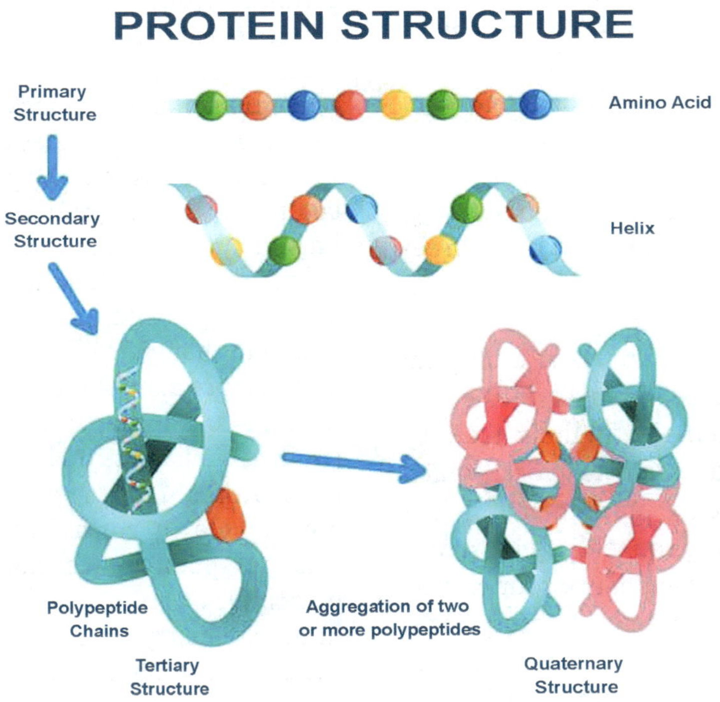

Figure 7.5. Levels of protein structure.

Source: https://biologydictionary.net/wp-content/uploads/2021/01/levels-of-protein-structure-1.jpg.

A change in just one amino acid in the primary structure can seriously affect how a protein functions or how stable it is, and may cause diseases such as sickle cell anemia. It is important to know this basic level, since it guides the formation of higher-level structures that control metabolic regulation and cellular signaling, connecting the protein sequence to how proteins and amino acids are used. The secondary structure describes how parts of the polypeptide chain are folded together, mostly due to hydrogen bonds between the backbone atoms. Alpha-helices and beta-pleated sheets are the types of secondary structures found most often. They help pack proteins in a cell and are important for their stability. The way these structures are formed depends on the side chains of amino acids, which allow for hydrophobic, hydrogen bonding, and electrostatic attractions to occur and hold the interactions together. When proteins fold, the secondary structure prepares the way for tertiary and quaternary structures that determine the functions of proteins. In the context of protein and amino acid metabolism, understanding secondary structures is vital for predicting how proteins interact with substrates and reagents, ultimately impacting metabolic pathways (Hedqvist, 2004). The tertiary structure of a polypeptide shows its three-dimensional shape, which includes both secondary structures and interactions between side chains. Stabilizing this structure depends a lot on hydrophobic interactions, ionic bonding, and disulfide bridges. Thanks to their three-dimensional shape, proteins can interact with substrates, cofactors, or other proteins, which helps them take part in important biological functions for metabolism. Moreover, the proper folding of some proteins into their tertiary structure is needed for them to work, which demonstrates why folding mechanisms in the cell are crucial. Targeting the tertiary structure helps in the development of pharmaceuticals, as this can lead to useful therapies. Subsequently, the quaternary structure emerges when multiple polypeptide chains come together to form a functional protein complex, revealing additional layers of regulation and activity within metabolic processes (Slavny, 2010) (Figure 7.5).

7.1.3. Role of Protein Folding in Function

Protein folding is very important for proteins and amino acids in the body since it decides how well a protein is built and how it can function. Misshapen proteins can result in many diseases, for example, Alzheimer's and Parkinson's. Proteins adopt a certain shape in space to be able to perform tasks such as acting as enzymes, sending signals, and transporting substances. Recent studies have stressed that molecular chaperones are required in the process, since they help fold proteins and stop them from clumping. Studies of various organisms, such as Chinook salmon, reveal a strong correlation between thermal exposure and protein folding responses, establishing a link between environmental stressors and maintenance of physiological function (Tomalty et al., 2015). If proteins are not folded correctly, cellular problems and disorders may take place. In addition, the evolutionary process of protein folding gives us an understanding of how metabolic processes develop in organisms. The RNA World hypothesis claims that the shift from RNA to proteins happened as amino acid coding increased gradually, which had a direct impact on proteins and their functions. This model suggests that the early recruitment of amino acids, such as alanine, was a pivotal moment that guided the evolution of protein architecture and folding mechanisms, ultimately leading to sophisticated metabolic pathways (Budisa et al., 2019). The formation of α-helices in proteins led to their folding playing a bigger role in controlling metabolism. From this perspective, we can see that the main principles of protein folding still play a key role in biochemistry in living organisms. Moreover, the connection between protein folding and cell function is important in modern biomedical research since it can help find new treatments. Researchers working on protein misfolding and aggregation are also trying to find ways to prevent the negative results caused by these processes. Several strategies, including using small molecules to protect or boost chaperones, show that it is possible to treat the results of misfolded proteins. Furthermore, exploring the pathways by which environmental stressors affect protein folding, as evidenced by the transcriptional analysis conducted in juvenile salmon exposed to thermal stress, underscores the necessity of protein stability for maintaining metabolic homeostasis (Tomalty et al., 2015). Because of these discoveries, there can be significant improvements in medical treatments, proving how important protein folding is for the overall protein and amino acid metabolism (Figure 7.6).

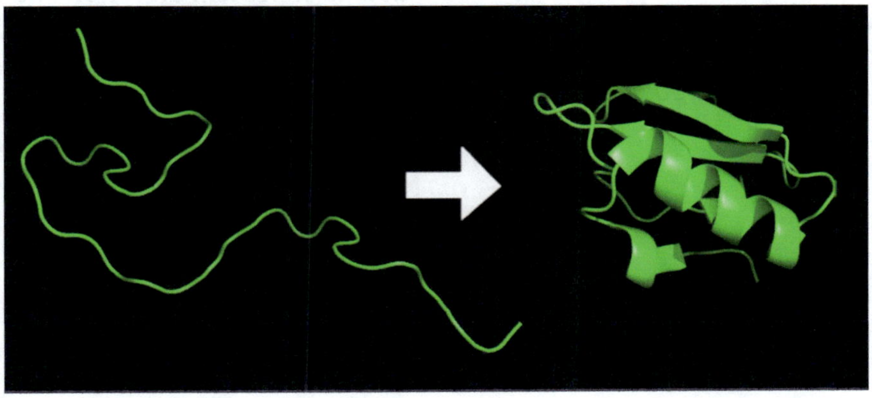

Figure 7.6. Protein before and after folding.

Source: https://upload.wikimedia.org/wikipedia/commons/a/a9/Protein_folding.png.

Test Your Knowledge

1. What is the composition of amino acids?
2. What are the 4 levels of protein structure?

7.2. Digestion of Proteins

Learning Outcome

1. Know the process of protein digestion in the gastrointestinal tract;
2. Describe the enzymes involved in protein breakdown;
3. Understand the absorption of amino acids in the small intestine.

The metabolism of amino acids depends on the complicated process of digesting proteins. The stomach is where the acid and pepsin help break down protein into smaller polypeptides. After this, the proteins that have been broken down are sent to the small intestine, where trypsin, chymotrypsin, and carboxypeptidase from the pancreas further break them into amino acids. For the body to use nutrients properly, it needs to digest food efficiently since amino acids are used for hormone, neurotransmitter, and muscle protein production. It is important to understand protein digestion to realize why some protein sources are better for our bodies than others. It has been found that the way we digest protein can change a lot based on what we eat and the type of protein we consume. It has been shown that refined diets usually result in better apparent fecal nutrient digestibility than high-fiber diets. Such differences make it hard to rely on the Atwater factors, which help predict how much energy comes from protein. Such differences point out that we need models that look at each nutrient and how it affects metabolism. How easy it is to digest food from different diets matters for energy as well as for nitrogen retention, which is essential for growing and repairing muscles. Consequently, it is essential to continue exploring these dynamics to optimize nutritional strategies tailored to specific populations, thereby enhancing overall health outcomes (Zou, 2007). In addition, protein metabolism researchers are now paying special attention to the use of protein hydrolysates instead of intact proteins. Scientific studies suggest that hydrolyzed proteins are absorbed faster than whole proteins, which might lead to more amino acids being available.

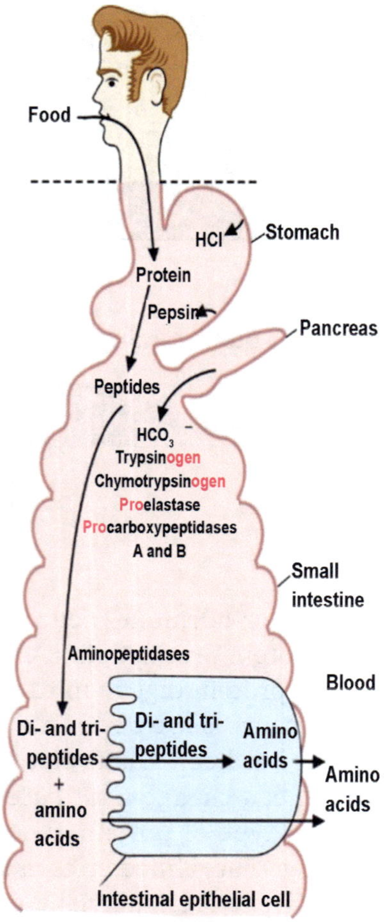

Figure 7.7. Digestion of proteins.

Source: https://i0.wp.com/basicmedicalkey.com/wp-content/uploads/2022/08/fig35-1.jpg?w=960.

When comparing the way nitrogenous metabolites are excreted in pigs, it was found that hydrolysates affected the pattern of metabolites. In particular, ammonia excretion dropped because the hydrolysates contained fixed cations. It proves that different protein sources are handled by the body in different ways and that it is important to know the details of protein digestion and absorption. The findings suggest that protein hydrolysates could be strategically utilized in dietary formulations, particularly in clinical settings, to optimize amino acid delivery and metabolic efficiency (Cintora et al., 2000) (Figure 7.7).

7.2.1. Process of Protein Digestion in the Gastrointestinal Tract

It takes many steps and is very carefully controlled for protein to be digested, starting in the stomach and ending in the small intestine. When dietary proteins enter the stomach, they are exposed to an acidic environment created by gastric acid (HCl), which denatures the protein structure, rendering it more accessible to enzymatic action. The acidity in the stomach causes pepsinogen to change into the enzyme pepsin. The action of pepsin allows proteins to be broken down into smaller polypeptides, which starts the digestion of proteins. This step is very important because it makes the proteins ready for digestion in the small intestine, where pancreatic proteases such as trypsin and chymotrypsin break them down into smaller peptides and amino acids, which is basic for their metabolism. In the digestive process, the small intestine is needed to break down and absorb peptides and amino acids that were created in the stomach. Proteolytic enzymes from the pancreas are secreted into the small intestine to keep breaking down proteins. They are able to split polypeptides into oligopeptides and then cut them into dipeptides and amino acids. Bile acids in the small intestine help break up fats and also make the environment right for enzymes to function well. After absorption, amino acids and peptides move through the intestinal wall with the help of special transporters, so they can enter the blood. Since amino acids are needed for protein synthesis and metabolic control, it is very important that the process happens efficiently. Not only do enzymes and gastric juices take part in protein digestion, but also important regulatory mechanisms that affect genes involved in digestion and metabolism. As an example, when nutrient levels change, genes responsible for digestion in the intestine are affected. At times , such as weaning, when there are changes in what a baby eats, the gut can be affected by these changes. When feed intake is reduced, it leads to changes in genes coding for digestive enzymes and proteins that help absorption, which improves the digestive process. Learning about these factors is important for making strategies that help improve digestion and the use of nutrients. As noted in the literature, there is potential for dietary interventions to enhance intestinal gene expression and alleviate weaning-associated disorders, thereby supporting cellular homeostasis and overall health (Bauer et al., 2011; Sarmidi, 2012) (Figure 7.8).

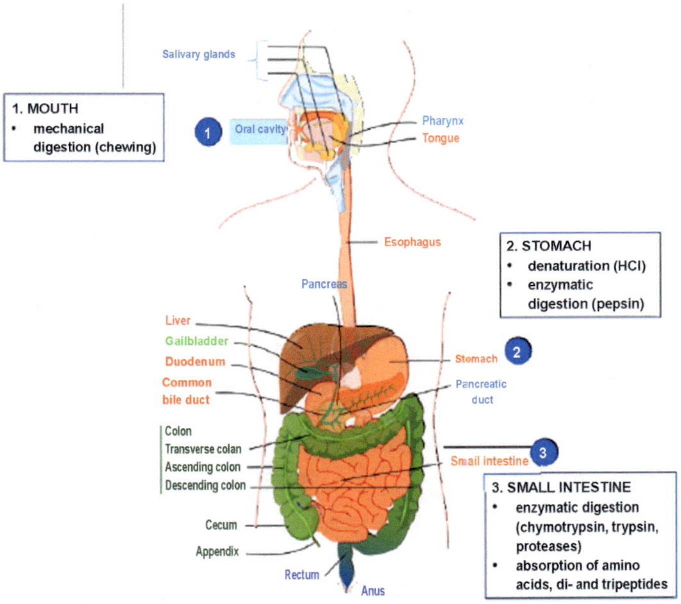

Figure 7.8. Protein digestion in the human GI tract.

Source: https://openoregon.pressbooks.pub/app/uploads/sites/98/2019/11/image5-3.png.

7.2.2. Enzymes Involved in Protein Breakdown

In the process of breaking down proteins and amino acids, it is enzymes that help make the amino acids available for different metabolic functions. For this breakdown to happen, proteases, which break down peptide bonds in proteins, are very important. They are organized into several categories depending on the way their active sites work, , such as serine, cysteine, aspartic, and metalloproteases. Proteases are controlled so that protein breakdown is efficient and does not happen too much. Maintaining cellular homeostasis depends on this regulation, because too little or too much proteolysis may result in either the buildup of misfolded proteins or the loss of important cellular materials. The involvement of proteases in several signaling pathways shows that they are important in both healthy and sick conditions. Serine proteases are especially remarkable because they are found in many places and play a major role in important metabolic processes. A serine residue in their active site is important for the way they work as catalysts. They help digest dietary proteins as well as take part in immune response, cell signaling, and apoptosis in the body. Trypsin is a serine protease produced by the pancreas and it helps break down proteins in the small intestine by cleaving peptide bonds. The process of trypsin and similar enzymes breaking down proteins proves that it is a well-regulated dance that makes sure there are enough amino acids for building proteins and producing energy. Besides digestion, enzymes are important for maintaining the proper level of amino acids in the body. The RidA proteins are important since they protect cells by breaking down imines that can be harmful during amino acid metabolism. The way they work with other enzymes, for example, threonine dehydratase, points out how metabolism includes steps for both breaking down and building up substances. Proper regulation of these enzymes is necessary because any problems with regulation can lead to metabolic diseases involving the buildup of harmful substances or the lack of important amino acids. By understanding the nuanced actions of these enzymes, researchers can develop targeted therapies for various conditions related to protein metabolism, providing valuable insights into both health and pathology (Dixon et al., 2009; Niehaus et al., 2015) (Figure 7.9).

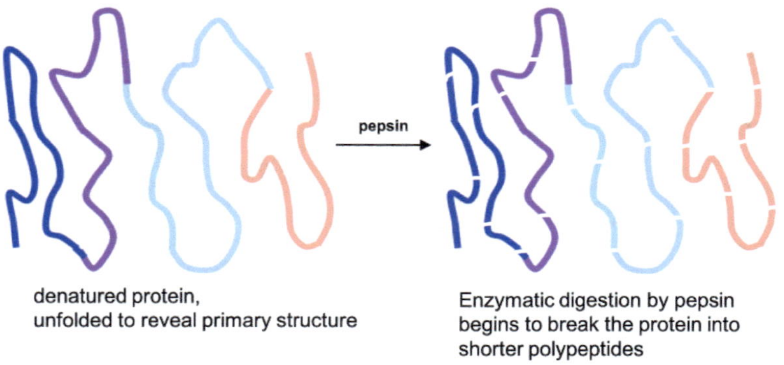

Figure 7.9. Enzymatic digestion of proteins begins in the stomach with the action of the enzyme pepsin.

Source: https://openoregon.pressbooks.pub/app/uploads/sites/98/2019/11/image1-3.png.

7.2.3. Absorption of Amino Acids in the Small Intestine

Protein and amino acid metabolism rely on the important process of absorbing amino acids in the small intestine, which has a big effect on metabolic health. Once dietary proteins are digested by enzymes into amino acids, the amino acids are able to enter the intestinal epithelium. The jejunum is the main place where amino acids are absorbed, followed by the ileum. Specific transporters, including the sodium-coupled neutral amino acid transporter 2 (SNAT2), play a vital role in this process by facilitating the uptake of essential and non-essential amino acids into enterocytes. The modulation of these transporters has profound implications for cellular amino acid availability, which in turn influences a range of vital cellular processes, including protein synthesis and cell proliferation, underscoring the importance of efficient amino acid absorption in maintaining homeostasis within the organism (Tang et al., 2018). When amino acids are taken up by enterocytes, they mainly go into the blood through the basolateral membrane of the intestinal epithelial cells. Afterward, they move to different body tissues to be turned into proteins or used to make energy. It helps with biosynthesis and metabolism and also affects the secretion of hormones and growth factors that oversee different body processes. It is shown by research that the intestinal epithelium contains many amino acid transporters, which help it absorb amino acids efficiently in different conditions. For example, certain transporters can adapt their activity based on dietary protein intake, contributing to the dynamic regulation of amino acid levels in the systemic circulation (Chen et al., 2020). Besides, the link between amino acid absorption in the small intestines and metabolic health is highlighted by the fact that amino acid deficiency can lead to several disorders. If a person does not get enough essential amino acids, it can slow down protein synthesis and impact muscle mass, the immune system, and the body's growth and repair. Besides, some disorders, , such as malabsorption syndromes, can interfere with digestion and result in health complications. The body must use amino acids efficiently to prevent problems that come with insufficient amino acids. Thus, understanding the regulatory mechanisms associated with amino acid transport and metabolism in the small intestine is vital for developing therapeutic strategies to address nutritional deficiencies and related health disorders (Tang et al., 2018).

Test Your Knowledge

1. What is the process of protein digestion in the gastrointestinal tract?
2. Which enzyme is involved in the breakdown of proteins?

7.3. Amino Acid Metabolism

Learning Outcome

1. Describe the metabolic processes of transamination and deamination;
2. Understand the role of amino acids in energy production;
3 Describe the synthesis of non-essential amino acids.

The breakdown and formation of amino acids in the body is called amino acid metabolism and is important for making proteins. It is important for the nitrogen metabolism in organisms, as it supports the balance of amino acids and delivers the necessary substances for making proteins. Most of the process is controlled by enzymes, which help convert amino acids into other substances that take part in metabolism. A main part of amino acid metabolism is the transamination and deamination reactions that allow amino acids to be converted and the creation of molecules that are part of the citric acid cycle, linking the process of protein metabolism to energy production. It proves that amino acids are involved in protein construction and also support the body's energy production. Apart from being part of proteins, amino acids also take part in signaling inside different metabolic pathways. For example, some amino acids, including arginine, can control how microorganisms' cells behave. It has been found that l-arginine is a sensor that regulates the amount of c-di-GMP, which is needed for bacteria like Pseudomonas aeruginosa to create biofilms. It appears that amino acids help maintain the structure of the cell and also control its processes. Therefore, exploring these interactions gives us a better idea of metabolism and shows us how amino acids can play a role in pathogenicity and microbial resistance, as seen in studies that study their effects on gene expression and metabolic processes in microbes. The fact that protein sources affect amino acid metabolism differently proves that these pathways are both complex and specific. For instance, studies that look at how soy and meat proteins affect various markers in the body show that the proteins have different effects. It has been found that eating a diet with more soy protein can help manage blood sugar and weight better than animal proteins. These differences prove that the different amino acid profiles in proteins can play a big role in maintaining metabolic health. It is clear that both types of proteins keep affecting the liver and lipid metabolism, as seen by changes in genes involved in lipid and energy metabolism pathways. Thanks to such connections, studies on amino acid metabolism can suggest helpful dietary guidelines for good health, which also support the proper balance of protein and amino acids in human nutrition and disease prevention (Figure 7.10).

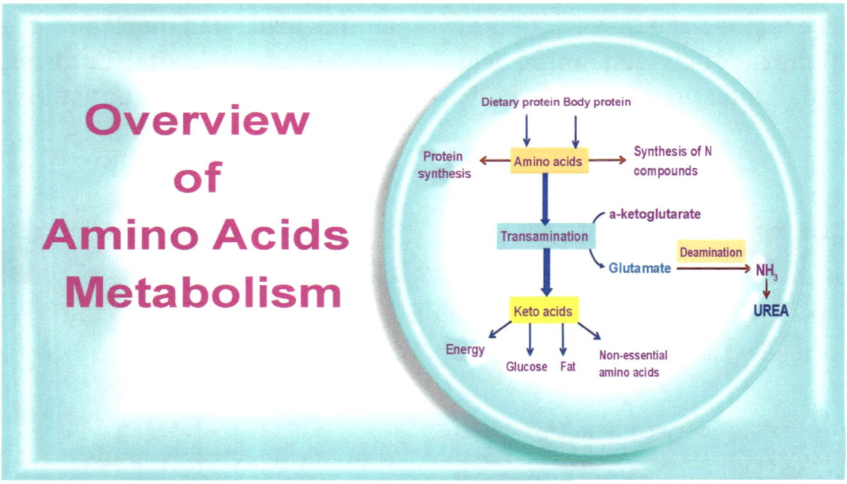

Figure 7.10. Overview of amino acid metabolism.

Source: https://i.ytimg.com/vi/Aa7aLhdFRJs/maxresdefault.jpg.

7.3.1. Transamination and Deamination Processes

The processes of transamination and deamination are key to protein and amino acid metabolism since they help convert and use amino acids in biochemical pathways. In transamination, the amino group is transferred from an amino acid to an α-keto acid, which leads to the creation of new amino acids and the creation corresponding α-keto acid. The main role of transaminases or aminotransferases is to help make alanine and aspartate from their α-keto acid precursors. It supports the right amount of amino acids in the body and helps move nitrogen to the urea cycle, which is important for maintaining the nitrogen balance needed for different physiological functions. The fact that transamination is dynamic makes it important for energy and biomolecule balance. Alternatively, deamination means removing an amino group from an amino acid, which usually creates ammonia and an α-keto acid. During times of energy shortage or when we eat too much protein, this process helps break down amino acids. Deamination helps amino acids become substrates that are used in energy-producing processes, for example, the citric acid cycle. In addition, the ammonia is then changed into urea by the urea cycle, which helps avoid the buildup of dangerous ammonia in the body. In specific contexts, , such as stress conditions or heavy metal exposure, variations in deamination rates can affect the overall metabolic response, illustrating the interconnected nature of these processes in maintaining homeostasis under varying environmental conditions (Vovchek et al., 2025). Scientific studies have pointed out that probiotic microorganisms are involved in regulating the breakdown and formation of amino acids. It has been found that having live bacteria , such as Lactobacillus and Bifidobacterium, in dietary supplements can help the host organism's functions and metabolism by increasing the availability of amino acids. The organic acids produced during probiotic fermentation can facilitate metabolic pathways, leading to the production of ATP and proteins (Mosyagin et al., 2024). With the help of these probiotics, amino acid formation and deamination happen, which ensures the body uses energy and nutrients well. Such findings point out the need to study the relationship between microbial activity and the metabolism of amino acids, which increases our knowledge of nutrients in the gut (Figure 7.11).

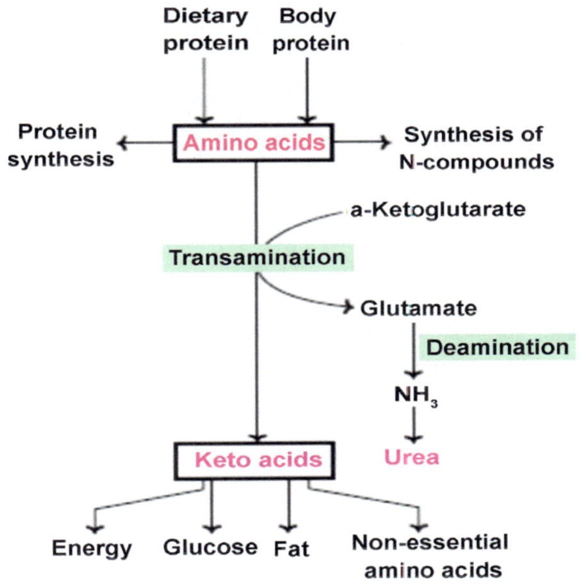

Figure 7.11. Transamination and deamination processes.

Source: https://encrypted-tbn0.gstatic.com/images?q=tbn:ANd9GcSw718hjXuyPj2UESJE2P_INxaSoj6WoQTj4Q&s.

7.3.2. Role of Amino Acids in Energy Production

Amino acids play key parts in making proteins and also help produce energy. If you fast or do a lot of exercise, amino acids are used to make glucose by the process of gluconeogenesis. In particular, glucogenic amino acids are turned into pyruvate or oxaloacetate, which can be used again by gluconeogenesis to make glucose. Meanwhile, BCAAs, , such as leucine, isoleucine, and valine, can be directly oxidized in muscle tissue to generate ATP, contributing to energy demands during prolonged exercise. In this role, it is highlighted that amino acids are key to maintaining the body's energy balance, especially when carbohydrates are limited or extra energy is needed. Apart from being used in gluconeogenesis, amino acids are essential in the citric acid cycle, which is important for making energy. The process of oxidative deamination in amino acids produces ammonia and keto acids that are able to join the citric acid cycle and help produce energy. As an illustration, glutamate is broken down to α-ketoglutarate, and alanine is changed into pyruvate, both of which are vital intermediates in the citric acid cycle. Besides, the products of these metabolic pathways, NADH and FADH2, are used in the electron transport chain to create ATP.

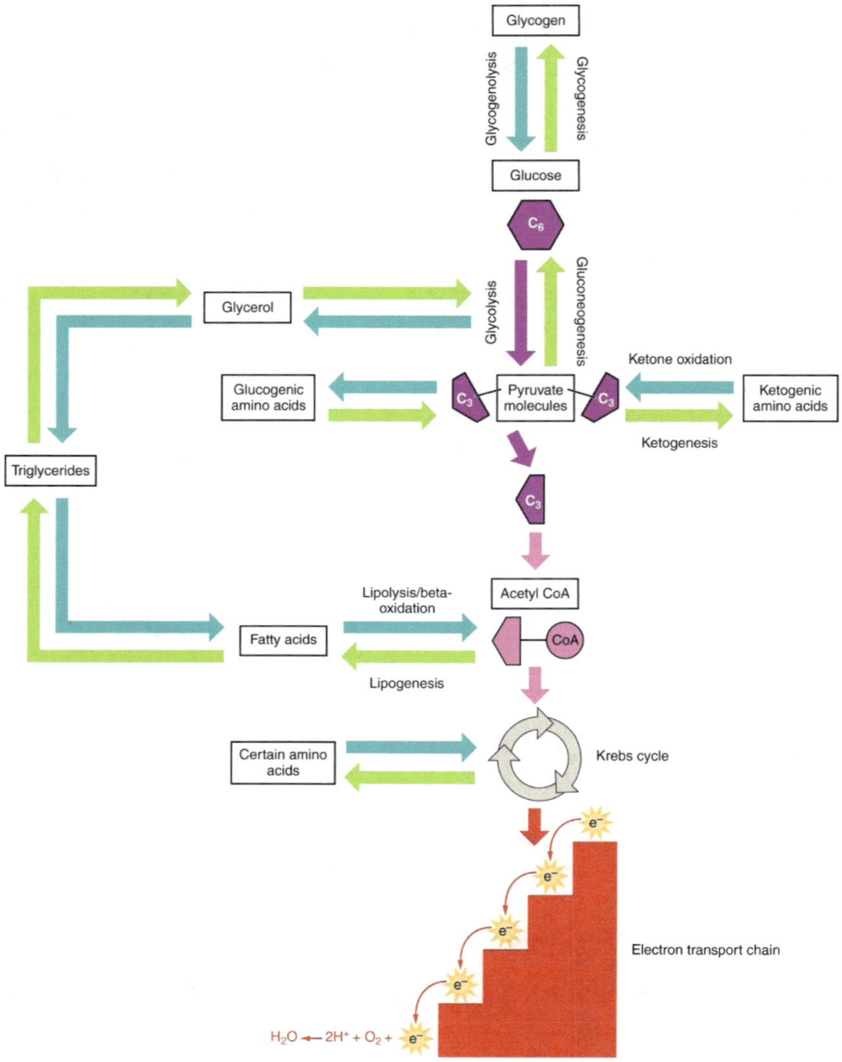

Figure 7.12. Nutrients follow a complex pathway from ingestion through anabolism and catabolism to energy production.

Source: https://s3-us-west-2.amazonaws.com/courses-images-archive-read-only/wp-content/uploads/sites/403/2015/04/21031818/2520_Catabolic_and_Anabolic-Pathways.jpg.

Therefore, amino acids play a key role in energy production by participating in different enzymatic processes and showing their importance as energy providers during metabolism. Studies done recently have pointed out the links between amino acid metabolism and energy production, mainly in microbial communities. It has been found through research that proteins connected to amino acid metabolism can affect both the development of biofilms and the amount of energy in Pseudomonas aeruginosa. Proteins involved in amino acid catabolism have been identified among those that differentially express and may affect energy metabolism, illustrating the critical link between amino acid availability and energy dynamics within microbial populations (Wu & Cheng, 2011). Furthermore, the role of amino acids in energy production is accentuated through their involvement in metabolic pathways that regulate biofilm formation, where energy metabolism significantly impacts the organism's capability to adapt to varying environmental conditions (Chen et al., 2013). The study shows that amino acids are vital nutrients and also active in energy production in various parts of the body (Figure 7.12).

7.3.3. Synthesis of Non-Essential Amino Acids

Non-essential amino acids are made by the body from simple substances, showing that the body can synthesize these molecules. Amino acids , such as alanine, aspartate, and glutamate are made from glycolysis and citric acid cycle intermediates through different metabolic processes. When this synthesis happens, amino groups are moved from one molecule to another through transamination reactions, which produce amino acids. As an example, the body changes α-ketoglutarate into glutamate to maintain nitrogen balance and support cells, without needing to get nitrogen from food. Since amino acids take part in protein synthesis and many metabolic reactions, learning more about their synthesis highlights the importance of all metabolic pathways in the body's balance. In some situations, , such as stress, disease, or fast growth, some non-essential amino acids may become essential, so the body needs to make them more quickly. If metabolic needs increase, it may cause a lack of necessary substances for producing amino acids, which can affect the body's overall metabolism. During illness, the body might not be able to make enough arginine and glutamine, which are important for both the immune system and repairing cells. Taking in these amino acids when the metabolism is high may support a faster and better recovery. For this reason, although the body is good at making non-essential amino acids, knowing how their synthesis can change is important for good health and disease control, because their availability can affect protein and body processes. Besides, the process of making non-essential amino acids is tied to cell signaling, mainly through the mTOR pathway. The mTOR complex is important for detecting nutrients and regulating the production of proteins, which shows that amino acid balance is crucial. Recent findings indicate that asparagine acts as an exchange factor in amino acid metabolism, influencing the uptake and availability of other amino acids , such as serine and arginine (Braas et al., 2016). This shows that the amount of amino acids in the body can impact the cellular processes that promote growth. So, the presence of non-essential amino acids in proteins is important for structure, but they also help regulate nutrient sensing and cell growth, proving their key role in maintaining a healthy metabolism in the body.

Test Your Knowledge

1. What is the process of transamination and deamination?
2. What is the role of amino acids in energy production?

7.4. Protein Synthesis

Learning Outcome

1. Give an overview of transcription and translation;
2. Understand the role of ribosomes in protein synthesis;
3. Describe the post-translational modifications (PTMs) of proteins.

Growth, repair, and metabolic control in living organisms depend on the process of protein synthesis. It involves the intricate interplay between deoxyribonucleic acid (DNA), messenger ribonucleic acid (mRNA), ribosomes, and transfer RNA (tRNA). At first, transcription happens in the nucleus, where a DNA template makes mRNA, which carries the genetic code to ribosomes in the cytoplasm. Ribosomes are the place where the mRNA sequence is translated and the amino acids are put together in a certain order to produce a polypeptide chain. Afterward, the chain becomes a protein that is important for the body's cells and health, proving that protein synthesis plays a key role in protein and amino acid metabolism. Moreover, the amount of protein synthesis is greatly affected by diet, mainly because of essential amino acids, which are used to make proteins. If the diet contains too little protein or has limited phenylalanine, it can greatly affect the body's metabolic processes. For example, if phenylalanine is eaten in smaller amounts, it may reduce the development of important proteins in the brains of infants and children. Studies show that the administration of chloramphenicol, an antibiotic that inhibits protein synthesis, can perturb amino acid metabolism and influence overall growth outcomes (Cockburn et al., 1966). This points out that the right amount of each amino acid in the diet is needed for proper protein synthesis, showing how nutrition and protein metabolism are related. Studies on the effects of protein intake and dietary rules on muscle composition show more about how protein synthesis works. For example, altering the protein content in the diets of growing pigs has been shown to correlate with intramuscular fat (IMF) deposits and the expression of various genes associated with lipid metabolism. Interestingly, a low protein diet was observed to increase IMF content while negatively impacting protein synthesis pathways, which could have broader implications for growth and development (Aslan et al., 2013). As a result, having enough essential amino acids is important for protein synthesis and the health of the body's metabolism. As restricting dietary protein causes stress and changes genes, studying these effects helps find the best ways to support growth and development (Figure 7.13).

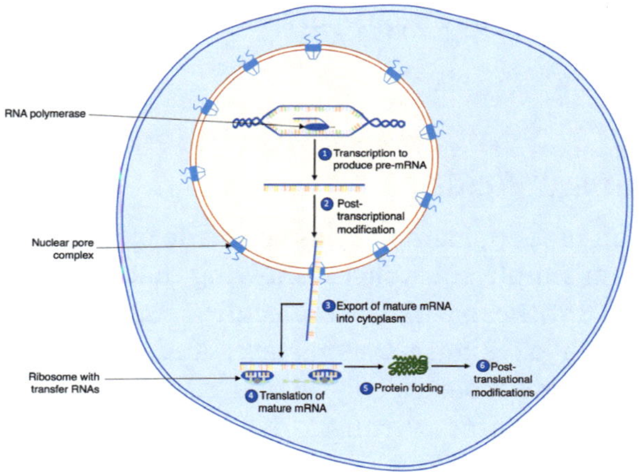

Figure 7.13. Protein synthesis.

Source: https://chemistrytalk.org/wp-content/uploads/2023/05/Summary_of_the_protein_biosynthesis_process.png.

7.4.1. Overview of Transcription and Translation

Transcription and translation help genes be expressed and proteins be synthesized, so that the DNA code can be used in the cell. During transcription, RNA polymerase binds to the promoter region of a gene in the DNA, unwinding the double helix and synthesizing a complementary strand of mRNA from the DNA template. It is the job of this mRNA to bring the genetic code from the nucleus to the ribosome, where it is translated.

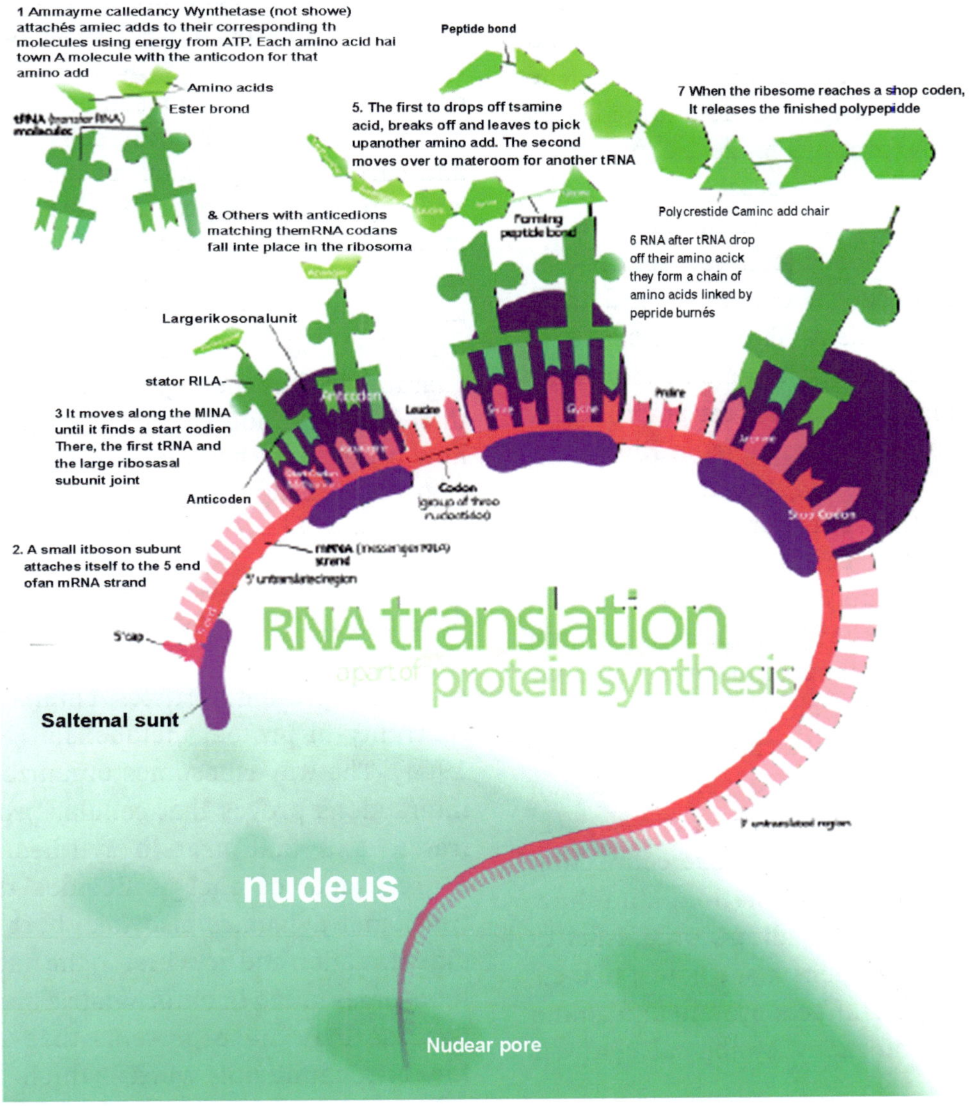

Figure 7.14. Transcription and translation process of protein synthesis.

Source: By Kelvinsong - Own work, CC BY 3.0, https://commons.wikimedia.org/w/index.php?curid=23198939

It is very important for transcription to be precise, since accurate mRNA production means the sequence of nucleotides matches the original gene, supporting correct protein synthesis and metabolic regulation needed for protein and amino acid metabolism. After mRNA is made in transcription, the ribosome uses the mRNA sequence to make a specific polypeptide chain in the next step, called translation. Transfer RNA (tRNA) plays a significant role in this process by bringing the appropriate amino acids to the ribosome, aligning with the mRNA codons through complementary base pairing. The matching of an anticodon on tRNA with a codon on mRNA guarantees that the right amino acid is included in the chain of amino acids. The process of translation is needed for cells to function, since the proteins made are important for different metabolic processes. Besides, the regulation of translation is determined by tRNA, regulatory proteins, and cellular conditions, which can influence protein levels and their function in metabolism. The significance of transcription and translation is also shown by how they respond to changes in the environment in many organisms. For example, in *Rhizobium leguminosarum* bv. *trifolii*, the transcriptional regulation of different genes is triggered by environmental conditions to support plant symbiosis and bacterial metabolism (Janczarek et al., 2019). Similarly, Yersinia enterocolitica demonstrates a cold response in which the transcription of specific genes is altered to enable survival at low temperatures, emphasizing the significance of gene expression modulation in adapting to external stressors (Li et al., 2020). They reveal the close connection among transcription, translation, and how proteins function, as this allows organisms to maintain a stable metabolism and adjust to their environments, which affects protein and amino acid metabolism in many biological contexts (Figure 7.14).

7.4.2. Role of Ribosomes in Protein Synthesis

Protein synthesis relies on ribosomes, as they help turn genetic information into useful proteins in the metabolism of proteins and amino acids. Ribosomes function as the cellular machinery where amino acids are assembled into polypeptide chains, following the instructions encoded in mRNA. It takes several actions to complete the process, , such as initiation, elongation, and termination. At the beginning of the process, the ribosome joins the mRNA so that it can choose the proper start codon. It proves that ribosomes are actively involved in the processes that control the functions of cells. How efficiently ribosomes work highlights their major role in helping cells remain stable and carry out important reactions for growth and repair. Once ribosomes are fully engaged in the translation process, they facilitate the recruitment of transfer RNA (tRNA) molecules that carry specific amino acids corresponding to the mRNA codons. The anticodon on each tRNA guarantees that the right amino acid is added to the polypeptide chain, which demonstrates how protein synthesis is faithful. At a fast pace, ribosomes change the genetic code into proteins, which shows how vital they are in biology.

Notably, extensive research has demonstrated that the incorporation of amino acids into proteins primarily occurs at these ribonucleoprotein particles, emphasizing their centrality in protein metabolism (Nicol et al., 1964). The way ribosomes organize molecular interactions proves that cellular processes are fragile and that protein synthesis requires a great deal of energy. Besides translation, ribosomal dynamics also take part in cellular differentiation and activities in the mitochondria. Ribosomes found in mitochondria are important because they make proteins that are needed for mitochondrial work, which helps the cell to produce energy. The morphological differentiation of mitochondria during early embryonic development remains reliant on mitochondrial ribosomal and transfer RNA synthesis, which underscores the significance of ribosomes in developing complex organisms (Chase et al., 1973). While cells are developing, the careful control of ribosomes goes along with the need for energy and metabolism, proving that ribosomes are involved in both protein production and the well-being of the cell. The way ribosomes work together in metabolism proves their importance for life at all levels of living organisms (Figure 7.15).

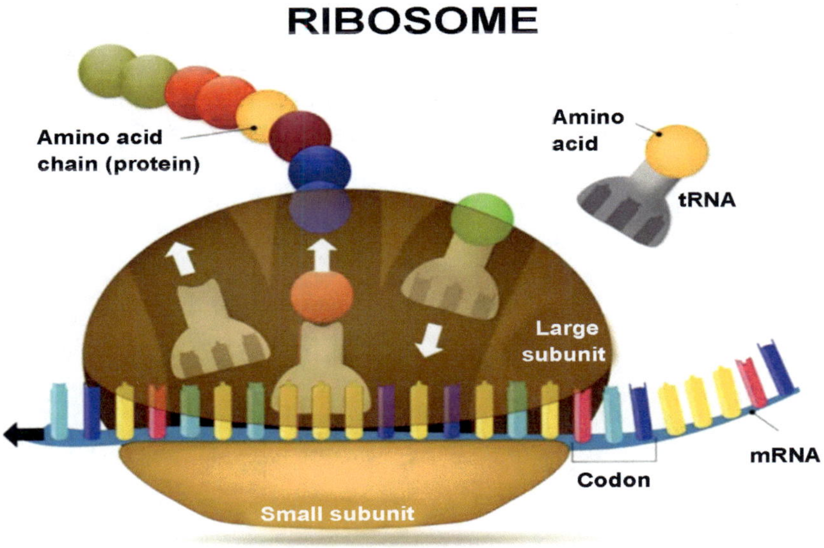

Figure 7.15. Ribosomes interact with mRNA to produce proteins in a process called translation.

Source: https://www.thoughtco.com/thmb/a8-nwCJRbFm90i4sXp8C1N_-FJE=/750x0/filters:no_upscale():max_bytes(150000):strip_icc():format(webp)/protein_synthesis-6c2ebf130fd141f3944ff88dbe4481c8.jpg.

7.4.3. Post-Translational Modifications of Proteins

Post-translational modifications (PTMs) of proteins play a critical role in expanding the functional diversity of the proteome, profoundly influencing protein activity, localization, stability, and interactions. After protein synthesis, these modifications happen and include phosphorylation, methylation, acetylation, and ubiquitination. Every PTM has its own role; for example, phosphorylation can control how enzymes and signaling pathways work, while acetylation can impact the stability of proteins and their ability to transcribe DNA. Because of how these modifications change, cells can react fast to changes within and around them, helping to control cellular metabolism. It is necessary to understand PTMs, since their disruption has been linked to several diseases and shows how important they are for maintaining the balance of proteins in metabolic pathways. The importance of PTMs goes further than just chemical changes; they are involved in basic biological activities, for example, gene expression and signaling between cells. Mitochondrial ribosomal protein (RP) MRPL12 is acetylated in mitochondria, which points to the role of PTMs in regulating the transcription of mitochondrial DNA. It has been found that acetylation can affect how much mitochondrial RNA polymerase binds to DNA, which changes the amount of mitochondrial transcripts. This regulation is especially crucial, as mitochondrial function is intimately tied to energy metabolism and overall cellular health (Katelynn et al., 2023). The results prove that PTMs are involved in regulating metabolism and are therefore an important part of protein and amino acid metabolism. Investigating the various PTMs helps us understand their general effects on the body, mainly in terms of health and disease. The attention to methylation and citrullination of amino acids like arginine and lysine is high because they take part in complex biological processes. For instance, citrullination can create new antigenic epitopes that may contribute to autoimmune diseases, including rheumatoid arthritis, highlighting the pathology stemming from aberrant PTMs (Tsikas, 2021). Besides, methylated proteins are related to nitric oxide synthesis, meaning PTMs can affect protein function and also produce important metabolites involved in health. They demonstrate the many roles PTMs have in proteins, which are linked to important metabolic processes and diseases in the body, so their study is necessary for finding better treatments (Figure 7.16).

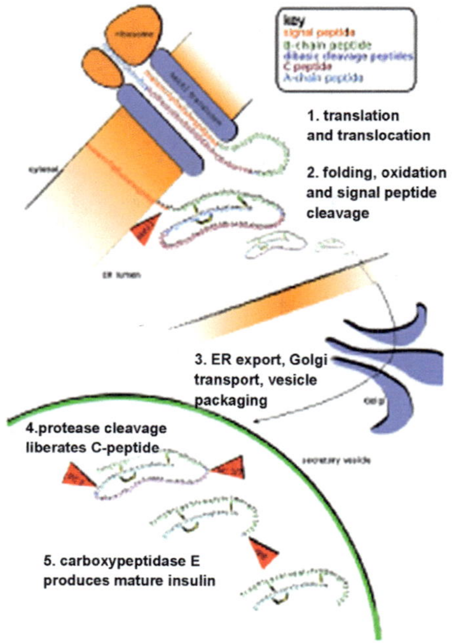

Figure 7.16. Post-translational modifications.

Source: https://chemistrytalk.org/wp-content/uploads/2023/05/800px-Insulin_path.svg.png.

Test Your Knowledge

1. What is transcription and translation?
2. What is the role of ribosomes in protein synthesis?

7.5. Regulation of Protein Metabolism

Learning Outcome

1. Understand the hormonal regulation of protein synthesis and degradation;
2. Describe the nutritional factors affecting protein metabolism;
3. Describe the impact of exercise on protein metabolism.

Many biological pathways are important in determining how proteins are made and broken down in protein metabolism. These processes rely mostly on signaling pathways that bring together several conditions, , such as the amount of nutrients and hormones in the body. As an illustration, insulin and glucagon control how protein is metabolized, mainly by guiding the movement of amino acids and protein breakdown. So, knowing the ways these hormones affect metabolism is necessary to grasp the main aspects of protein and amino acid metabolism. Also, studies show that the way soy and meat proteins are expressed in the body adds to the complexity of this mechanism. The findings suggest that distinct protein sources can invoke unique physiological responses, thereby influencing overall metabolic health in significant ways (Hagiwara et al., 2016). Another important part of regulating protein metabolism is the role played by some amino acids as signals. Certain amino acids, especially BCAAs, have been implicated in metabolic regulation by activating key signaling pathways related to growth and nutrient sensing. For instance, BCAAs can stimulate the mammalian target of rapamycin (mTOR) pathway, which is pivotal for protein synthesis and muscle growth. In situations , such as working out and muscle recovery, this regulatory mechanism plays a key role since nutrients greatly influence the body's anabolic processes. Such studies also reveal that changes in protein metabolism can be the result and the cause of various health problems. Understanding the differential responses in amino acid metabolism under stress conditions can pave the way for targeted nutritional interventions (Tischler et al., 2025). The kind and quality of proteins in the diet play a major role in how the body handles and controls protein metabolism. The way proteins affect the body and genes highlights the role of food in keeping people healthy. Research has demonstrated that soy protein might make insulin function better and reduce body fat more than meat proteins, pointing out the different ways these proteins affect metabolism. Researchers can use these results to learn more about how dietary proteins can help with both immediate metabolic effects and long-term health problems connected to metabolic syndrome (MS) and obesity. The nuanced regulatory effects of different proteins on metabolic pathways accentuate the importance of personalized nutrition strategies aimed at optimizing protein intake for improved metabolic health and overall well-being (Hagiwara et al., 2016).

7.5.1. Hormonal Regulation of Protein Synthesis and Degradation

The way hormones interact is key to overseeing both the creation and breakdown of proteins in organisms, which plays a major role in controlling metabolic activities. Hormones control which genes are active to support both the building up and breaking down of proteins. As an example, insulin and growth hormone are anabolic hormones that encourage amino acids to enter cells and stimulate the ribosome, which leads to more protein production. On the other hand, hormones , such as glucagon and cortisol help break down proteins and supply amino acids for energy or glucose production during stressful situations. Keeping the balance between anabolic and catabolic activities is important for maintaining cells' normal functions and meeting the body's needs. Because of hormonal regulation, proteins are produced or broken down in an exact amount that matches the organism's needs at any given time. The process includes certain endocrine factors that affect pathways that control translation and the breakdown of proteins. For example, the mTOR pathway is a critical regulator of protein synthesis, integrating signals from nutrients and growth factors.

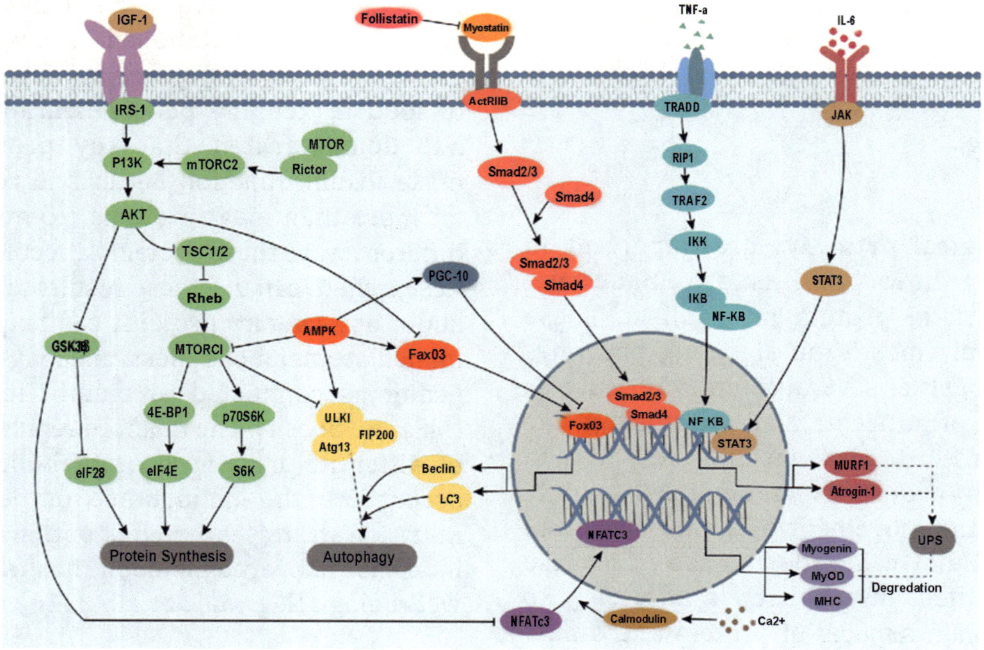

Figure 7.17. Regulation of protein synthesis and degradation pathways.

Source: https://www.researchgate.net/profile/Hanbing-Li-6/publication/364638091/figure/fig1/AS:11431281167504207@1686661185870/Regulation-of-protein-synthesis-and-degradation-pathways-1-Protein-synthesis-The-Akt.png.

When insulin is present, mTOR turns on protein synthesis by making certain translation and RPs active. If energy is limited or stress exists, hormones like glucagon stimulate systems that cause the body to break down protein and release amino acids for energy or gluconeogenesis. Hormones can change the activity of these pathways, leading to major shifts in protein metabolism and maintaining a proper balance between making and breaking down proteins needed for adjusting to different situations. It has been found that hormones affect not only the short-term metabolic process but also contribute to long-term changes in protein and muscle growth. Having anabolic stimuli, , such as growth factors and hormones, can cause protein synthesis to rise and, at the same time, decrease the rate of proteolysis. Besides, using insulin and growth hormone has been found to boost muscle mass, which points to their ability to change how fast proteins are used and made in the body. Alternatively, situations that raise catabolic hormone levels, , such as fasting for a long time or dealing with chronic stress, cause the body to break down proteins through increased activity of lysosomes and proteasomes. Thus, the hormonal regulation of protein metabolism is a complex network that plays a crucial role in growth, adaptation, and recovery during metabolic challenges, as seen in studies exploring various hormonal interactions with amino acid metabolism (Wang et al., 2023; Zhang et al., 2024) (Figure 7.17).

7.5.2. Nutritional Factors Affecting Protein Metabolism

The metabolism of proteins and amino acids depends a lot on the nutrients you consume. The kind and quality of protein in your diet can have a strong impact on your metabolism. Quality proteins that have essential amino acids are used in building proteins and help maintain the body's nitrogen balance. Eating a diet low in quality protein may result in less than enough amino acids, which can negatively affect muscle health and hormone regulation. In addition, how nutrients are absorbed into the body, influenced by methods of food processing and preparation, is important for proper protein metabolism. For example, cooking changes proteins and removes harmful substances, which results in better absorption and use of amino acids. Certain parts of the diet can also impact protein metabolism by changing hormones and enzymes in the body. Carbohydrates and fats work together with proteins to affect the hormones that control anabolism and catabolism. A sufficient intake of carbohydrates can cause insulin to be released, which makes it possible for amino acids to be absorbed and for muscle protein to be formed using the mTOR pathway. Also, some micronutrients , such as vitamins and minerals, help enzymes work in the metabolism of amino acids. Not having enough of these micronutrients can negatively affect metabolic reactions, which can affect the body's overall metabolism. Hence, it is important to get enough macronutrients and micronutrients to support healthy protein metabolism and different metabolic processes. Furthermore, the influence of chronic conditions, including chronic kidney disease (CKD), underscores the significance of nutritional factors in protein metabolism. In patients with CKD, alterations in metabolic pathways, , such as increased inflammatory cytokines and disrupted anabolic hormone signaling, can severely impact protein utilization and muscle health (Slee et al., 2012). Dietary restrictions can cause a person's nutrition to suffer, which may result in muscle loss and additional problems. In such cases, dietary advice that fits the patient's needs can help reduce problems with protein synthesis. Additionally, emerging research highlights the role of diet in modulating mesenchymal stem cell activity, where specific nutrients facilitate beneficial differentiation pathways that may influence overall metabolic health (Ammendola et al., 2018). As a result, it is very important to pay attention to nutrition when aiming to optimize protein metabolism in healthy people and those with long-term health problems.

7.5.3. Impact of Exercise on Protein Metabolism

Exercise and protein metabolism are closely connected, as they both play a big role in building and breaking down muscle proteins. Resistance training causes small tears in muscle fibers, which then lead to various changes in the body to help it heal and get stronger. This happens when the body increases the rate at which it builds muscle proteins, which can only be possible if the rate of synthesis is higher than the rate of breakdown. For this reason, the changes in metabolism after resistance exercise can last for 48 hours after the workout. So, how much amino acid you eat after exercise and your body's high metabolic state are very important for building muscle and aiding recovery. Evidence suggests that a robust response in muscle protein metabolism is contingent upon the availability of amino acids during this window, further highlighting the importance of post-exercise nutrition in promoting muscle anabolism (Tipton et al., 2001). Besides, the type and source of dietary protein play a key role in how muscle protein is affected after exercise. It has been found that different sources of protein differ in their ability to stimulate muscle protein synthesis due to the unique amino acid content and how fast they are absorbed. For example, proteins containing important amino acids, mainly leucine, are more helpful in building muscle tissue after exercise. Even so, eating protein as part of a whole food or alone can make a difference in its effectiveness. Although there is a lot of research on isolated proteins, recent studies indicate that proteins in whole foods can impact postmeal metabolism and, as a result, muscle recovery and development. This complexity emphasizes the necessity for future research focused on understanding how protein form and processing techniques impact protein quality and metabolic outcomes (West et al., 2023). Besides the effects of exercise on muscle protein, hormones also help control the impact of exercise on protein metabolism. Insulin and testosterone help the body build muscle proteins and slow down the breakdown of muscle proteins. After exercising, the release of these hormones is increased, and this, together with enough protein, helps create the best conditions for muscle growth. While insulin is mainly known for assisting amino acids into muscle cells, it also prevents the breakdown of proteins, which helps build muscle after exercising. Therefore, understanding the intricate interplay between exercise, dietary protein intake, and hormonal regulation is fundamental for devising effective nutrition and training strategies aimed at optimizing muscle health and performance (Tipton et al., 2001) (Figure 7.18).

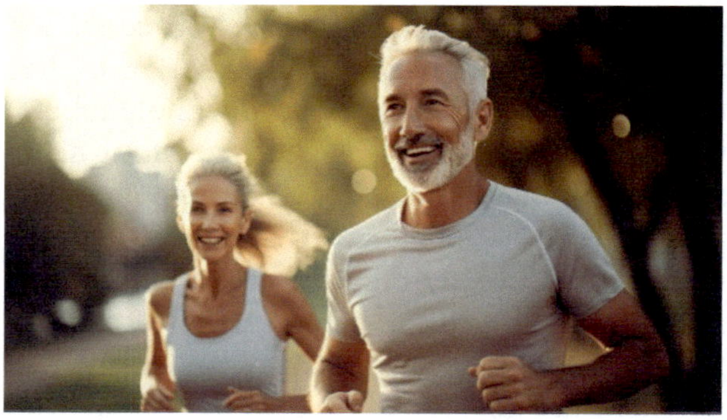

Figure 7.18. Active older adults jogging outdoors, representing healthy aging and wellness.

Source: https://www.matakanasuperfoods.com/cdn/shop/articles/AdobeStock_649377955_578ad881-d106-4049-bcc1-5160453c9333.jpg?v=1710895120&width=1200.

Test Your Knowledge

1. What are the nutritional factors affecting protein metabolism?
2. What effect does exercise have on protein metabolism?

7.6. Disorders Related to Protein Metabolism

Learning Outcome

1. Describe the inborn errors of metabolism;
2. Learn about protein-energy malnutrition;
3. Describe the effects of excessive protein intake.

Disturbances in protein metabolism are gaining notice because of their strong effects on people's health. As a result of problems in protein and amino acid pathways, these disorders cause various medical issues. One such disorder, Peutz-Jeghers syndrome (PJS), exemplifies the intricate relationship between genetic mutations and protein function. The serine-threonine kinase 11 (STK11) gene, a critical tumor suppressor involved in various cellular processes, showcases how specific single amino acid substitutions can disrupt its activity. The resultant dysfunction fosters disease susceptibility and underscores the need for a deeper understanding of the molecular implications of these mutations, particularly in how they destabilize pivotal protein structures and influence enzymatic efficiency in metabolic pathways (Md. Islam et al., 2019). Protein metabolism disorders can have cascading effects on several physiological systems, potentially manifesting in conditions , such as myalgic encephalomyelitis/chronic fatigue syndrome (ME/CFS). This disease causes lasting tiredness and other serious symptoms that are related to metabolic problems. Studies done recently suggest that pathways for energy and amino acid processing are altered in people with ME/CFS. Importantly, alterations in taurine and glycerophospholipid metabolism, along with others, show the many aspects of this disorder. By examining how genetic and metabolic factors intertwine to contribute to symptoms, researchers advance the understanding of the biological underpinnings of ME/CFS, revealing potential targets for therapeutic interventions (Germain et al., 2016). In addition, examining protein metabolism disorders points out their effects on the health of the public. These disorders impact a person's daily life and also put pressure on healthcare systems because they require special care and multiple therapies. To deal with these problems, researchers, clinicians, and policymakers should work together to improve how diseases are diagnosed and how they can be treated. With the help of genomics and metabolomics, scientists may be able to recognize important biomarkers and pathways related to these disorders, giving a better insight into their causes and how to deal with them. This comprehensive approach to studying protein metabolism disorders is essential as it not only enhances scientific knowledge but also informs clinical practice and improves patient outcomes in the long term (Germain et al., 2016; Islam et al., 2019) (Figure 7.19).

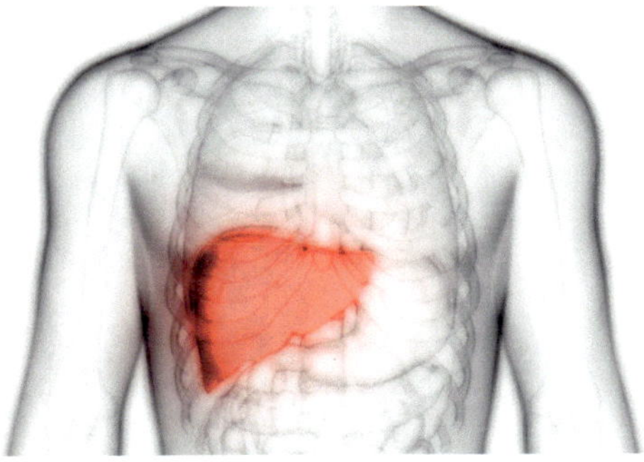

Figure 7.19. Protein metabolism disorder.

Source: https://static.ticimax.cloud/cdn-cgi/image/width=540,quality=99/32584/uploads/blog/what-is-the-protein-metabolism-disorder-058c.jpg.

7.6.1. Inborn Errors of Metabolism (e.g., Phenylketonuria)

The metabolic pathways that govern protein and amino acid metabolism are subject to a variety of genetic anomalies known as inborn errors of metabolism (IEMs). One prominent example is phenylketonuria (PKU), a condition caused by a deficiency in the enzyme phenylalanine hydroxylase, which is necessary for the conversion of phenylalanine to tyrosine. As a result of this enzyme problem, phenylalanine builds up in the blood, endangering the nervous system if it is not treated. The way enzymes work with amino acids clearly shows that genetics is very important for metabolic health. Recognizing the fundamental role of such enzymes is essential for understanding how their malfunction can trigger a cascade of metabolic disturbances that affect overall health and development in affected individuals (Ismail et al., 2019). Treating PKU reminds us that finding and treating the condition as soon as possible is very important. Thanks to newborn screening, metabolic disorders are often found before the patient shows any symptoms. Using targeted metabolic assays, it is possible to screen newborns for PKU and other IEMs, which helps begin proper treatment early to avoid health problems. Still, there is a chance that targeted assays can produce false results. So, scientists have suggested using untargeted metabolomics to improve the efficiency of screening. By utilizing untargeted analyses, it is possible to detect a wider array of metabolites, thereby providing a more comprehensive understanding of metabolic disorders and improving diagnostic accuracy for various IEMs, , such as PKU, and their management strategies (Martins et al., 1999). Besides controlling what people eat, new discoveries about the biochemical pathways of IEMs have encouraged the search for new treatments. For PKU, where sticking to a strict diet is always necessary, research on enzyme and gene therapies looks promising for finding better treatment. The purpose of these advancements is to treat the enzyme issues and also help patients enjoy more freedom in their diets. The field of metabolic disorder treatment is now focused on the need for continuous research and cooperation among various experts. This multidisciplinary approach is crucial in developing innovative solutions that can potentially transform the prognosis for individuals living with IEMs, thereby enhancing outcomes and quality of life (Martins et al., 1999) (Figure 7.20).

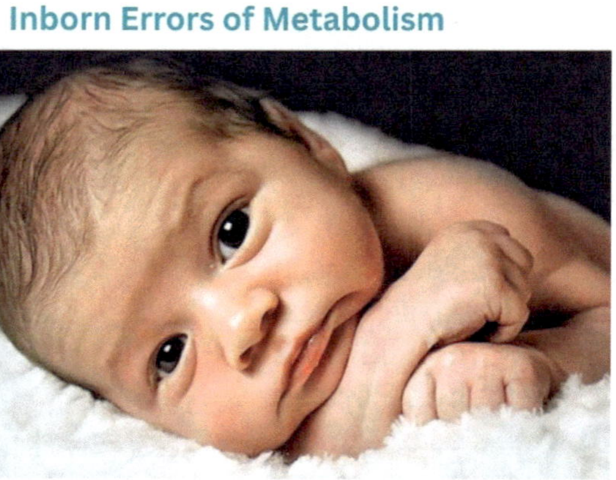

Figure 7.20. Inborn errors of metabolism.

Source: https://www.diagnopein.com/img/BlogImages/Inborn%20Errors%20of%20Metabolism.jpg.

7.6.2. Protein-Energy Malnutrition (e.g., Kwashiorkor and Marasmus)

Protein-energy malnutrition (PEM) significantly impacts global health, presenting primarily in two forms: kwashiorkor and marasmus. Kwashiorkor is mostly seen in children who get enough calories but not enough protein, which results in major physical and immune problems. Signs of the disease are swelling, changes in skin color, and a bloated stomach, all caused by metabolic problems made worse by not getting enough essential amino acids and problems with protein formation. Alternatively, marasmus happens when a person does not get enough calories, resulting in a lot of muscle and fat loss. When this condition occurs, the body starts using its own tissues as a source of energy, which seriously affects both amino acid metabolism and the balance of nutrients. Both forms highlight the importance of dietary protein in maintaining metabolic health and illustrate how deficiency leads to multifaceted disruptions in bodily functions and growth (Carolyn et al., 2021).

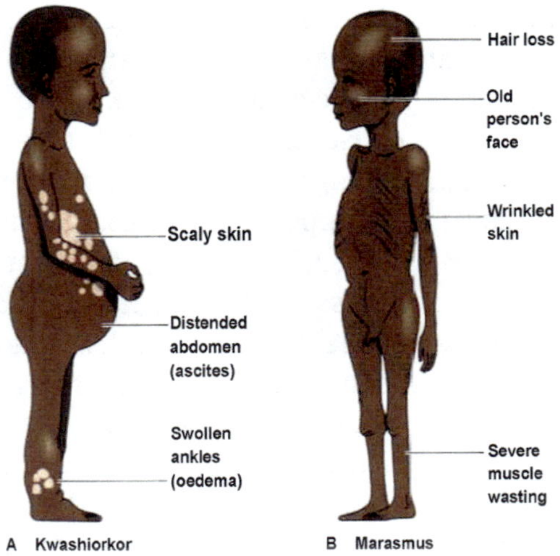

Figure 7.21. Protein-energy malnutrition: (A) kwashiorkor; and (B) marasmus.

Source: https://www.w3schools.blog/wp-content/uploads/2019/09/unnamed-jpg-1.jpeg.

Kwashiorkor and marasmus are caused by the way energy is used, how protein is processed, and the work of hormones in the body. When protein is lacking in kwashiorkor, albumin is not produced enough, which causes hypoalbuminemia, low oncotic pressure, and edema. Having infections also makes the problem worse since the inflammatory response can stop protein production and increase breakdown, causing malnutrition to continue. In marasmus, the body lacks fuel in general, and it uses amino acids to produce glucose for essential functions, which weakens the muscles and the whole metabolism. A thorough understanding of these metabolic alterations can inform effective nutritional interventions and therapeutic strategies aimed at restoring health in affected individuals, emphasizing the critical role that balanced protein intake plays in recovery from PEM (Dioguardi et al., 2011). To deal with PEM, different actions are needed, , such as improving nutrition through diets and public health measures. In most cases, kwashiorkor is treated by increasing protein slowly, usually with special formulas or foods that are fortified to help the patient's body without causing more stress. When a child has marasmus, it is important to feed them slowly, since fast re-nourishment may cause metabolic problems. It is important to keep an eye on micronutrients, hydration, and other possible health problems in both conditions. Ultimately, the intersection of protein and amino acid metabolism with broader nutritional support strategies underscores the importance of tailored nutritional care in reversing the effects of PEM and restoring optimal biochemical function (Dioguardi et al., 2011) (Figure 7.21).

7.6.3. Effects of Excessive Protein Intake

Having too much protein may cause several negative effects, mainly related to metabolism. If the body gets more protein than it can use for repair and growth, the extra protein usually goes through deamination, which creates ammonia. The liver is put under greater pressure since it has to change ammonia into urea and remove it through the kidneys. Repeatedly high levels of urea may lead to hyperuricemia, which can worsen gout or cause problems with the kidneys. Besides, the extra nitrogen may negatively affect the kidneys, especially in those who already have kidney problems. This points out that it is important to eat protein in balanced amounts based on your health and how active you are. Along with issues in the kidneys and liver, eating too much protein may harm bone health. Some studies indicate that too much protein can cause the body to take calcium from the bones in order to balance the acid produced by protein. Although protein is believed to help bones, having too much in the diet may cause harm, mainly for people who are already at risk of osteoporosis. It is important to consume enough calcium and other nutrients along with protein to avoid any problems linked to excessive consumption. So, knowing the details of protein metabolism and its effects on bones is necessary for creating dietary advice that supports good health and reduces health problems in the future. Excessive protein intake may also lead to problems with how the body uses energy and keeps its metabolism stable. When people eat a lot of protein, they usually eat less carbohydrate and fat, which are needed for good energy and metabolism. If a person's diet is not balanced, it may lead to poor performance in sports and make them feel tired. Eating a lot of protein for a long period may result in more insulin resistance and changes in glucose metabolism, making metabolic health worse. Thus, it is imperative to consider not only the total protein consumed but also the balance of macronutrients in the broader context of protein and amino acid metabolism to ensure that health and performance goals are met without incurring detrimental effects on overall health (Bauer et al., 2009; Kwakkel et al., 2011) (Figure 7.22).

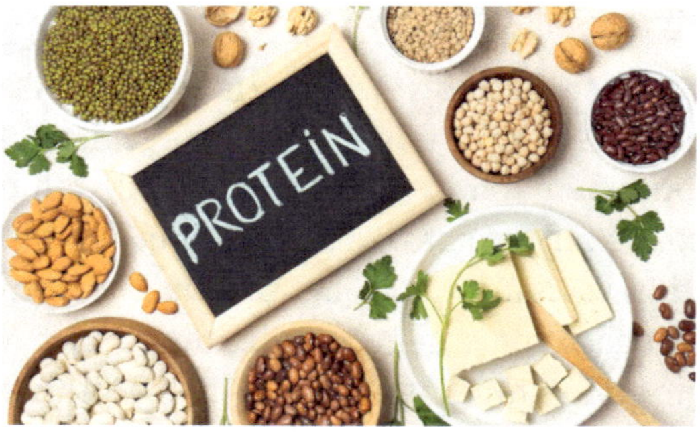

Figure 7.22. Effects of excessive protein intake on the body.

Source: https://assets.thehansindia.com/h-upload/2024/03/24/1433167-protine.webp.

Test Your Knowledge

1. What are the most common inborn errors of metabolism?
2. What is protein-energy malnutrition?

SUMMARY

To conclude, protein and amino acid metabolism is important for the proper functioning of the body. When proteins are digested into amino acids, the body helps build and repair tissues and also manages several metabolic processes necessary for the body's stability. Apart from being building blocks, amino acids are important in making neurotransmitters, sending cellular signals, and producing energy. Since new research is revealing many roles of amino acids, it is essential to understand metabolic processes thoroughly. Thus, this information might help choose treatments for metabolic disorders and improve general health. It is also becoming clear that amino acid metabolism is connected to several health conditions, mainly mental health and problems of the nervous system. The kynurenine pathway has been linked to psychiatric diseases, implying that metabolism can play a role in mental health. Studies have pointed out that working on this pathway may lead to new drugs for preventing or reducing diseases. Learning more about amino acid metabolism helps create solutions for specific problems, which proves the importance of biochemistry in medical settings. Pointing out the links among metabolism, physiology, and pharmacology can result in stronger treatment approaches and better health results. Research should keep evolving so that scientists consider both the chemical processes and the health and disease outcomes. Investigations ahead should pay attention to the processes that control amino acid metabolism as well as how the environment can shape them. The way nutrition and metabolism affect diseases is very important for designing successful interventions. Giving importance to the overall process of protein and amino acid metabolism helps researchers and clinicians discover more about its complicated aspects and develop new solutions for health management. In the end, this work is important for education as well as for improving the health and well-being of people.

It is important to know the details of protein and amino acid metabolism to see how organisms rely on these macromolecules to survive. The process relies on making and breaking proteins, which are formed by linking amino acids with peptide bonds. Catabolic reactions split protein into amino acids, which may be used for energy or changed into glucose or fatty acids according to what the cell needs. Additionally, protein synthesis, regulated by ribosomes, involves translating mRNA sequences into polypeptides, which fold into functional proteins. Thanks to this relationship, amino acids are important for both energy and for the body's repair, enzyme activity, and hormone signaling. In addition, controlling metabolic pathways helps the body adjust to different demands on the body. If the body is starving or doing intense exercise, it breaks down skeletal muscle proteins to produce amino acids that enter gluconeogenesis to keep blood glucose levels steady. Depending on nutrition and hormones, important enzymes control the changes in metabolism. It is the liver's job to handle amino acids, remove ammonia from them, and convert the ammonia to urea to be excreted. Also, the link between amino acid metabolism and the Krebs cycle demonstrates that the body is focused on energy production. When someone has cancer, changes in amino acid metabolism can strongly affect the growth and actions of the tumor. Cancerous cells usually need more certain amino acids to grow fast, showing how metabolism and signaling pathways for growth are linked. The environment around the tumor can greatly affect these needs, deciding on the amount of nutrients and oxygen present. For this reason, knowing more about amino acid use in cancer has encouraged researchers to find therapies that attack the specific metabolic processes of cancer cells. Such insights underscore the significant role of protein and amino acid metabolism not only in cellular function and energy management but also in the development of therapeutic strategies, emphasizing its relevance across various biological and clinical contexts, as highlighted by Vazquez et al. (2016).

KEY TERMS FROM THIS CHAPTER

- Amino acid metabolism
- Beta-pleated sheets
- Carbon
- Carboxypeptidase
- Chinook salmon
- Chymotrypsin
- Hydrogen
- Hydrophobic interactions
- Ionic bonding
- Lactococcus lactis
- Metabolic regulation
- Nitrogen
- Oxygen
- Protein metabolism
- Trypsin

CRITICAL THINKING QUESTIONS

1. **The primary site of protein metabolism in the body is:**
   a. Kidney
   b. Liver
   c. Muscle
   d. Adipose tissue
2. **The process of removing an amino group from an amino acid is called:**
   a. Transamination
   b. Deamination
   c. Decarboxylation
   d. Oxidation
3. **The urea cycle occurs in the:**
   a. Mitochondria and cytoplasm of liver cells
   b. Cytoplasm of muscle cells
   c. Plasma
   d. Mitochondria of kidney cells
4. **The enzyme that catalyzes the conversion of glutamate to alpha-ketoglutarate is:**
   a. Glutamate dehydrogenase
   b. Alanine aminotransferase
   c. Aspartate aminotransferase
   d. Carbamoyl phosphate synthetase
5. **Which amino acid is the primary carrier of nitrogen in the blood?**
   a. Glutamate
   b. Glutamine
   c. Alanine
   d. Serine

Answers to Critical Thinking Questions

1. (b); 2. (b); 3. (a); 4. (a); 5. (b)

Short Answer Questions

1. What is a protein and amino acid?
2. What is the structure of the protein?
3. Why is protein metabolism important in the body?
4. What is the regulation of protein metabolism?
5. What are the disorders of protein metabolism?

REFERENCES

1. Dioguardi F. S. (2011). Clinical use of amino acids as dietary supplement: pros and cons. *Journal of cachexia, sarcopenia and muscle*, *2*(2), 75–80. https://doi.org/10.1007/s13539-011-0032-8 (accessed on 11th June 2025).
2. Li, C., Murugaiyan, J., Thomas, C., Alter, T., & Riedel, C. (2020). Isolate Specific Cold Response of *Yersinia enterocolitica* in Transcriptional, Proteomic, and Membrane Physiological Changes. *Frontiers in microbiology*, *10*, 3037. https://doi.org/10.3389/fmicb.2019.03037 (accessed on 11th June 2025).
3. Ammendola, S., Cocchiola, R., Lopreiato, M., Scotto D'Abusco, A., et al. (2018). Effects of nutrients, mainly from Mediterranean dietary foods, on mesenchymal stem derived cells: Growth or differentiation. https://core.ac.uk/download/188823135.pdf (accessed on 11th June 2025).
4. Argano, V., Balistreri, C. R., Giarratana, R. M., Lio, D., et al. (2019). On the road to accurate biomarkers for cardiometabolic diseases by integrating precision and gender medicine approaches. https://core.ac.uk/download/268910274.pdf (accessed on 11th June 2025).
5. Aslan, O., Hamill, R. M., McBryan, J., Morris, D. W., et al. (2013). Transcriptome analysis of porcine *M. semimembranosus* divergent in intramuscular fat as a consequence of dietary protein restriction. https://core.ac.uk/download/16431846.pdf (accessed on 11th June 2025).
6. Avilla, M. N., Malecki, K. M. C., Hahn, M. E., Wilson, R. H., & Bradfield, C. A. (2020). The Ah Receptor: Adaptive Metabolism, Ligand Diversity, and the Xenokine Model. *Chemical research in toxicology*, *33*(4), 860–879. https://doi.org/10.1021/acs.chemrestox.9b00476(accessed on 11th June 2025).
7. Ayuso, M., Barragán, C., Benítez, R., Cánovas, Á., et al. (2015). Comparative analysis of muscle transcriptome between pig genotypes identifies genes and regulatory mechanisms associated to growth, fatness and metabolism. https://core.ac.uk/download/323071060.pdf (accessed on 11th June 2025).
8. Tomalty, K. M., Meek, M. H., Stephens, M. R., Rincón, G., Fangue, N. A., May, B. P., & Baerwald, M. R. (2015). Transcriptional Response to Acute Thermal Exposure in Juvenile Chinook Salmon Determined by RNAseq. *G3 (Bethesda, Md.)*, *5*(7), 1335–1349. https://doi.org/10.1534/g3.115.017699(accessed on 11th June 2025).
9. Bauer, E., Metzler-Zebeli, B. U., Mosenthin, R., Verstegen, M. W. A., et al. (2011). Intestinal gene expression in pigs: Effects of reduced feed intake during weaning and potential impact of dietary components. https://core.ac.uk/download/pdf/29230036.pdf (accessed on 11th June 2025).
10. Bauer, K., Böhles, H., Fusch, C., Jochum, F., et al. (2009). Neonatologie/Pädiatrie–Leitlinie Parenterale Ernährung, Kapitel 13. https://core.ac.uk/download/14527634.pdf (accessed on 11th June 2025).
11. Bender, D. A., & Cunningham, S. M. C. (2020). *Introduction to Nutrition and Metabolism*. CRC Press eBooks. https://doi.org/10.1201/9781003139157 (accessed on 11th June 2025).
12. Berdanier, C. D., & Berdanier, L. A. (2021). *Advanced Nutrition: Macronutrients, Micronutrients, And Metabolism*.
13. Bogart, E., & Myers, C. R. (2015). Multiscale metabolic modeling of C4 plants: Connecting

nonlinear genome-scale models to leaf-scale metabolism in developing maize leaves. http://arxiv.org/abs/1502.07969 (accessed on 11th June 2025).

14. Braas, D., Christofk, H. R., Graeber, T. G., Krall, A. S., et al. (2016). Asparagine promotes cancer cell proliferation through use as an amino acid exchange factor. https://core.ac.uk/download/323077084.pdf (accessed on 11th June 2025).

15. Budisa, N., & Kubyshkin, V. (2019). The Alanine World model for the development of the amino acid repertoire in protein biosynthesis. https://core.ac.uk/download/287885179.pdf (accessed on 11th June 2025).

16. Chase, D. G., & Pikó, L. (1973). Role of the mitochondrial genome during early development in mice. https://core.ac.uk/download/10210347.pdf (accessed on 11th June 2025).

17. Chen, A., Kalai, M., Ni, M., Tian, Y., et al. (2013). The effect of *mucA* allele on biofilm architecture and the biofilm-related proteomes. https://core.ac.uk/download/478326911.pdf (accessed on 11th June 2025).

18. Chen, Anqun; Xie, Linka; Mathee, Kalai; and Tian, Deying, "The effect of mucA allele on biofilm architecture and the biofilm-related proteomes" (2011). *HWCOM Faculty Publications.* 80. https://digitalcommons.fiu.edu/com_facpub/80(accessed on 11th June 2025).

19. Chen, P., Jez, J. M., Krishnan, H. B., Liu, Y., et al. (2017). β-N-oxalyl-L-α,β-diamino propionic acid (β-ODAP) content in *Lathyrus sativus*: The integration of nitrogen and sulfur metabolism through β-cyanoalanine synthase. https://core.ac.uk/download/83100997.pdf (accessed on 11th June 2025).

20. Chen, Y., Cramer, S. E., Dinges, M. M., Green, D. M., et al. (2020). Absorptive transport of amino acids by the rat colon. https://core.ac.uk/download/305124405.pdf (accessed on 11th June 2025).

21. Cintora, M. E. Q. (2000). *The Effect of Enzymatic Hydrolysis of a Dietary Protein on The Excretion of Urinary Nitrogen Metabolites: A Thesis Submitted in Partial Fulfilment of The Requirements for The Degree of Master of Science in Nutritional Science at Massey University, Palmerston North, New Zealand.* https://core.ac.uk/download/148645530.pdf (accessed on 11th June 2025).

22. Cockburn, F. (1966). Phenylalanine–Its role in infant nutrition and disease. https://core.ac.uk/download/429733732.pdf (accessed on 11th June 2025).

23. Niehaus, T. D., Gerdes, S., Hodge-Hanson, K., Zhukov, A., Cooper, A. J., ElBadawi-Sidhu, M., Fiehn, O., Downs, D. M., & Hanson, A. D. (2015). Genomic and experimental evidence for multiple metabolic functions in the RidA/YjgF/YER057c/UK114 (Rid) protein family. *BMC genomics, 16*(1), 382. https://doi.org/10.1186/s12864-015-1584-3(accessed on 11th June 2025).

24. Cutruzzolà, F., Giardina, G., Janson, G., Leoni, L., et al. (2018). A novel bacterial L-arginine sensor controlling c-di-GMP levels in *Pseudomonas aeruginosa*. https://core.ac.uk/download/188824095.pdf (accessed on 11th June 2025).

25. Dixon, R. A., Gang, D. R., He, J., Marks, M. D., et al. (2009). Identification of candidate genes affecting Delta9-tetrahydrocannabinol biosynthesis in *Cannabis sativa*. https://core.ac.uk/download/323070626.pdf (accessed on 11th June 2025).

26. Ismail, I. T., Showalter, M. R., & Fiehn, O. (2019). Inborn Errors of Metabolism in the Era of

Untargeted Metabolomics and Lipidomics. *Metabolites, 9*(10), 242. https://doi.org/10.3390/metabo9100242(accessed on 11th June 2025).

27. Gao, C., Liu, P., Li, W., Chen, W., Zhang, Z., Wu, D., Huang, J., et al. (2025). Preparation of *Morchella esculenta* protein and its preventive effect on nonalcoholic fatty liver disease in mice. *Food & Function*. https://www.semanticscholar.org/paper/7f4104a0451908d71b884a9f1aed0cc0d6515a5a (accessed on 11th June 2025).
28. Germain, A., Ruppert, D., Levine, S., & Hanson, M. R. (2016). Metabolic profiling of a myalgia encephalomyelitis/chronic fatigue syndrome discovery cohort reveals disturbances in fatty acid and lipid metabolism. *Molecular Biosystems, 13*, 371–379. https://doi.org/10.1039/c6mb00600k (accessed on 11th June 2025).
29. Vazquez, A., Kamphorst, J. J., Markert, E. K., Schug, Z. T., Tardito, S., & Gottlieb, E. (2016). Cancer metabolism at a glance. *Journal of cell science, 129*(18), 3367–3373. https://doi.org/10.1242/jcs.181016(accessed on 11th June 2025).
30. Hagiwara, A., Lass, A., Shukla, A., Subramanian, A., Uhe, A. M., He, B., Albert, B. B., et al. (2016). Dietary soy and meat proteins induce distinct physiological and gene expression changes in rats. https://core.ac.uk/download/41992685.pdf (accessed on 11th June 2025).
31. Hedqvist, H. (2004). Metabolism of soluble proteins by rumen microorganisms and the influence of condensed tannins on nitrogen solubility and degradation. https://core.ac.uk/download/11694797.pdf (accessed on 11th June 2025).
32. Islam, M. J., Khan, A. M., Parves, M. R., Hossain, M. N., & Halim, M. A. (2019). Prediction of deleterious non-synonymous SNPs of human *STK11* gene by combining algorithms, molecular docking, and molecular dynamics simulation. *Scientific Reports, 9*. https://doi.org/10.1038/s41598-019-52308-0 (accessed on 11th June 2025).
33. Janczarek, M., Lipa, P., Vinardell González, J. M. (2019). Transcriptomic studies reveal that the *Rhizobium leguminosarum* serine/threonine protein phosphatase PssZ has a role in the synthesis of cell-surface components, nutrient utilization, and other cellular processes. https://core.ac.uk/download/222572771.pdf (accessed on 11th June 2025).
34. Ji, P., Li, G., Li, J., Tan, B., et al. (2018). The regulatory role of MeAIB in protein metabolism and the mTOR signaling pathway in porcine enterocytes. https://core.ac.uk/download/323069261.pdf Tang, Y., Tan, B., Li, G., Li, J., Ji, P., & Yin, Y. (2018). The Regulatory Role of MeAIB in Protein Metabolism and the mTOR Signaling Pathway in Porcine Enterocytes. *International journal of molecular sciences, 19*(3), 714. https://doi.org/10.3390/ijms19030714 (accessed on 11th June 2025).
35. Kwakkel, R. P., Syafwan, W., & Verstegen, M. W. A. (2011). Heat stress and feeding strategies in meat-type chickens. https://core.ac.uk/download/pdf/29231768.pdf (accessed on 11th June 2025).
36. Mahley, R. W. (2016). Apolipoprotein E: From cardiovascular disease to neurodegenerative disorders. https://core.ac.uk/download/323073264.pdf (accessed on 11th June 2025).
37. Martins, A. M. (1999). Inborn errors of metabolism: A clinical overview. https://core.ac.uk/download/37704201.pdf (accessed on 11th June 2025).
38. Moore, I. L. (1994). Peptide metabolism in the lactococci and its regulation: A thesis presented in partial fulfilment of the requirements for the degree of Master of Science in Biochemistry

at Massey University. https://core.ac.uk/download/157568895.pdf (accessed on 11th June 2025).

39. Mosyagin, V. V., Popov, V. S., Svazlyan, G., & Naumov, N. M. (2024). The effect of organic acids and amino acids of a probiotic dietary supplement on metabolism in animals. *Agrarian Scientific Journal.* https://www.semanticscholar.org/paper/147af83481ba898963a64771f9e73a7b3c829250 (accessed on 11th June 2025).

40. Nicol, S. (1964). Nucleic acids and protein synthesis. https://core.ac.uk/download/59211234.pdf (accessed on 11th June 2025).

41. Niu, R. C., Meng, F. X., Zeng, Q. H., Wang, Y. J., Liu, T. X., Chu, D., & Zhang, S. Z. (2025). Comprehensive transcriptomic analyses of silk-associated genes and functional characterization of key silk fibroins in *Plutella xylostella*. *International Journal of Molecular Sciences, 26.* https://www.semanticscholar.org/paper/90922eb83fd41cd01bd14927414f529506db1eb2 (accessed on 11th June 2025).

42. Paluch, K. V., Platz, K. R., Rudisel, E. J., Erdmann, R., Laurin, T. R., & Dittenhafer-Reed, K. E. (2023). The role of lysine acetylation in the function of mitochondrial ribosomal protein L12. *Proteins: Structure, 92*, 583–592. https://www.semanticscholar.org/paper/62613c52df8dd3f27b566251aed370a99b7302a9 (accessed on 11th June 2025).

43. Sarmidi, M. R. (2012). *Food is Our Medicine.* https://core.ac.uk/download/11801185.pdf (accessed on 11th June 2025).

44. Schwarcz, R., & Stone, T. W. (2017). The kynurenine pathway and the brain: Challenges, controversies and promises. https://core.ac.uk/download/46559921.pdf (accessed on 11th June 2025).

45. Slavny, P. (2010). *Role of the PAS2 Domain of the NifL Regulatory Protein in Redox Signal Transduction.* https://core.ac.uk/download/2769012.pdf (accessed on 11th June 2025).

46. Slee, A. D. (2012). Exploring metabolic dysfunction in chronic kidney disease. https://core.ac.uk/download/17352998.pdf (accessed on 11th June 2025).

47. Tipton, K., & Wolfe, R. R. (2001). Exercise, protein metabolism, and muscle growth. https://core.ac.uk/download/9549081.pdf (accessed on 11th June 2025).

48. Tischler, M. E. (2025). *Skeletal Muscle Metabolism in Hypokinetic Rats.* https://core.ac.uk/download/pdf/42788263.pdf (accessed on 11th June 2025).

49. Tsikas, D. (2021). Post-translational modifications (PTM): Analytical approaches, signaling, physiology and pathophysiology—Part I. *Amino Acids, 53*, 485–487. https://www.semanticscholar.org/paper/b3a4c77a9c858fc5b6df8306b01a0dc34658d245 (accessed on 11th June 2025).

50. Vovchek, N. O., Markiv, V. S., Khomenchuk, V. O., & Kurant, V. Z. (2025). Activity of transamination processes in freshwater fishes under the cobalt ions impact. *Hydrobiological Journal.* https://www.semanticscholar.org/paper/36d68182d98bc7e578aeba3e35acb2847e43f3cb (accessed on 11th June 2025).

51. Wang, C., Zhang, P., He, Y., Huang, F., Wang, X., Li, H., Yuan, L., et al. (2023). Exogenous spraying of IAA improved the efficiency of microspore embryogenesis in *Wucai (Brassica campestris L.)* by affecting the balance of endogenous hormones, energy metabolism, and

cell wall degradation. *BMC Genomics, 24.* https://www.semanticscholar.org/paper/0a23d2b5a4cd9df7e59ab433086a5bce35bdbd98 (accessed on 11th June 2025).

52. West, S. (2023). *Dietary Protein Form and Postprandial Protein Metabolism.* https://core.ac.uk/download/595479234.pdf (accessed on 11th June 2025).

53. Zhang, Q., Zhu, L., Li, H., Chen, Q., Li, N., Li, J., Zhao, Z., et al. (2024). Insights and progress on the biosynthesis, metabolism, and physiological functions of gamma-aminobutyric acid (GABA): A review. *PeerJ, 12.* https://www.semanticscholar.org/paper/f73ddc358b44522f114fff571c236e5565efb0de (accessed on 11th June 2025).

54. Zou, M. L. (2007). *Variation in the Apparent Fecal Digestibility of Macronutrients and Urinary Energy Excretion for Three Diets Varying in Fat and Fiber Content—Assessment of The Atwater Factors and Related Energy Conversion Factors: A Thesis Presented in Partial Fulfillment of The Requirements for The Degree of Master of Science in Nutritional Science at Massey University, Palmerston North, New Zealand.* https://core.ac.uk/download/162617248.pdf (accessed on 11th June 2025).

NUCLEOTIDE METABOLISM

8

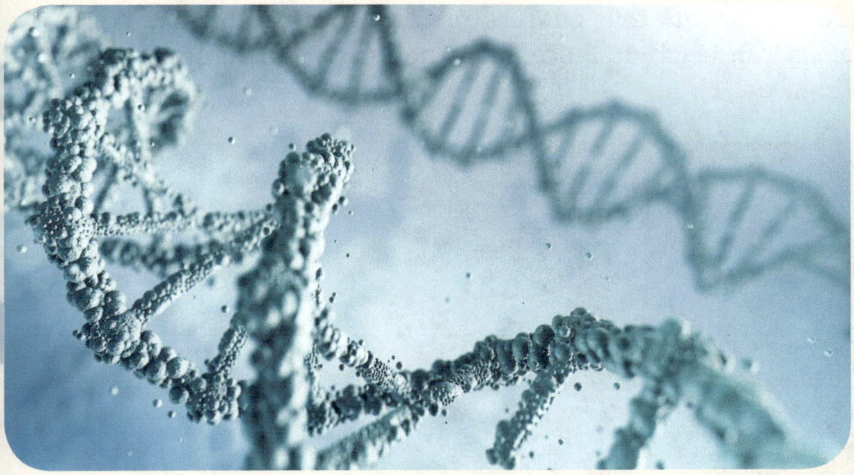

LEARNING OBJECTIVES

After studying this chapter, you will be able to:

1. Describe the structure of nucleotides;
2. Know the nucleotide synthesis pathways;
3. Describe the purine metabolism;
4. Understand the pyrimidine metabolism;
5. Describe the process of nucleotide interconversion;
6. Describe the nucleotide metabolism and disease.

Introduction

The proper function and structure of cells depend on the careful process of nucleotide metabolism. Nucleotides are vital parts of nucleic acids and take part in DNA replication, RNA transcription, and the transfer of energy by ATP. The breakdown and building up of these molecules use both anabolic and catabolic pathways that are controlled to meet the needs of the cell. Problems in nucleotide metabolism can be serious, as they may lead to metabolic problems as well as the development of diseases , such as cancer. By closely studying these metabolic pathways, scientists can learn about cellular machinery and how it changes in different situations, which may lead to new medicines for metabolic diseases. Gaining knowledge about nucleotide metabolism has revealed that cancer cells undergo important changes in their metabolism. Increased glycolysis and production of lactate under oxygen are part of the Warburg effect, which is only one of the many ways cancer cells change their metabolism. It has become clear that cancer cells use alterations in nucleotide production and breakdown to support their growth and stop apoptosis. As described in the literature, cancer cells manipulate their metabolic networks to create a favorable environment for tumor growth, largely via intercellular communication mediated by microRNAs (miRNAs), which influence both their own behavior and that of surrounding cells (Conti et al., 2020). They point out the need to consider nucleotide metabolism together in cancer, which helps find new ways to treat the disease. Nucleotide metabolism is important for many functions in the body, not only cancer. Problems with nucleotide synthesis can result in several diseases, , such as immunodeficiency and neurodegenerative conditions, proving that different metabolic pathways are linked. Furthermore, the advent of omics technologies enables researchers to explore the complexities of nucleotide metabolism with unprecedented detail, aiding in the contextualization of metabolic alterations observed in various diseases (Yizhak et al., 2015). With the help of these maps, scientists can come up with new treatments that address problems in metabolism. As a result, looking into nucleotide metabolism can teach us more about how cells function and may lead to new ways to handle diseases (Figure 8.1).

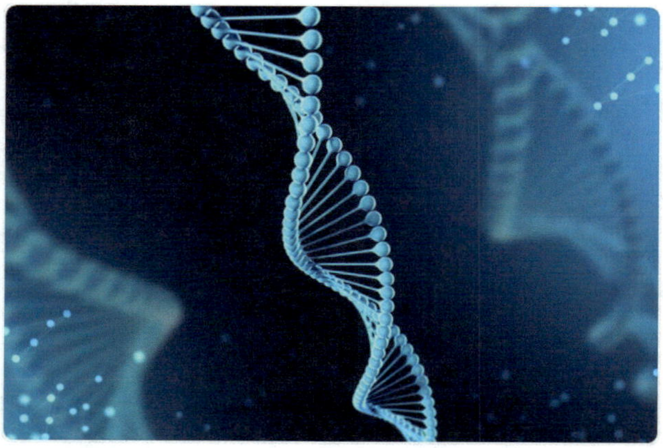

Figure 8.1. 3D illustration of a DNA double helix structure.

Source: https://www.news-medical.net/image-handler/ts/20201222090503/ri/673/picture/2020/12/shutterstock_1267516252.jpg.

Definition of Nucleotides

The definition of nucleotides includes an important part of molecular biology that helps explain nucleotide metabolism. Nucleotides are made up of three things: a nitrogenous base, a pentose sugar, and one or more phosphate groups. Because of this structure, nucleotides are different from other biomolecules and play many roles in the cell. The nitrogenous bases can be classified into two categories—purines (adenine and guanine) and pyrimidines (cytosine, thymine, and uracil)—which play a significant role in the formation of nucleic acids. Ribose is the sugar in RNA, and deoxyribose is the sugar in DNA, so the type of sugar helps to separate nucleotides into RNA and DNA types. Apart from their structure, nucleotides are vital parts of nucleic acids that are essential for life. When nucleotides are polymerized, they form DNA and RNA, and the sequences in the nucleotides hold the genetic code. Yet, nucleotides have a big impact on cellular energy movement and signaling processes. For instance, ATP, a nucleotide, functions as the primary energy currency in the cell, facilitating various biochemical reactions necessary for sustaining life. In addition, nucleotides, including cyclic AMP (cAMP) help carry out signals that control a wide range of cellular actions. So, although nucleotides are first understood in terms of their structure, their role in metabolism and cellular functions makes them even more important in biology. Biochemical pathways oversee the way nucleotides are produced, broken down, and recycled. Nucleotide metabolism mainly involves two pathways called *de novo* synthesis and salvage pathways. Nucleotides are made in the *de novo* pathway using basic metabolic precursors and then used to form the needed nucleotides for nucleic acid production. Unlike the other ways, the salvage pathway takes nucleotides from broken nucleic acids, saving both energy and materials. As nucleotides are not kept in the cell, knowing these metabolic pathways is important to understand how cells maintain enough nucleotides for important jobs , such as DNA replication, transcription, and signaling. Disruptions in nucleotide metabolism can have profound implications, ranging from genetic disorders to MSs, further highlighting the significance of nucleotides in both health and disease, a notion that is elaborated upon in studies discussing viral interactions with cellular pathways (Ebenhoeh et al., 2008) and evolutionary contexts involving cellular domains (Claudiu, 2009) (Figure 8.2).

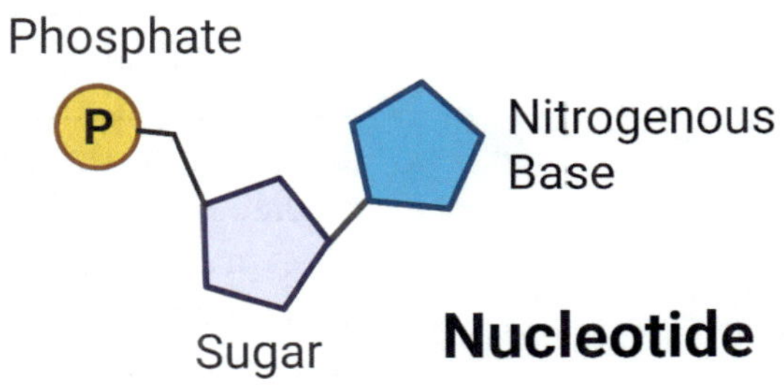

Figure 8.2. Nucleotide.

Source: https://microbenotes.com/wp-content/uploads/2022/03/Nucleotide.jpeg.

Importance of Nucleotide Metabolism in Cellular Functions

Nucleotide metabolism is very important for cells since it supports many key processes needed for life. Nucleotides are important parts of nucleic acids and take part in energy transfer, signaling, and controlling cell functions. There are special pathways that control the synthesis and breakdown of nucleotides to maintain cellular stability. A disturbance in these pathways can result in serious problems; for example, cells cannot divide or survive properly, so nucleotide metabolism relates to the well-being of the entire cell. For example, in rapidly dividing cells, including those in embryos and tissues that repair, the need for nucleotides rises a lot, showing the connection between these metabolic processes and the cell cycle and other growth signals. In addition, scientists have paid more attention to how changes in nucleotide metabolism relate to various diseases, mainly cancer. The increased synthesis of nucleotides in cancer cells helps them grow without control. As a result, the cells' metabolism is altered to support both the making of DNA and RNA and the production of chemicals that assist in cell growth and survival. In some cases, cancer cells depend on certain metabolic routes, for example, those using glutamine, to maintain their nucleotides and keep their functions in check when under stress. Such metabolic adaptations underscore the critical nature of nucleotide metabolism in cancer progression and raise important considerations for therapeutic strategies aimed at targeting these metabolic networks in tumor cells, thereby potentially hindering their growth and survival (Jiang et al., 2019). Nucleotide metabolism is important for more than cancer, since it also plays a role in virology. It has been discovered that several viruses interfere with the host's nucleotide metabolism to help them replicate and survive inside cells. Hijacking the machinery for nucleotide synthesis, viruses secure enough nucleotides for their DNA or RNA, which makes them more dangerous and harmful. Gaining knowledge about how viruses use nucleotide metabolism helps develop effective strategies against viruses. Moreover, elucidating the mechanisms through which viral infections alter host cellular metabolism can inform broader cancer research, as some oncogenic viruses share similar strategies to induce metabolic rewiring in host cells (Thaker et al., 2019). Such a relationship between nucleotide metabolism, viral infections, and cancer proves that more research is needed to learn about the connections between metabolic needs and disease.

8.1. Structure of Nucleotides

Learning Outcome

1. Describe the components of nucleotides;
2. Differentiate between DNA and RNA nucleotides;
3. Understand the role of nucleotide structure in metabolism.

Nucleotides form the basic structure of nucleic acids and are needed for both DNA and RNA creation. A nucleotide is made up of three main things: a nitrogenous base, a five-carbon sugar, and one or more phosphate groups. The base in the nitrogenous group is either a purine, for example, adenine or guanine, or a pyrimidine , such as cytosine, thymine, or uracil. Ribose in RNA and deoxyribose in DNA make the sugar moiety the feature that separates these two types of nucleic acids. Besides, phosphate plays a key role in holding the structure of nucleotides together and joining them to build the nucleic acid backbone. As essential agents in metabolic regulation and the storage and retrieval of genetic information, understanding the detailed structure of nucleotides is crucial for comprehending their role in cellular metabolism and function (Bowater et al., 2005). The processes that make nucleotides are complicated and are closely managed. Nucleotides are produced in the body by two main ways: *de novo* synthesis and salvage pathways. In the *de novo* pathway, nucleotides are built from amino acids and carbon dioxide, which shows that the process depends on the cell's metabolism. On the other hand, the salvage pathway recycles free nucleotides or nucleosides to help save energy. The presence and control of these pathways make sure that cells have the right amount of nucleotides needed for DNA and RNA replication, transcription, and signaling. If there is a problem with nucleotide metabolism, it can result in different disorders, proving their importance for keeping cells in balance. Therefore, a comprehensive understanding of nucleotide structures enhances the depth of knowledge regarding their metabolic roles (Fonteh, 2018). It is especially important to mention that orotic acid is needed for the synthesis of pyrimidines in nucleotide metabolism. Orotic acid helps in the process where carbamoyl phosphate and aspartate are turned into orotate, which is then changed into pyrimidine nucleotides. The process ends with the formation of important nucleotides, for example, cytidine and uridine. Problems in the enzymes of this pathway may result in orotic aciduria, which is characterized by increased orotic acid levels in the urine. This condition points out that correct cellular function depends on efficient nucleotide metabolism. Early diagnosis of problems related to nucleotide synthesis is necessary in clinical practice since late treatment may cause serious issues , such as developmental delays and anemia. Consequently, ongoing research into these pathways enhances the potential for targeted therapeutic strategies in managing related metabolic diseases (Fonteh, 2018) (Figure 8.3).

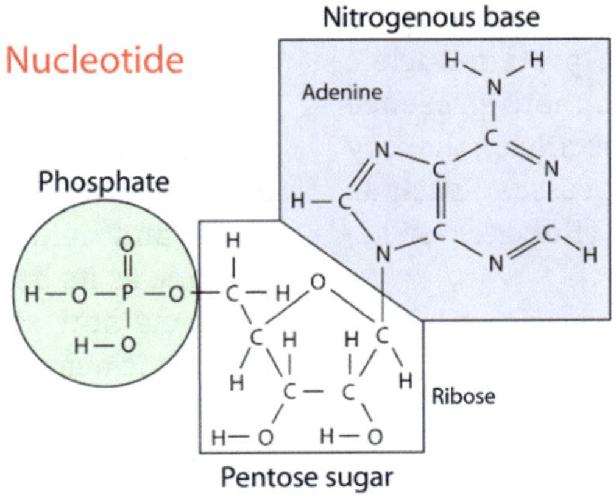

Figure 8.3. Structure of nucleotides.

Source: https://lh6.googleusercontent.com/proxy/I6STlKkfXdfHEwgbIsytVUIsz8YwoyCEwjqpeJ-NmX3J0FkPS1xXYj9m8bxG9V0jeF-3sTBtbiHcnyM8f9zBmMRtVnAIwXF-WNJWecOTQCwujmwbwcN-fA.

8.1.1. Components of Nucleotides: Nitrogenous Bases, Sugars, and Phosphate Groups

Nucleotides are essential in cellular metabolism because their main components—nitrogenous bases, sugars, and phosphate groups—work together. Each nucleotide consists of a nitrogenous base, , such as adenine, guanine, cytosine, or thymine (in DNA), or uracil (in RNA), a five-carbon sugar (ribose in RNA and deoxyribose in DNA), and one or more phosphate groups. They are necessary for storing genetic information since they take part in base pairing during DNA replication and RNA transcription, supporting molecular recognition and interaction. The various properties of bases, due to their structures, ensure that the right base pair, which is necessary for accurate transfer of genetic information in the cell. Therefore, these molecules interact to keep the genetic material safe and functioning, which supports the basic metabolism of cells. Nucleotides' structure and functions in the body are strongly affected by the sugar part they contain. The pentoses ribose and deoxyribose in RNA and DNA nucleotides add to the stability and reactivity of nucleic acids. The presence or absence of specific hydroxyl groups (-OH) on ribose as compared to deoxyribose plays a critical role in the chemical behavior of the nucleic acids they compose. Since ribose has a hydroxyl group, RNA is more active and less stable than DNA, which is required for its tasks in transcription and translation, but DNA's stability allows it to store information for a longer time. As a result, learning about sugar structure gives us an idea of how nucleotides are processed and how nucleic acids play many roles in the body, which explains their importance in evolutionary biology and biochemistry. Phosphate groups help nucleotides carry energy and regulate their structure and how they function in the body. The presence of one or more phosphate units can modify the nucleotide energy state and play a critical role in energy transfer within the cell, particularly in ATP. Phosphate groups in DNA are very energetic, so breaking them provides energy for different cellular activities , such as making and breaking molecules. Also, when phosphate groups are added or removed, they can control metabolism through several signaling methods. For this reason, it is very important to understand how the phosphate groups are involved in nucleotide function and interactions with other biomolecules. This interplay is notably observed in studies of protein-nucleic acid interactions, where phosphate presence impacts binding affinity and specificity, thereby influencing crucial cellular processes , such as replication and transcription (Bowater et al., 2015) (Figure 8.4).

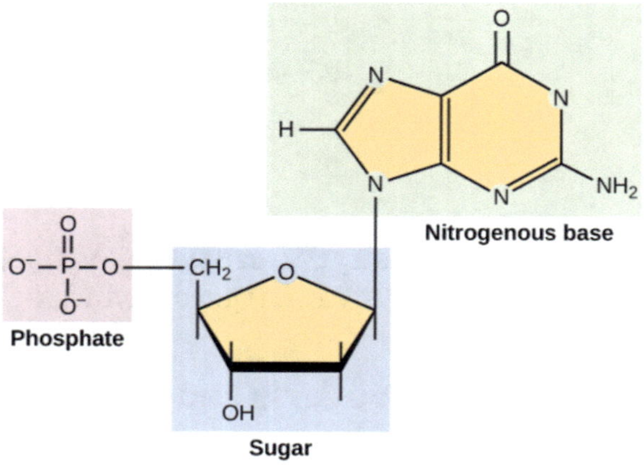

Figure 8.4. A nucleotide is made up of three components: A nitrogenous base, a pentose sugar, and a phosphate group.

Source: https://s3-us-west-2.amazonaws.com/courses-images/wp-content/uploads/sites/198/2016/11/23212722/3-1-10.jpeg.

8.1.2. Differences Between DNA and RNA Nucleotides

The key differences between DNA and RNA nucleotides show why they have different roles in the cells. These differences mainly come from the type of sugar each nucleotide contains. DNA has deoxyribose with no hydroxyl group at the 2 carbons, but RNA includes ribose with a hydroxyl group at this spot. The different structure of DNA and RNA makes DNA more stable, which makes it less likely to undergo hydrolysis. Also, DNA's stability is necessary for it to hold genetic information for a long time, while RNAs can react quickly and take part in several cellular activities, like making proteins and carrying out chemical reactions. Because of this, sugar has a major effect on the physical and biological activities of nucleotides. A further important difference is found in the nitrogenous bases that are part of DNA and RNA nucleotides. DNA is made up of adenine, thymine, cytosine, and guanine, but RNA replaces thymine with uracil and holds adenine, uracil, cytosine, and guanine as its bases. The change is not random; it affects how stable and how they are coded in nucleic acids. The presence of uracil in RNA and its absence in DNA ensures that RNA can participate in a variety of transient roles, , such as mRNA, transfer RNA (tRNA), and ribosomal RNA (rRNA). Alterations in the base composition have an effect on how faithfully the genetic code is copied and the mutations that can develop during replication, demonstrating that nucleotides evolve to better function in their roles in nucleotide metabolism. Besides, the way DNA and RNA nucleotides are arranged and configured is another way to tell them apart.

Because DNA is a double-stranded helix, it allows complementary base pairing that is needed for replication and transcription. Unlike DNA, RNA is mostly single-stranded, so it can form different secondary and tertiary structures that help it take part in many cellular processes. Because RNA can change its shape, it can carry genetic information and also take part in biochemical reactions, increasing what it can do. Besides, how RNA works with proteins and other cellular parts demonstrates its active role in cellular functions. As research progresses, the understanding of nucleotide variations and their implications for metabolic pathways, , such as those discussed by SLC25A33 and SLC25A36 in transporting nucleotides across mitochondrial membranes (Agrimi et al., 2014), continues to evolve, further elucidating the intricacies of nucleotide metabolism (Figure 8.5).

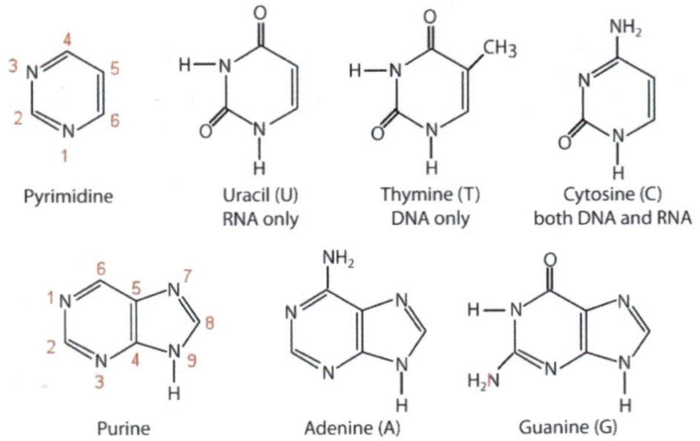

Figure 8.5. The nitrogenous bases found in DNA and RNA.

Source: https://s3-us-west-2.amazonaws.com/courses-images/wp-content/uploads/sites/3101/2018/03/21200728/dc9df397a1d1801eb3c21a8630c64325.jpg.

8.1.3. Role of Nucleotide Structure in Metabolism

Nucleotides are important for many metabolic pathways because they affect energy transfer and the building of biomolecules. Nucleotides are made up of a nitrogenous base, a pentose sugar, and one or more phosphate groups and serve both as the building blocks of nucleic acids and as key parts of metabolic reactions. The energy-rich phosphate bonds, particularly in ATP, are vital for cellular functions, providing the necessary energy for enzymatic reactions, muscle contractions, and active transport mechanisms. Besides, nucleotides are important in signaling and metabolism because their shape allows them to interact with many enzymes and proteins. One important thing about nucleotide metabolism is that the structure of its components plays a key role in regulating metabolic processes, especially in cases of disorders. For example, any changes in nucleotides can affect the activities of enzymes involved in lipid metabolism and signaling in cells. It has been found that by controlling certain microRNAs, the metabolism of nucleotides can be altered, which may result in the onset of obesity and diabetes. The inhibition of microRNA-378 has emerged as a significant area of study, showing promise for treating such conditions through the modulation of lipid processing pathways and overall energy homeostasis (Carrer et al., 2014). Because nucleotide structure affects metabolic regulation, targeting nucleotide metabolism could help treat various metabolic diseases. Because nucleotides have diverse structures, they are useful in medicine by developing small molecules that regulate their metabolism. New studies have proven that blocking certain enzymes in nucleotide synthesis can help in treating cancer. For example, inhibiting deoxycytidine kinase has shown effectiveness in combating acute lymphoblastic leukemia, with advancements reflecting the intricate relationship between nucleotide structure and cellular metabolism (Rosser et al., 2020). When researchers understand how changes in structure affect nucleotides and enzymes, they can design new treatments that rely on these discoveries, proving that nucleotide structure is important in metabolic processes.

Test Your Knowledge

1. What are the three components of nucleic acids?
2. What are the differences between DNA and RNA nucleotides?

8.2. Nucleotide Synthesis Pathways

Learning Outcome

1. Describe the de novo synthesis pathway and salvage pathway;
2. Understand the regulation of nucleotide synthesis.

Nucleotide synthesis pathways are important for nucleotide metabolism because they supply what is needed for nucleic acid synthesis and many cellular functions. Nucleotides are mainly made using the *de novo* pathway or the salvage pathway. The *de novo* pathway begins by making nucleotides from simple molecules, and a series of enzymatic reactions is needed to change ribose-5-phosphate into purine and pyrimidine nucleotides. The DNA and RNA inside cells are made possible during rapid cell division thanks to this pathway. On the other hand, the salvage pathway gathers nucleotides from damaged DNA and RNA, which helps save energy and resources. All of these pathways together help cells keep enough nucleotides, which are necessary for energy use, communication, and cell division.

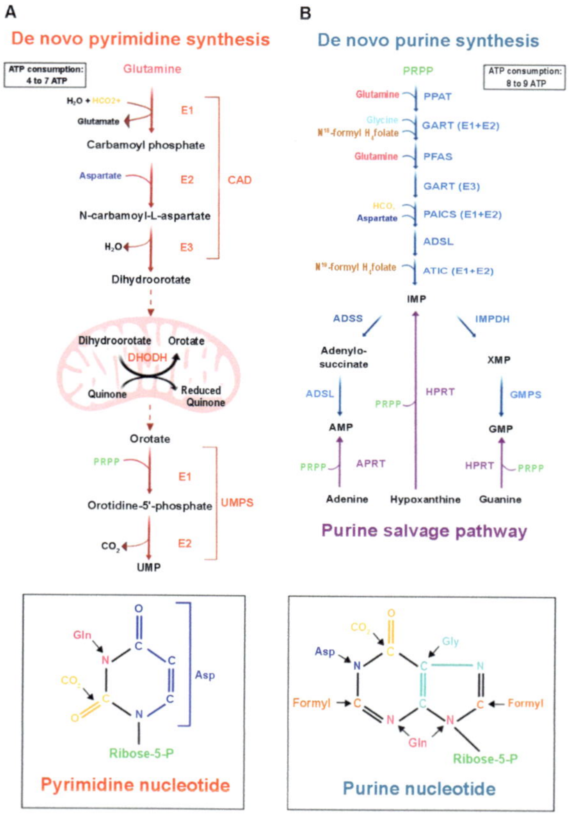

Figure 8.6. The *de novo* pyrimidine and purine synthesis pathways. (A) Schematic of the *de novo* pyrimidine synthesis pathway; and (B) schematic of the *de novo* and purine salvage pathways.

Source: https://www.researchgate.net/publication/333181709/figure/fig1/AS:11431281210527058@1702049047462/The-de-novo-pyrimidine-and-purine-synthesis-pathways-A-Schematic-of-the-de-novo.tif.

The role of nucleotide metabolism is most noticeable when there is muscle atrophy in a disease. It has been found that a significant decrease in adenine nucleotides, like ATP, happens in atrophic skeletal muscle in cancer and chronic diseases.

The degradation of these nucleotides correlates with increased activities of adenine nucleotide-degrading enzymes and the accumulation of degradation products, like inosine monophosphate (IMP) and hypoxanthine. An interruption in the processes that produce and break down nucleotides plays a role in muscle atrophy, since this can cause a shortage of energy and add to health complications. Therefore, investigating nucleotide metabolism not only sheds light on normal cellular physiology but also unveils potential therapeutic targets for reversing or mitigating muscle atrophy in various disease contexts, as highlighted by studies exploring the metabolic consequences of nucleotide degradation in atrophic tissues (Brault et al., 2019). Besides, knowing how nucleotides are made is very important in medicine, especially when dealing with diseases and treatments.

The study of a biochemical reaction network of platelet metabolism shows that the metabolism of nucleotides is closely connected to many disorders. By combining proteomic information, this study has shown that nucleotide metabolism is related to many diseases and drugs, stressing how metabolic pathways are connected throughout the body. With the help of computational models, researchers have studied how changes in nucleotide metabolism can influence cell behavior in cases of aspirin resistance, showing that nucleotide flow is related to disease development. Such insights contribute to the broader understanding of pathophysiological conditions, including coagulopathies, reflecting the essential role that nucleotide synthesis pathways play in both health and disease (Bordbar et al., 2014) (Figure 8.6).

8.2.1. De Novo Synthesis Pathway

The process of *de novo* synthesis of nucleotides is very important for cells since it helps produce purines and pyrimidines needed for DNA and RNA production. The first part of this pathway is when ribose-5-phosphate is formed by the pentose phosphate pathway. After that, enzymes take part in complex reactions that result in the formation of the nucleotide structure. In the case of purine nucleotides, the initial product is IMP, from which adenine and guanine nucleotides are derived. This network makes it clear that the pathways are vital for genes and also for many cell activities, , such as producing energy and sending signals, which are all important for life. As outlined in recent industrial biotechnology studies, the manipulation of the *de novo* synthesis pathway can significantly enhance nucleotide production, particularly with IMP. Targeted genetic engineering has resulted in much larger amounts of IMP inside the cells. As an example, blocking the ways that AMP and GMP are broken down has been found to boost IMP levels by 45 times in some microorganisms. However, the overall control of the purine biosynthetic pathway remains tightly regulated due to its interconnectedness with broader metabolic networks, indicating that strategic metabolic engineering could further enhance nucleotide yields for both biotechnological applications and research purposes (Barduhn et al., 2012). Apart from its usual functions in cells, the creation of nucleotides from scratch is linked to diseases , such as cancer. It has been found through research that some cancer cells depend mainly on serine for making nucleotides. This is important since serine aids in making one-carbon units that are needed for making nucleotides. When serine is not available, cancer cells cannot grow and also have problems creating nucleotides. It is interesting that glycine cannot take the place of serine in these pathways, which underlines the importance of detailed control over nucleotide metabolism in different metabolic states, mainly in cancer. Moreover, restoring the one-carbon cycle through additional supplementation can rescue nucleotide synthesis, reinforcing the significance of the *de novo* synthesis pathway in both normal and pathological cellular activities (Labuschagne et al., 2014) (Figure 8.7).

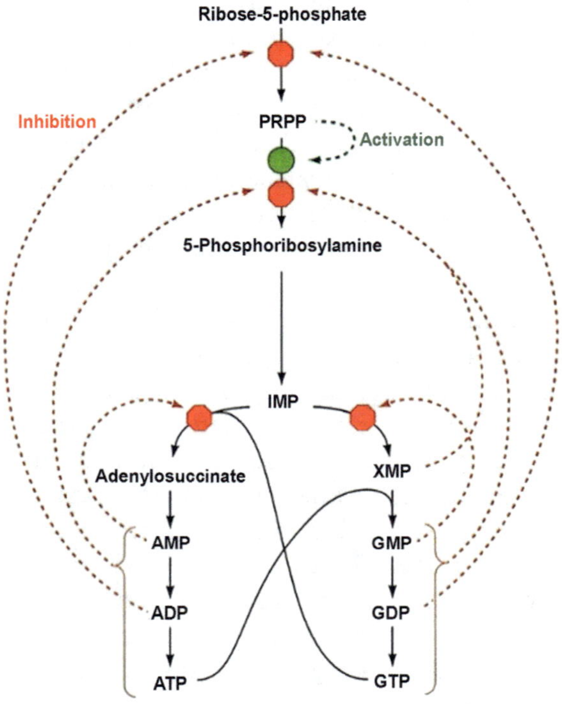

Figure 8.7. *De novo* nucleotide synthesis.

Source: https://upload.medbullets.com/topic/102004/images/26-007.jpg.

8.2.2. Salvage Pathway

The salvage pathway is vital in nucleotide metabolism since it allows nucleotides to be made from existing nucleosides and nucleobases. While *de novo* synthesis uses a lot of energy and complex materials, the salvage pathway efficiently uses the components found in cells to make new nucleotides. Rapidly dividing immune cells and cancer cells need a lot of nucleotides, so this is especially important for them. Enzymes , such as deoxycytidine kinase and adenine phosphoribosyl transferase help change nucleobases into nucleotides, so the body can maintain a good supply of nucleotides without requiring lots of metabolic activity. Hence, the salvage pathway helps cells save energy and keeps the nucleotides required for DNA and cell reproduction. The relationship between salvage and *de novo* pathways has been made clear by research, especially in leukemia cells that depend on both ways to produce dNTPs. Studies indicate that inhibiting the ataxia telangiectasia and Rad3-related protein (ATR), a key regulator in the replication stress response, impacts the activity of both pathways. Inhibiting such enzymes as ribonucleotide reductase and deoxycytidine kinase improves the cell's ability to cope with various metabolic difficulties. Still, although ATR is needed for nucleotide synthesis, some activity in both pathways is enough to keep the cell alive. This idea is important for therapy, as focusing on salvage activities could cause replication stress that kills leukemia cells and brings new approaches for treatment. Besides its role in immediate cellular processes, the salvage pathway has a wider effect on metabolic and therapeutic situations. For instance, in biotechnological applications, the manipulation of purine nucleotide biosynthesis has been emphasized, given its substantial impact on producing valuable compounds like IMP. When degradation of IMP is stopped, the levels of IMP rise and this can lead to improved yields in metabolic engineering. It reveals the main processes in nucleotide metabolism and also points out possible ways to improve microbial strains. As our understanding of the salvage pathway deepens, it becomes increasingly clear that its role is multifaceted, bridging fundamental biology and practical applications in health and industry, as highlighted in recent exploration of microbial production systems (Barduhn et al., 2012) (Figure 8.8).

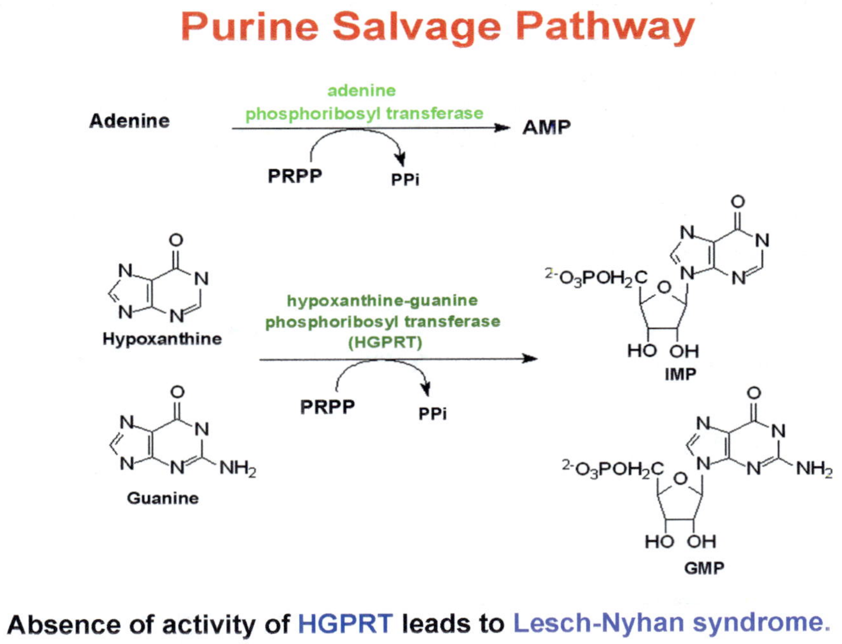

Figure 8.8. Salvage pathway.

Source: https://i1.wp.com/imedscholar.com/wp-content/uploads/2018/05/slide_35.jpg?fit=960%2C720&ssl=1.

8.2.3. Regulation of Nucleotide Synthesis

The process of making nucleotides is very important for nucleotide metabolism and impacts DNA replication, RNA transcription, and energy use in cells. The regulation mainly depends on the amount of precursors, the activity of enzymes, and the responses of signaling pathways to the cell's condition. To allow for fast cell division, nucleotide pools have to be maintained by both making new nucleotides and recovering those that are broken down. Thanks to ribonucleotide reductase, enzymes control the process of making deoxyribonucleotides from ribonucleotides, which links the metabolism of nucleotides with the metabolism of the whole cell. The way these enzymes interact with other metabolic regulators points out how important it is for nucleotide synthesis to be regulated for cellular balance and effective response to metabolism. In addition, asparagine, a kind of amino acid, is known to regulate the process of nucleotide synthesis. The amino acid asparagine helps make proteins and also helps control the uptake of other essential amino acids. As of late, it has been found that the intracellular amount of asparagine may manage the synthesis of nucleotides by influencing serine uptake, which is key for a variety of metabolic processes. In cancer cells, asparagine is very important because it helps control mTORC1 and protein production, which are needed for their fast growth. This connection suggests that asparagine acts as a metabolic bridge between amino acid availability and nucleotide synthesis, further underscoring its significance in the context of cellular metabolism and growth (Braas et al., 2016). In addition, the availability of nutrients has a major effect on regulating the synthesis of nucleotides, which is clear from studies in bacterial models. When *Escherichia coli* was deprived of inorganic nitrogen, the amount of RNA and nucleotides produced went down due to stringent control. The accumulation of guanosine-5′-diphosphate-2′- or 3′-diphosphate (ppGpp) showcased the intricate regulatory pathways activated during nutrient deprivation. It points out that how nutrients are present in the body can directly influence the production of important metabolites during RNA synthesis. These findings not only contribute to a better understanding of bacterial adaptation but also highlight the conserved nature of stress responses across organisms, suggesting that similar regulatory mechanisms may operate in eukaryotic cells, thereby enriching our comprehension of nucleotide metabolism (Irr et al., 1972).

Test Your Knowledge

1. What is the de novo synthesis pathway?
2. What is the salvage pathway?

8.3. Purine Metabolism

Learning Outcome

1. Understand the synthesis of purine nucleotides;
2. Know the degradation of purines and uric acid formation;
3. Describe the disorders related to purine metabolism.

Because it contributes to the formation and breakdown of ATP, ADP, and AMP, purine metabolism is very important for nucleotide metabolism. Adenine nucleotides are needed for many cellular actions , such as moving energy, transmitting signals, and managing protein metabolism. It is clear from observing atrophic skeletal muscle in cancer and diabetes that having enough adenine nucleotides is important. Under these conditions, the amount of adenine nucleotides often decreases, which goes along with higher activity of enzymes that break them down. Consequently, the dysregulation of purine metabolism can result in elevated levels of degradation products like IMP and hypoxanthine, further illuminating the complex interplay between nucleotide metabolism and cellular health, particularly in muscle atrophy (Brault et al., 2019). At the cellular level, purine metabolism consists of many pathways that help in the synthesis of nucleotides or their breakdown. In the *de novo* synthesis pathway, purine nucleotides are made from simpler materials, but the salvage pathway reuses purines from broken-down nucleotides to keep the cell's supply of nucleotides. The two processes should be carefully balanced to ensure enough energy for the cell and the production of nucleic acids. If the pathways are not regulated properly, it can result in problems that spread outside of muscle tissue. As an example, when macrophages are exposed to different types of signals, both those that promote and those that suppress inflammation, their purine metabolism is affected and this changes how the immune system responds. The interaction between multiple metabolic pathways signifies the broader implications of purine metabolism in systemic health and disease (Achcar et al., 2018). Purine metabolism is connected to many other aspects of the body, including normal and abnormal functions. Adenine nucleotide breakdown that occurs during atrophy reduces energy and also disrupts vital pathways needed for growth and repair. As new studies are carried out, exploring the link between purine metabolism and muscle wasting may uncover new therapies. Investigating changes in metabolism during disease could help scientists find out if treating low adenine nucleotide levels with drugs could reduce muscle loss and improve health. Thus, continued investigation into purine metabolism is vital for both fundamental biochemistry and the development of treatments that address metabolic dysfunctions associated with various diseases (Brault et al., 2019) (Figure 8.9).

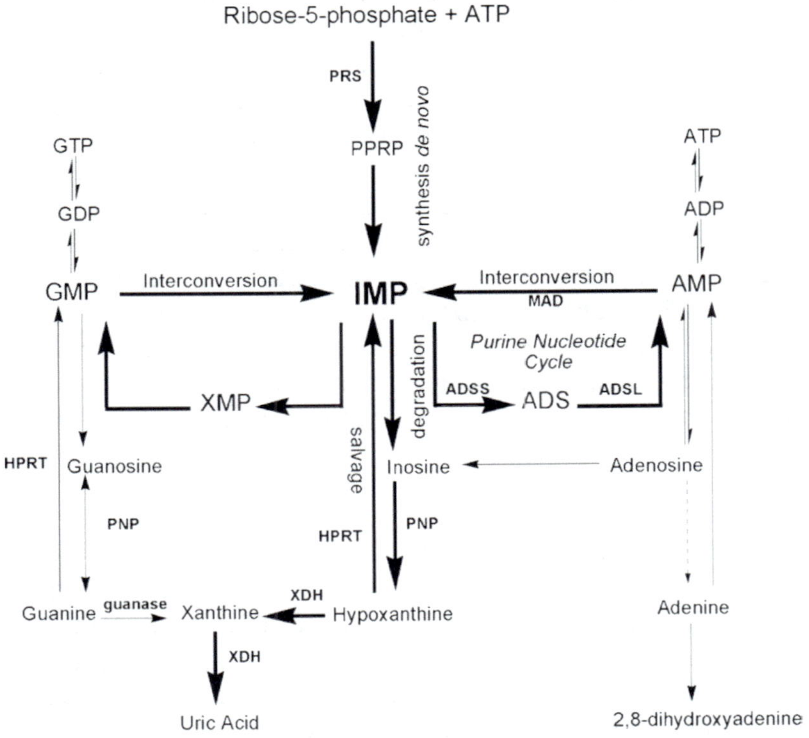

Figure 8.9. Human purine metabolism. Pertinent pathways: Formation of the purine nucleotide inosine monophosphate (IMP) from non-purine precursors (synthesis *de novo*), or purine bases (salvage reactions); purine nucleotide interconversion reactions; degradation to the end product uric acid (catabolic reactions).

Source: https://www.researchgate.net/profile/Maria-Lucia-De-Oliveira/publication/6313058/figure/fig1/AS:372622505332737@1465851536165/Human-purine-metabolism-Pertinent-pathways-formation-of-the-purine-nucleotide-inosine.png.

8.3.1. Synthesis of Purine Nucleotides

The formation of purine nucleotides is a vital part of nucleotide metabolism, which is necessary for many cell activities, , such as making DNA and RNA. The main ways to synthesize purine nucleotides are called the *de novo* synthesis pathway and the salvage pathway. The first step of the *de novo* pathway is to use ribose-5-phosphate, and then it uses amino acids and carbon dioxide to make purine structures. The pathway is tightly controlled to respond to a cell's needs, mainly when there is a lot of cell division. On the other hand, the salvage pathway uses degraded nucleic acids to provide cells with purines, saving them from using lots of resources. This points out that purine metabolism is vital in both healthy and diseased cells, as cancer cells require a lot more nucleotides. Cancer biologists have given special attention to purine nucleotide synthesis since it is important for tumor development and survival. Because of changes in their metabolic pathways, tumor cells can grow uncontrollably, so they become possible targets for treatment. When enzymes involved in nucleotide synthesis are not working properly, cancer cells can balance their growth and the process of cell death. It is especially important that the salvage pathway enzymes assist in making the nucleotides required for quick cell division. As an implication of this, a disruption or inhibition of purine synthesis can trigger cellular stress responses, leading to apoptosis in cancer cells that are already predisposed to mutations affecting apoptotic pathways (Bayram et al., 2024). Knowing about these metabolic changes is important for making cancer therapies that can target the special needs of cancer cells. Studies have been done to evaluate how stopping purine nucleotide synthesis can be used to treat cancer. Chemicals that interfere with specific enzymes in the purine metabolism, , such as those in the salvage pathway, may successfully cause apoptosis in tumor cells since they need these pathways to survive. For example, when adenosine deaminase is blocked, toxic metabolites build up, disrupting how nucleotides are balanced and affecting the cells' survival. Furthermore, innovative methods , such as isotope tracing techniques have provided insights into how tumor cells metabolize these substrates, revealing how glutamine, a key nitrogen donor, can impact purine synthesis during times of glutamine deprivation (Bayram et al., 2024). This shows that targeting purine metabolism could be a useful method for designing better cancer treatments.

8.3.2. Degradation of Purines and Uric Acid Formation

The process of breaking down purines is very important and ends with the production of uric acid, which plays many important roles in the body. The liver and kidneys mainly break down purines like adenine and guanine by using enzymes. Xanthine oxidase is important in this pathway because it helps break down hypoxanthine and xanthine to uric acid, which controls the amount of these metabolites in the body. If uric acid levels become too high, people may develop gout or uric acid kidney stones, which underlines the need to know about this process in nucleotide metabolism. The delicate control of enzymes in purine breakdown affects uric acid levels and also influences overall metabolic functions, so we should look more closely at these mechanisms and their effects on human health. Having high uric acid levels can greatly increase the chances of gout and kidney stones in humans. When the concentration of uric acid in the body goes above normal levels, it becomes insoluble and settles in the joints and kidneys. While some species, like lower apes and *D. melanogaster*, possess the enzyme urate oxidase, allowing them to further metabolize uric acid into allantoin—a more soluble form—humans lack this capability (Lu et al., 2015). As a result, gaining knowledge about the reasons behind high serum uric acid can guide the creation of helpful prevention and treatment methods for these conditions. Moreover, knowing how diet affects purine metabolism can direct actions that help regulate uric acid and reduce the risk of diseases related to it. Researchers are now focusing on how neopterin and other metabolites regulate the activities of enzymes and the body's response to stress when uric acid is formed. Neopterin, an intermediate in biopterin synthesis, has been shown to inhibit xanthine oxidase, potentially serving as a natural regulatory mechanism for uric acid levels (Ebong et al., 1996). The way enzymes respond to neopterin in stress suggests that it may help treat conditions marked by too much uric acid. Therefore, looking into neopterins along with traditional treatments might lead to new ways of handling gout and uric acid-related problems. To advance treatments in nucleotide metabolism and handle the health problems linked to purine imbalance, it is necessary to know how purines are degraded and how uric acid is formed (Figure 8.10).

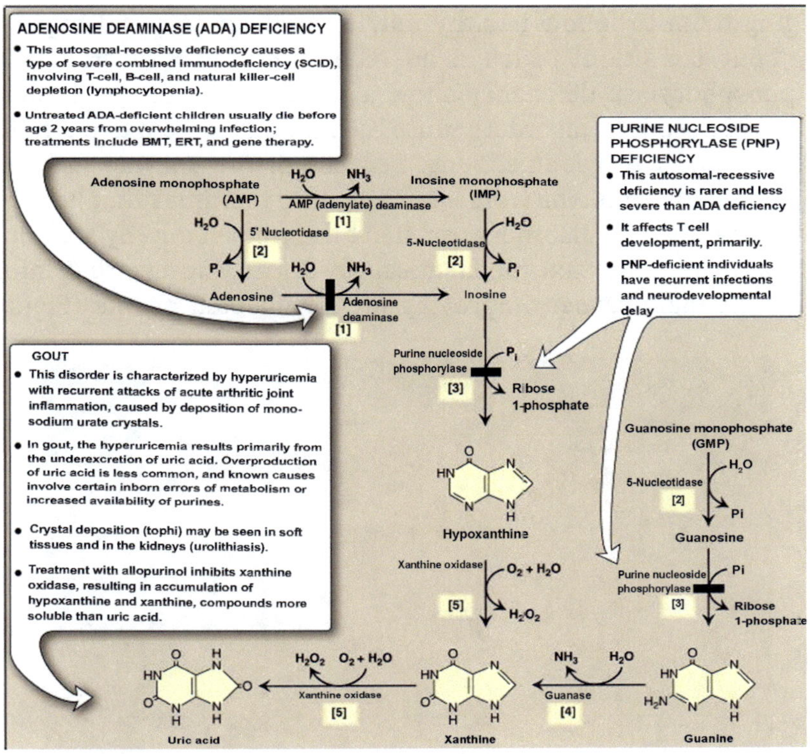

Figure 8.10. The degradation of purine nucleotides to uric acid illustrates some of the genetic diseases associated with this pathway.

Source: https://almerja.com/medea/images/7_34.jpg.

8.3.3. Disorders Related to Purine Metabolism

There are several medical conditions under purine metabolism disorders, and these are marked by problems in purine synthesis, breakdown, and elimination. As a result of these disorders, the body may produce dangerous metabolites that can cause major problems. In particular, any disturbance in how nucleotides are recycled can lead to changes in cell function and may cause different symptoms. A main part of purine metabolism is breaking down nucleotides with the help of enzymes that ensure the right balance of nucleotides in cells. For example, studies have shown that deoxyribonucleoside triphosphate pyrophosphohydrolases have crucial roles in metabolizing various nucleotide substrates, including ITP and dITP, underscoring the complexity and significance of these enzymatic processes (Davies et al., 2011). If these enzymes do not function properly, diseases may develop and affect the whole cellular and body's health. A well-known consequence of altered purine metabolism is gout, a disease where uric acid crystals in the joints bring about inflammation and pain. Gout is caused by several things, and what you eat, especially purine, is a major factor. It is shown in research that high levels of purines in foods like red meat and certain seafood can lead to higher uric acid levels, which is part of the disease's development. A study conducted in Masohi Town revealed strong associations between the incidence of gouty arthritis and purine-rich diets, highlighting a substantial odds ratio for those consuming such foods (Amiruddin et al., 2012). It shows that public health efforts should focus on teaching people about unhealthy foods and encouraging them to follow healthy nutrition advice to avoid hyperuricemia and gout attacks. Apart from gout, conditions , such as adenine phosphoribosyl transferase deficiency and purine nucleoside phosphorylase deficiency show a wide variety of symptoms related to purine metabolism problems. Such genetic disorders cause the immune system to malfunction, slow growth, and make people more likely to get infections. Because of the enzyme deficiencies, metabolites build up and make the health problems worse. Looking into therapies that help restore metabolism points out how purine metabolism disorders can affect the whole body. By studying these conditions further, we can find out the important biochemical processes and use that information to design treatments that treat the main causes, improving life for affected people (Figure 8.11).

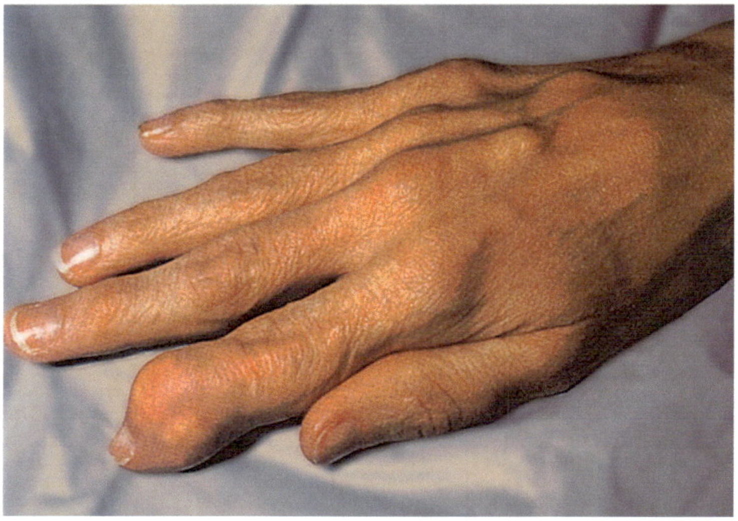

Figure 8.11. Tophaceous gout.

Source: https://www.pharmacy180.com/media/imgph02/aXSGnx7.jpg.

Test Your Knowledge

1. What is the synthesis of purine nucleotides?
2. What are the disorders of purine metabolism?

8.4. Pyrimidine Metabolism

Learning Outcome

1. Describe the synthesis of pyrimidine nucleotides;
2. Understand the degradation of pyrimidines;
3. Know the clinical implications of pyrimidine metabolism disorders.

Nucleotides, which are needed for DNA and RNA, are made with the help of pyrimidine metabolism. The process of making pyrimidines starts when carbamoyl phosphate is formed, then dihydroorotate is produced with the help of the enzyme dihydroorotase. It is important in the process because dihydroorotate is needed as an intermediate. The subsequent transformation of dihydroorotate into orotic acid is catalyzed by the mitochondrial enzyme dihydroorotate dehydrogenase (DHODH). This reaction demonstrates how pyrimidine metabolism is complicated and emphasizes the role of mitochondria, because disturbances in mitochondrial pathways can decrease the supply of pyrimidines, which can negatively affect nucleic acid production and may cause problems in the entire body.

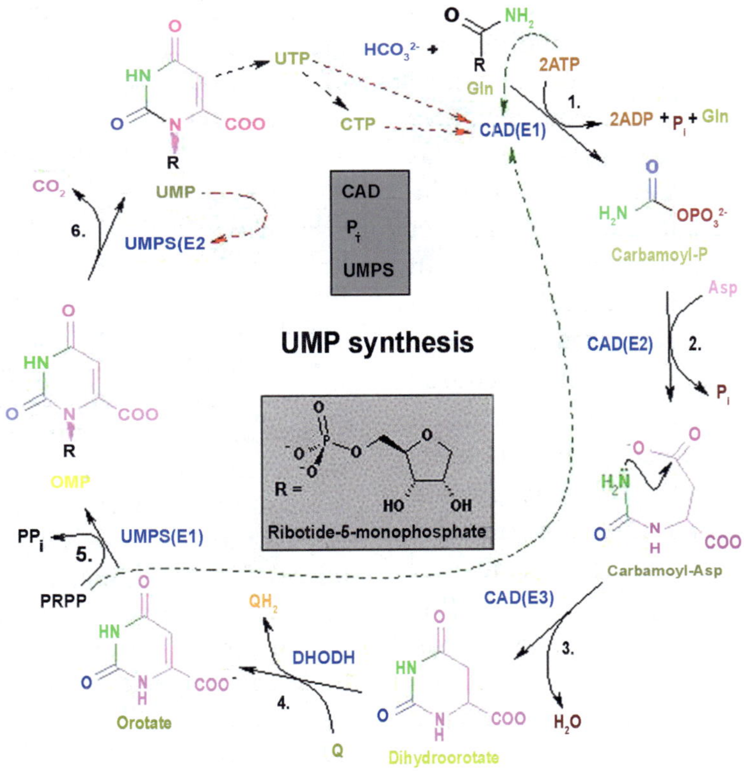

Figure 8.12. Pyrimidine metabolism.

Source: https://s3.amazonaws.com/static.wd7.us/6/6b/Nucleotides_syn2.png.

Orotic acid, which appears during pyrimidine metabolism, is important for cellular metabolism and health, not only a waste product. Elevated levels of orotic acid can indicate underlying metabolic conditions, , such as orotic aciduria, which may arise from genetic defects in enzymes , such as

UMPS. Those suffering from this disorder usually experience major symptoms like megaloblastic anemia and developmental delays, proving that pyrimidine metabolism is vital. The process of turning orotic acid into nucleotides shows how the amino acid and urea cycle are linked. Problems with pyrimidine metabolism may cause different clinical symptoms, showing that it is important for both basic cell functions and human health. Its importance is also shown by the way it affects both pyrimidine metabolism and the immune system. Studies done recently found that both pro-inflammatory and anti-inflammatory stimuli can change macrophage metabolism, especially in nucleotide synthesis. The use of metabolomics in studies has found that the quantity of different metabolites can change in the presence of these stimuli, which indicates that immune cells are very sensitive to metabolic changes. Besides, the fact that these interactions are complex means that the metabolic state of cells can have a big impact on how they react to diseases and changes in their environment. This understanding of how pyrimidine metabolism is regulated in immune cells contributes to the broader discourse surrounding metabolic reprogramming in health and disease, particularly in the context of host-pathogen interactions and immune system functionality, as noted in studies that examine immune-metabolism interactions (Achcar et al., 2018). Applying findings from pyrimidine metabolism and immunology may greatly help in designing new treatments for disorders related to metabolism and the immune system (Figure 8.12).

8.4.1. Synthesis of Pyrimidine Nucleotides

The process of synthesizing pyrimidine nucleotides is very important in nucleotide metabolism because it mainly results in the production of cytosine, thymidine, and uracil. This process begins with the formation of carbamoyl phosphate, which is synthesized from ammonia and bicarbonate in the mitochondria, catalyzed by carbamoyl phosphate synthetase II (CPSII). After that, dihydroorotate is created through several enzymatic reactions, which ends in the formation of orotic acid. It is important at this stage for the cell to produce the nucleotides needed for the creation of RNA and DNA. The regulation of this pathway is very strict, so cells can respond to changes in the need for nucleotides, especially when they divide quickly, for example, during development or during the immune response. Orotic acid serves as an essential intermediate in the pyrimidine synthesis pathway, where it undergoes further biochemical transformations to generate uridine monophosphate (UMP). The enzyme orotate phosphoribosyl transferase helps the process by adding a ribose-phosphate group to orotic acid. The conversion needs to happen so that more pyrimidine nucleotides are available. When there is a disorder like orotic aciduria, it shows how important it is to have proper pyrimidine nucleotide synthesis. Orotic aciduria manifests due to defects in the UMPS enzyme, which plays a pivotal role in this biosynthetic pathway. Clinical manifestations can be severe, impacting neural and developmental health, highlighting the need for understanding the underlying mechanisms of pyrimidine metabolism and the importance of early diagnosis and treatment for related metabolic disorders (Fonteh, 2018). Studies carried out recently have shown how pyrimidine synthesis pathways are closely balanced, especially in cases of leukemia. In these malignancies, cells exhibit a heightened dependency on both *de novo* and salvage pathways to synthesize deoxyribonucleoside triphosphates (dNTPs) necessary for their rapid proliferation. Disruptions in the way nucleotides are made in cells can be used as a treatment approach, since targeting the main enzymes can cause cancer cells to replicate uncontrollably and die. As an example, inhibiting ribonucleotide reductase and deoxycytidine kinase changes the production of pyrimidine nucleotides, which offers new ways to fight certain leukemias. This dual approach of targeting nucleotide metabolism not only emphasizes the integral role in maintaining cellular homeostasis but also opens avenues for innovative cancer therapies that exploit these metabolic vulnerabilities (Le et al., 2017).

8.4.2. Degradation of Pyrimidines

The breakdown of pyrimidines is very important in nucleotide metabolism because it helps maintain the balance of necessary molecules in the cell. Most of the breakdown of pyrimidines happens with uracil and cytosine, producing substances that can be used in different metabolic processes. This process starts when dihydropyrimidine dehydrogenase enzyme helps to change uracil into dihydrouracil. It means that organisms can use pyrimidines more efficiently because of a specific metabolic response. For instance, in plants, the catabolic pathway is activated under nitrogen-limited conditions, allowing them to recycle pyrimidine nitrogen and maintain metabolic equilibrium, showcasing the adaptability of biological systems in nutrient-scarce environments (Abramoff et al., 2009).

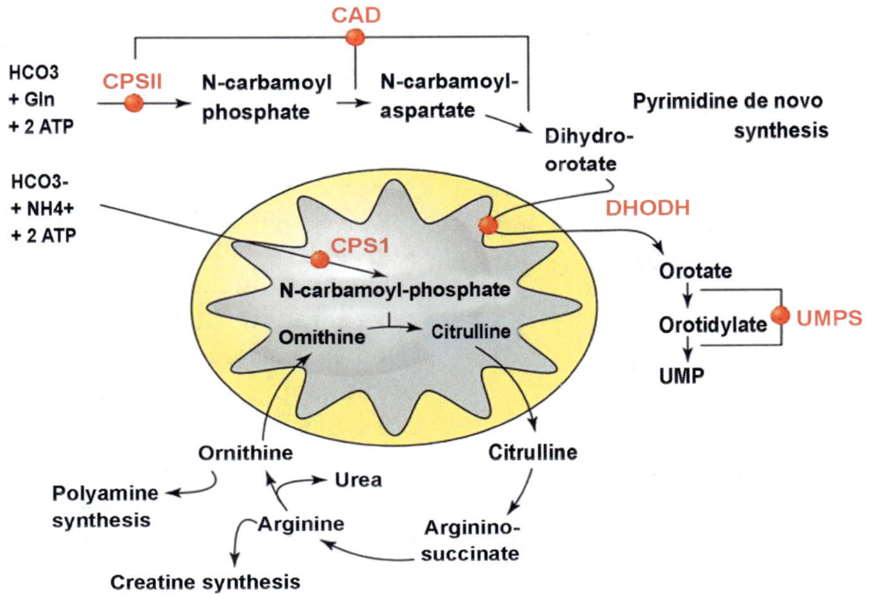

Figure 8.13. Pyrimidine metabolism pathways: synthesis and degradation.

Source: https://www.creative-proteomics.com/blog/wp-content/uploads/2024/09/pyrimidine-metabolism-synthesis-degradation-pic1.jpg.

As the process of pyrimidine degradation continues, it produces β-alanine, which is needed for making neurotransmitters and other metabolic substances. The catabolic pathway is especially complex because dihydropyrimidinase and β-ureidopropionase enzymes act in sequence to break uracil into smaller nitrogenous compounds. They show that pyrimidine metabolism is closely controlled and has effects on cellular functions. In Arabidopsis studies, mutations in these enzymes have led to a diminished ability to utilize uracil as a nitrogen source, emphasizing the importance of this pathway in plant nitrogen utilization and suggesting evolutionary adaptations to optimize nutrient usage under varying environmental conditions (Abramoff et al., 2009). In addition, damage to pyrimidines can change the way cells react to stresses , such as viruses. In the case of influenza virus infection, research has found that metabolite levels in the body, especially those related to pyrimidine and purine, are disrupted and match the severity of the disease and lung injury. Since more than 100 metabolites have been found to change during viral infections, the body's response to viruses can likely impact how nucleotides are metabolized and affect the host's general health. The way pyrimidine degradation affects the host's response demonstrates that metabolic pathways are connected and play a role in keeping the body stable in stressful situations. So, knowing about pyrimidine degradation goes further than just biochemical reactions and shows its importance in both normal and abnormal body functions (Figure 8.13).

8.4.3. Clinical Implications of Pyrimidine Metabolism Disorders

These disorders can lead to serious health problems since they affect the production of nucleic acids and cell functions. Such disorders may result in different health complications, including problems with metabolism and serious neurological symptoms. For example, if pyrimidine metabolism is not normal, it can lead to orotic aciduria, where there is too much orotic acid in the urine and this is connected to delays in development and hematological issues. It is important for clinicians to notice these disorders early so they can use the best treatment and diagnostic methods. Also, since nucleotide metabolism is closely connected, any disturbance in pyrimidine pathways can lead to other metabolic problems, showing why it is important to test the metabolism of affected patients. The fact that pyrimidine metabolism disorders are related to neurological conditions demonstrates how complicated their clinical effects can be. Because neurons rely on pyrimidines for DNA and RNA production, they could be easily harmed by metabolic problems. Patients with these disorders usually experience cognitive problems, seizures, and weakness in their movements. When the levels of nucleosides and nucleotides in the brain change, it may result in diseases affecting the central nervous system. As shown in the literature, region-specific distribution of nucleotides affects physiological processes; for example, adenosine and other nucleosides influence functions ranging from sleep to memory and mood regulation, suggesting that pyrimidine metabolism disorders may have broad effects on mental health and cognitive functions (Dobolyi et al., 2013). Emerging research also indicates that pyrimidine metabolism disorders may play a role in the pathogenesis of age-related conditions, , such as age-related macular degeneration (AMD). These disorders have been implicated in the metabolic dysfunction of retinal pigment epithelial (RPE) cells, which are crucial for maintaining vision. Studies have shown that disturbances in cellular metabolism, including alterations in nucleotide metabolism, may lead to the accumulation of metabolic waste products and increased oxidative stress in RPE cells (Alamri et al., 2019). Such oxidative stress can be a reason for the deterioration of these cells, which is typical in AMD. As a result, studying the pathways of pyrimidines may help find new treatments by controlling these pathways to slow down AMD, and hence improve clinical outcomes for patients with these conditions (Figure 8.14).

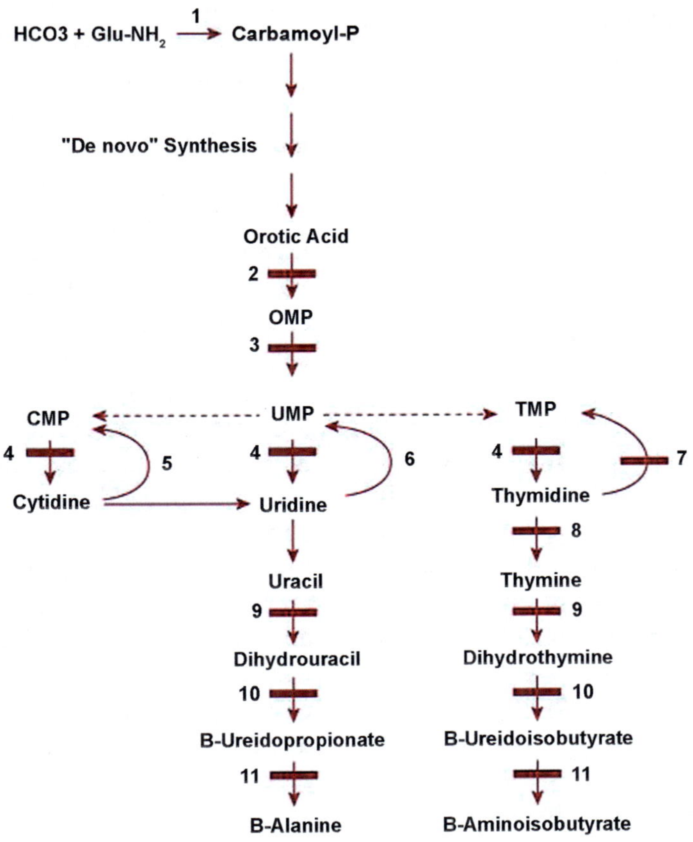

Figure 8.14. Disorders of pyrimidine metabolism.

Source: https://obgynkey.com/wp-content/uploads/2017/01/00453.jpg.

Test Your Knowledge

1. What is the synthesis of pyrimidine nucleotides?
2. What is pyrimidine degradation?

8.5. Nucleotide Interconversion

Learning Outcome

1. Describe the role of nucleoside diphosphate kinases;
2. Understand the importance of nucleotide triphosphate interconversion;
3. Describe the impact on energy metabolism and signaling.

The process of changing one nucleotide into another is very important for nucleotide metabolism, since it allows ATP, ADP, and AMP to balance each other. Changes in phosphorylation and dephosphorylation affect the cell's energy level and the use of energy-releasing pathways. As cellular energy fluctuates, the adenylate energy charge (AEC), a measure proposed by Atkinson, provides a critical framework for understanding these transitions. The cells are able to adjust their metabolism when the concentration of nucleotides changes. Experimental studies have revealed that cells across various organisms are capable of preserving this energy charge, suggesting evolutionary conservation of the mechanism that governs nucleotide interconversion (Biegniewska et al., 2014). For this reason, the way nucleotides interact is vital for cellular functions. Apart from ATP, ADP, and AMP, purine nucleotides are important in cellular metabolism because they help with energy transfer and signaling. Enzymes mainly help in changing one nucleotide to another, , such as ATP to ADP and AMP, and AMP to ATP. Cells depend on the reversibility of these reactions to keep their energy levels in check according to what is needed. Moreover, the synthetic pathways leading from IMP provide further complexity; disruptions in these pathways, , such as blocking degradation reactions, can significantly influence intracellular nucleotide pools. For instance, targeted genetic engineering can optimize strains for increased IMP accumulation, thereby enhancing their utility in biotechnological applications (Barduhn et al., 2012). Such results prove that nucleotide interconversion is linked to other parts of the metabolic system. Nucleotide interconversion is important not only for energy balance but also for keeping the metabolism of cells stable. All these processes are closely watched by the body, so cells can react to changes in their environment, including what nutrients are available or how much stress they face. For instance, the pathways that convert nucleotides are involved in central metabolism, showing how many different and important controls help the body function well. It is clear from adenylate energy models that cells rely on feedback to regulate the various steps in metabolism. In addition, finding out how purines are synthesized and broken-down highlights the complexity of these networks, showing that carefully adjusting enzyme activity can help cells use their nucleotides effectively. Such insight is essential for biochemistry and cellular biology, illustrating how nucleotide interconversion serves as a foundational element of cellular metabolism (Barduhn et al., 2012; Biegniewska et al., 2014).

8.5.1. Role of Nucleoside Diphosphate Kinases (NDPKs)

Nucleoside diphosphate kinases (NDPKs) play a pivotal role in the intricate web of nucleotide metabolism, particularly in the synthesis and interconversion of nucleotides. These enzymes facilitate the transfer of phosphate groups from nucleoside triphosphates (NTPs) to nucleoside diphosphates (NDPs), thus enabling the regeneration of important nucleotide pools within the cell. Besides supporting the growth and energy needs of cells, this flexibility is important for keeping the right balance of nucleotides, which is necessary for DNA and RNA production. In tumors and during embryonic development, when cell division is fast, the work of NDPKs is very important due to the high demand for nucleotides. Thus, knowing how NDPKs work can show possible ways to treat cancer by targeting nucleotide metabolism. In the context of oncological therapies, NDPKs are increasingly recognized for their significance in the effectiveness of nucleoside analogues (NAs), which are employed in cancer treatment. The breakdown of NAs depends on several enzymes, among them are NDPKs. Once inside cancer cells, NAs are phosphorylated to become active and stop the usual metabolism of nucleosides as well as block the production of DNA and RNA. The effectiveness of these drugs depends on how active and present NDPKs are since this affects the amount of nucleotides available for nucleotide pools. Besides, changes in NDPK can result in different reactions to medication, showing why personalized treatment is important.

Therefore, looking into the link between NDPKs and NAs could help find ways to deal with drug resistance in cancer therapy. Studies done recently have pointed out the important connection between NDPKs and the various stress responses in cells, mainly when replication stress is present in cancer cells. For instance, the inhibition of replication stress-sensing kinases, , such as ataxia telangiectasia and Rad3-related protein (ATR), has been shown to affect the output of nucleotide biosynthetic pathways reliant on NDPKs. Blocking ATR shows that NDPKs are needed not only for maintaining the amount of nucleotides in cells but also for handling genotoxic stress. Therefore, strategies that influence the interactions between NDPKs and the nucleotide biosynthetic pathways may be used to weaken cancer cells. This complex interdependency emphasizes the potential for innovative treatments that disrupt nucleotide metabolism, shedding light on critical mechanisms that underpin the progression and treatment resistance of cancers (Balzarini et al., 2014; Le et al., 2017) (Figure 8.15).

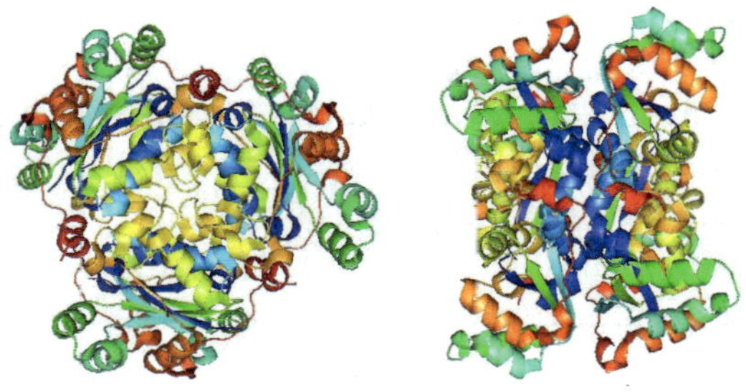

Figure 8.15. Nucleoside diphosphate kinases.

Source: https://upload.wikimedia.org/wikipedia/commons/c/ce/NDPK_structure_.jpg.

8.5.2. Importance of Nucleotide Triphosphate Interconversion

The interconversion of nucleotide triphosphates (NTPs) plays a pivotal role in cellular metabolism by regulating energy dynamics and facilitating various biochemical reactions. NTPs, primarily ATP, guanosine triphosphate (GTP), cytidine triphosphate (CTP), and uridine triphosphate (UTP), serve as critical energy currency within cells. Because of this process, cellular energy can change quickly, which is key to keeping metabolic balance. When cellular energy demands fluctuate, the rapid conversion of ATP to ADP or AMP, and vice versa, ensures that the AEC remains within narrow physiological limits, which is essential for sustaining cellular functions (Biegniewska et al., 2014). So, the ability of cells to adjust NTPs by converting them is important for their metabolism and survival. Additionally, the exchange of NTPs is essential in different metabolic pathways since it helps determine the synthesis of biomolecules. ATP is important because it provides energy and also acts as a substance in reactions that produce nucleic acids and amino acids. For example, turning ATP to GTP is important for both protein synthesis and signal transduction, demonstrating that nucleotide metabolism is linked to many cellular processes. Since nucleotides are versatile, cells can handle changes in the environment and energy stress, while still maintaining their important metabolic activities. Thus, understanding the biochemical routes and reactions governing NTP interconversion reveals the complexity and adaptability inherent in cellular metabolism, which is critical for both unicellular and multicellular organisms (Mills et al., 2020). As well as regulating metabolism, the interchange of NTPs is important for cellular signaling and communication. NTPs give energy and also signal cells to respond to different stimuli. Changing levels of ATP, ADP, and AMP in cells allow them to sense their energy situation and respond in the right way. This phenomenon, termed homeorhesis, underscores the importance of maintaining a stable AEC and ultimately the survival of the organism (Biegniewska et al., 2014). Researchers can learn more about the main principles of nucleotide metabolism by using computational models to show these energy transactions. Ultimately, this knowledge serves as a basis for potential biotechnological applications, helping to harness the metabolic pathways of organisms like cyanobacteria for renewable energy production and other innovative uses (Mills et al., 2020) (Figure 8.16).

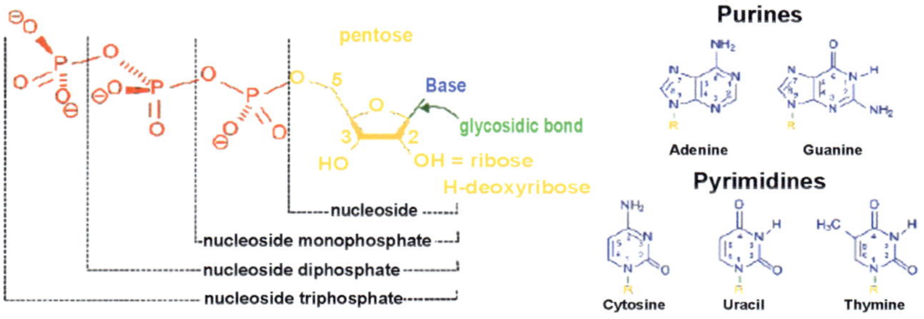

Figure 8.16. Schematic showing the structure of nucleoside triphosphates.

Source: https://upload.wikimedia.org/wikipedia/commons/e/e2/Nucleotides_1.svg.

8.5.3. Impact on Energy Metabolism and Signaling

Cellular homeostasis depends greatly on the connection between nucleotide metabolism and energy signaling. They work as energy carriers and are also important for managing different metabolic processes. They play a role in signaling that controls how cells react to having too enough or not enough energy. For instance, a decline in ATP levels can trigger AMP-activated protein kinase (AMPK), which promotes catabolic processes to restore energy balance. In pathological conditions , such as skeletal muscle atrophy, there is a significant depletion of adenine nucleotide levels, which hampers energy metabolism and exacerbates muscle degradation (Brault et al., 2019). When AdNs are reduced, it changes the cell's energy situation, connecting the metabolism of nucleotides to the control of cell functions and survival in stressful situations. When cancer occurs, energy metabolism is changed so that the cells use more glutamine and other alternative sources. As a result of this change, cells can produce more energy and also build the substances needed for fast cell division and tumor growth. Since these cells use a lot of nucleotides, the production of adenine nucleotides is increased to help them divide. The dependency on glutamine further complicates the relationship between nucleotide metabolism and energy signaling, as it is utilized not merely for energy but also as a critical building block for nucleotides and other macromolecules (Jiang et al., 2019). Therefore, exploring the effects of nucleotide metabolism on signaling pathways in cancer could lead to the discovery of new ways to stop tumors from being flexible in their metabolism. What's more, the decrease in adenine nucleotides in atrophic tissues greatly affects both signaling and metabolic control. A substantial decrease in AdN levels, , such as ATP and ADP, is observed in various diseases, including muscle atrophy, where the degradation enzymes become increasingly active (Brault et al., 2019). Therefore, this situation shows that as nucleotides break down, the pathways responsible for cell repair and growth also deteriorate, causing negative changes in the body. It is important to look at the link between energy metabolism and signaling to understand the causes of these conditions. Exploring the causes behind nucleotide degradation could result in methods to boost cell signaling and fix energy levels in diseases, making them useful for muscle-wasting syndromes and similar conditions.

Test Your Knowledge

1. What is the role of nucleoside diphosphate kinases?
2. What is the importance of nucleotide triphosphate interconversion?

8.6. Nucleotide Metabolism and Disease

Learning Outcome

1. Describe the relationship between cancer and altered nucleotide metabolism;
2. Know the genetic disorders affecting nucleotide metabolism;
3. Explore the therapeutic targets in nucleotide metabolism.

It is clear from the relationship between nucleotide metabolism and diseases that understanding how nucleotide levels affect cells is very important. Nucleotides, important for DNA and RNA synthesis, are also important for signaling and energy transfer since they help make ATP. Any disturbance in the metabolism of nucleotides may result in different diseases, , such as metabolic and neurological disorders. Notably, recent studies indicate that low nucleotide levels may contribute to the development of autoimmune diseases , such as multiple sclerosis (MS). Therefore, changes in genes responsible for nucleotide synthesis and breakdown may influence a person's risk of disease, showing the importance of learning more about the genetic factors of nucleotide metabolism and health in various populations. Of all the diseases connected to nucleotide metabolism, diabetes mellitus is notable because it greatly affects the heart and blood vessels. Diabetic patients exhibit higher incidences of ischemic heart disease (IHD), which is intricately connected to the metabolic disturbances associated with diabetes. Nucleotide metabolism is important for ATP-dependent potassium channels, which help determine the energy levels in the heart and manage blood circulation. If these metabolic pathways change, it can worsen myocardial ischemia, as there is a complicated relationship between energy metabolism, ion channels, and the development of the disease. As studies on these metabolic pathways progress, scientists are expected to focus on using nucleotide metabolism to help manage the complications of diabetes, mainly those that result in serious cardiovascular problems. Besides, certain genetic variants in genes that handle nucleotides, including those linked to vitamin D, explain why diseases , such as MS have many contributing factors. Scientists are paying close attention to the Klotho gene since it may explain how genetic changes can affect serum vitamin D levels and the development of diseases. It has been found that particular alleles of Klotho might be linked to vitamin D changes, meaning that nucleotide metabolism can be influenced by genes. With further research on nucleotide metabolism, it is apparent that both genes and metabolic pathways are important in making people more susceptible to and affected by diseases, so it is necessary to use different approaches in disease prevention and therapy (Figure 8.17).

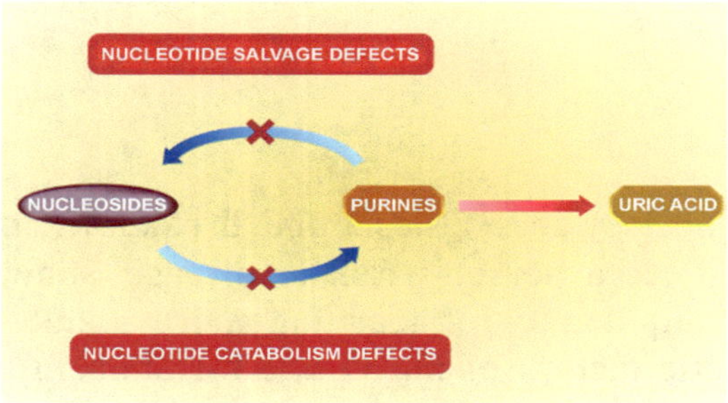

Figure 8.17. Diseases of nucleotide metabolism.

Source: https://reactome.org/download/current/ehld/R-HSA-9735804.svg?title=false.

8.6.1. Cancer and Altered Nucleotide Metabolism

The link between cancer and how nucleotide metabolism is altered is very important for learning about tumor growth and cancer progression. Since cancer cells grow and divide very quickly, they require more nucleotides and must change how their metabolism works. Thus, there are changes in how nucleotides are made and broken down, which increases the amount of DNA and RNA building blocks. It has been found that cancer cells rely on changes in metabolic pathways to live and adapt in various conditions. Besides, the relationship between nucleotide metabolism and certain cancer pathways points to possible therapies that target these processes. Learning about the metabolic effects of oncogenes shows how cancer cells use nucleotide metabolism to their benefit, so it is an important area in cancer research and treatment. Estrogen receptor α (ERα) in breast cancer exemplifies how altered nucleotide metabolism can influence cancer progression through metabolic reprogramming. ERα is known to control many metabolic functions in cancerous breast cells, mainly affecting the ways nucleotides are made. The presence of estrogen that activates ERα prompts a rise in aerobic glycolysis, which is important for creating ATP and other substances needed for nucleotide formation. In this case, CHPT1 genes are upregulated by ERα, which causes an increase in phosphatidylcholine synthesis and affects both the cell membrane and its signaling routes. If these processes are disrupted, it can reduce cell growth and resistance to treatment, so it is important to study these metabolic networks in breast cancer to find new treatment methods. It is also clear from pancreatic cancer that changes in the metabolism of nucleotides are related to how aggressive and metastatic the tumor is. It is found through research that MUC16 plays a key role in changing the metabolism of pancreatic adenocarcinoma.

When MUC16 is knocked down, cancer cells take up less glucose and make less lactate, which points to a decrease in aerobic glycolysis, which is crucial for cancer cells. After mTOR activity is stopped, there is a decrease in c-MYC, which is very important for cell growth and proliferation. Metabolomic studies also confirm these results by revealing that nucleotide metabolites are less available in cancer cells without MUC16. All in all, this points out that MUC16 is important for cancer cell movement, invasion, and the unusual metabolism that helps them survive and grow, making it a suitable target for treating pancreatic cancer (Figure 8.18).

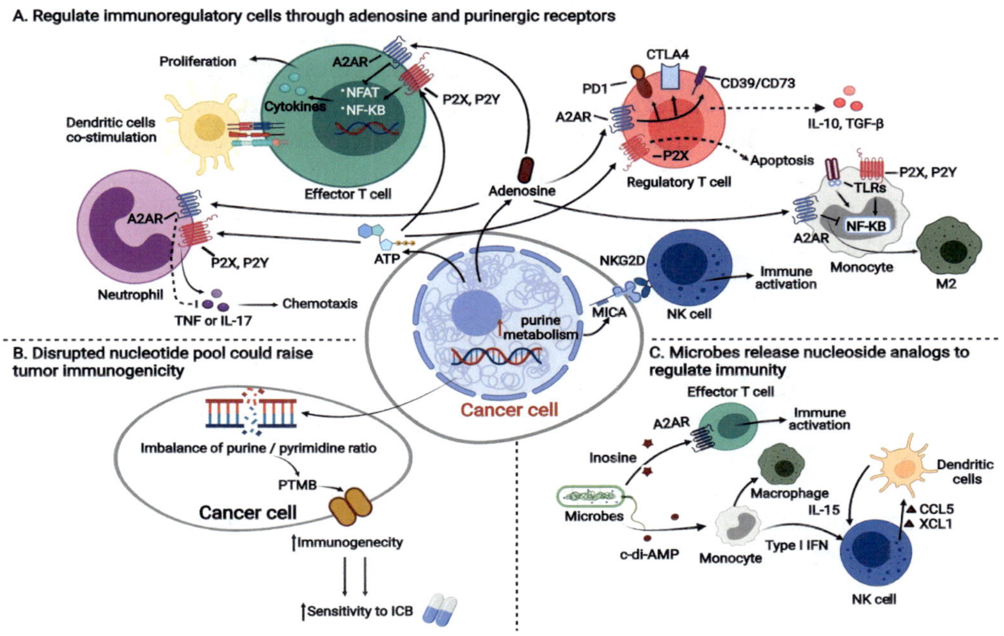

Figure 8.18. Interactions between nucleotide metabolism and host immunity. Cancer cells could release metabolites from nucleotide metabolism, , such as ATP, adenosine to (A) regulate immunoregulatory cells through adenosine and purinergic receptors; (B) in cancer cells, a disrupted nucleotide pool could raise tumor immunogenicity; and (C) microbes release nucleoside analogs to regulate immunity.

Source: https://media.springernature.com/full/springer-static/image/art%3A10.1186%2Fs13045-022-01263-x/MediaObjects/13045_2022_1263_Fig2_HTML.png?as=webp.

8.6.2. Genetic Disorders Affecting Nucleotide Metabolism

Looking at genetic disorders involving nucleotide metabolism teaches us a lot about cells and the reasons behind diseases. The metabolism of nucleotides covers the chemical reactions that produce and break down nucleotides, which are needed for nucleic acids. Disorders in this area can happen when genes responsible for metabolism are changed, which can result in different health problems. As an example, people with purine metabolism disorders can develop serious health problems , such as gout or a weak immune system. Knowing about these genetic bases is important for creating treatments that fix the main metabolic problems and the associated symptoms. Also, problems involving nucleotide metabolism usually have a mix of genetic and environmental factors. It has been found that variations in the genes that make certain enzymes can increase a person's chance of getting certain diseases. A lack of enzymes , such as adenine deaminase causes the body to build up toxic substances, which seriously reduces the immune system and leads to severe combined immunodeficiency. Such genetic disorders point out the vital role of nucleotide metabolism in keeping cells healthy and also indicate that treating these diseases can be personalized by targeting the metabolic pathways changed by genetic mutations. Besides their clinical effects, studies of genetic disorders involving nucleotide metabolism may help us better understand several MSs. As shown in recent research, health issues related to metabolism can trigger obesity and diabetes in the body by affecting metabolic processes. A possible approach is to change the levels or roles of certain microRNAs, as seen in studies about miR-378 and its part in metabolic disorders. Thus, the intersection of genetic research and nucleotide metabolism not only enhances our understanding of fundamental biological processes but also paves the way for novel treatments aimed at improving health outcomes in patients afflicted by related genetic conditions (Carrer et al., 2014; Ferraguti et al., 2015).

8.6.3. Therapeutic Targets in Nucleotide Metabolism

Looking into therapeutic targets in nucleotide metabolism has gained a lot of interest because it may help treat different metabolic disorders. Researchers are especially interested in how microRNAs, for example, miR-378, affect the metabolism of cells. It has been found that changing the level of miR-378 can affect fatty acid metabolism, which might provide new treatments for obesity and MS. When scientists use miR-378 inhibitors, they hope to correct metabolic issues, pointing out the close link between nucleotide metabolism and other metabolic pathways.

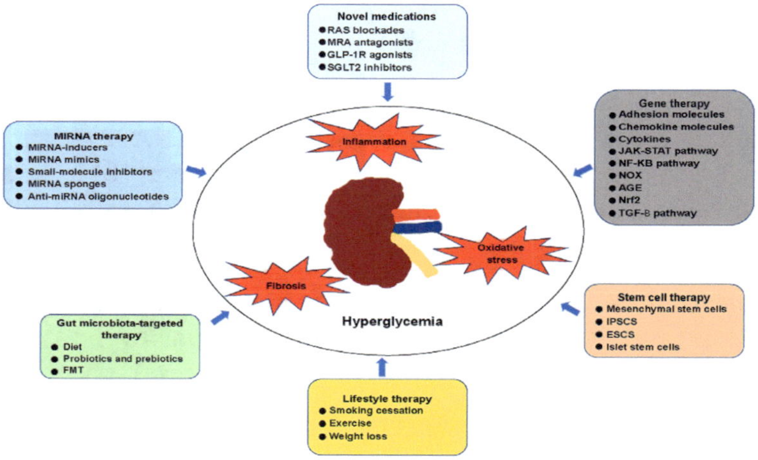

Figure 8.19. Current and potential targets for therapeutic interventions of diabetic kidney disease (DKD).

Source: Guo, M.; He, F.; Zhang, C. Molecular Therapeutics for Diabetic Kidney Disease: An Update. *Int. J. Mol. Sci.* **2024**, *25*, 10051. https://doi.org/10.3390/ijms251810051

This way of thinking highlights the importance of looking at nucleotide metabolism in several ways, so that medicines can be developed to fix specific problems in the metabolism, leading to better results for related diseases. Chronic kidney disease (CKD) serves as another compelling context for targeting nucleotide metabolism therapeutically. Many people with CKD are more likely to develop serious vascular disease and other major health problems early in life. Studies carried out recently have shown that epigenetic factors are important in the development of diseases, as they affect the synthesis and breakdown of nucleotides. By changing the expression of genes in nucleotide metabolism, epigenetic modifications underline the significance of these processes in dealing with CKD. With knowledge of epigenetics and its impact on nucleotides, scientists might create new ways to diagnose and treat patients that consider their unique differences. They could greatly improve the care given to patients with CKD and their general health, helping to establish personalized medicine. It is necessary to use all available research information when dealing with the therapeutic issues linked to diseases of nucleotide metabolism. Because nucleotide metabolism and epigenetic modifications are linked, as we have discussed, there are new opportunities for treating metabolic disorders and renal diseases. For example, stopping the action of certain metabolic pathways could help a lot in treating CKD and its complications. As more studies are done, it is necessary to consider both genetic and epigenetic aspects in the study of nucleotide metabolism. With the help of new discoveries in molecular biology and genetics, researchers can find new treatments for metabolic disorders that meet the needs of each patient (Figure 8.19).

Test Your Knowledge

1. Describe the genetic disorders affecting nucleotide metabolism.
2. What are the therapeutic targets in nucleotide metabolism?

SUMMARY

In short, knowing about nucleotide metabolism is necessary for understanding basic cellular functions and for spotting how metabolic problems contribute to several diseases. Nucleotide metabolism supports cell growth, repair, and replication, so it is important in healthy and unhealthy situations. If there are changes in nucleotide levels, it can result in many conditions , such as cancer and genetic disorders, which shows that more research is needed on the pathways that control nucleotide synthesis and degradation. In addition, what we learn about nucleotide metabolism can guide treatments by targeting particular metabolic paths, possibly opening up new ways to treat diseases. Maintaining the right amount of nucleotides in the cell depends on many enzymes and regulatory factors that are involved in nucleotide metabolism. It has been suggested by new studies that the restriction on DNA coding and noncoding parts gives insights into the evolutionary stresses affecting metabolic pathways. For example, the presence of many restricted noncoding sites, most in intergenic regions, suggests that these regions might help regulate metabolic activities. Understanding these subtleties can significantly enhance our comprehension of cellular responses to metabolic changes and the evolutionary adaptations that have emerged over time, as illuminated by research findings in murids that indicate a higher occurrence of constrained sites in developmental and neuronal genes compared to metabolic process genes (Altschul et al., 2006). More study of nucleotide metabolism highlights the important connection between nucleotides and cell cycle regulators, proving how vital these processes are for cells. The way cAMP signaling is described in archaea indicates that this process is similar in many living organisms and helps control the cell cycle, showing how important nucleotide metabolism is for evolution. Nucleotides play a key role in keeping metabolism healthy and also affect the overall health of the organism. Future research focusing on these connections will undoubtedly deepen our insight into the metabolic framework that underpins cellular life, paving the way for advancements in biotechnology and medicine (Baumann et al., 2007).

The process of nucleotide metabolism is important for many cellular activities, including making DNA and RNA needed for cell growth and division. A major feature of this pathway is that certain cancer cells rely on certain nutrients to make their nucleotides. Evidence shows that serine is more important than glycine for cancer cells in making nucleotides. Serine coming from the environment is especially important for cancer cells since it is changed into glycine and one-carbon units needed for making nucleotides. Conversely, while glycine can be utilized by cancer cells, it fails to adequately replace serine in supporting their growth, underscoring the selective importance of serine in this context (Labuschagne et al., 2014). The regulation and presence of one-carbon units are important for the process of nucleotide metabolism. It is clear from the relationship between serine and glycine metabolism that what a cell prefers to eat can have a major effect on its function and growth. If serine is not present, glycine does not help make nucleotides and may even stop cell proliferation because there are not enough one-carbon molecules. The result points out that the supply of certain substrates in a cell can impact how nucleotides are produced and, as a result, whether the cell lives or dies. The revelation that formate can rescue nucleotide synthesis in glycine-fed cells emphasizes the critical role of one-carbon units in sustaining metabolic processes (Labuschagne et al., 2014). Besides the interactions between amino acids, nucleotide metabolism also plays a role in wider ecological areas, for example, microbes affecting human health. Studies of the gut microbiome have shown that many microbes work together, affecting the production of nucleotides. Researchers found that specific microbial functions are important for human health based on a study that found a core metatranscriptomic profile in various individuals. In addition, the metatranscriptome was different from one individual to another, showing that metabolic interactions in the microbiome can change a lot. Studying the influence of microbial communities on nucleotide metabolism increases the area of research and suggests new ways to treat metabolic disorders with drugs.

KEY TERMS FROM THIS CHAPTER

- Adenine
- Cellular proliferation
- Cytosine
- Guanosine triphosphate
- Inosine monophosphate
- Nucleotides
- Pyrimidine metabolism
- Uridine triphosphate
- Cancer cells
- Cytidine triphosphate
- Guanine
- Hypoxanthine
- Nucleotide metabolism
- Purine metabolism
- RNA synthesis

CRITICAL THINKING QUESTIONS

1. **Nucleotides are composed of all the following EXCEPT:**
   a. Nitrogenous base
   b. Pentose sugar
   c. Phosphate group
   d. Amino acid
2. **The *de novo* synthesis of purine nucleotides begins with which molecule?**
   a. Ribose-5-phosphate
   b. PRPP (Phosphoribosyl pyrophosphate)
   c. UMP (Uridine monophosphate)
   d. GMP (Guanosine monophosphate)
3. **Which enzyme catalyzes the conversion of ribose-5-phosphate to PRPP?**
   a. PRPP synthetase
   b. Ribonucleotide reductase
   c. Adenylate kinase
   d. Carbamoyl phosphate synthetase
4. **In purine metabolism, the first purine nucleotide formed is:**
   a. AMP (Adenosine monophosphate)
   b. GMP (Guanosine monophosphate)
   c. IMP (Inosine monophosphate)
   d. XMP (Xanthosine monophosphate)
5. **Pyrimidine nucleotide synthesis requires which of the following amino acids?**
   a. Glycine
   b. Glutamine
   c. Aspartate
   d. Both b and c

Answers to Critical Thinking Questions

1. (d); 2. (b); 3. (a); 4. (c); 5. (d)

Short Answer Questions

1. What is nucleotide metabolism?
2. Why is nucleotide metabolism important in cellular functions?
3. What is the structure of nucleosides?
4. What is purine metabolism?
5. What is the pyrimidine metabolism?

References

1. Bowater, R.P., Cobb, A.M., Pivonkova, H. *et al.* Biophysical and electrochemical studies of protein–nucleic acid interactions. *Monatsh Chem* **146**, 723–739 (2015). https://doi.org/10.1007/s00706-014-1405-4 (accessed on 11th June 2025).
2. Shukla, S. K., Gunda, V., Abrego, J., Haridas, D., Mishra, A., Souchek, J., Chaika, N. V., Yu, F., Sasson, A. R., Lazenby, A. J., Batra, S. K., & Singh, P. K. (2015). MUC16-mediated activation of mTOR and c-Myc reprograms pancreatic cancer metabolism. *Oncotarget*, *6*(22), 19118–19131. https://doi.org/10.18632/oncotarget.4078 (accessed on 11th June 2025).
3. Le, T.M., Poddar, S., Capri, J.R. *et al.* ATR inhibition facilitates targeting of leukemia dependence on convergent nucleotide biosynthetic pathways. *Nat Commun* **8**, 241 (2017). https://doi.org/10.1038/s41467-017-00221-3(accessed on 11th June 2025).
4. Abu-Ali, G. S., Branck, T., Chan, A. T., et al. (2018). Meta transcriptome of human fecal microbial communities in a cohort of adult men. https://core.ac.uk/download/286364483.pdf (accessed on 11th June 2025).
5. Achcar, F., Barrett, M. P., Goodyear, C. S., et al. (2018). Metabolomic profiling of macrophages determines the discrete metabolomic signature and metabolomic interactome triggered by polarizing immune stimuli. https://core.ac.uk/download/153444716.pdf (accessed on 11th June 2025).
6. Agrimi, G., Cirigliano, A., Di Noia, M. A., et al. (2014). The human SLC25A33 and SLC25A36 genes of solute carrier family 25 encode two mitochondrial pyrimidine nucleotide transporters. https://core.ac.uk/download/54505794.pdf (accessed on 11th June 2025).
7. Alamri, A., Biswas, L., Watson, D. G., & Shu, X. (2019). Deletion of TSPO resulted in change of metabolomic profile in retinal pigment epithelial cells. *International Journal of Molecular Sciences, 20*(6), 1387. https://doi.org/10.3390/ijms20061387 (accessed on 11th June 2025).
8. Allegrini, S., Camici, M., Garcia-Gil, M., Pesi, R., & Tozzi, M. G. (2019). Purine-metabolizing enzymes and apoptosis in cancer. https://core.ac.uk/download/286467281.pdf (accessed on 11th June 2025).
9. Amiruddin, R., Arsin, A. A., & Talarima, B. (2012). Risk factors in the incidence of gouty arthritis in Masohi Town, Central Maluku Regency in 2010. https://media.neliti.com/media/publications/149736-EN-risk-factors-in-the-incidence-of-gouty-a.pdf (accessed on 11th June 2025).
10. Andreassen, T., Bathen, T. F., Cao, Y., et al. (2016). Estrogen receptor α promotes breast cancer by reprogramming choline metabolism. https://core.ac.uk/download/646196450.pdf (accessed on 11th June 2025).
11. Balzarini, J., Liekens, S., & Vande Voorde, J. (2014). Mycoplasmas and cancer. https://core.ac.uk/download/46915803.pdf (accessed on 11th June 2025).
12. Bandea, C. I. (2009). A unifying scenario on the origin and evolution of cellular and viral domains. https://core.ac.uk/download/pdf/288874.pdf (accessed on 11th June 2025).
13. Barduhn, T., Heinzle, E., Peifer, S., Schneider, et al. (2012). Metabolic engineering of the purine biosynthetic pathway in *Corynebacterium glutamic* results in increased intracellular

pool sizes of IMP and hypoxanthine. https://core.ac.uk/download/14526749.pdf (accessed on 11th June 2025).

14. Barr, E. W., Bollinger, J. M., Brown, D. M., et al. (2008). Lethal mutagenesis of picornaviruses with N-6-modified purine nucleoside analogues. https://core.ac.uk/download/4877318.pdf (accessed on 11th June 2025).

15. Baumann, A., Lange, C., & Soppa, J. (2007). Transcriptome changes and cAMP oscillations in an archaeal cell cycle. https://core.ac.uk/download/14500832.pdf (accessed on 11th June 2025).

16. Bayram, Ş. (2024). Analysis of the glutamine dependent transaminases as possible therapeutic targets in colon cancer cells. https://core.ac.uk/download/614349539.pdf (accessed on 11th June 2025).

17. Biegniewska, A., Eke, A., García-Muñoz, A., Goldbeter, A., Gottlieb, A., Kahru, A., et al. (2014). On the dynamics of the adenylate energy system: Homeorhetic vs homeostasis. https://core.ac.uk/download/74389839.pdf (accessed on 11th June 2025).

18. Bordbar, A., Jamshidi, N., Palsson, B. Ø., et al. (2014). Network reconstruction of platelet metabolism identifies metabolic signature for aspirin resistance. https://core.ac.uk/download/323077862.pdf (accessed on 11th June 2025).

19. Bowater, R. P. (2005). *Nucleotides: Structure and Properties.* https://core.ac.uk/download/2776256.pdf (accessed on 11th June 2025).

20. Braas, D., Christofk, H. R., Graeber, T. G., Krall, et al. (2016). Asparagine promotes cancer cell proliferation through use as an amino acid exchange factor. https://core.ac.uk/download/323077084.pdf (accessed on 11th June 2025).

21. Brault, J. J., Hafen, P. S., & Miller, S. G. (2019). Increased adenine nucleotide degradation in skeletal muscle atrophy. https://core.ac.uk/download/299809081.pdf (accessed on 11th June 2025).

22. Carlson, J. E., Geib, S. M., Hoover, K., McKenna, et al. (2014). Functional genomics and microbiome profiling of the Asian long horned beetle (*Anoplophora glabripennis*) reveal insights into the digestive physiology and nutritional ecology of wood feeding beetles. https://core.ac.uk/download/33142967.pdf (accessed on 11th June 2025).

23. Carrer, M., & Olson, E. N. (2014). Regulation of metabolism by miR-378. https://core.ac.uk/download/211342145.pdf (accessed on 11th June 2025).

24. Thaker, S. K., Ch'ng, J., & Christofk, H. R. (2019). Viral hijacking of cellular metabolism. *BMC biology*, *17*(1), 59. https://doi.org/10.1186/s12915-019-0678-9(accessed on 11th June 2025).

25. Chan, T. K., Chen, J., Cui, L., et al. (2015). Metabolomics investigation reveals metabolite mediators associated with acute lung injury and repair in a murine model of influenza pneumonia. https://core.ac.uk/download/83227123.pdf (accessed on 11th June 2025).

26. Yizhak, K., Chaneton, B., Gottlieb, E., & Ruppin, E. (2015). Modeling cancer metabolism on a genome scale. *Molecular systems biology*, *11*(6), 817. https://doi.org/10.15252/msb.20145307(accessed on 11th June 2025).

27. Conti, I., Laface, I., Milani, D., et al. (2020). miRNAs as influencers of cell-cell communication in tumor microenvironment. https://core.ac.uk/download/286469910.pdf (accessed on 11th June 2025).

28. Davies, O., Malys, N., Mendes, P., et al. (2011). Characterization of multiple substrate-specific (d)ITP/(d)XTPase and modelling of deaminated purine nucleotide metabolism. https://core.ac.uk/download/9323820.pdf (accessed on 11th June 2025).

29. De Marchis, M., D'Amato, A., Fedele, F., et al. (2018). Diabetes mellitus and ischemic heart disease: The role of ion channels. https://core.ac.uk/download/159269109.pdf (accessed on 11th June 2025).

30. Dobolyi, Á., Juhász, G., Kovács, Z., et al. (2013). 5'-Nucleotidases, nucleosides and their distribution in the brain: Pathological and therapeutic implications. https://core.ac.uk/download/42928318.pdf (accessed on 11th June 2025).

31. Ebenhoeh, O., Matthaeus, F., & Salazar, C. (2008). Biosynthetic potentials of metabolites and their hierarchical organization. https://core.ac.uk/download/25497442.pdf (accessed on 11th June 2025).

32. Ebong, S. J. (1996). Possible role for neopterin: Control of purine metabolism. https://core.ac.uk/download/617783487.pdf (accessed on 11th June 2025).

33. Ekström, T. J., Nordfors, L., Shiels, P. G., Stenvinkel, et al. (2017). Current epigenetic aspects the clinical kidney researcher should embrace. https://core.ac.uk/download/84340482.pdf (accessed on 11th June 2025).

34. Ferraguti, G., Lucarelli, M., & Pascale, E. (2015). Alcohol addiction: A molecular biology perspective. https://core.ac.uk/download/54518723.pdf (accessed on 11th June 2025).

35. Fonteh, Aliah L. (2018) "Orotic Aciduria," *Fidei et Veritatis: The Liberty University Journal of Graduate Research*: Vol. 2: Iss. 1, Article 1. Available at: https://digitalcommons.liberty.edu/fidei_et_veritatis/vol2/iss1/1(accessed on 11th June 2025).

36. Gaffney, D. J., & Keightley, P. D. (2006). Genomic selective constraints in murid noncoding DNA. *PLoS Genetics*, *2*(11), e204. https://doi.org/10.1371/journal.pgen.0020204 (accessed on 11th June 2025).

37. Irr, J. D. (1972). Control of nucleotide metabolism and ribosomal ribonucleic acid synthesis during nitrogen starvation of *Escherichia coli*. https://core.ac.uk/download/213082730.pdf (accessed on 11th June 2025).

38. Jiang, J., Srivastava, S., & Zhang, J. (2019). Starve cancer cells of glutamine: Break the spell or make a hungry monster? https://core.ac.uk/download/228066288.pdf (accessed on 11th June 2025).

39. Labuschagne, C. F., van den Broek, N. J., Mackay, G. M., Vousden, K. H., & Maddocks, O. D. (2014). Serine, but not glycine, supports one-carbon metabolism and proliferation of cancer cells. *Cell reports*, *7*(4), 1248–1258. https://doi.org/10.1016/j.celrep.2014.04.045(accessed on 11th June 2025).

40. Mills, L. A., McCormick, A. J., & Lea-Smith, D. J. (2020). Current knowledge and recent advances in understanding metabolism of the model cyanobacterium Synechocystis sp. PCC 6803. *Bioscience reports*, *40*(4), BSR20193325. https://doi.org/10.1042/BSR20193325(accessed on 11th June 2025).

41. Lo Sasso, B., Gambino, C. M., Bellia, C., Scazzone, C., Iacolino, G., Bivona, G., Salemi, G., et al. (2020). Klotho and vitamin D in multiple sclerosis: An Italian study. https://core.ac.uk/download/287858100.pdf (accessed on 11th June 2025).

42. Lu, H. T. H. (2015). Modeling uric acid kidney stones disease in *D. melanogaster* using RNAi and dietary modulation. https://core.ac.uk/download/215554481.pdf (accessed on 11th June 2025).

43. Rosser, E. (2020). Identification, development, and evaluation of small-molecule modulators of nucleotide metabolism. https://core.ac.uk/download/324161468.pdf (accessed on 11th June 2025).

44. Zrenner, R., Riegler, H., Marquard, C. R., Lange, P. R., Geserick, C., Bartosz, C. E., Chen, C. T., & Slocum, R. D. (2009). A functional analysis of the pyrimidine catabolic pathway in *Arabidopsis*. *New Phytologist*, *183*(1), 117–132. https://doi.org/10.1111/j.1469-8137.2009.02843.x (accessed on 11th June 2025).

VITAMINS AND COENZYMES

9

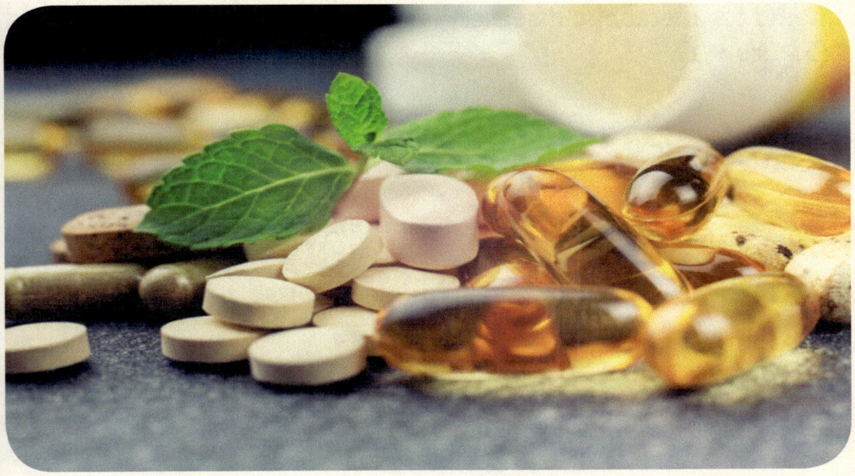

LEARNING OBJECTIVES

After studying this chapter, you will be able to:

1. Describe the types of vitamins;
2. Know the functions of coenzymes;
3. Understand the sources of vitamins;
4. Know the deficiency and excess of vitamins;
5. Describe the research and advances in vitamin and coenzyme studies.

Introduction

The way vitamins and coenzymes interact is essential in biochemistry because it shows how different organic compounds cooperate to help life. Vitamins are important micronutrients that organisms need in small amounts for basic biochemical activities, but the body cannot produce them in enough quantity. Unlike enzymes, coenzymes are organic substances that help enzymes function better and are important for the progress of metabolism. To see the importance of vitamins, one must realize that they are often used in the process of making coenzymes for metabolic reactions. It highlights the main role that these molecules have in keeping metabolism healthy and efficient. When we look further into this topic, we realize that having a good understanding of vitamins and coenzymes helps us understand metabolic processes better. Making coenzymes from vitamins is an active process that clearly shows the role of biochemistry in metabolism. Vitamins , such as B vitamins take part in making coenzymes like NAD+, FAD, and coenzyme

A, which are important for metabolizing carbohydrates, proteins, and lipids. Cellular respiration and the building of macromolecules in cells are mostly supported by coenzymes. If the body does not get enough vitamins, the way enzymes function can suffer, which could result in metabolic disorders and less efficient cells. It shows that vitamins are necessary for more than nutrition, since a lack of one can result in many other body problems. Exploring how vitamins and coenzymes interact also helps us understand bigger biological processes, for example, cell growth, aging, and cell signaling. For instance, the physiological mechanisms underpinning cellular aging, particularly in fungi like *Saccharomyces cerevisiae* and *Schizosaccharomyces pombe*, are pertinent areas of research (Boswell et al., 2017). Looking at these organisms helps scientists see how vitamins and other nutrients impact cell metabolism and division. Looking at apoptosis, we can see that vitamins affect the cell's ability to use energy and also its lifespan. That's why, to learn more about life-sustaining biological changes and to develop treatments for metabolic diseases, it's important to understand how vitamins and coenzymes function (Figure 9.1).

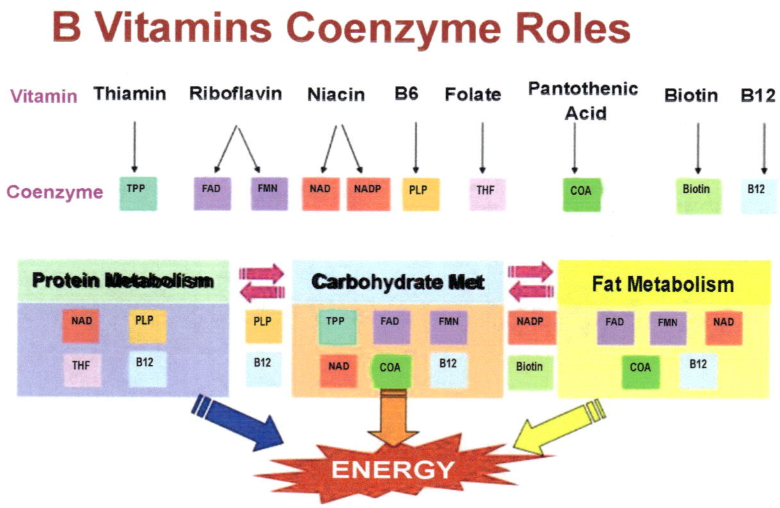

Figure 9.1. B vitamins: coenzyme roles.

Source: https://image1.slideserve.com/3300492/b-vitamins-coenzyme-roles-n.jpg.

Definition of Vitamins

To define vitamins, you need to know their biochemical roles and how they are organized among other nutrients. Vitamins are necessary for many body functions and mainly work by serving as coenzymes or providing materials needed for coenzymes to take part in metabolic processes. The body does not make enough of these nutrients and we must get them through our meals. Because of their differences in absorption, storage, and effects on the body, vitamins A, D, E, and K are called fat-soluble, while the B-complex and vitamin C are water-soluble. By dividing nutrients, it points out that eating a variety of foods is important for good health since too little or too much of certain vitamins can create serious health problems. The latest studies have explained in greater detail the many functions of vitamins in the body, mainly as coenzymes. A lot of the reactions that sustain life, from making energy to creating DNA, depend on coenzymes. B vitamins are a good example because they usually help enzymes in transforming substances needed for cellular activities and metabolism. Learning how vitamins are available and used in the body has important effects on human health, the environment, and farming. For instance, Colinas & Fitzpatrick (2022) discuss the critical regulation of coenzyme supply concerning metabolic demands, highlighting the intricate relationships between primary and specialized metabolism in organisms. In addition, vitamins are important not only for nutrition, but also for many biological processes. Vitamins are important for the way microbial communities interact and are arranged in various ecosystems. Recent studies have found that some phytoplankton need certain B vitamins, proving that the supply of vitamins can affect the makeup and behavior of aquatic communities. It shows that vitamin metabolism should be fully understood in ecological research. As Allen et al. (2017) illustrate, the complexity of vitamin cycling in ecosystems and the versatile metabolic strategies employed by phytoplankton highlight the broader implications of vitamins in nutrient cycling and the maintenance of biodiversity. Exploring these factors gives us a clearer picture of health and the environment (Figure 9.2).

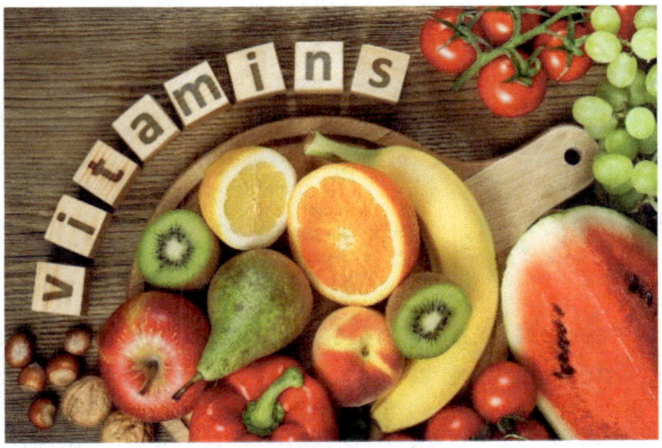

Figure 9.2. Vitamins.

Source: https://images.squarespace-cdn.com/content/v1/606fa67ad10220013b33bb0e/1712650181329-95DP218G55HLRSO3Y3FM/shutterstock_417009853.jpg.

Definition of Coenzymes

To know how vitamins function in living organisms, we need to understand coenzymes. Coenzymes help enzymes perform their duties in catalyzing different biochemical reactions. Most of them come from vitamins and help various metabolic activities, mainly those linked to energy production and the making of molecules. While substrates are changed by enzymes, coenzymes do not change and are able to take part in several different reactions. Thanks to this property, cells can handle changing conditions without always having to make new enzymes. Coenzymes help us understand how metabolic regulation works, showing that each coenzyme works with enzymes to help important reactions and keep life going. The way vitamins and coenzymes work together is a well-developed evolutionary process that is very important for cells. Since vitamins are important nutrients, the body does not make enough of them and they must be taken from foods. Certain vitamins that are ingested are used to produce coenzymes that are vital for many metabolic processes. As an illustration, vitamin B-based coenzymes are necessary for breaking down carbohydrates and fats, which helps produce energy. These linkages reveal that if vitamins are available, they can increase coenzyme levels and thus affect the overall course of metabolism. This relationship points out that vitamins are necessary and that they help in the formation of coenzymes needed for enzymes to work. A closer look at coenzymes' role in regulation shows that they play a major part in metabolic networks. Studies carried out lately suggest that coenzymes are responsible for both driving certain enzymatic reactions and helping maintain balance in metabolism. As an illustration, coenzymes made from vitamin B compounds have been found to control the movement of metabolites in different biosynthetic pathways and also join processes , such as cellular signaling and energy management. Because the body's needs can change, it is important to regulate the supply of coenzymes to make sure enzymes are well supported. In light of synthetic biology advancements, recognizing the importance of coenzymes in metabolic engineering opens pathways for enhancing biochemical processes, suggesting that coenzymes should be at the forefront of future metabolic research and applications in biotechnology (Kun et al., 2008; Colinas & Fitzpatrick, 2022) (Figure 9.3).

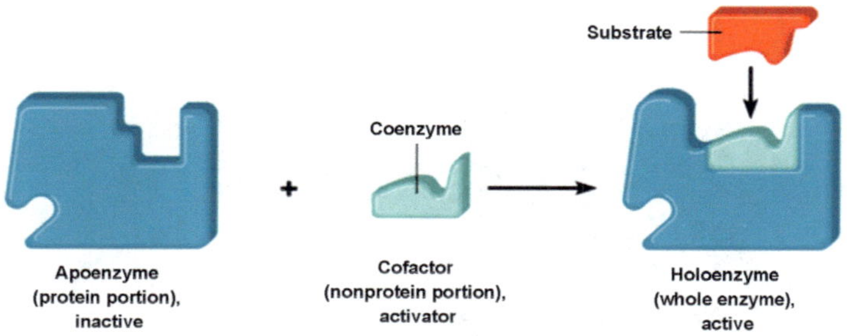

Figure 9.3. A cofactor is a non-protein chemical compound that is required for the protein's biological activity. Many enzymes require cofactors to function properly.

Source: https://cdn-ildfibj.nitrocdn.com/qaWeLntkRcyxNUcEoWbLpZLQkcgLFsiJ/assets/images/optimized/www.biologyonline.com/wp-content/uploads/2019/10/Cofactor-and-apoenzyme.png.

9.1. Types of Vitamins

Learning Outcome

1. Describe the water-soluble vitamins and fat-soluble vitamins;
2. Understand the role of vitamins in human health.

Understanding the roles of vitamins in the body is based largely on how vitamins are classified, especially when it comes to enzymes. Vitamins are mainly sorted into water-soluble and fat-soluble groups. Vitamins B and C, which can be dissolved in water, are important for energy production and the production of red blood cells. Because the body does not keep much of these vitamins, you need to eat them regularly to avoid deficiency. Since they can be dissolved easily, hormones are carried and excreted without affecting the body's metabolic balance. Alternatively, vitamins A, D, E, and K are fat-soluble and need to be eaten with dietary fat to be well absorbed; they are stored in the liver and fatty tissues. This difference is very important when thinking about vitamins, as water-soluble vitamins usually act as coenzymes in metabolism, while fat-soluble ones generally have a role in regulating and building cells. The B-complex group of vitamins is significant because it plays a big role in metabolism that depends on coenzymes. Thiamine, riboflavin, niacin, and biotin from the B vitamin group are essential for enzymes that turn macronutrients into energy. In this way, thiamine helps the enzyme pyruvate dehydrogenase convert pyruvate into the citric acid cycle. It shows that vitamins are important for the body not only as part of the diet but also because they enable enzymes to function properly. Lacking just one B vitamin can result in metabolic problems, which shows how important all of them are together. Because of this, B vitamins play an important role of vitamins in helping coenzymes maintain good metabolism and support general health. Fat-soluble vitamins are important for many body functions, not only for metabolism, but also for various cellular activities. Vitamin D is important for calcium regulation and bone health since it acts as a hormone that oversees calcium absorption in the intestines and its reabsorption in the kidneys. This illustrates that fat-soluble vitamins assist the body's metabolism and also act as signals that direct the actions of cells. Likewise, vitamin A is required for vision and the immune system, and vitamin E works as an antioxidant to protect the cells. Because fat-soluble vitamins have many roles, they clearly demonstrate how vitamins, enzymes, and the body's functions are closely connected. Studying these relationships helps build a base for more work in nutritional biochemistry and its impact on human health, mainly for prevention (Figure 9.4).

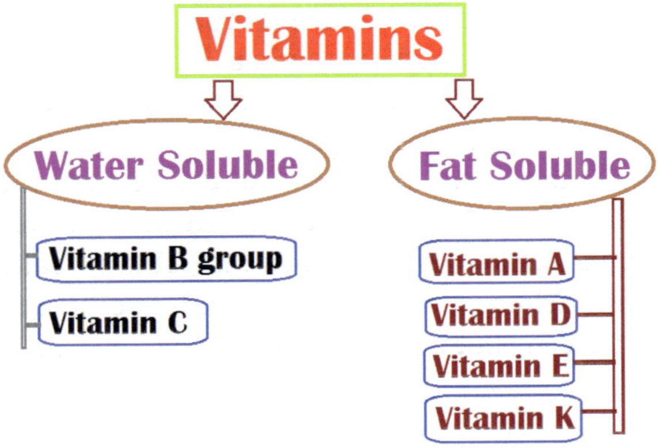

Figure 9.4. Types of vitamins.

Source: https://www.uaex.uada.edu/counties/miller/images/AtoZFitness-Vitamins.png.

9.1.1. Water-Soluble Vitamins

The B-complex vitamins and vitamin C are important for many processes in the human body since they are water-soluble. Since they are water-soluble, these vitamins are easily absorbed and carried by the blood. Since water-soluble vitamins are not stored well, you must include them in your diet regularly to keep your level high. Vitamins , such as B1 (thiamine),

B2 (riboflavin), and B6 (pyridoxine) are essential for energy metabolism, participating in enzymatic reactions that convert nutrients into usable energy. Besides, certain water-soluble vitamins act as coenzymes, which help enzymes in speeding up biochemical reactions and supporting cell functions. Apart from helping the body use energy, water-soluble vitamins contribute to DNA production, fixing damaged cells, and keeping the body healthy. Folate, which is vitamin B9, is very important for DNA synthesis and methylation, both of which are necessary for correct cell division and avoiding genetic problems. When these vitamins are lacking, people may suffer from anemia, problems with their nervous system, and a weak immune system. Vitamin B6 has been found to play a key part in immune control and reducing inflammation, making it important for warding off diseases. This interconnection between vitamins and metabolic pathways emphasizes the necessity of a balanced diet rich in complex carbohydrates, fruits, and vegetables to ensure adequate intake of these essential nutrients (Ibrahim et al., 2018). In addition, studies have pointed out the effects of water-soluble vitamin deficiencies on human health, mainly when it comes to chronic diseases. An example is that a lack of vitamin B6 may cause a higher risk of type 1 diabetes and rheumatoid arthritis, proving how important these vitamins are for a healthy body. It appears that when water-soluble vitamins are low, the body's inflammation increases, especially among those who are at risk. Noticing these effects shows that following nutritional recommendations and learning about nutrition is important for good health. Notably, the classification and understanding of vitamins continue to evolve, as indicated by the historical naming systems documented by researchers, which reflect the dynamic nature of nutritional science and its application in health communication (Williams, 2015) (Figure 9.5).

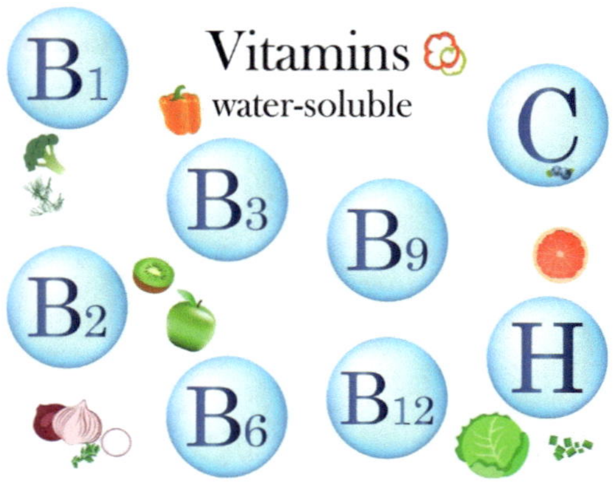

Figure 9.5. Water-soluble vitamins.

Source: https://purayati.com/cdn/shop/articles/SATtdQEtsV.jpg?v=1611754938.

9.1.2. Fat-Soluble Vitamins

Among vitamins, fat-soluble vitamins are important because of their special chemical features and important functions. The body can use vitamins A, D, E, and K best when there is fat present in the diet. Unlike water-soluble vitamins, fat-soluble vitamins are stored in the body's fatty tissues and liver, so they can act for a longer time and may cause toxicity if eaten in large amounts. Their role in metabolism makes it important to store them in the right amounts, so a proper diet is needed to avoid excessive intake and its possible side effects. The historical development of vitamin nomenclature reflects the ongoing discovery of their functions and roles, contributing to our understanding of these essential micronutrients (Williams, 2015). Fat-soluble vitamins play many roles in the body, helping to maintain different important functions for good health. An example is that vitamin A is needed for good vision and a strong immune system, and vitamin D is essential for controlling calcium levels and maintaining healthy bones. Besides, vitamin E shields cell membranes from damage by free radicals, and vitamin K is important for the process of blood clotting. Since these vitamins work together in metabolism, it shows how vital they are and why we should pay attention to their role in the diet and in the body. As we continue to explore the intricate relationships between vitamins and overall well-being, the scientific community notes that knowledge gaps regarding optimal levels and synergies remain a topic of investigation (Cooper et al., 2025).

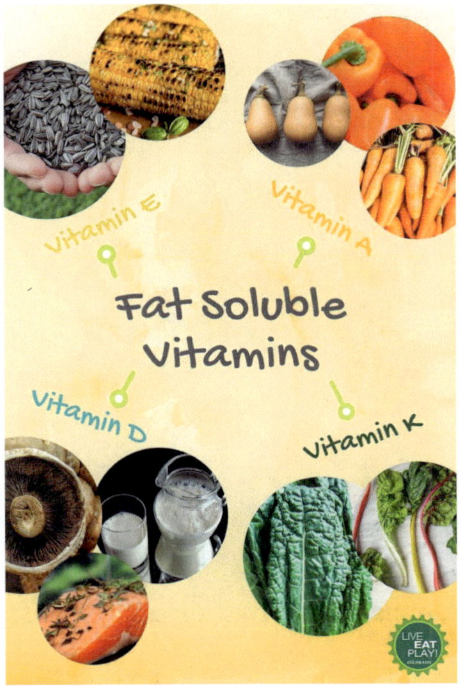

Figure 9.6. Fat-soluble vitamins.

Source: https://i.pinimg.com/736x/9e/5f/98/9e5f9826ccde903a1f4bea7178f9a3f5.jpg.

Also, including fat-soluble vitamins in nutrition strategies is very important for ensuring good health for people everywhere. But, because there are many factors to consider and everyone's needs are not the same, this task is more complicated. For example, age, sex, and any health problems may determine how much of these vitamins a person should get. These initiatives should manage these challenges and clearly advise people on how to get enough nutrients through their diets. Teaching people about fat-soluble vitamins through nutrition education is important for preventing shortages and boosting general health. Ultimately, the ongoing research into the roles of these vitamins within broader nutritional frameworks continues to illuminate their critical importance in human physiology (Williams, 2015) (Figure 9.6).

9.1.3. Role of Vitamins in Human Health

It is well-known that vitamins are important for human health, mainly because they take part in many metabolic functions. Vitamins help enzymes do their work, which is important for the body's overall stability. B6, B12, and folate from the B-complex group are important for amino acid metabolism and making neurotransmitters, which affects both mental function and mood. They help prevent the health problems that can happen if you don't get enough of these vitamins. Additionally, vitamin D and calcium work closely together, showing that vitamins are important for healthy bones and the whole body. It has been found that vitamins work with oxidative stress and neurodegenerative diseases in a complex way. It has been pointed out that oxidative stress plays a major role in the development of Alzheimer's disease, which leads to damage to brain cells and cognitive decline. Some recent studies suggest that vitamins C and E have antioxidant effects that minimize the harm caused by free radicals. In this context, the modulation of poly (ADP-ribose) polymerase 1 (PARP-1) activity by specific nutrients has gained attention, suggesting a potential therapeutic avenue for managing oxidative stress in neurodegenerative conditions. This means that getting enough vitamins is important and that they may also help prevent diseases, showing their key role in maintaining human health. Vitamins help the body function properly and also support good health and the prevention of long-term diseases. It has been found through epidemiological studies that having enough vitamins reduces the chances of getting cardiovascular diseases (CVDs) and certain cancers. For instance, vitamins A, C, and E are antioxidants that have been related to less oxidative damage in cells, which can help lower inflammation and the risk of diseases. Vitamin K's part in blood coagulation and its new role in bone health show how vitamins have many important functions in our health. As we learn more about vitamins, it is obvious that they are important in many biological functions and help maintain health by preventing diseases (Figure 9.7).

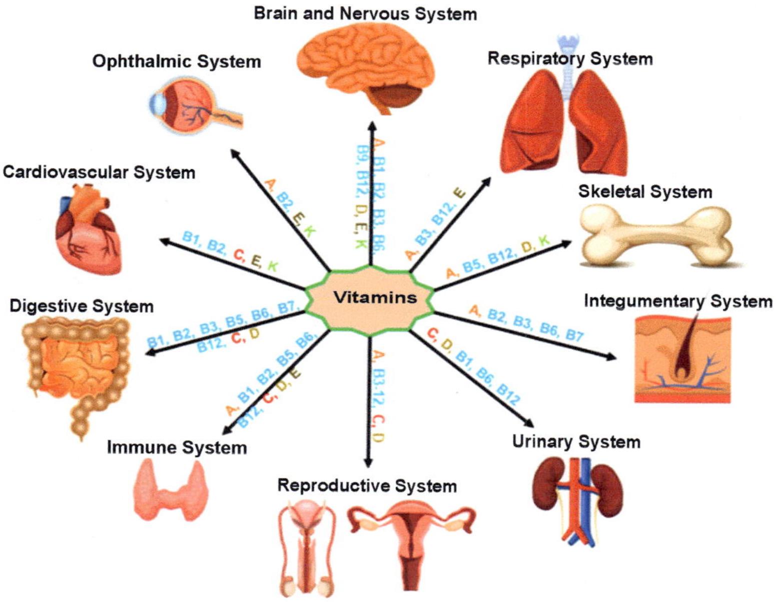

Figure 9.7. A diagram illustrating the roles of various vitamins in different organ systems.

Source: https://www.researchgate.net/publication/358902039/figure/fig3/AS:11431281211992909@1702515794551/A-diagram-illustrating-the-roles-of-various-vitamins-on-different-organ-systems-All-of.tif.

Test Your Knowledge

1. What are the water-soluble vitamins?
2. What is the role of vitamins in human health?

9.2. Functions of Coenzymes

Learning Outcome

1. Understand the role of vitamins and coenzymes in enzymatic reactions;
2. Describe the examples of common coenzymes;
3. Understand the importance of coenzymes in metabolism.

Coenzymes play a key role in enzymatic reactions by greatly boosting how active the enzymes are. They are usually made from vitamins and help with biochemical reactions by supporting the activation of substances and offering structure. It is most noticeable in metabolic reactions that coenzymes often function as electron carriers or transfer groups. For example, NAD+ and FAD coenzymes take part in redox reactions to help change the energy present in nutrients into ATP. If coenzymes were missing, metabolic pathways would not work well, which would affect cell functions and the well-being of the organism. So, knowing the roles of coenzymes highlights the importance of these compounds in keeping life functions running properly. Apart from assisting in energy production, coenzymes also play a vital part in making important cellular molecules. Coenzymes help in different synthetic processes, for example, the production of nucleotides, amino acids, and lipids. For example, coenzyme A (CoA) is paramount in fatty acid metabolism and the Krebs cycle, enabling the breakdown of fatty acids to generate energy. In addition, coenzymes play a key role in cell reproduction by taking part in DNA replication and repair. The relationship between coenzymes and enzymes points to the precise way metabolic pathways are regulated, with each coenzyme's action affecting the chemistry of the cell. For this reason, coenzymes aid in the use of energy and also help maintain the overall health and stability of cells. Studies are revealing that coenzymes have a long history in metabolic pathways and are very important for their functions. Researchers now believe that the first core metabolism might have worked without phosphate-based coenzymes. This points out that coenzymes can be used in different ways in various biochemical reactions. Because of these findings, we now realize that fungi-like coenzymes may help ancient organisms take in nutrients and deal with their surroundings. In the context of fungal physiology, the reliance on various coenzymes showcases how these molecules facilitate essential processes, , such as growth and nutrient assimilation, contributing to a deeper understanding of coenzyme functions beyond conventional metabolic pathways (Boswell et al., 2017; Goldford et al., 2017) (Figure 9.8).

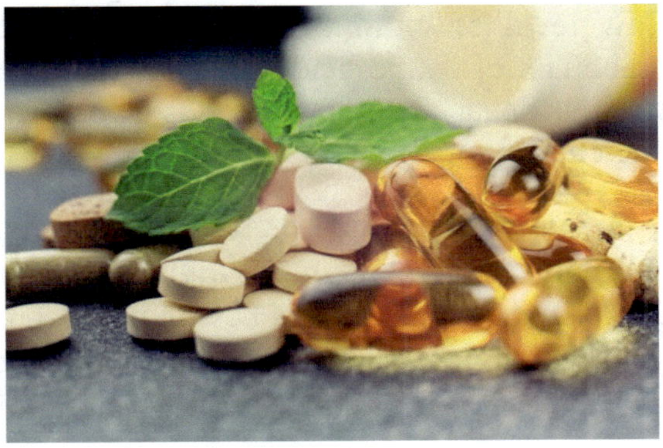

Figure 9.8. Assorted dietary supplements and coenzyme-rich capsules.

Source: https://www.sciencing.com/sciencing/functions-coenzymes-5070676/063deec45f72444eb5e97169a116ff44.jpg.

9.2.1. Role in Enzymatic Reactions

Enzymatic reactions are greatly improved and better regulated by the way vitamins and coenzymes interact. Enzymes act as biological catalysts by helping reactions to proceed faster by stabilizing the transition states and lowering how much of energy needed to begin the reaction. Still, most enzymes work best when they have additional molecules besides proteins. Vitamins, being organic substances required in small amounts, help in the creation of coenzymes, which play a role in enzymatic activities. As an example, riboflavin and niacin are B vitamins that play a key role in making flavin adenine dinucleotide (FAD) and nicotinamide adenine dinucleotide (NAD^+), respectively. They are important in helping with oxidation-reduction reactions that play a key role in energy and metabolism. Coenzymes that come from vitamins are important for enzyme functions and also help maintain the proper workings of metabolic pathways. They allow the movement of important groups or atoms between the enzyme and the substrate. It demonstrates that when there are not enough vitamins, metabolic functions may be disrupted and this can cause different health problems. A low level of vitamin B6 can disrupt the metabolism of amino acids since its coenzyme form, pyridoxal phosphate, is not available in sufficient amounts.

For this reason, the link between vitamins, coenzymes, and enzymes highlights how metabolism is regulated and how important it is to have enough micronutrients for good health. It is also clear from the study of metabolic networks in different living organisms that vitamins and their coenzymes play an important role in enzymatic reactions. Recent research posits that early biochemical processes may have operated through phosphate-independent mechanisms, suggesting that alternative metabolic networks could have existed before phosphate incorporation into biological systems (Goldford et al., 2017). The hypothesis suggests that complex changes in metabolic pathways during evolution could have made thioester-based metabolism important for the development of today's enzymes. By exploring the intricacies of these biochemical interactions, we gain deeper insights into the foundational aspects of life and the critical roles vitamins and coenzymes play in sustaining metabolic homeostasis and facilitating evolutionary survival (Chen et al., 2017).

9.2.2. Examples of Common Coenzymes

Among the plethora of coenzymes identified in biological systems, NAD+ stands out as a pivotal player in cellular metabolism. Since NAD+ is related to niacin, one of the B vitamins, it mostly helps in redox reactions, allowing electrons to move during glycolysis and the citric acid cycle. It is important for the body to make ATP, the energy that cells use, by converting food into energy. Because NAD+ is involved in oxidation-reduction reactions, it helps with energy metabolism and also supports DNA repair and the regulation of apoptosis, showing that it has many roles. Another prominent coenzyme is coenzyme A (CoA), which is vital in the metabolism of fatty acids and the synthesis of acetyl-CoA, a crucial substrate for the citric acid cycle. It comes from pantothenic acid, or vitamin B5, which shows how vitamins and coenzymes are connected. CoA carries acyl groups, which help in the reactions needed for making fatty acids, cholesterol, and steroid hormones. Besides, the addition of coenzyme A to metabolic pathways demonstrates the link between primary and specialized metabolism in organisms. As recent studies suggest, understanding the regulation of coenzyme supply relative to metabolic demands can significantly enhance our knowledge of metabolic engineering and synthetic biology, emphasizing CoAs beyond mere metabolic function (Colinas & Fitzpatrick, 2022). Another key coenzyme is FAD, which plays a crucial role in various oxidation-reduction reactions within the cell. FAD is created from riboflavin, which is vitamin B2, and helps move electrons in the metabolism of carbohydrates and fats. The fact that it participates in the citric acid cycle and fatty acid oxidation proves its role in producing energy for the body. FAD also helps enzymes called flavoproteins, which are needed for several metabolic processes, , such as those involving amino acids. The versatility of FAD in facilitating redox reactions illustrates its significance in biochemical pathways and highlights how vitamins, through their roles as precursors of coenzymes, contribute to the intricate network of metabolism and energy regulation within cells (Boswell et al., 2017) (Figure 9.9).

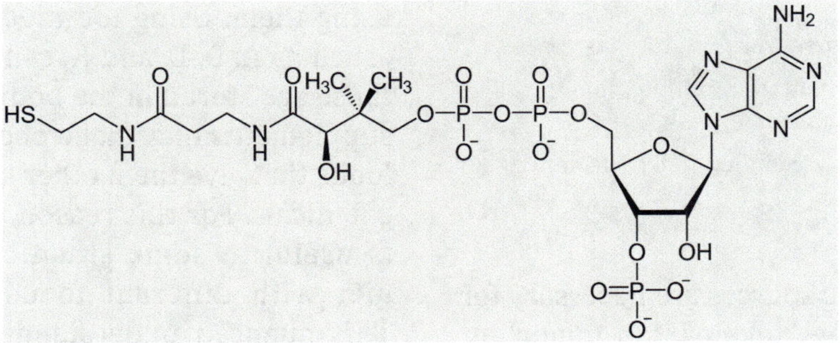

Figure 9.9. Coenzyme A.

Source: By NEUROtiker - Own work, Public Domain, https://commons.wikimedia.org/w/index.php?curid=1555660

9.2.3. Importance of Coenzymes in Metabolism

Coenzymes are important in metabolism because they help in many biochemical reactions needed for the cell's function. Usually, these organic molecules, which are often from vitamins, help enzymes to speed up different metabolic processes. As an illustration, B vitamins are coenzymes that help break down carbohydrates, fats, and proteins, making sure energy is produced and the needed biomolecules are made. Besides helping reactions, coenzymes help direct metabolic pathways so that cells can react to changes in the environment. If the body lacks enough coenzymes, the metabolic pathways can slow down, which may result in a lack of energy and nutrients throughout the body. Coenzymes take part in many crucial metabolic reactions, which help maintain stability in the body. One notable example is the involvement of NAD+ (derived from niacin, a B vitamin) in oxidation-reduction reactions, crucial for the generation of ATP through cellular respiration. Coenzymes , such as coenzyme A (CoA) are instrumental in the Krebs cycle, where they assist in the acetylation of substrates, playing a key role in fat, carbohydrate, and protein metabolism. The way coenzymes and enzymes work together demonstrates a well-organized metabolic system that, if interrupted, may cause several health problems. Therefore, it is important to eat enough vitamins to provide enough coenzymes, which help maintain normal metabolism and energy supply in different parts of the body. Coenzymes affect many aspects of biology, , such as the environment and the causes of diseases. Studies done recently have found that the metabolic role of coenzymes can affect whole ecosystems, mainly in aquatic areas where the presence of phytoplankton is affected by vitamins. The interplay of vitamins as coenzymes is crucial for sustaining phytoplankton productivity, which serves as the foundation for aquatic food webs (Allen et al., 2017).

Test Your Knowledge

1. How are vitamins involved in enzymatic reactions?
2. What is the role of coenzymes in metabolism?

9.3. Sources of Vitamins

Learning Outcome

1. Describe the dietary sources of vitamins;
2. Explore the supplementation options for vitamins and coenzymes;
3. Understand the recommended daily allowances (RDAs).

Vitamins from various sources are necessary for people's health, as they take part in important biochemical activities. Fruits and vegetables are the main sources of vitamins, full of nutrients that help the body's metabolism. A good example is citrus fruits, which are rich in vitamin C that helps make collagen and supports the immune system. Vitamins A, K, and many B vitamins are found in large amounts in leafy greens, making them good for your overall health. Whole grains are rich in B vitamins, which take part in the process of generating energy. More people choosing energy drinks and flavored waters as beverages allows them to get vitamins in a new way. As these drinks are marketed heavily to various demographics, particularly youth, understanding their nutritional implications and how they contribute to vitamin consumption is crucial in contemporary dietary practices (Becker et al., 2014). Animal products are important because they contain vitamins that are easy for the body to absorb. Meat, fish, eggs, and dairy provide a lot of vitamins B12, D, and A, which are important for the body's cells and health. Vitamin B12 is needed for healthy red blood cells and nerves, and it is mostly available in animal products, creating difficulties for people who do not eat meat. This points out that those with particular dietary needs should try to find alternative ways or supplements. Additionally, nutritional education must address the varied absorption rates of vitamins from plant versus animal sources, ensuring that individuals make informed choices about their diets based on their nutritional needs (Williams, 2015). What's more, dietary supplements have made it easier for people to get the vitamins they need each day. Even though these supplements help fill nutritional gaps, you should be careful when using them. Using too much of some vitamins, , such as A, D, E, and K, can cause toxicity since these are stored in the body. In addition, taking supplements may make people less likely to eat foods that give them other nutrients and helpful chemicals. For this reason, taking supplements is useful in some situations, but a balanced diet with different foods is still necessary. This nuanced understanding is necessary for optimizing vitamin intake and ensuring overall well-being (Becker et al., 2014; Williams, 2015) (Figure 9.10).

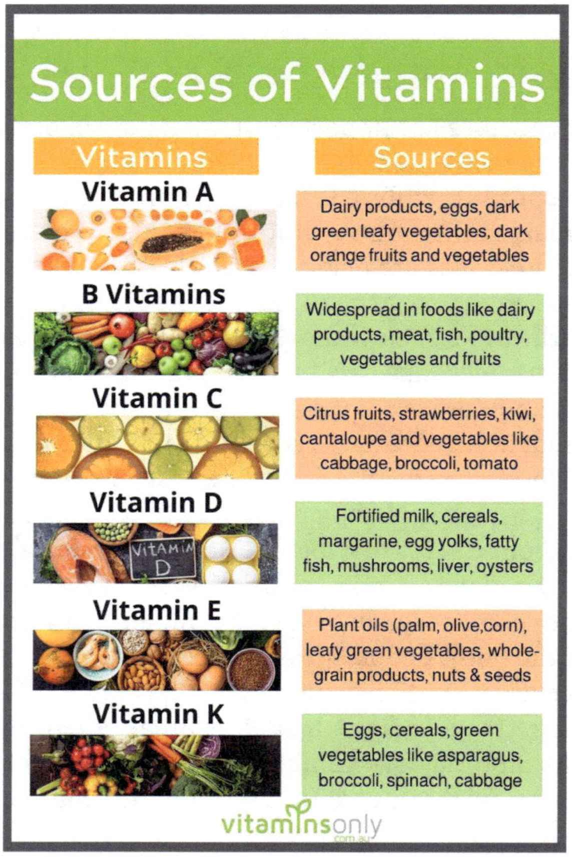

Figure 9.10. Sources of vitamins.

Source: https://i.pinimg.com/736x/d6/b8/28/d6b82803669bed0f574536757f064c6d.jpg.

9.3.1. Dietary Sources of Vitamins

Vitamins are mainly found in different foods that help keep our health in good condition. Fruits and vegetables serve as rich sources of vitamins, with citrus fruits like oranges and grapefruits high in vitamin C, while leafy greens , such as spinach and kale contain ample amounts of vitamins A and K. Additionally, different food groups contribute to a well-rounded intake of vitamins; for instance, whole grains are significant sources of B vitamins, especially B1 (thiamine), B2 (riboflavin), and B3 (niacin). Since people have many different dietary needs, it is important to eat a variety of foods to make sure the body gets enough vitamins for good health. Animal products give us important vitamins, which are sometimes hard to get from plants. A good example is vitamin B12, which helps with blood cell growth and brain function, and it is mostly found in animal foods , such as meat, fish, dairy, and eggs. Liver, fatty fish, nuts, and avocados are foods that contain fat-soluble vitamins A, D, E, and K. They are important for various functions in the body, for example, vision, bone strength, and antioxidants. For the best nutrient balance, people should eat both plant and animal foods since each type offers different vitamins that help keep the body healthy. With this approach, you help your body function properly and also prevent any deficiencies. To provide good nutrition education and health advice, it is important to know the foods that contain vitamins. Even so, the names and groupings of vitamins may confuse both people who take them and those who prescribe them. For instance, old ways of naming vitamins and new alphabetical names create difficulties in explaining them. Studies have cataloged numerous vitamin names, revealing over 67 different alphabet-based designations in the scientific literature (Williams, 2015). Because things are so complex, it is important to have clear guidelines about vitamins that are both accurate and helpful. As research continues to unveil the intricate roles of vitamins and minerals in human health, effective nutrition communication is essential for promoting informed dietary choices that support well-being, including the interaction between vitamin levels and optimal physiological performance (Cooper et al., 2025) (Figure 9.11).

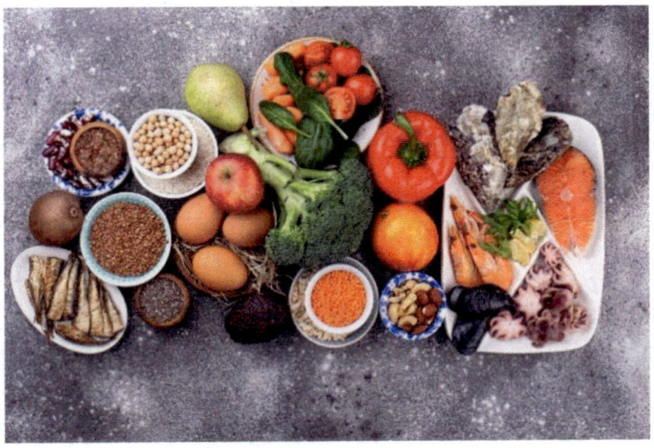

Figure 9.11. An assortment of nutrient-rich foods including seafood, legumes, fruits, and vegetables.

Source: https://e4tb2ebssiw.exactdn.com/wp-content/uploads/2024/04/pescetarian-diet-with-seafood-fruit-and-vegetable-2023-11-27-05-02-50-utc.jpg?strip=all&lossy=1&ssl=1.

9.3.2. Supplementation Options

Investigating ways to add vitamins and coenzymes to the diet shows the important relationship between nutritional science and public health. Notably, riboflavin (vitamin B2) acts as a vital cofactor in various biochemical reactions, particularly in the context of intermediary metabolism. More people are now using vitamin D supplements, mainly because the elderly are at risk of lacking this vitamin. Inadequate riboflavin intake in older adults can lead to disruptions in metabolic pathways, potentially exacerbating the prevalence of chronic diseases, including CVD and cataracts, which are significant health concerns in developed countries. Giving riboflavin supplements to people at risk might help prevent these health concerns. Furthermore, public health strategies to improve riboflavin status may consider the development of food fortification programs targeting vulnerable groups, thereby enhancing community health outcomes and overall quality of life (Tavares et al., 2009). Also, the fact that riboflavin supplementation can be influenced by genes highlights that personalized nutrition is not simple. The common C677T polymorphism in the methylenetetrahydrofolate reductase (MTHFR) gene has been associated with increased risk for hypertension and CVD in certain populations. According to studies, riboflavin is important in managing the effects of this genetic condition. Studies suggest that those with two copies of the polymorphism may see a big drop in their systolic blood pressure after taking riboflavin, showing that dietary changes can be tailored. Using supplements that match a person's genes could improve the ability of riboflavin to lower the health risks of CVD. Hence, these insights into supplementation options inform the design of more personalized nutritional guidelines, bridging the gap between genetic predisposition and dietary practices (Hughes et al., 2016). In addition, riboflavin supplementation is important for international efforts to deal with vitamin deficiencies. Even though clinical deficiencies are scarce in developed countries, many individuals have insufficient riboflavin, so more attention and actions are needed. Erythrocyte glutathione reductase is a useful biomarker for checking riboflavin levels, but information about it is still scarce. Studying riboflavin levels in different groups of people can help create better public health measures. As riboflavin is shown to help with health, especially blood pressure, it is crucial to develop supplementation plans for people with a genetic risk. Overall, addressing the multifaceted aspects of riboflavin supplementation can contribute significantly to enhancing community health and reducing the burden of chronic diseases (Tavares et al., 2009) (Figure 9.12).

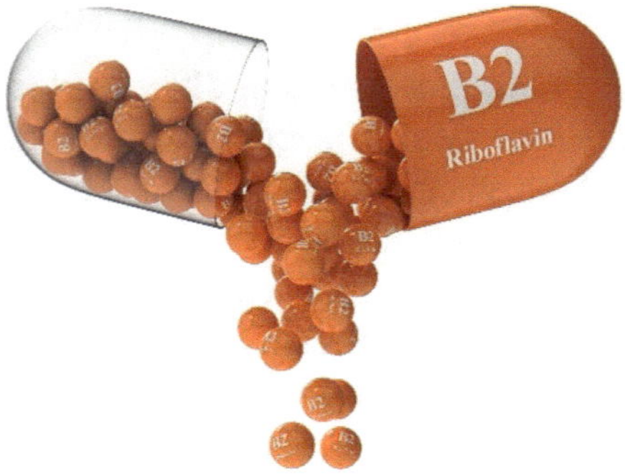

Figure 9.12. Vitamin B2 (riboflavin).

Source: https://cdn.mos.cms.futurecdn.net/ybcJw9Y8EFGjBmdKd5g3dF.jpg.

9.3.3. Recommended Daily Allowances

Navigating the complexities of nutrition requires an understanding of recommended daily allowances (RDAs), particularly for vitamins, which play crucial roles as coenzymes in various metabolic processes. RDAs are defined as the daily dietary intake levels sufficient to meet the nutrient requirements of nearly all (97–98%) healthy individuals in a specific life stage and gender group. They help people get enough of the essential vitamins, which reduces the risk of serious health problems. B vitamins, which help with energy and brain function, are included in RDAs that are different for people of different ages, sexes, and physical conditions , such as pregnancy. This method shows that having dietary advice that fits each person's health is important for good health. Vitamins and their RDAs must interact, since not having enough of these nutrients can be harmful to your health. According to research, many people suffer from vitamin deficiency diseases, which proves that clear dietary advice is needed. As an illustration, RDA values reveal that vitamin C is needed in large amounts to ward off scurvy, whereas vitamin D is vital for healthy bones and avoiding rickets when it is consumed enough. According to a study that compiled extensive data on vitamin deficiencies and food sources rich in these nutrients, it was determined that approximately 1,912 foods contain at least one vitamin (Sarkar et al., 2015). It points out the wide range of foods you can choose and invites you to include different and nutritious foods in your diet to fulfill the RDAs. Besides, as fortified drinks are becoming more popular, it is important to know how they affect vitamin intake according to RDAs. Added vitamins in fortified beverages are usually aimed at improving the health and wellness of people, mainly children and adolescents. Nevertheless, an increase in the consumption of these beverages raises concerns regarding their overall healthfulness, especially in light of the obesity epidemic prevalent among children (Becker et al., 2014). Even though these drinks give you some vitamins, they might cause you to miss out on the nutrients found in real foods. Since people's eating habits are changing, it is necessary to review the role of fortified foods in meeting RDAs, as the relationship between getting enough vitamins and leading a healthy lifestyle is still a major concern in nutrition.

Test Your Knowledge

1. What is the main dietary source of vitamins?
2. What are the recommended daily allowances?

9.4. Deficiency and Excess of Vitamins

Learning Outcome

1. Know the consequences of vitamin deficiency;
2. Understand the symptoms of vitamin excess;
3. Describe the public health implications surrounding vitamins and coenzymes.

Proper levels of vitamins in the body are necessary to avoid serious health problems due to either a lack or an excess of these nutrients. In most cases, a lack of vitamins happens when someone does not eat enough of them, has trouble absorbing nutrients, or has certain health problems. Many people lack vitamins A, C, D, and B1, which can cause different health problems. If someone lacks vitamin A, it may result in visual problems, while lacking vitamin C can cause scurvy and tiredness, as well as gum disease. Moreover, the prevalence of fortified beverages in the market raises concerns, particularly among youth, as excessive consumption could lead to vitamin imbalances that negatively impact their growth and development (Becker et al., 2014). It stresses that we should know the roles of vitamins and also eat healthily to avoid any shortages. At the same time, having too many of the fat-soluble vitamins A, D, E, and K can also cause health problems. Water-soluble vitamins are removed from the body through urine, but fat-soluble ones build up in the body, which could lead to dangerously high levels. As an example, if a person takes too much vitamin A, it can lead to hypervitaminosis A, which may bring about nausea, headaches, and liver problems. In the same way, having too much vitamin D can result in hypercalcemia, which is marked by high blood calcium, and may cause problems in the digestive tract and kidneys. These possible problems stress the importance of having a balanced amount of vitamins, since having too much may not be good. Understanding the intricate balance of vitamins and their biochemical roles as coenzymes is therefore essential for maintaining health and preventing adverse effects from either deficiency or excess (Ankita et al., 2018). To ensure a balanced diet, people should pay attention to both low and high levels of vitamins, because this balance directly affects the body's metabolism. A lot of individuals believe that supplements can make up for any dietary imbalance or surplus, but this is not true because vitamins have their own unique roles in the body. For instance, the increasing popularity of fortified beverages, often laden with added vitamins, encourages consumers to overlook the potential risks of excessive intake while neglecting whole foods rich in necessary nutrients (Becker et al., 2014). It is important to teach people about balanced nutrition so they can avoid both shortages and overdoses and focus on eating good foods first. Ultimately, ongoing research into the diverse roles and effects of vitamins is essential to foster informed dietary choices, thereby enhancing public health outcomes and mitigating the risks associated with vitamin imbalances (Ankita et al., 2018) (Figure 9.13).

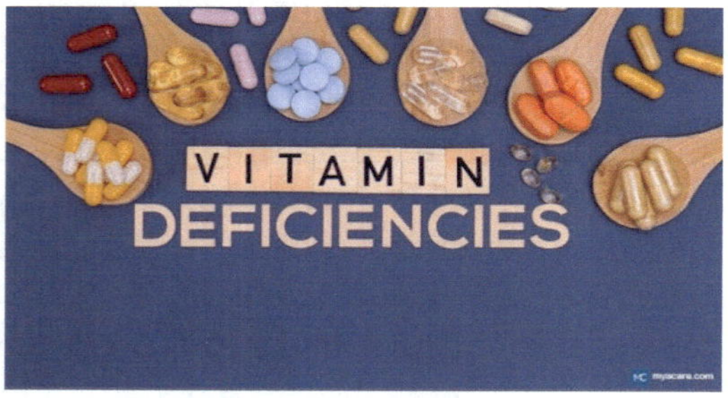

Figure 9.13. Vitamins deficiency.

Source: https://images.myacare.com/uploads/AdminBlogs/eaac3ad558594620a81d8423d5f046f1.webp.

9.4.1. Consequences of Vitamin Deficiency

Having vitamin deficiency can affect both the body and the mind, influencing several body systems. Vitamins are involved in important biochemical reactions, so their absence may cause cells to function improperly. Not having enough B3, B6, and B9 vitamins has been associated with different diseases and faster aging. A lack of water-soluble vitamins in the diet can disrupt the body's metabolism, leading to problems with DNA and affecting the health of genes, which may result in various diseases. The inability to effectively carry out these functions can contribute to the onset and progression of chronic diseases, underscoring the critical role of vitamins in maintaining health and well-being (Martire & Fuso, 2015). In addition, studies continue to show that not having enough of these nutrients can worsen oxidative stress and negatively affect how cells work and live. Older people are especially at risk of cognitive decline due to vitamin deficiency. For good neurological health, it is important to have vitamins B12 and folate. A lack of these vitamins may increase the chances of developing neurodegenerative diseases, for example, Alzheimer's disease. It is well known that oxidative stress can cause damage to neurons, and this is shown by the fact that vitamin deficiencies can result in neuronal death and impairments in thinking. The accumulation of oxidative damage also disrupts essential intracellular processes, including mitochondrial function, further complicating the health of the affected cells (Martire & Fuso, 2015). When there are vitamin deficiencies, the brain is not able to fight oxidative stress, which may be a major cause of Alzheimer's disease and similar conditions, showing why good nutrition is necessary for brain health. In addition, not getting enough vitamins can result in poor health, causing problems with body processes and making a person more prone to infections. If Vitamin D is lacking, the immune system is not as strong, which increases the risk of serious infections, mainly those affecting the lungs. When vitamin C is not present in sufficient amounts, it can stop the production of antimicrobial proteins, which makes people more at risk for infections. Likewise, Vitamin C is needed for the formation of collagen and the health of the skin and immune system. If there are nutrient deficiencies, people may notice their immune system does not work as well, it takes them a long time to recover from illnesses, and they are more likely to suffer from chronic diseases. The multifaceted consequences of these deficiencies emphasize the intricate relationship between vitamins, coenzyme functions, and the holistic health of individuals, further advocating for the need for well-rounded dietary sources and fortification strategies (Ibrahim et al., 2018) (Figure 9.14).

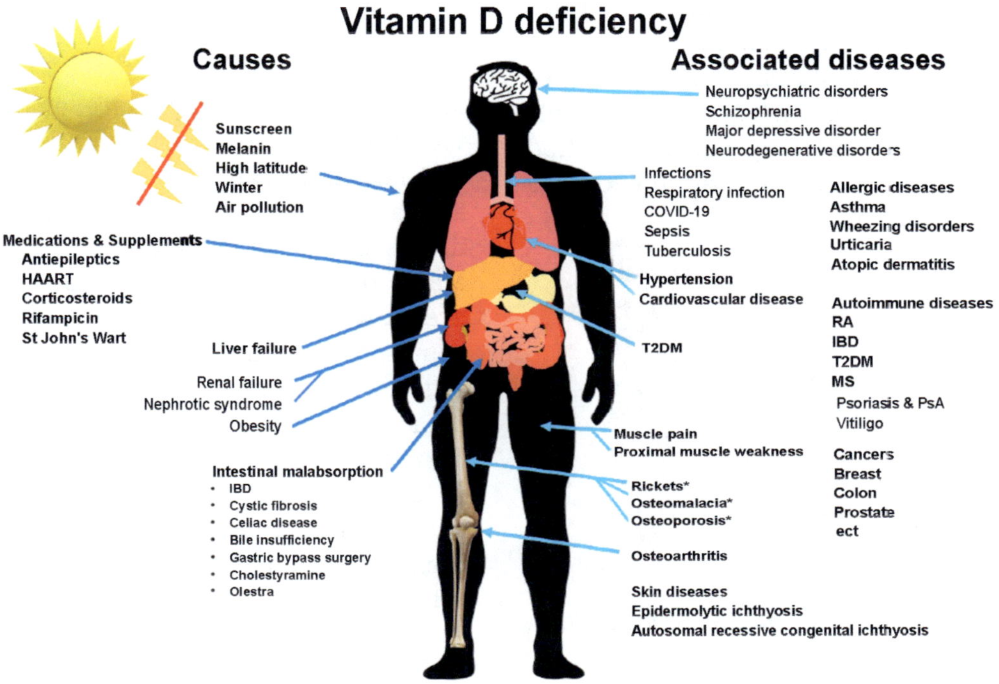

Figure 9.14. Summary of causes of vitamin D deficiency and diseases and disorders associated with vitamin D deficiency.

Source: Charoenngam, N.; Holick, M.F. Immunologic Effects of Vitamin D on Human Health and Disease. *Nutrients* **2020**, *12*, 2097. https://doi.org/10.3390/nu12072097

9.4.2. Symptoms of Vitamin Excess

Most of the time, people focus on vitamin deficiencies instead of the risks of getting too much. At the same time, taking more vitamins than needed can cause some serious problems. If too much of the fat-soluble vitamins A, D, E, and K is taken in, they may build up in the body and become harmful. An example of this is that hypervitaminosis A can bring about nausea, headaches, and blurred vision, while too much vitamin D may lead to hypercalcemia and cause weakness and problems with the kidneys. This points out that it is important to control vitamin intake, especially for people who get most of their vitamins from supplements. Given the popularity of fortified beverages and dietary supplements, becoming aware of potential vitamin excess symptoms is crucial for maintaining optimal health and avoiding adverse effects (Becker et al., 2014). Although water-soluble vitamins are less likely to be toxic right away, taking a lot of them can still cause problems. Taking too much vitamin C may cause diarrhea and stomach cramps, whereas high amounts of vitamin B6 may damage the nerves and result in neuropathy. This calls for paying extra attention to vitamin intake, especially since many people are choosing supplements for their health. The fact that children and adolescents are often the target of strong marketing for fortified products makes the problems of vitamin excess especially important for them. Understanding these risks is essential to ensure a balanced approach to nutrition and prevent potential health issues stemming from overconsumption (Tahir et al., 2024). Besides, the growing use of fortified drinks creates worries about vitamin overdose in people of different ages.

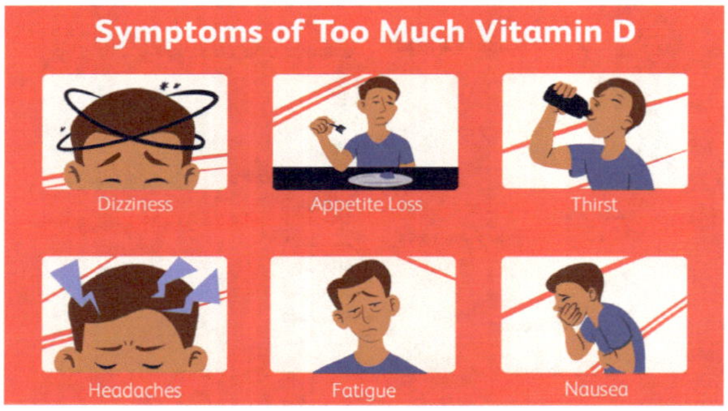

Figure 9.15. Symptoms of too much vitamin D.

Source: https://www.verywellmind.com/thmb/GHYUnOsM8Yc69Xm1wQ-8fN3OgZc=/1500x0/filters:no_upscale():max_bytes(150000):strip_icc()/symptoms-of-too-much-vitamin-d-5105134_final1-eb2f19a74bd54a80950644df25ccb5b2.png.

A lot of these products are promoted for their health effects, but usually not enough attention is given to their vitamin content. It is concerning, since young people might be more easily affected by the risks of high levels of vitamins. It is important to look at the health effects and the risk of vitamins becoming too high when people drink more energy drinks, sports drinks, and similar beverages. Promoting safe consumption and spreading awareness about the dangers of vitamin excess among people should be given priority. This shared responsibility between manufacturers, health professionals, and consumers is essential to navigate the complex landscape of vitamins and coenzymes effectively, ensuring that healthful practices are adhered to without falling victim to the dangers of excess (Becker et al., 2014) (Figure 9.15).

9.4.3. Public Health Implications

More and more, people are discussing how vitamins and coenzymes affect public health and nutrition. Lately, more and more children and adolescents have been drinking fortified drinks that have extra vitamins and minerals. Many of these products show that people are now choosing to get healthier through commercial products instead of natural foods. This development causes concern about the possible health and nutrition effects of such beverages, mainly for people who are already at risk. Because these drinks are aimed at young people, who are easily influenced by advertising, their effects on childhood obesity and health-related problems should be carefully checked. Addressing these implications necessitates a collective effort among public health officials and educators to promote informed choices about nutritional intake and the consumption of fortified beverages (Becker et al., 2014). Additionally, the intersection of vitamin intake with the use of oral contraceptives (OCs) also highlights essential public health considerations. Even though OCs empower women and help them be involved in society, their possible negative effects on nutrition are often ignored by doctors. Researchers believe that women who take OCs may lose important vitamins and minerals, so healthcare providers should be more aware of this risk. Therefore, public health programs should give detailed information on the risks of long-term OC use and advise women to look for nutritional supplements to make up for the missing nutrients. By fostering awareness among both healthcare providers and patients, the health community can better address the nutritional needs of women utilizing these contraceptive methods, ultimately fostering improved health outcomes across the population (Sanchez et al., 2022). Also, public health strategies should focus on encouraging people to eat foods rich in vitamins each day. If people often drink fortified beverages, it would be wise to encourage them to eat whole foods as a better way to get vitamins and coenzymes. Teaching families to focus on fruits, vegetables, and whole grains can make their diets better and help them eat less of processed foods. It deals with current nutritional concerns and also helps people adopt better eating habits for many years. When farmers markets and school programs are included in the community, it becomes easier for people to find and use nutritious foods, which benefits community health. Ultimately, public health frameworks must adopt a holistic perspective on nutrition, ensuring that education and accessibility come together to combat nutritional deficiencies effectively (Becker et al., 2014) (Figure 9.16).

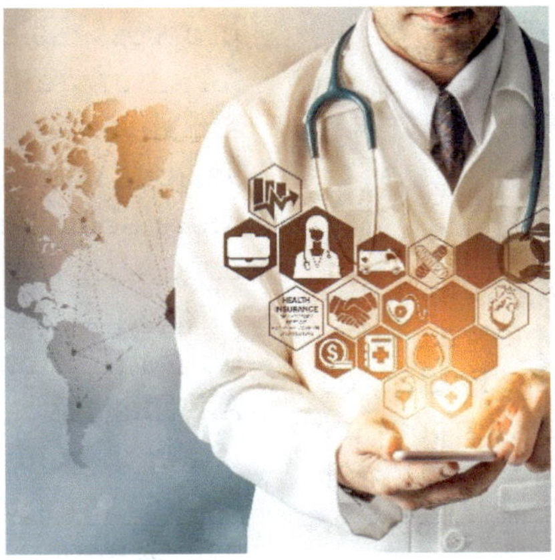

Figure 9.16. Conceptual image of a doctor interacting with digital health technology.

Source: https://www.climateone.org/files/images/media/Pod-Implications%20for%20Public%20Health.jpg.

Test Your Knowledge

1. What is the consequence of vitamin deficiency?
2. What are some of the major implications for public health?

9.5. Research and Advances in Vitamin and Coenzyme Studies

Learning Outcome

1. Describe the recent findings in vitamin research;
2. Know the innovations in coenzyme applications;
3. Understand the future directions in nutritional science.

Over the last few decades, there have been major developments in exploring vitamins and coenzymes. A thorough study has pointed out that vitamins are important and play a major role in our nutrition. As defined by Paulraj et al. (1987), vitamins are organic compounds necessary for various metabolic processes and exist in minor quantities within foodstuffs. Because of this, scientists have carried out many studies to find out which vitamins there are and how they function in the body. Besides, vitamins acting as nutrients, they are also coenzymes in many biochemical reactions, which has encouraged new approaches to studying their effects on both humans and animals. With further research, new ideas keep changing how we understand the way these compounds work with other nutrients and support our bodies. Research on B vitamins is especially revealing since they are important in key metabolic processes. It has been found by recent studies that these water-soluble molecules are coenzymes inside cells, essential for making energy and biomolecules. Significantly, Allen et al. (2017) reveal how certain eukaryotic algae, which cannot synthesize certain B vitamins, rely on environmental availability and intricate acquisition strategies. Because of this, people are now paying more attention to vitamin changes in aquatic environments. How the B vitamins cycle in these areas helps explain the structures of phytoplankton and how the entire ecosystem works. Studies on algae genetics can help explain how vitamins are processed, which may lead to new solutions for problems in biotechnology and environmental care. Besides, when vitamin research meets modern technology, it creates new opportunities in the field of nutrition. With the help of high-throughput screening and metabolomics, scientists can now study vitamin precursors and metabolites with great accuracy. As a result of this technological progress, scientists have discovered different forms of vitamins and found out how well they are absorbed by the body, revealing the details of various metabolic processes. As scientists learn more about vitamins' wide range of functions, especially in organisms that were once thought to need them from outside sources, our view of both nutrition and biology is greatly affected. All this research improves our knowledge of vitamins and coenzymes and leads us to ask important questions about their effects on health and disease, so more studies are needed in this field of biochemistry.

9.5.1. Recent Findings in Vitamin Research

New studies have revealed how vitamins are linked to human health, especially when there is a lack of them. A thorough study applied computational tools to explain vitamin deficiency diseases and identified 41,584 links between different vitamins and the related illnesses reported in the literature. Using this method, big data helps to analyze a large amount of information and find out the impact of certain vitamins on preventing diseases. The new knowledge points out that increasing vitamin intake through public health efforts can greatly reduce the risk of diseases caused by deficiency. This proves that vitamins are essential for health, not only as dietary supplements, but also as important parts of any health-related research. Besides, the study has examined the nutritional information of plant-based foods by using the United States Department of Agriculture Standard Reference database. The findings show that the amount of vitamins in these foods varies a lot. Vitamin B12 and Vitamin D are not as common in foods, and this is a problem for people who eat only plant-based meals. Therefore, it is necessary to talk about fortification and supplementation to ensure that people who are at risk get enough vitamins. Such results prompt nutritionists and public health policymakers to find ways to promote various foods and also deal with the shortcomings in certain diets. Because of these findings, dietary advice and health policies everywhere have been strongly affected. The link between vitamin shortages and certain health problems shows that we need to organize nutrition education and food availability better. When we know which foods contain important vitamins, we can try to help vulnerable people eat more healthily. In addition, this research forms a key base for further studies that look into the metabolic functions of vitamins as coenzymes in biochemical reactions. With the connection between vitamins and health becoming more obvious, it encourages researchers to explore how to improve nutrition for each individual. The call for integrated approaches to dietary health further cements the relevance of vitamins in contemporary nutritional science and public health discourse (Johnson et al., 2000; Sarkar et al., 2015) (Figure 9.17).

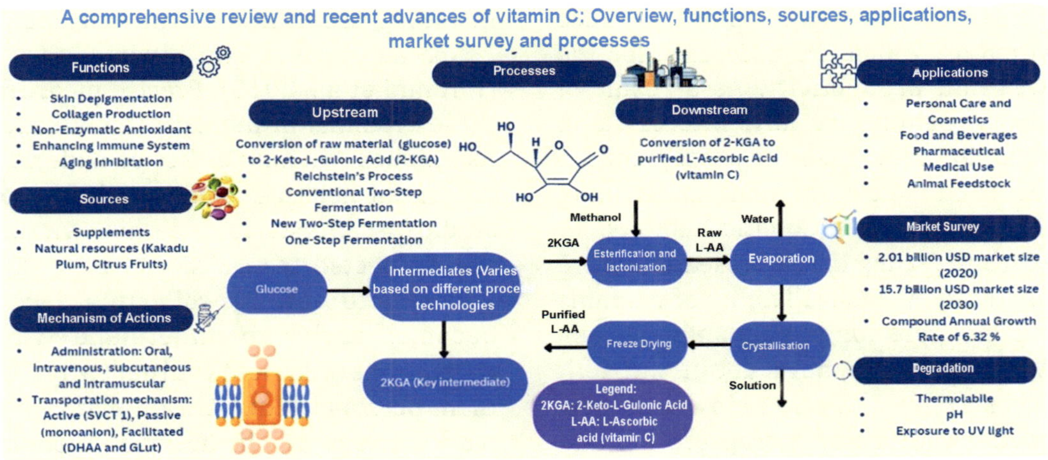

Figure 9.17. A comprehensive review and recent advances of vitamin C: Overview, functions, sources, applications, market survey, and processes.

Source: https://ars.els-cdn.com/content/image/1-s2.0-S026387622400251X-ga1_lrg.jpg.

9.5.2. Innovations in Coenzyme Applications

Biotechnology progress has made it possible to use coenzymes in new ways, mainly in metabolic engineering. Thanks to coenzymes, researchers are now able to improve the way metabolism happens to produce more valuable compounds. For example, genetically engineering microorganisms to make more B vitamins, especially their coenzyme forms, has attracted a lot of interest in industrial biotechnology. This method helps produce more bioactive substances and also supports sustainable ways of production that reduce the environmental problems linked to old methods. This shows that coenzymes are important not only for biochemical reactions but also for creating sustainable bioproduction systems that fit today's sustainability goals. Also, better knowledge of coenzymes in the body has led to new efforts in developing new treatments. Since coenzymes , such as coenzyme A are important for many metabolic activities, they have been studied for use in drug development and regenerative medicine. Scientists are coming up with new treatments for metabolic disorders and diseases by studying the roles of coenzymes in certain pathways. Studies done recently have proven that some coenzyme forms can greatly improve health, showing they are more important than just vitamins. As time goes on, this research may help doctors provide personalized medicine by using coenzyme profiles to guide effective treatments for health and disease prevention. Besides, new uses of coenzymes are being found in agriculture, as their role in plant metabolism is now being noticed. Many research studies have shown that eukaryotic algae cannot produce some B vitamins, which are necessary for the best growth and productivity. As a result of this discovery, people are now interested in altering vitamin metabolism in phytoplankton with genetics and the environment, underlining the role of coenzymes in aquatic habitats. To boost the carbon cycling in seas, researchers are trying to increase the bioavailability of vitamins and their precursors for phytoplankton. They contribute to learning more about nutrient cycles in ecosystems and also help create new farming methods that boost crop growth and toughness, helping to solve global food security issues.

9.5.3. Future Directions in Nutritional Science

With the progress of nutritional science, more attention will be given to the connections between vitamins, coenzymes, and health. It is important to know how these nutrients work in the body to create useful dietary advice and special interventions. For instance, research has shown that vitamins are important in many metabolic functions, so it is necessary to study how a lack of them can cause chronic illnesses. Recent studies have utilized computational approaches to identify associations between vitamin deficiency diseases and vitamin-rich plant foods, establishing a knowledge base for enhancing nutritional recommendations through food sources (Sarkar et al., 2015). Through this approach, nutritional biochemistry and public health are connected, which makes it easier to develop solutions for vitamin deficiencies that match each population's needs and eating habits. Future advancements in nutritional science will also leverage emerging technologies, , such as high-performance liquid chromatography coupled with mass spectrometry (HPLC/LC-MS/MS), to profile vitamin levels in diverse populations accurately. The importance of water-soluble vitamins, including B3, B6, and B9, has been established in various health contexts, including associations with chronic ailments, , such as diabetes and inflammatory diseases (Ibrahim et al., 2018). Precise measurement of these vitamins in human plasma using certain techniques will help us better understand their effects on health and illness. With population studies, scientists can see how vitamin levels are connected to health and suggest the best amounts to eat. By collecting such data, it becomes easier to understand why people metabolize nutrients differently and offer them personalized nutrition plans. In addition, working together in nutrition, genomics, and public health will be necessary to turn scientific results into useful dietary plans. With the shift to a more holistic approach, researchers will pay attention to the disease-preventing as well as the therapeutic roles of vitamins and coenzymes. Research on the role of genes and epigenetics in nutrient processing will give us a better understanding of how people react to what they eat. Moreover, investigating vitamin-rich foods, mainly from plants, can result in a healthier and more sustainable way of eating. Learning about the interaction of micronutrients in various diets will improve the ability of nutritional science to solve global health problems and help people live longer and healthier lives (Figure 9.18).

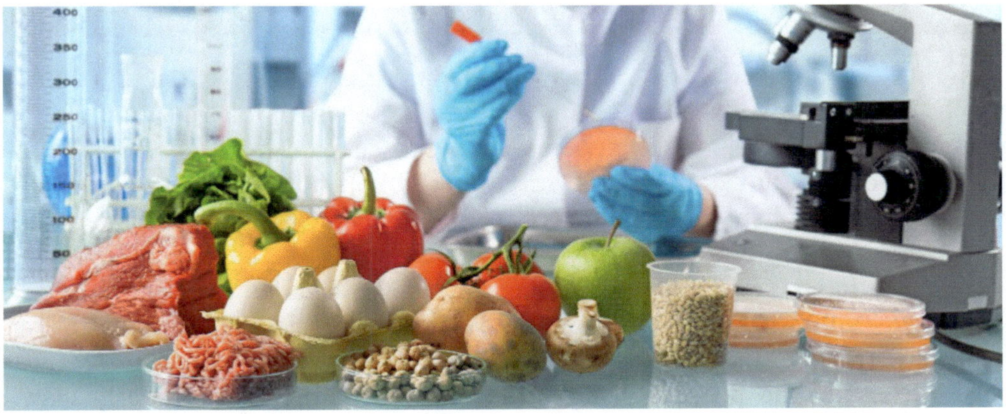

Figure 9.18. A food scientist conducting laboratory testing on various food samples.

Source: https://thinkmagazine.mt/wp-content/uploads/2023/07/food-science-banner.jpg.

Test Your Knowledge

1. Describe the innovations in coenzyme application.
2. What is the future of nutrition science?

SUMMARY

When summing up the connection between vitamins and coenzymes, it is important to point out their basic roles in keeping cells healthy and maintaining overall health. Vitamins are necessary for the body because they take part in biochemical processes and help create coenzymes that aid enzymes. If someone does not get enough vitamins, the body cannot produce these coenzymes, which leads to poor metabolism and a higher chance of deficiency-related diseases. This highlights why it is important to eat a diet rich in different vitamins, since they help each other and play a key role in maintaining the body's metabolism and cells. Besides affecting how adequate our nutrition is, the way vitamins and coenzymes interact also affects cellular growth, reproduction, and the length of life. For example, *Saccharomyces cerevisiae* and *Schizosaccharomyces pombe* are used as models to study the process of aging and how cells die in an orderly way. How these biochemical partners interact gives insight into the mechanisms that control cell development and longevity, which are becoming more important in biological research. Therefore, vitamins and coenzymes play a major role in explaining the details of how cells function and stay healthy. To conclude, it is important to know about vitamins and coenzymes to support good health and avoid deficiency problems. When these nutrients are balanced well, it helps the body's metabolism work properly and also supports important cell processes like growth and repair. With more research, it is becoming obvious that vitamins and coenzymes influence many aspects of cellular activity, including aging. Therefore, future studies should continue to explore these relationships, providing deeper insights that could inform dietary guidelines and therapeutic strategies aimed at enhancing health and longevity, enriching our understanding of the mineral-rich tapestry of life (Boswell et al., 2017; Chen et al., 2017).

Vitamins and coenzymes work together in a keyway in the biochemistry of living beings. Since the body cannot produce enough vitamins, we have to get them from our diet. They mainly take part in metabolism by serving as precursors or catalysts for coenzymes. Coenzymes are not proteins, but they are needed by enzymes to be active and to affect biochemical reactions. Without vitamins, many enzymes would not work, which would cause different problems in the body. This highlights the importance of adequate vitamin intake in maintaining metabolic health and homeostasis, reiterating how the interplay between vitamins and coenzymes facilitates energy production and nutrient utilization in the body, as exemplified in comprehensive studies of animal nutrition that emphasize the biochemical pathways reliant on these micronutrients, including the summaries provided in "A Guide to Principles of Animal Nutrition" (Cherian, 2020). Vitamins are important in both metabolism and in regulating and sending signals in cells. Water-soluble vitamins, for example, the B-complex group and vitamin C, support cell activities by helping form important coenzymes used to produce biomolecules. For example, thiamine (B1) is integral to the conversion of carbohydrates into glucose, while vitamin C plays a crucial role in the synthesis of collagen, an essential protein in connective tissues. Alternatively, fat-soluble vitamins A, D, E, and K help with vision, protect bones, act as antioxidants, and blood clotting. Therefore, understanding the multifaceted roles of various vitamins in supporting coenzyme function is essential for professional fields concerned with nutrition and health, particularly as disparities in micronutrient availability can lead to deficiencies impacting overall well-being (Berger et al., 2021). In addition, deficiencies in vitamins and coenzymes can affect the health of the general public as well as individuals. Emerging research has established a clear connection between micronutrient deficiencies and conditions , such as acute kidney injury, especially regarding the lack of guidance for supplemental nutrition during renal replacement therapies (Berger et al., 2021). It shows that we should keep looking into the effects of losing micronutrients and keep checking the blood of vulnerable people for important vitamins and trace elements. It is important to use detailed strategies to deal with these issues to avoid complications and ensure better nutrition. With new information on how vitamins and coenzymes are important in the body, we can better focus on using this knowledge to improve the nutritional health of whole populations.

KEY TERMS FROM THIS CHAPTER

- Apoptosis
- Biosynthesis
- Coenzymes
- Flavin adenine dinucleotide
- Niacin
- Saccharomyces cerevisiae
- Vitamin deficiency
- Water-soluble vitamins
- B-complex vitamins
- Biotin
- Fat-soluble vitamins
- Krebs cycle
- Riboflavin
- Schizosaccharomyces pombe
- Vitamins

CRITICAL THINKING QUESTIONS

1. **Which of the following is a fat-soluble vitamin?**
   a. Vitamin B12
   b. Vitamin C
   c. Vitamin D
   d. Vitamin B6
2. **Vitamin B1 is also known as:**
   a. Riboflavin
   b. Thiamine
   c. Niacin
   d. Pyridoxine
3. **Which vitamin acts as a coenzyme in carboxylation reactions?**
   a. Vitamin K
   b. Biotin
   c. Riboflavin
   d. Vitamin C
4. **Which vitamin is essential for the synthesis of collagen?**
   a. Vitamin A
   b. Vitamin D
   c. Vitamin C
   d. Vitamin E
5. **Which coenzyme is derived from niacin (Vitamin B3)?**
   a. FAD (Flavin adenine dinucleotide)
   b. NAD+ (Nicotinamide adenine dinucleotide)
   c. TPP (Thiamine pyrophosphate)
   d. Coenzyme A

Answers to Critical Thinking Questions

1. (c); 2. (b); 3. (b); 4. (c); 5. (b)

Short Answer Questions

1. Define the vitamin.
2. What is the concept of a coenzyme?
3. List the types of vitamins.
4. What is the function of coenzymes?
5. What are the main sources of vitamins?

REFERENCES

1. Tahir, N. T., Alkubaisi, M. R., Elias, N. G., & Al-Auqbi, T. F. R. (2024). Reflection of Vitamins and Mineral Deficiency in General Health Condition: Article Review. *Journal for Research in Applied Sciences and Biotechnology*, *2*(6), 184–193. https://doi.org/10.55544/jrasb.2.6.27 (accessed on 11th June 2025).
2. Becker, C., Crawford, P. B., & Pirotin, S. (2014). Looking beyond the marketing claims of new beverages: Health risks of consuming sports drinks, energy drinks, fortified waters, and other flavored beverages. https://core.ac.uk/download/75778515.pdf (accessed on 11th June 2025).
3. Berger, M. M., Broman, M., De Waele, E., Forni, et al. (2021). Nutrients and micronutrients at risk during renal replacement therapy: A scoping review. https://core.ac.uk/download/479273744.pdf (accessed on 11th June 2025).
4. Chen, L., Jiang, X., Liu, Y., et al. (2017). Effects and mechanisms of a new multivitamin on chronic metabolic syndromes and aging. https://core.ac.uk/download/478371166.pdf (accessed on 11th June 2025).
5. Cherian, G. (2020). *A Guide to The Principles of Animal Nutrition*. https://core.ac.uk/download/622361034.pdf (accessed on 11th June 2025).
6. Colinas, M., & Fitzpatrick, T. B. (2022). Coenzymes and the primary and specialized metabolism interface. *Current opinion in plant biology*, *66*, 102170. https://doi.org/10.1016/j.pbi.2021.102170(accessed on 11th June 2025).
7. Cooper, S. C. (2025). Effects of vitamin and mineral nutriture on systemic and visual function: A review. https://core.ac.uk/download/pdf/212798978.pdf (accessed on 11th June 2025).
8. Fuso, A., & Martire, S. (2015). Nutrition-based modulation of poly-ADP-ribosylation and its possible role in Alzheimer's disease. https://core.ac.uk/download/54516110.pdf (accessed on 11th June 2025).
9. Goldford, J. E., Hartman, H., Smith, T. F., & Segrè, D. (2017). Remnants of an Ancient Metabolism without Phosphate. *Cell*, *168*(6), 1126–1134.e9. https://doi.org/10.1016/j.cell.2017.02.001(accessed on 11th June 2025).
10. Helliwell, K. E. (2017). The roles of B vitamins in phytoplankton nutrition: New perspectives and prospects. *New Phytologist*, *216*(1). https://doi.org/10.1111/nph.14669 (accessed on 11th June 2025).
11. Hughes, C. F., McAuley, E., McNulty, H., et al. (2016). Riboflavin status, MTHFR genotype and blood pressure: Current evidence and implications for personalized nutrition. https://core.ac.uk/download/287020908.pdf (accessed on 11th June 2025).
12. Johnson, C. (2000). The nutritional impact of fortified ready-to-eat cereals on the diets of school age children. https://core.ac.uk/download/5065640.pdf (accessed on 11th June 2025).
13. Kola, A., Nencioni, F., & Valensin, D. (2023). Bioinorganic chemistry of micronutrients related to Alzheimer's and Parkinson's diseases. https://core.ac.uk/download/576879437.pdf (accessed on 11th June 2025).
14. Ankita A. Mojad et al / International Journal of Advances in Pharmaceutics 2018; 07(02): 05-09. (accessed on 11th June 2025).

15. Kun, Á., Papp, B., & Szathmáry, E. (2008). Computational identification of obligatorily autocatalytic replicators embedded in metabolic networks. https://core.ac.uk/download/pdf/8064287.pdf (accessed on 11th June 2025).

16. Paulraj, R. (1987). Vitamin requirements of finfish and prawns. https://core.ac.uk/download/33015162.pdf (accessed on 11th June 2025).

17. Sanchez, L. Z. (2022). Navigating potential nutrient depletions in college women taking birth control pills and creation of a booklet guide "Eat for your hormones." https://core.ac.uk/download/552768049.pdf (accessed on 11th June 2025).

18. Sarkar, I. N., & Yu, C. (2015). A computational approach for identifying plant-based foods for addressing vitamin deficiency diseases. https://core.ac.uk/download/215152787.pdf (accessed on 11th June 2025).

19. Shafiek Ibrahim, G. R. M. (2018). LC-MS/MS based analysis of vitamins B3 and B6 in healthy and obese Emirati population. https://core.ac.uk/download/402107210.pdf (accessed on 11th June 2025).

20. Tavares, N. A. R. (2009). Riboflavin status and effects of supplementation on biomarkers of cardiovascular disease in the elderly. https://core.ac.uk/download/143378212.pdf (accessed on 11th June 2025).

21. Walker, G. M., & White, N. A. (2017). Introduction to fungal physiology. In *The Mycota: A Comprehensive Treatise on Fungi as Experimental Systems for Basic and Applied Research*. https://onlinelibrary.wiley.com/doi/pdf/10.1002/9781119374312.ch1 (accessed on 11th June 2025).

22. Williams, P. G. (2015). The missing vitamin alphabet. https://core.ac.uk/download/37029464.pdf (accessed on 11th June 2025).

HORMONES AND SIGNAL TRANSDUCTION

10

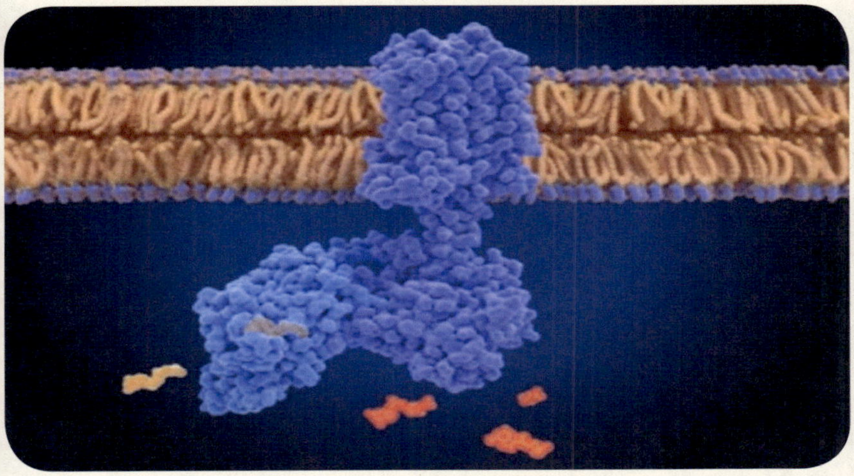

LEARNING OBJECTIVES

After studying this chapter, you will be able to:

1. Describe the types of hormones;
2. Know the mechanisms of hormone action;
3. Understand the signal transduction pathways;
4. Understand the hormonal regulation of metabolism;
5. Describe the hormones and homeostasis;
6. Learn about disorders related to hormonal imbalance.

Introduction

Hormones and signal transduction are necessary parts of biology that control many functions in animals and plants. Since hormones act as messengers, they make it possible for cells to connect over different distances, which is vital for organizing activities needed for survival, growth, and reproduction. Among mammals, estradiol and progesterone are important hormones that control the cycles of reproduction and development. The many connections between hormones and metabolism reveal that these systems are very complex and require further study of how hormones are sent and understood by cells. Thanks to recent progress in genomics and molecular biology, researchers are able to study these signaling pathways and learn about their control and possible effects on health and disease management in different settings. The role of hormone signaling is most noticeable when we look at certain case studies involving various species. In dairy cattle, hormones play a key role in regulating estrous behavior and, as a result, the animals' reproductive performance. According to what is found in the literature, having less estrous behavior in cows leads to increased milk yield, proving the link between hormones and animal farming. Key hormones , such as estradiol (E2), along with various regulatory genes, orchestrate the behavioral and physiological changes during the estrous cycle. However, the complexities involved in these hormonal interactions remain somewhat enigmatic, as a comprehensive understanding of signaling pathways and their influence on reproductive traits is still evolving, calling for continued research in this vital area of animal biology (Boer et al., 2010). Hormone signaling is also important in helping plants deal with changes in their environment. Like mammals, plants have advanced ways of sensing and responding to things happening around them. The mechanism of protein phosphorylation/dephosphorylation stands out as a central process in signal transduction, allowing plants to relay messages across membranes into their cellular nuclei to instigate appropriate developmental responses (Manuela, 2011). The research on receptor-like kinases in plants shows that they are similar to mammalian systems, as different receptors help control the balance of hormones. With the development of knowledge about these networks, joining insights from plant and animal research will explain how hormones manage living processes, and this will benefit both farming and medicine (Figure 10.1).

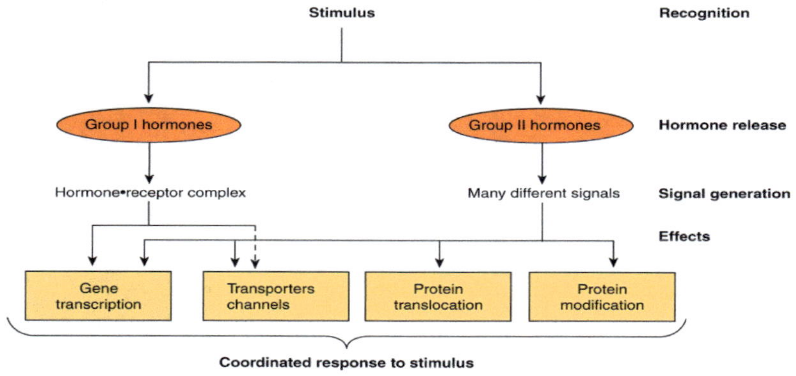

Figure 10.1. Hormonal involvement in responses to a stimulus. A challenge to the integrity of the organism elicits a response that includes the release of one or more hormones. These hormones generate signals at or within target cells, and these signals regulate a variety of biological processes that provide for a coordinated response to the stimulus or challenge.

Source: https://basicmedicalkey.com/wp-content/uploads/2017/02/image02222.gif.

Definition of Hormones

Hormones are chemicals that help the body communicate and control various bodily activities. Hormones are mainly defined as substances made by endocrine glands, which are released directly into the blood to travel and affect cells in other parts of the body. Chemical signals in the body are necessary for keeping the body stable, controlling metabolism, supporting growth, reproduction, and dealing with stress. Hormones are organized into steroid, peptide, and amine groups, and every type of hormone binds to its receptor differently. Such interactions are important for signal transduction, which changes hormonal signals into cellular actions, proving how hormones can affect many biological activities and health. Hormones are known to be complex, and they activate different pathways when they reach the target cells. After a hormone binds to its receptor, it can start a series of events inside the cell through signal transduction. These pathways often involve second messengers, , such as cyclic AMP (cAMP) or inositol triphosphate (IP3), which amplify the hormonal signal, leading to diverse cellular outcomes. For instance, corticotropin-releasing hormone (CRH) illustrates this dynamic interplay, as it plays a critical role in the stress response within the hypothalamic-pituitary-adrenal axis. Studies indicate that the signaling mechanisms of CRH not only activate stress-related responses but also influence behaviors through neuromodulatory pathways, thus underscoring the multifaceted impact that hormones exert on both physiological and psychological processes (Armando et al., 2017).

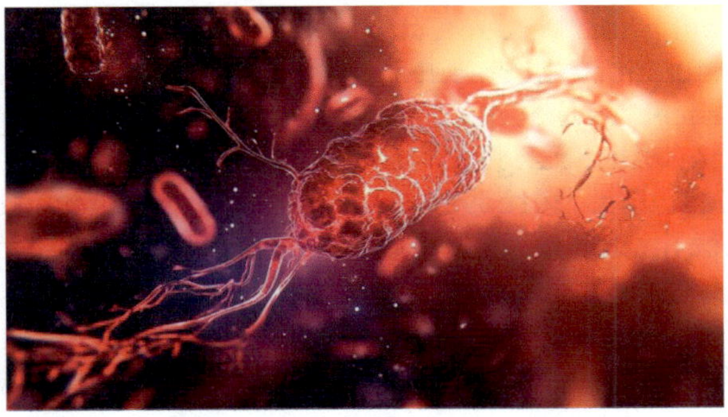

Figure 10.2. Hormones.

Source: https://www.yourhormones.info/media/gpviecwm/hormones4.jpg.

Additionally, hormones are important because they work together with different signaling pathways to show how the body's systems are connected. For growth, the immune system, and reproduction to work properly, hormonal regulation is necessary. For example, hormones play a role in guiding the biochemical changes that change the taste, texture, and general quality of ripening fruit. This process illustrates a broader perspective on hormonal action, revealing how hormones drive developmental programs through gene expression and regulatory mechanisms (Bouzayen et al., 2010). Such knowledge of hormones helps explain how hormones play a key role in important changes in both individuals and the environment. Therefore, studying hormones and the pathways they use to send signals improves our understanding of how the body works and how it gets affected by diseases (Figure 10.2).

Overview of Signal Transduction

Signal transduction helps cells react correctly to things happening outside the body. First, signaling molecules called hormones attach to particular receptors found on the cell surface. Such interactions start a series of events inside the cell that strengthen the signal and cause the cell to alter gene expression, metabolism, or grow. Signal transduction is not simple because it includes several routes and loops that help keep an organism's stability. In hormone signaling, transduction pathways closely interact with regulating various physiological processes, which highlights their role in keeping the body healthy and working well. Therefore, any disturbance or poor regulation of these pathways may bring about serious health problems, for example, metabolic disorders and challenges with reproduction. Hormones in mammals play a key role in connecting the endocrine system with the way genes are expressed. For example, estrogen is a main hormone that controls many body functions by working on its target cells. It has been found that estrogens affect both genes and the brain's connections, which in turn control the estrous behavior of dairy cows. Studies indicate that estradiol (E2) acts as a key regulator by modulating gene expression, particularly in the hypothalamus, impacting physiological processes related to fertility and overall reproductive health in these animals (Boer et al., 2010). With this knowledge, scientists are able to study how different hormone pathways interact and influence the activities of cells in many parts of the body. In addition to traditional hormonal influences, recent advancements in molecular biology have highlighted the role of small RNAs (sRNAs) in signal transduction, especially in plant systems. sRNAs, including microRNAs and small interfering RNAs, actively participate in gene regulation through mechanisms that often intersect with hormonal pathways. For instance, specific sRNAs have been shown to mediate responses to stress by interacting with phytohormones, thereby influencing plant growth and development (Li et al., 2020). From these findings, it appears that hormonal signaling and small RNA pathways work together, adding more detail to how organisms react to changes in their environment. Exploring the ways hormones work in plants increases our knowledge of signal transduction and also helps in developing better stress responses and crop yields through biotechnology.

10.1. Types of Hormones

Learning Outcome

1. Understand the peptide hormones;
2. Define the steroid hormones;
3. Describe the amine hormones.

Hormones take part in many important bodily functions, and they can be sorted by their chemical structure and ability to dissolve in water. Out of the main types, peptide hormones are made up of amino acids linked together, for example insulin and glucagon. These hormones can dissolve in water and thus travel through the bloodstream and connect to the receptors on target cells. This interaction sets off signal transduction processes that usually cause cells to respond fast. Because peptide hormones can change quickly, they are important for regulating metabolic activities and glucose metabolism. They demonstrate the important role that hormones play in cellular communication, which controls the body's functions. Unlike peptide hormones, steroid hormones, which are made from cholesterol, can easily go through cell membranes because they are fat-soluble. Once inside the target cells, steroid hormones attach to receptors inside the cell and change gene activity by interacting with the DNA. By this mechanism, protein production is affected, leading to results that last longer than those caused by peptide hormones. As an illustration, cortisol and the sex hormones testosterone and estrogen help control metabolism, support reproduction, and play a part in handling stress. Being able to contact the cell's transcriptional machinery, hormones are important for many processes that need continuous action, showing the wide range of their roles in biological signaling. Moreover, the roles of hormones are not limited to their classical functions; they also display unique non-genomic effects, particularly exemplified by dihydrotestosterone (DHT). Studies have pointed out that DHT acts quickly on skeletal muscle by helping amino acids enter the cells through particular signaling pathways that do not alter the genes. The fact that DHT can stimulate cellular responses through epidermal growth factor receptor (EGFR) activation and the subsequent involvement of the MAPK pathway showcases a layer of complexity within hormonal signaling. This proves that hormones can act quickly and strongly without interacting with DNA, so we now understand their role in muscle physiology and growth better. This multifaceted nature of hormonal action is critical to advancing our knowledge of signal transduction and its implications for health and disease (Bouzayen et al., 2010) (Figure 10.3).

Hormone Class	Components	Example(s)
Amine Hormone	Amino acids with modified groups (e.g. norepinephrine's carboxyl group is replaced with a benzene ring)	Norepinephrine 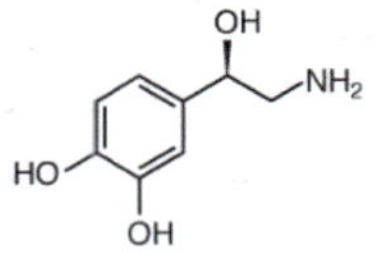
Peptide Hormone	Short chains of linked amino acids	Oxytocin 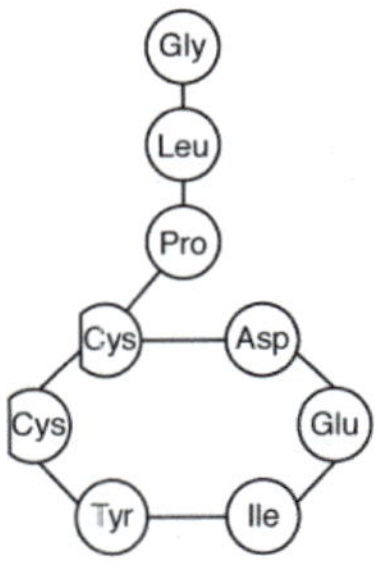
Protein Hormone	Long chains of linked amino acids	Human Growth Hormone 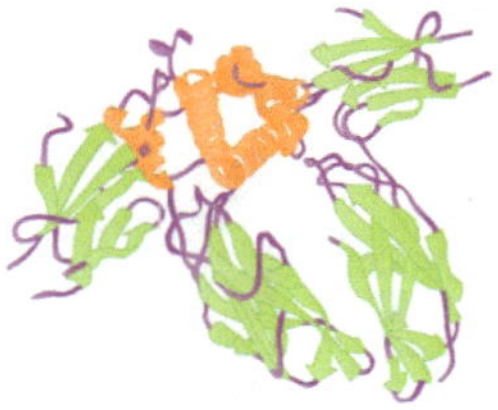
Steroid Hormones	Derived from the lipid cholesterol	Testosterone 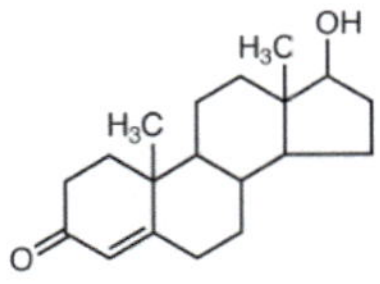 Progesterone 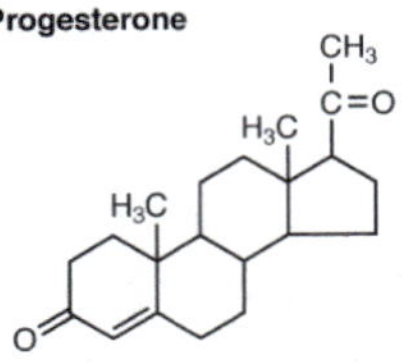

Figure 10.3. Amine, peptide, protein, and steroid hormone structure.

Source: https://s3-us-west-2.amazonaws.com/courses-images/wp-content/uploads/sites/3047/2018/03/26184130/1802_Examples_of_Amine_Peptide_Protein_and_Steroid_Hormone_Structure.jpg.

10.1.1. Peptide Hormones

Peptide hormones are important signaling molecules in the endocrine system because they are made from amino acids. Since they are soluble in water, these hormones usually bind to certain receptors on the membrane of target cells and trigger a series of reactions within the cells. Peptide hormones are different from steroid hormones because the latter can diffuse into cells since they are lipid soluble. Peptide hormones usually cause a quick release of second messengers , such as cAMP or inositol trisphosphate (IP3), which results in quick changes in the body. These detailed pathways point out that peptide hormones play a key role in regulating metabolism, growth, and reproductive functions, which helps keep the body's systems balanced and allows them to talk to each other. In the kidney, peptide hormones have a major influence through detailed signaling processes that respond to both outside and inside factors. A salient example is the interaction of atrial natriuretic peptide (ANP) and the renin-angiotensin system, which demonstrates the complexity of these hormonal networks. ANP encourages natriuresis, which helps regulate the amount of sodium in the blood and the body's water level. When sodium levels in the body shift, the kidneys react with the help of peptide hormones to maintain fluid balance. Research indicates that the balance between natriuretic and antinatriuretic factors is essential for maintaining renal health, and disruptions in this balance are often linked to pathological conditions , such as hypertension and nephrotic syndrome, highlighting the profound implications of peptide hormones in human health (Choi et al., 2014).

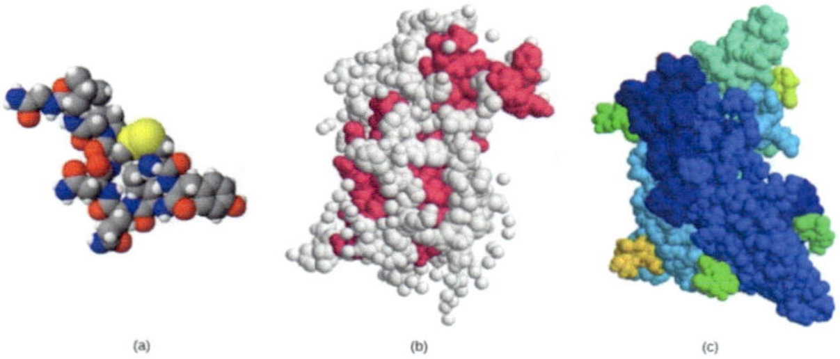

Figure 10.4. The structures of peptide hormones – (a) oxytocin; (b) growth hormone; and (c) follicle-stimulating hormone are shown. These peptide hormones are much larger than those derived from cholesterol or amino acids.

Source: https://s3-us-west-2.amazonaws.com/courses-images/wp-content/uploads/sites/1223/2017/02/07225200/Figure_37_01_03abc-1024x434.jpg.

Further emphasizing the biological significance of peptide hormones, follicle-stimulating hormone (FSH) exemplifies their role in reproductive physiology. Made by the anterior pituitary gland, FSH helps with the development of gametes and follicles in both men and women. FSH connects with certain receptors that start signal pathways, leading to effects , such as sperm production in males and ovarian follicle growth in females. Still, there are difficulties in measuring FSH since the traditional radioimmunoassay does not accurately reflect what the hormone can do in the body. The use of cell lines expressing human FSH receptors to check bioactivity is a major development in learning about the detailed actions of peptide hormones like FSH. This evolving research underlines the complexity and critical functions of peptide hormones, which are vital for various hormonal interactions and maintaining overall health (Young et al., 2000) (Figure 10.4).

10.1.2. Steroid Hormones

Steroid hormones are important in endocrinology since they greatly affect growth, metabolism, and reproductive functions. Made from cholesterol, these hormones are able to go through cell membranes and interact with receptors inside the cells. As a result of this interaction, complicated pathways are set in motion that change gene activity and cell behavior. It is well known that testosterone and estrogen, types of steroid hormones, have a big impact on the health of the cardiovascular system. For instance, testosterones can induce relaxation in coronary arteries, which is critical for maintaining adequate blood flow, highlighting the intricate relationship between steroid hormones and cardiovascular physiology (Madanu et al., 2012). This shows that it is important to know about steroid hormones in detail since they influence more than just reproductive health. Their effects can be seen in reproductive organs, but they also play a major role in brain and mental functions. Pregnenolone sulfate (PregS), a precursor to steroid hormones, exemplifies this multifaceted role by modulating synaptic activity in the brain. Produced in neurons, PregS is critically involved in developmental stages, with its levels peaking during key periods , such as infancy and adolescence (Webster, 2019). PregS's ability to modulate neurotransmitters by binding to receptors in the brain shows that steroid hormones have a complex effect on the nervous system. PregS helps boost signaling in synapses by working with receptors like TrpM3, which in turn helps produce calcium transients required for changes in the brain and memory formation. It appears that steroid hormones are important in controlling both physical and mental development. Also, steroid hormones are important because they have many functions in both healthy and unhealthy conditions. A problem with steroid hormone levels can cause several health problems. For example, reduced PregS production has been associated with neurodegenerative disorders, highlighting the hormones' protective role in neural integrity (Webster, 2019).

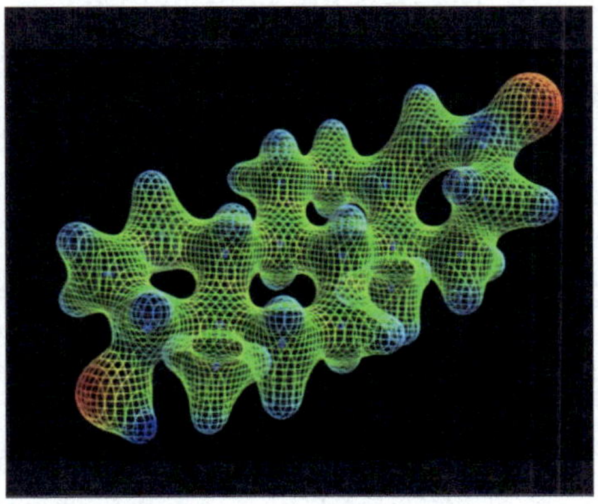

Figure 10.5. 3D mesh model of the testosterone molecule.

Source: https://www.thoughtco.com/thmb/RE1dLsjavYqikO3Fs9FtYkY8tGY=/750x0/filters:no_upscale():max_bytes(150000):strip_icc():format(webp)/testosterone_molecule-5c365dd6c9e77c00018ab0ef.jpg.

The fact that coronary arteries react differently to testosterone points out how complicated steroid hormone signaling is, especially with regard to CVD risk factors. The pathways that steroid hormones turn on in the body show how they help with immediate and long-term responses. Knowing about these interactions is very important to design treatments that address steroid hormone signaling in diseases, proving their significance in clinical settings and human health (Figure 10.5).

10.1.3. Amine Hormones

Amine hormones, for instance, catecholamines and thyroid hormones (THs), are very important for controlling many processes in the body. Being amines made from single amino acids, these hormones activate certain reactions in target cells by using signal transduction pathways. Catecholamines , such as adrenaline help the body get ready for action by increasing the heart rate and energy supply. Amine hormones usually bind to membrane receptors, start a sequence of events within cells, and use secondary messengers to make the response to the hormone stronger and faster. The way amine hormones work shows how important they are for keeping the body stable and able to adjust to outside changes. Amine hormones are synthesized and work based on both outside and inside factors. For example, THs are produced in a way that is controlled by the body's energy and growth needs, and feedback systems keep the levels at the right amounts. Gaspar et al. (2003) emphasize the idea that the physiological activity of hormones cannot be viewed in isolation; rather, it involves a complex interplay of concentrations, sensitivities, and systemic interactions. Amine hormones are able to affect the activity of certain genes and the production of other hormones, showing that they coordinate different metabolic signals. Amine hormones help in maintaining balance in the body by triggering important changes in response to the different influences in the environment. Amine hormones have effects that go beyond the basic actions of the body. The fact that they take part in stress adaptation and growth regulation makes them important in hormonal communication. For example, amine hormones in plants regulate copper levels to show how they can respond to the availability of elements. Andrés et al. (2015) discusses how hormonal pathways interact with circadian rhythms to optimize nutrient acquisition, showcasing the temporal and spatial dimensions of hormonal action. This interaction shows that amine hormones are needed for both the regulation and the coordination of growth and adaptability. Because hormones take part in many different signaling pathways, the regulation of these chemicals is both complex and very important for the body.

Test Your Knowledge

1. What are peptide hormones?
2. What are amine hormones?

10.2. Mechanisms of Hormone Action

Learning Outcome

1. Describe the process of receptor binding;
2. Know the intracellular signaling pathways;
3. Understand the gene expression modulation.

The way hormones work in the body is mainly controlled by signal transduction, which is vital for triggering reactions to hormones. Hormones attach to certain receptors on cells and start a sequence of reactions that turn the signal into a useful response. As an illustration, estradiol and other steroid hormones enter cells using the membrane and then bind to receptors inside, influencing the expression of genes. As a result of this binding, the transcription of certain genes is changed, which brings about changes in the body. It is also seen in reproductive biology, as the actions of hormones and their receptors oversee activities , such as estrous behavior in dairy cows. As noted in recent literature, understanding the gene expression changes underlying these processes can aid in linking hormonal signaling to behavioral outcomes, highlighting the breadth of hormone action in modulating physiological and behavioral responses in animals (Boer et al., 2010). Changes in hormones also play a key role in biochemical and physiological changes that happen during different life processes, for example, fruit ripening. This process shows how hormones help control the development of different parts of the body by influencing genes. The hormone ethylene is responsible for a series of changes in the fruit's color, texture, and flavor, caused by certain genes. The proteins made by these genes direct the changes in the plant, which lead to better fruit and also indicate the start of cell death. This illustrates how hormonal mechanisms are not only pivotal in regulating growth and development but also play vital roles in programmed physiological processes (Bouzayen et al., 2010). The accurate regulation of these hormonal pathways proves the link between hormone signaling and the main control of biological systems. In addition, the process of understanding how hormones function is always advancing, and current improvements in systems biology are giving us new knowledge. Researchers can use physiological, genomic, and mathematical methods to design detailed models that show how hormonal signaling pathways interact. As an example, understanding how estrous behavior is regulated in cows requires looking at the influence of hormones and genes on their fertility. When data sets are combined into models, it becomes easier to see how the endocrine system affects reproduction and behaviors. As this field progresses, the ability to harness genomic information and computational tools will be instrumental in addressing challenges related to fertility and hormone action, thus making significant contributions to both agricultural and biological sciences (Boer et al., 2010) (Figure 10.6).

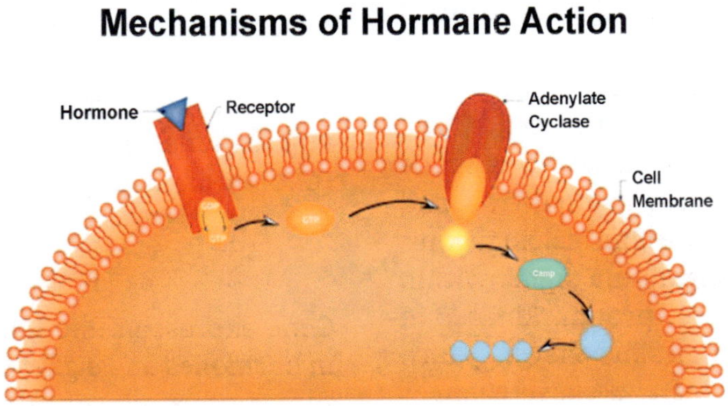

Figure 10.6. Mechanisms of hormone action.

Source: https://img.freepik.com/premium-vector/mechanisms-hormone-action_33402-1253.jpg.

10.2.1. Receptor Binding

Receptor binding is an important step in explaining how hormones work in signal transduction. As soon as hormones are released into the blood, they go to various tissues and attach to the receptors found either on the cell surface or inside the cell. This link is essential since it triggers a series of reactions inside the cell that cause the body to react. The shape of receptors is designed to recognize and link with hormones very accurately and strongly. Such interactions prove that receptor systems have evolved to send exact signals needed for keeping the body in balance and reacting to its needs. Besides, the process of receptor binding involves several structural and functional features. Usually, a receptor has an extracellular part that detects hormones, a middle portion that goes through the cell membrane, and an intracellular region that works with signaling molecules. For example, the glycoprotein hormone receptors in vertebrates, together with their lamprey homologs, have been found to keep similar structural features even after long periods of evolution. Some studies show that the way these domains interact is essential for hormone-receptor binding and for triggering the proper signals. This complexity emphasizes the important role of receptor binding in the modulation of hormonal activity and suggests that perturbations in these interactions can lead to dysregulations in physiological processes, , such as the estrous cycle in livestock, as mentioned by Boer et al. (2010). Studying how hormones bind to receptors reveals both the usual functions of the body and possible ways to treat hormone-related illnesses. As an example, how hormone receptors from different domains interact can change the sensitivity of the receptors and the ligands they respond to. Research on lamprey glycoprotein hormone receptors illustrates how evolutionary adaptations in receptor structure facilitate nuanced hormonal communication in response to environmental and physiological conditions (Freamat et al., 2010). As a result, it becomes possible to use knowledge about receptors to build therapies that either change the way receptors communicate or stop abnormal signaling. For this reason, further research on how receptors bind can greatly help boost fertility and address metabolic issues that are common in both agriculture and medicine.

10.2.2. Intracellular Signaling Pathways

Hormones affect target cells by using intracellular signaling pathways to control many body processes. The pathways depend on hormone receptors on the cell surface that send signals to the inside of the cell. Upon activation, these receptors initiate a cascade of intracellular events, often involving second messengers , such as cAMP and calcium ions, which amplify and propagate the signal within the cell. The importance of protein kinases in phosphorylation is very high since they help turn on or off different proteins and cause changes in the cell. If these signaling pathways do not work properly, it can result in diseases, proving that careful control of hormone signaling is very important for cells. Tight junctions (TJs) exemplify how intracellular signaling pathways can regulate membrane integrity and cellular communication. It has been demonstrated in recent studies that TJs act as barriers as well as take part in internal signaling in response to hormones. For example, protein kinase C and mitogen-activated protein kinase are among the signaling pathways that adjust TJs in response to things happening outside the cell. They demonstrate how the structure of cells and their signaling processes are closely related, mainly in epithelial cells. Furthermore, the regulatory effects of hormones on TJs emphasize their significance in maintaining homeostasis across different tissues, as evidenced by pathological conditions where TJ functionality is compromised, leading to issues , such as inflammation and disease progression (Himi et al., 2014). Intracellular signaling pathways are important in the kidneys, mainly by controlling sodium excretion and fluid balance. How cells maintain homeostasis is shown by the way they respond to different hormonal signals , such as angiotensin II and ANP. The kidneys work better at managing electrolytes because of the influence of hormones on their function. It is important for renal health that the balance between prooxidants from the renin-angiotensin system and antioxidants , such as dopamine is kept. Disruptions in this balance can lead to conditions like nephrotic syndrome and hypertension, underscoring the importance of understanding these intracellular pathways in the context of hormone action and their broader implications on renal function and pathology (Choi et al., 2014).

10.2.3. Gene Expression Modulation

Gene expression modulation is very important in hormones and signal transduction since these systems are closely linked to regulating the body's responses. Most hormones influence the body by sending messages to genes that cause them to be turned on or off. It is possible for modulation to occur at the start of transcription, during mRNA processing, or after the transcription is done. Significantly, small RNAs (sRNAs), , such as microRNAs (miRNAs) and small interfering RNAs (siRNAs), play an essential role in the post-transcriptional silencing of genes. These sRNAs can bind to mRNAs and promote their degradation or inhibit their translation, thereby fine-tuning gene expression in response to hormonal signals. As highlighted in recent studies, this interplay between hormones and sRNAs is particularly evident in plants, where hormonal pathways are regulated by sRNA responses to environmental stimuli (Li et al., 2020). Also, hormones do not only control gene expression by turning genes on or off; they also take part in complex feedback loops and signaling chains. Neurosteroids, , such as Pregnenolone sulfate (PregS), illustrate this phenomenon effectively. PregS is made first in the body and then acts as a precursor to many steroid hormones. It is regulated by brain activity and changes a lot during important growth periods. As a positive allosteric modulator of NMDA and TrpM3 receptors, it demonstrates its ability to affect pathways that cause changes in gene expression. For example, activation of TrpM3 by PregS results in calcium-dependent transcription of early immediate genes, highlighting how hormonal influences can have lasting effects on cellular function and gene expression during development (Webster, 2019). This shows how hormones play many roles in influencing the activity of genes. Also, the way hormones, genes, and environmental factors interact is necessary for plants and animals to adapt. The control of sRNAs by phytohormones in plants shows how several signaling pathways are brought together to deal with various stresses. The sRNA pathways in plants help change gene expression and also help the plant adjust to different environmental conditions. PregS and other neurosteroids in animals show that hormones can direct both quick changes in the body and long-term developmental changes by affecting gene expression. This duality in hormonal action emphasizes the importance of gene expression as a central element of hormone signaling and suggests potential avenues for research aimed at understanding these complex interactions in a broader biological context (Webster, 2019; Li et al., 2020).

Test Your Knowledge

1. What is a binding receptor?
2. What are intracellular signaling pathways?

10.3. Signal Transduction Pathways

Learning Outcome

1. Understand the role of G-protein coupled receptors (GPCRs) in hormone signaling and transduction;
2. Describe the receptor tyrosine kinases (RTKs);
3. Know the ion channel receptors.

Signal transduction pathways are made up of many biochemical stages that allow hormones to work on target cells. With the help of these pathways, cells are able to respond to their surroundings in the right way. These pathways are started when hormones attach to particular receptors found on the surface of the target cell. This interaction of receptor and ligand sets off a series of events inside the cell, like the activation of second messengers and protein kinases, which change gene expression, enzyme activity, and cellular metabolism. They are important because they change hormone signals into actions that keep the body balanced and regulate different functions. Research has increasingly uncovered the multifaceted roles of small RNAs (sRNAs), primarily microRNAs (miRNAs) and small interfering RNAs (siRNAs), in regulating signal transduction pathways, particularly within plant systems. They play an important role in controlling how genes work in response to hormones and stress. It has been found in recent studies that phytohormones are key to how plants respond to stress, and new research suggests that sRNAs are deeply involved in these processes too. Understanding these regulatory mechanisms enhances our knowledge of how cells, particularly in plants, adapt to environmental changes and hormonal signals, thus highlighting the importance of sRNAs in hormone-mediated signal transduction (Li et al., 2020). Besides, the way hormones affect estrous behavior in mammals through endocrinology proves the importance of signal transduction in animal physiology. Estradiol (E2), a key hormone in regulating the estrous cycle, orchestrates an array of endocrine and behavioral events through complex signaling mechanisms. It has been found that E2 is able to control gene activity in the brain regions needed for estrous behavior. It is also interesting to note how E2 works with progesterone and insulin-like growth factor-1 in different reproductive processes. As investigations continue to reveal the genetic and molecular underpinnings of these pathways, it becomes increasingly evident how vital they are for understanding fertility and reproductive health in high-yield dairy cattle, emphasizing the necessity for multidisciplinary approaches to today's biological challenges (Boer et al., 2010) (Figure 10.7).

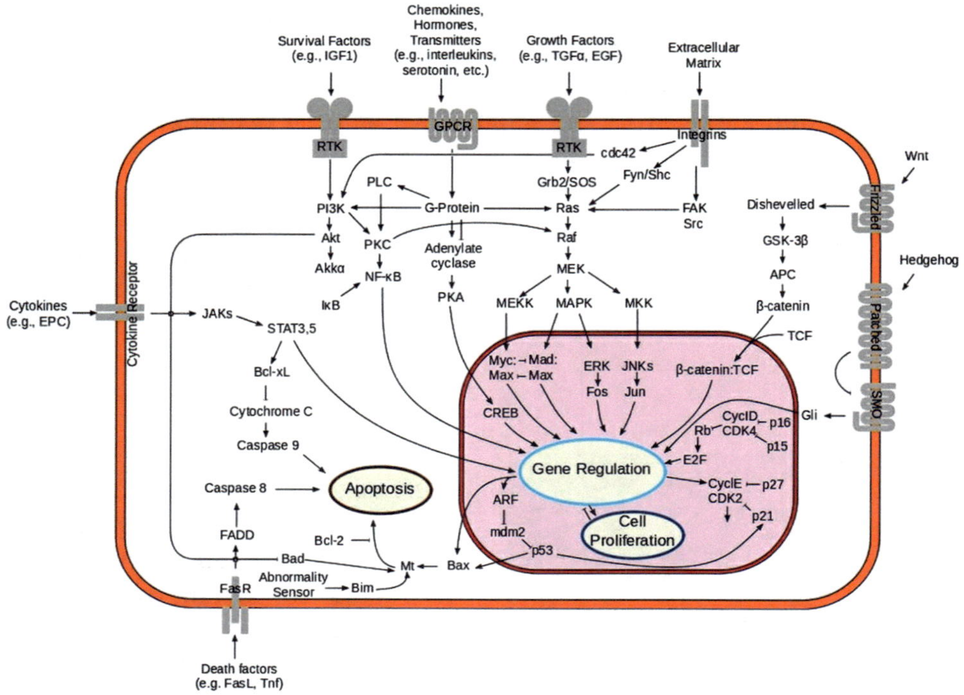

Figure 10.7. Signal transduction pathways.

Source: https://biologydictionary.net/wp-content/uploads/2018/03/Signal-transduction-pathways.jpg.

10.3.1. G-Protein Coupled Receptors (GPCRs)

G-protein coupled receptors (GPCRs) play a critical role in hormone signaling and transduction, acting as essential mediators for numerous physiological processes. These receptors are found in the cell membrane and are turned on by several ligands, for example, hormones, neurotransmitters, and stimuli from the environment. As soon as a ligand binds, GPCRs change shape, making it possible for them to interact with G-proteins inside the cell. This interaction initiates a cascade of intracellular signaling pathways that include the activation of enzymes and the generation of secondary messengers , such as cAMP. Thanks to these processes, GPCRs are important for many functions, including regulating metabolism and responses in the nervous and endocrine systems. An exemplar of GPCR functionality is the corticotropin-releasing hormone receptor (CRHR), which is pivotal in the hypothalamic-pituitary-adrenal axis. CRHR1 and CRHR2 are GPCRs that help control the body's response to stress and how it reacts to changes. New studies have explained the detailed pathways that follow CRHR activation, which go against the traditional concepts of GPCR signaling. For instance, novel insights into cAMP generation and extracellular signal-regulated kinase (ERK1/2) activation highlight the nuanced roles these receptors play in both basal and stress-induced conditions.

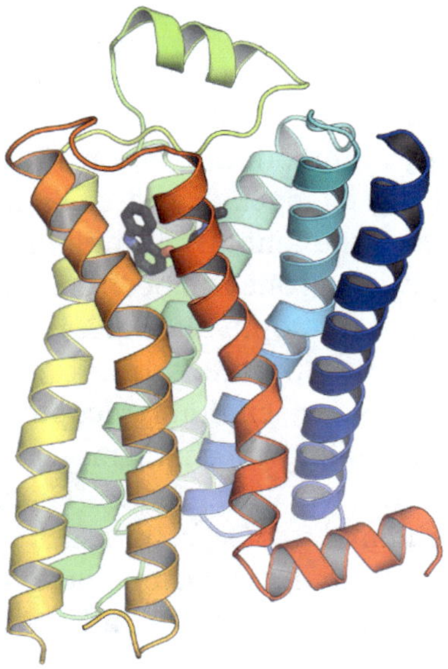

Figure 10.8. Ribbon diagram of the β_2-adrenergic receptor, a G protein-coupled receptor.

Source: https://upload.wikimedia.org/wikipedia/commons/6/6a/Beta-2-adrenergic-receptor.png.

Understanding the molecular intricacies of CRHR signaling is vital for identifying potential therapeutic targets for stress-related disorders and evaluating the broader implications of GPCR function in neuroendocrinology, as indicated by contemporary studies (Armando et al., 2017). Another noteworthy GPCR is the melanocortin-4 receptor (MC4R), which has garnered attention for its role in energy homeostasis and obesity regulation. Activated by melanocyte-stimulating hormones (MSH), MC4R mediates signals related to appetite suppression. In contrast, the endogenous antagonist agouti-related peptide (AgRP) counteracts this effect, leading to increased food intake. Because MC4R signaling is complex, it highlights the receptor's role in metabolism and how hard it is to create drugs that target only this receptor. Understanding how MC4Rs binds to other molecules and forms its three-dimensional structure is crucial for finding out how it signals and can be used in treating obesity. The prevalence of naturally occurring MC4R mutations, linked to monogenic obesity, further emphasizes the need for in-depth research into the signaling mechanisms of this vital GPCR (Biebermann et al., 2019) (Figure 10.8).

10.3.2. Receptor Tyrosine Kinases (RTKs)

Receptor tyrosine kinases (RTKs) are integral components of cellular signal transduction pathways, playing a crucial role in regulating various physiological processes , such as growth, metabolism, and differentiation. When these transmembrane proteins bind to growth factors, they get activated and trigger a series of related events. As soon as ligands bind to RTKs, they dimerize and autophosphorylate, which leads to their kinase being activated and in turn causes tyrosine residues on RTKs and other proteins to be phosphorylated. The phosphorylation process gives a place for downstream molecules to bind, which triggers the Ras/MAP kinase cascade and the PI3K/AKT pathway. Dysregulation of RTK signaling is frequently implicated in a range of diseases, particularly cancer, thus highlighting their significance as therapeutic targets in modern medicine (Regad, 2015). Overactivation or increased expression of RTKs helps cancer development because they encourage cells to divide and live longer than usual. When RTKs and their downstream parts are altered by mutations, it can result in constant signaling, which causes cancer cells to grow and spread further. For instance, mutations in genes encoding RTKs, like the EGFR, have been extensively documented in various cancers, driving therapeutic strategies aimed at targeting these pathways. Among the strategies used against cancer, the development of RTK inhibitors, including monoclonal antibodies and small-molecule tyrosine kinase inhibitors, is very important. These agents aim to block the aberrant signals initiated by RTKs, presenting new avenues for personalized treatment (Mattila et al., 2009). Besides their role in cancer, RTKs are important for normal body functions, revealing that they can help or harm the body. RTKs help with embryonic development, the repair of tissues, and differentiation, and each RTK has a particular function in these processes. For example, the vascular endothelial growth factor receptor (VEGFR) is crucial for angiogenesis and tissue vascularization, while the platelet-derived growth factor receptor (PDGFR) has a significant role in cell migration and proliferation during tissue maintenance and repair. For this reason, we must study the complicated ways RTKs are regulated, especially by protein tyrosine phosphatases that balance their signaling. Understanding these regulatory dynamics can inform the development of novel therapeutic strategies and improve existing treatment paradigms targeting RTK-mediated signal transduction (Regad, 2015) (Figure 10.9).

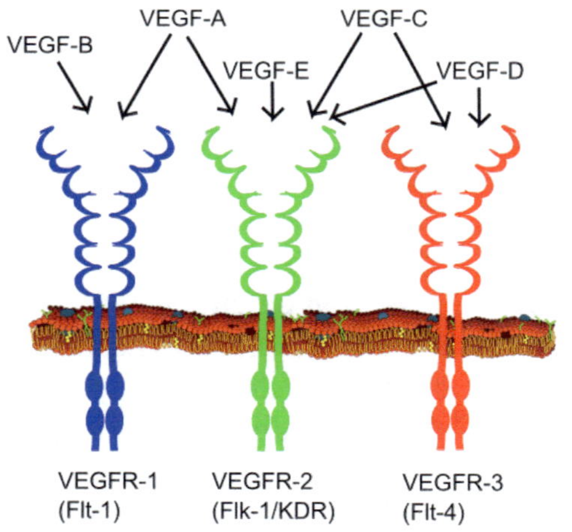

Figure 10.9. VEGF receptors and ligands.

Source: https://upload.wikimedia.org/wikipedia/commons/c/c8/VEGF_receptors.png.

10.3.3. Ion Channel Receptors

Ion channel receptors are important parts of cellular pathways that control how cells react to hormones. The receptors found in cell membranes are special because they can quickly allow ions like sodium, potassium, calcium, and chloride to move through the membrane when certain stimuli are present. The opening and closing of these channels are usually controlled by hormones, which results in big changes in the cell's membrane potential and the amount of ions inside it. For instance, progesterone has been shown to evoke immediate electrophysiological alterations in thymic epithelial cells, underscoring the nuanced roles ion channel receptors play in the rapid signaling mechanisms of endocrine functions (Brucker et al., 1999). Thanks to this fast movement of ions, cells react quickly to hormones and manage various body functions, for example, muscle activity and the release of neurotransmitters. How ion channel receptors work to activate reveals that hormones have many ways to affect cellular signaling. Hormones may connect with different ion channels, which leads to the activation of complex signaling pathways. G protein-coupled receptors (GPCRs) are notably influential in this context, as they can trigger the opening of ion channels through secondary messengers. For example, the binding of a hormone to a GPCR can lead to the activation of phospholipase C, resulting in the generation of IP3 and diacylglycerol (DAG), which subsequently promote calcium release from intracellular stores (Costanzo et al., 2015). Increased calcium inside the cells can also open calcium-dependent ion channels, showing that different signaling pathways interact and ion channels are essential for hormones to work. Besides their usual hormone roles, ion channel receptors are now being studied for their part in detecting lipid signaling molecules. They reveal that ion channel receptors are flexible and significant in reacting to a wide range of chemicals apart from typical hormones. Studies carried out recently suggest that CD36 and G protein-coupled receptor 120 may help detect fatty acids, which could make fat a new main taste. The ability of ion channel receptors to react to a variety of signaling molecules proves their vital part in hormone-triggered signaling, which helps us understand energy control and metabolism. As research uncovers more about the connections between ion channels, hormones, and cell signaling, the implications for health and disease are profound, particularly regarding conditions like obesity and MS (Brucker et al., 1999) (Figure 10.10).

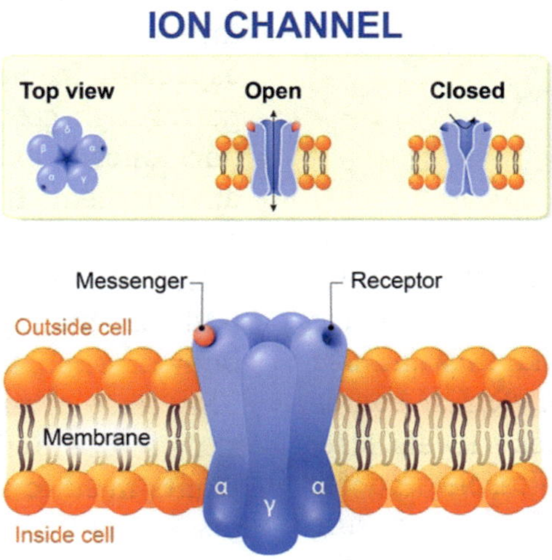

Figure 10.10. Ion channel receptors.

Source: https://www.news-medical.net/image-handler/ts/20181026120124/ri/673/picture/2018/10/shutterstock_479593594.jpg.

Test Your Knowledge

1. What are G protein coupled receptors?
2. What are ion channel receptors?

10.4. Hormonal Regulation of Metabolism

Learning Outcome

1. Understand the role of insulin in glucose metabolism;
2. Understand the role of glucagon in energy mobilization;
3 Describe the thyroid hormones and metabolic rate.

The way hormones affect metabolism is detailed and very important for the body to maintain balance. Insulin, glucagon, and cortisol are important for handling the availability and use of energy in the body. Insulin, which comes from the pancreas when glucose levels rise, encourages glucose to enter muscle and fat tissues and also stops the liver from producing more glucose. On the other hand, glucagon, which the pancreas produces, helps raise blood glucose by encouraging glycogenolysis and gluconeogenesis, mainly when there is no food in the body. Cortisol, which is a glucocorticoid from the adrenal glands, controls metabolism when stress occurs and affects both gluconeogenesis and lipolysis. Learning about these interactions and their signaling is necessary, as they affect both quick changes in metabolism and may lead to obesity and diabetes in the future. There is a link between hormonal regulation and metabolic health, which also involves the balance between reproductive health and metabolism. An example in dairy cattle is that higher milk production can cause reduced fertility, partly because hormone signaling is changed. Estradiol (E2) emerges as a central player in regulating the estrous cycle by influencing gene expression related to reproductive behavior and metabolic adaptation. The higher demand for energy to produce milk may upset the endocrine system and cause fertility problems. The relationship between insulin-like growth factor-1 and E2 is further complicated since metabolic stress can have a negative effect on reproductive hormones. The exploration of these connections through both physiological studies and systems biology models will provide deeper insights into the regulatory mechanisms governing reproductive metabolism and overall health in livestock and potentially in humans as well (Boer et al., 2010). Hormones not only affect metabolism but also take part in seasonal changes for organisms, especially in plants. The way perennial plants go through growth and dormancy shows how hormones help them respond to changes in the environment. In poplar, buds are made to go from growing to resting through the coordinated action of light, ethylene, and abscisic acid. Every pathway manages particular functions in the body that help animals survive climate changes. This close communication between hormones shows the wider changes in metabolism plants need to survive in different seasons. By dissecting these hormonal pathways and their influence on metabolism, particularly through systems biology approaches, researchers uncover a wealth of information that can inform agricultural practices and enhance our understanding of plant resilience to climate change (Arend et al., 2007).

10.4.1. Insulin and Glucose Metabolism

Insulin is very important for glucose metabolism since it helps regulate blood sugar levels. Insulin made in the pancreas allows tissues like skeletal muscle and adipose tissue to take in glucose, which helps maintain the body's metabolism. Upon the binding of insulin to its receptor, a cascade of signaling events occurs, which includes the activation of the insulin receptor substrate (IRS) proteins. This subsequently leads to the mobilization of glucose transporters (GLUT4) to the cell membrane, enhancing glucose uptake. Besides, insulin encourages the body to make glycogen and lipids while at the same time stopping the production of glucose from non-carbohydrate sources and the breakdown of fats. In this way, glucose is used efficiently, pointing out the close relationship between insulin signaling and energy metabolism for keeping the body healthy. Insulin affects cells in ways beyond glucose uptake by also regulating a number of metabolic processes important for energy balance.

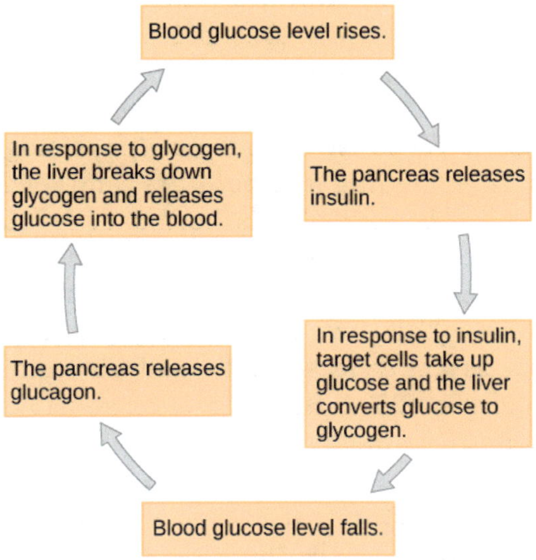

Figure 10.11. Insulin and glucagon regulate blood glucose levels.

Source: https://s3-us-west-2.amazonaws.com/courses-images/wp-content/uploads/sites/1223/2017/02/07230445/Figure_37_03_05.png.

After insulin is activated, the process of lipogenesis in adipose tissues is started, so any extra glucose can be turned into lipids and stored. At times when there is a lot of glucose, insulin directs the body to store more fat and prevents the breakdown of stored fats. In addition, insulin's actions are supported by other pathways that involve glucagon and epinephrine, highlighting its role in lowering high blood sugar. For example, glucagon works oppositely to insulin by releasing glucose from the liver into the blood. The balance between these hormones is essential for achieving metabolic equilibrium and reflects the complexity of hormonal signaling in glucose metabolism, as shown in studies involving beta-cell morphology and signaling mechanisms (Lee et al., 1995). New studies show that insulin has many effects and that insulin analogs can differently impact glucose metabolism. As an example, insulin glargine and its metabolites attach differently to insulin receptors than regular human insulin, which affects their metabolic and growth activities. Although these analogs control blood sugar well, their lower growth-promoting effects are helpful in clinical practice for people who may develop cancer or other conditions where cells grow too rapidly. Looking at the metabolites of insulin glargine reveals how insulin works with cell growth and why careful planning is needed in medicine. Understanding these dynamics not only enhances the grasp of its role in glucose metabolism but also underscores the importance of further investigating the signaling pathways involved to optimize treatments for metabolic disorders (Habermann et al., 2010) (Figure 10.11).

10.4.2. Glucagon and Energy Mobilization

Besides increasing blood glucose, glucagon is involved in guiding different metabolic processes as needed by the body. When produced by the alpha cells in the pancreas, glucagon mainly influences the liver to break down glycogen and make new glucose. At times when you are fasting or doing strenuous exercise, your blood glucose needs to be well-maintained to supply the body with energy. Glucagon signaling is primarily mediated through the cAMP (cyclic adenosine monophosphate) pathway, which amplifies the hormonal signal, facilitating swift metabolic responses that ensure glucose availability, thereby attesting to the importance of glucagon in energy homeostasis during energy-demanding situations (Furman et al., 2010). Also, glucagons affect energy mobilization by working together with other hormones like vasopressin. Research highlights that arginine vasopressin (AVP) can enhance both insulin and glucagon release from pancreatic cells, showcasing a glucose-dependent dynamic. At high glucose levels, AVP increases insulin production, while low glucose levels leads to glucagon release, showing that there is a complex way this is controlled. This process points out that glucagon is important for producing glucose and can also be adjusted to address low blood sugar levels. The glucagon release mechanism, influenced by AVP, exhibits how hormonal signaling is integral to managing blood glucose levels, further underscoring the importance of glucagon in the energy mobilization process (Abu-Basha et al., 2002). cAMP serves as a crucial second messenger in glucagon signaling, amplifying its metabolic effects. The elevation of cAMP levels within target cells leads to the activation of protein kinase A (PKA), which in turn stimulates processes like glycogen breakdown and the release of glucose into the bloodstream. It is shown that more cAMP in cells amplifies the effects of glucagons on glucose and helps release secretory granules for hormone secretion. Because of this connection, the body can mobilize energy in the right amount at any given time. Such intricate regulation illustrates how glucagon, through cAMP signaling pathways, plays a pivotal role in maintaining metabolic balance and responding to energetic demands (Furman et al., 2010).

10.4.3. Thyroid Hormones and Metabolic Rate

It is important in endocrinology to study the relationship between THs and the metabolic rate since these hormones control energy use and overall metabolism. THs, primarily thyroxine (T4) and triiodothyronine (T3), influence metabolic processes by modulating the activity of various enzymes involved in the cellular respiratory chain and carbohydrate metabolism. The hormones help mitochondria in oxidative phosphorylation, which boosts heat production. THs regulate metabolic rate in the body, but also through receptors inside cells, pointing out that signal transduction is essential for hormone function. The synthesis and release of these hormones themselves are influenced by glycosylation processes that enhance their functional activity, underlying the importance of cellular signaling pathways in shaping metabolic outcomes (Ząbczyńska et al., 2018). Furthermore, the hypothalamus-pituitary-thyroid (HPT) axis orchestrates the regulation of thyroid hormone levels in response to various physiological stimuli, including temperature and energy demands. As part of this hormonal feedback system, thyrotropin-releasing hormone (TRH) stimulates the secretion of thyroid-stimulating hormone (TSH), which in turn promotes the synthesis and release of T4 and T3 from the thyroid gland. The HPT axis is responsible for managing the metabolism of many organisms, as proven by studies on how birds regulate their temperature. In precocial and altricial birds, differences in the timing of HPT axis activity play a crucial role in the emergence of thermoregulation and metabolic adjustment to environmental temperature (Baarendse et al., 2008). They reveal the relationship between hormones and metabolism and show how this affects comparative endocrinology. Disruptions in how THs work and regulate metabolism can have serious effects on a patient's health. In hypothyroidism, when the thyroid hormone is not produced enough, metabolism slows, weight increases, and heat production drops. On the other hand, hyperthyroidism, which means too much thyroid hormone, can make metabolism faster and increase the breakdown of tissues. Key to understanding these pathologies is the recognition of the significance of glycan structures in thyroid hormone biology; alterations in glycosylation patterns can affect hormone transport and receptor binding, ultimately influencing metabolic clearance rates and physiological function (Ząbczyńska et al., 2018). Because THs and signal transduction pathways are connected, it is clear that the regulation of metabolism requires careful study, as this understanding helps address thyroid-related issues and their effects on metabolic health (Figure 10.12).

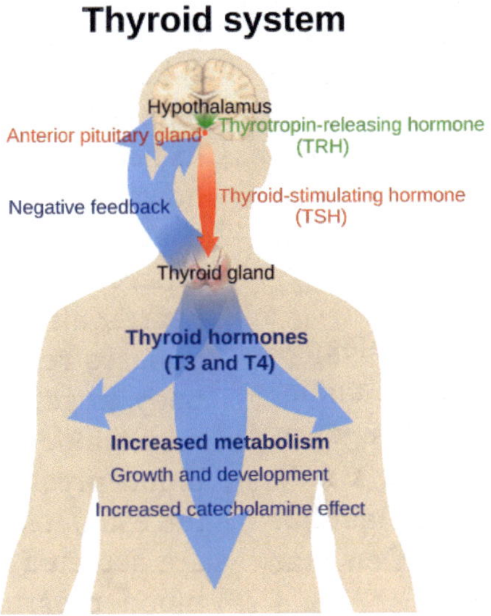

Figure 10.12. The thyroid system of the thyroid hormones T3 and T4.

Source: https://upload.wikimedia.org/wikipedia/commons/d/d1/Thyroid_system.svg.

Test Your Knowledge

1. What is the role of insulin in glucose metabolism?
2. What is the role of glucagon in energy mobilization?

10.5. Hormones and Homeostasis

Learning Outcome

1. Describe the role of hormones in maintaining blood pressure;
2. Know the hormonal control of water balance;
3. Understand the regulation of calcium levels.

Hormones and homeostasis are closely linked, which helps maintain the proper functioning of an organism's body. Hormones help control different activities in the body, for example, metabolism, growth, and reproduction. In this situation, the hypothalamus is key in linking hormones that help maintain balance in the body. As an example, leptin and insulin are adiposity signals that share information about how much energy and food is available. Adipose tissue produces leptin to decrease appetite, and insulin is mainly responsible for glucose regulation. All of these hormones contribute to the body's energy balance, proving the need for hormones to be stable for the body's health and stability. Homeostasis is controlled by hormones as well as by the complex pathways they use for communication. How leptin and insulin act as signals shows how the body can control and balance energy use. It has been found through research that Siberian hamsters' hormones are regulated with the seasons, meaning that their effect on weight management is affected by external conditions. In particular, the hormones can cause changes in signaling pathways that are sensitive to both light and temperature, proving the key role of neuroendocrine pathways in seasonal weight control. Being adaptable, hormones show that they are closely connected to the environment, helping organisms adjust and survive.

Besides, leptin resistance adds a deeper insight into how hormones work in maintaining homeostasis. It has been found that changes in the leptin signal transduction pathways may result in obesity and the health problems that come with it. It is important to mention that the hypothalamic reaction to leptin is guided by factors , such as the regulation of pathways that are downstream from the leptin receptor. It seems that, contrary to earlier thoughts, leptin and insulin do not always act together to control appetite and body weight. Gaining knowledge about these mechanisms reveals important aspects of homeostasis and offers possible ways to treat metabolic disorders, pointing out the crucial role hormones play in signal transduction and homeostasis.

10.5.1. Role of Hormones in Maintaining Blood Pressure

The way hormones maintain blood pressure is a very detailed part of human physiology that depends on the interaction among different hormones. Chief among these is the renin-angiotensin-aldosterone system (RAAS), a critical regulator of blood pressure that responds to changes in blood volume and electrolyte balance. When blood pressure decreases, renin from the kidneys starts the process of turning angiotensinogen into angiotensin I. After that, the inactive precursor is changed into angiotensin II, which is a strong constrictor of blood vessels that increases blood pressure. In addition, angiotensin II prompts the adrenal glands to release aldosterone, which helps the kidneys keep more sodium. It helps increase the amount of blood in the body and also plays a key part in raising blood pressure, which highlights the many ways the body regulates its heart health. In conjunction with RAAS, other hormones , such as ANP and catecholamines contribute to blood pressure regulation through different mechanisms. ANP is produced by the heart's atria when blood volume rises and it opposes renin and aldosterone by causing the body to get rid of sodium through urine. As a result, blood volume decreases and so does the blood pressure. Alternatively, catecholamines, for example, epinephrine and norepinephrine, are secreted by the adrenal medulla and raise blood pressure by increasing the heart rate and how much the heart contracts. The balance between natriuretic and antinatriuretic factors, as discussed in the context of renal physiology, highlights the delicate equilibrium maintained by these hormones under normal physiological conditions (Choi et al., 2014). If the balance is disturbed, people may develop diseases , such as hypertension and chronic kidney disease (CKD). Also, the connection between these hormones and cellular signaling is important for understanding blood pressure control in different health situations. Pathological scenarios, , such as hypertension or CKD, illustrate how dysregulation in hormonal signaling can exacerbate health issues. For instance, excessive activation of the renin-angiotensin system is often observed in hypertensive patients, leading to end-organ damage in the kidneys and other organs (Eckardt et al., 2019). In addition, the way angiotensin II signaling influences cellular responses, , such as hypoxia-induced activation of hypoxia-inducible factors, shows that these pathways have many sides. A thorough knowledge of these hormonal interactions and their results allows researchers to design special therapies for treating hypertension and CKD (Figure 10.13).

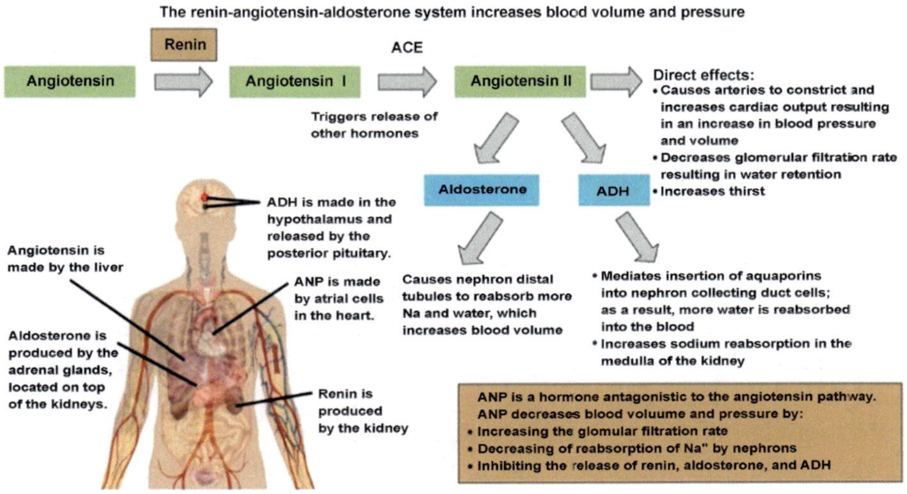

Figure 10.13. The renin-angiotensin-aldosterone system increases blood pressure and volume. The hormone ANP has antagonistic effects.

Source: https://s3-us-west-2.amazonaws.com/courses-images/wp-content/uploads/sites/1223/2017/02/09003431/Figure_41_07_01-1024x554.jpg.

10.5.2. Hormonal Control of Water Balance

Maintaining water balance in the body is very important and is controlled by hormones. Central to this regulation are hormones , such as antidiuretic hormone (ADH), aldosterone, and ANP. ADH, which comes from the hypothalamus and is secreted by the posterior pituitary, helps the kidneys keep water. Thanks to ADH, more water is kept in the body when the kidneys are not getting enough fluid. Alternatively, ANP made in the cardiac atria helps get rid of sodium through urine, which lowers blood volume by causing water loss. The way water balance is handled by the body points out the important interactions between hormones and the processes that control these interactions. There are other factors in the body's systems that affect the way hormones manage water retention and excretion. Aldosterone, which is made in the adrenal cortex and is a steroid hormone, plays a big role in regulating sodium and water in the kidneys. When sodium is reabsorbed with the help of aldosterone, water also remains in the body because water is drawn along with sodium. In the case of hypertension, the balance of fluids is very important since it affects how the blood vessels respond and the pressure within them. The interaction between aldosterone and the RAAS illustrates a complex feedback mechanism that regulates not only blood volume but also vascular health. All these hormones together represent a key part of signaling pathways that help maintain the body's water balance and homeostasis in various conditions. Besides, problems with hormones that control water balance can have major clinical effects, showing how vital these mechanisms are. It has been found by recent research that CKD is often made worse by hormonal imbalances , such as those in the RAAS. It demonstrates that the kidneys' function and fluid balance are affected by systemic signaling pathways, which is why hypertension is related to kidney damage. It is especially important to note that angiotensin II signaling links hormonal regulation with the development of diseases caused by imbalances in these signals. Understanding how hormonal control mechanisms intersect with various cellular pathways assists in the development of targeted therapies for managing conditions like CKD and hypertension, underscoring the relevance of studying signal transduction in the context of water balance (Eckardt et al., 2019).

10.5.3. Regulation of Calcium Levels

Calcium regulation is necessary for muscle movement, the sending of signals by nerves, and the secretion of hormones. Calcium ions (Ca^{2+}) serve as important second messengers in signal transduction pathways, where fluctuations in intracellular calcium concentrations can trigger diverse cellular responses. Calcium in the body is controlled by letting it in from the outside and releasing it from storage organelles, mainly the endoplasmic reticulum (ER). Hormones , such as parathyroid hormone (PTH) and calcitonin play significant roles in maintaining calcium homeostasis by modulating the activity of bone, kidney, and intestinal cells to regulate calcium absorption, resorption, and excretion. The way these hormones work together demonstrates the important role of endocrine regulation and signal transduction in maintaining cells and the body's stability. Also, the way hormones and calcium work together shows how complicated signal transduction networks can be. For example, PTH prompts osteoclasts to work, so calcium is released from bones and enters the bloodstream. At the same time, calcitonin helps calcium be deposited in bones and reduces the amount of calcium reabsorbed by the kidneys.

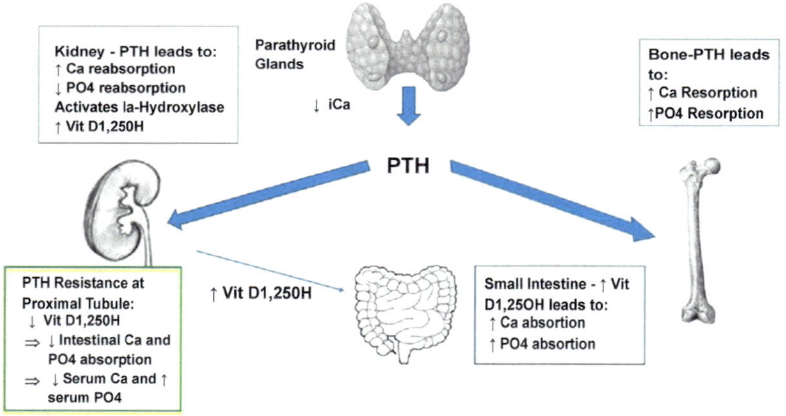

Figure 10.14. Regulation of calcium homeostasis.

Source: https://www.researchgate.net/publication/338193278/figure/fig1/AS:840724262174721@1577455692254/Regulation-of-calcium-homeostasis.png.

The antagonism between hormones shows a smart system that helps keep calcium in the body within a safe and narrow range. Vitamin D shows that mineral metabolism is closely connected to the signals sent by the endocrine system. The way these hormones work together highlights that problems with calcium signaling may cause diseases , such as osteoporosis or hypercalcemia, and therefore, proper hormone control is needed for calcium homeostasis and health. Several things can influence how well these regulatory mechanisms work, , such as age, what a person eats, and hormonal changes during their life. As an example, when growth is fast or hormones are changing, , such as at puberty or menopause, the body's need for calcium and how it responds to hormones may also change. Scientific studies suggest that if PTH and vitamin D levels change, it can result in either poor calcium absorption or too much bone loss. In addition, recent findings on how some signaling pathways, for example, the phosphoinositide cascade, control calcium balance in cells, point to the role of hormones in this process. Understanding the complexities of these interactions not only reveals the significance of calcium in human physiology but also points to potential interventions for calcium-related disorders (Young et al., 2000; Albrecht et al., 2002) (Figure 10.14).

Test Your Knowledge

1. What is the role of hormones in maintaining blood pressure?
2. Which hormones control water balance?

10.6. Disorders Related to Hormonal Imbalance

Learning Outcome

1. Learn about diabetes mellitus;
2. Describe hyperthyroidism and hypothyroidism;
3. Describe Cushing's syndrome.

It is clear from the connection between hormonal imbalance and different disorders that hormones are very important in the human body, especially for signal transduction. The proper functioning of metabolism, growth, and reproduction largely depends on insulin, cortisol, THs, and sex hormones. When hormone levels are not within their normal ranges, they may lead to many changes in the body and metabolism. As an example, when someone becomes insulin resistant due to hormonal changes, their glucose metabolism becomes abnormal, which increases their risk of type 2 diabetes. Gaining knowledge about such disruptions is crucial for designing proper treatment plans, since hormones and their signals can greatly shape a person's health and well-being. Problems caused by hormonal imbalance can show up in various ways and have a major impact on patients' well-being. Among these conditions, diabetes can cause sexual problems in patients because it affects their hormones and blood circulation. It has been found through research that women with diabetes regularly deal with sexual health issues due to the connection between metabolism, hormones, and sexual health. Since these issues are complex, healthcare providers should be proactive in their actions. For instance, since nurses often look after diabetes patients, they should understand the link between hormones and sexual health. Such awareness can enhance patient education and facilitate early identification of potential complications, thereby allowing for timely interventions that address both metabolic and psychosocial aspects of diabetic care (Phillips et al., 2015). Besides, adenylate kinase and its influence on cellular energy are additional factors to consider when managing disorders. Adenylate kinase helps the body sense and control important signals that affect hormones. In particular, when AMP levels change, due to adenylate kinase, it affects several signaling pathways, for example, those involved in hormonal secretion and metabolism. It has been found that changes in adenylate kinase activity may be related to disorders , such as obesity and type 2 diabetes, proving that hormone regulation and cellular energy are closely linked. Furthermore, disturbances in adenylate signaling can complicate hormone actions and increase risks of further imbalances, thereby necessitating an integrated approach that addresses both hormonal disorders and their metabolic consequences (Dzeja & Terzic, 2009) (Figure 10.15).

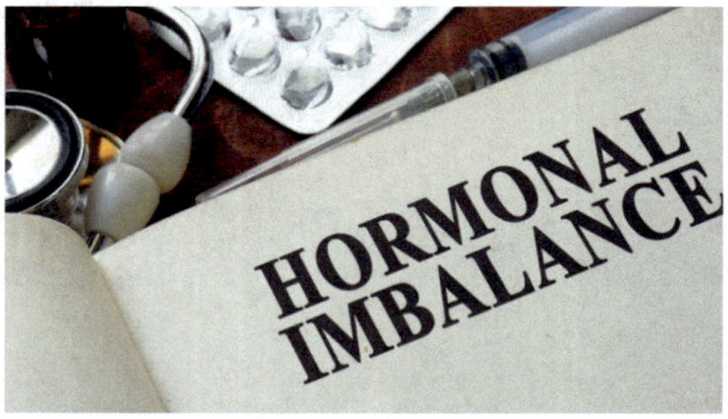

Figure 10.15. Conceptual image representing hormonal imbalance with medical tools in the background.

Source: https://aminoco.com/cdn/shop/articles/FeaturedImage_Hormones_2fb39633-c10e-44da-aa33-e031a4ac90c6.jpg?v=1739944721.

10.6.1. Diabetes Mellitus

This disease is called diabetes mellitus and is caused when the body doesn't make enough insulin or when insulin doesn't work properly. The condition is mainly described as Type 1 diabetes, where the immune system attacks insulin-producing cells in the pancreas, and Type 2 diabetes, where the body does not respond well to insulin and there is not enough insulin produced. The process of diabetes is related to the disruption of many hormones and signaling pathways, especially insulin and glucagon. In this case, insulin is important for glucose balance, and glucagon works to balance insulin and keep blood glucose levels steady. It is very important to know about these hormonal interactions since they play a key role in developing treatments for diabetic patients. According to research, hormones that are altered by diabetes can also bring about problems , such as heart and kidney complications. In particular, the fibroblast growth factor 23 (FGF23) and klotho axis has been observed as crucial in the pathophysiology of diabetes-related complications. Elevated levels of FGF23 in patients with diabetes have been linked to increased risk of bone fractures, particularly in the setting of CKD. This correlation suggests a complex interaction between endocrine signaling and metabolic health in diabetes, indicating that hormonal dysregulation contributes not only to hyperglycemia but also to secondary complications, thereby heightening the need for targeted therapeutic strategies that address these interrelated pathways (Lu et al., 2020). In addition, the way diabetes and placental hormones are connected adds more difficulty to the situation.

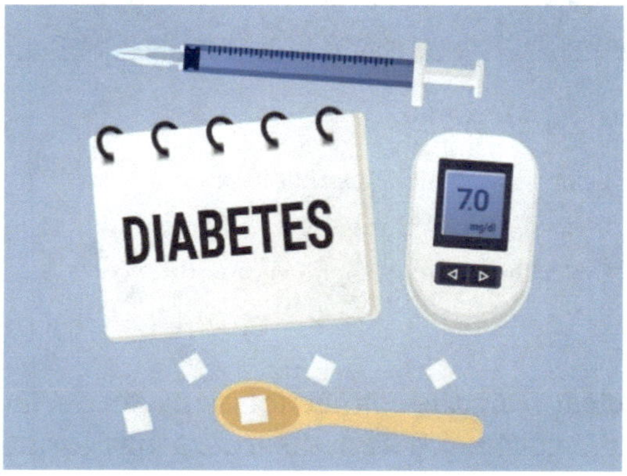

Figure 10.16. Diabetes mellitus.

Source: https://www.omegahospitals.com/blog/storage/2024/09/109c8350-786b-4a71-a406-da787e50cac0-1200x900.jpg.

The hormones released by the placenta play a role in changing a mother's metabolism during pregnancy. Gestational diabetes mellitus shows that problems in hormone signaling can be harmful to both the mother and her baby. When a pregnancy is healthy, placental hormones help control a mother's insulin sensitivity and glucose metabolism so that the fetus receives the needed nutrients. Still, in gestational diabetes, these hormones do not maintain a stable balance, which results in high blood sugar. Investigating the gene expression programs of the placenta through advanced transcriptomic approaches sheds light on the pathogenic mechanisms involved and highlights the necessity of understanding these hormonal interactions throughout pregnancy (Mege et al., 2018). So, diabetes mellitus highlights the key role hormones and their signals play in controlling metabolism and related health issues (Figure 10.16).

10.6.2. Hyperthyroidism and Hypothyroidism

The thyroid gland plays a critical role in regulating metabolism and overall bodily function through the secretion of hormones , such as thyroxine (T4) and triiodothyronine (T3). Both hyperthyroidism and hypothyroidism are thyroid problems that lead to major changes in the body's metabolism. Hyperthyroidism is caused by too many THs in the body, which bring about symptoms , such as weight loss, a higher heart rate, and anxiety. This heightened hormonal activity can disrupt various physiological processes, influence not only energy utilization but also impact the hypothalamic-pituitary-thyroid (HPT) axis, a crucial component of hormonal signal transduction. It is important to know these pathways to realize how thyroid problems can cause changes in many other systems, highlighting the role of the thyroid in keeping the body stable. Alternatively, hypothyroidism is caused by producing too little thyroid hormone, which brings about symptoms , such as tiredness, weight gain, and a depressed mood.

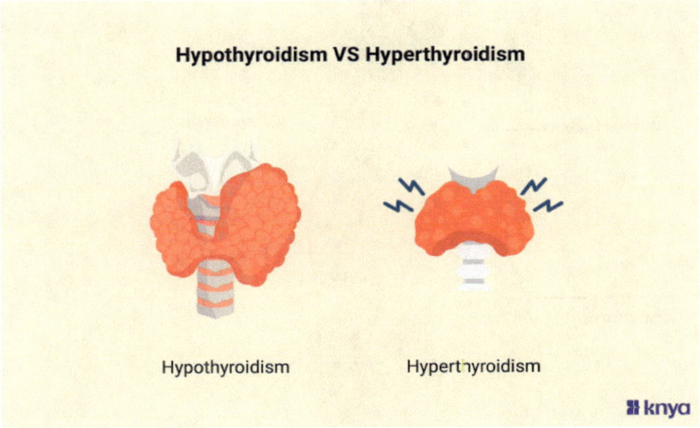

Figure 10.17. Hyperthyroidism and hypothyroidism.

Source: https://knyamed.com/cdn/shop/articles/Hypothyroidism-VS-Hyperthyroidism.jpg?v=1707743997.

One of the causes of this condition is autoimmune diseases, for example, *Hashimoto's thyroiditis*, where the immune system harms the thyroid gland. When thyroid hormone levels go down, it can slow down metabolism and worsen other health problems, including those of the heart and the mind. In hypothyroidism, the hormonal system usually causes changes in hormones and neurotransmitters to help the body maintain its energy balance. When THs interact with other signaling molecules, it becomes clear that problems with hormone levels can cause major changes in the body, so a thorough approach to diagnosis and treatment is required. A number of recent studies have pointed out that glycosylation plays a key role in how THs function, mainly in the cases of hyperthyroidism and hypothyroidism. Research has shown that glycosylated proteins, , such as thyroglobulin and TSH, are crucial for proper hormone synthesis and secretion. Alterations in glycan structures can lead to abnormal thyroid function, contributing to the progression of metabolic disorders and autoimmune conditions related to thyroid health (Ząbczyńska et al., 2018). Furthermore, within the framework of hyperthyroidism, the modulation of signaling pathways involving thyrotropin and its receptors reflects how hyperactive thyroid function can interfere with normal hormonal balance, particularly during critical physiological states , such as pregnancy and lactation (Jahn et al., 2017). These results point out that learning about the biochemical and molecular mechanisms of thyroid hormone action is necessary for a full picture of how the endocrine system is regulated (Figure 10.17).

10.6.3. Cushing's Syndrome

Cushing's syndrome, which happens because of too much cortisol, greatly affects both hormone messages and metabolic functions. Cortisol is commonly called the stress hormone because it has major effects on glucose metabolism, immune system control, and maintaining blood pressure. Cushing's syndrome is caused by cortisol dysregulation that can be due to pituitary adenomas, adrenal tumors, or ACTH secretion from a different part of the body.

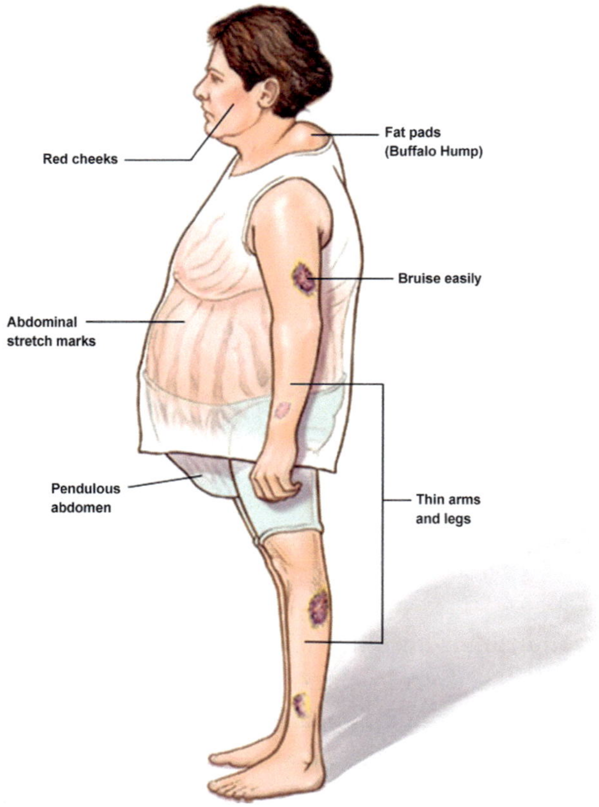

Figure 10.18. Cushing's syndrome.

Source: https://www.mayoclinic.org/-/media/kcms/gbs/patient-consumer/images/2013/08/26/10/11/ds00470_im00313_r7_cushingssyndromethu_jpg.jpg.

As a result of hypercortisolism, the body may experience several changes, , such as difficulty in processing carbohydrates, which makes it more likely to get infections. Exploring the reasons behind these changes gives important knowledge about how hormones shape health and diseases. At the cellular level, Cushing's syndrome presents unique challenges related to molecular signaling pathways, particularly those involving adrenocorticotropic hormone (ACTH) and its receptor pathways. Exposure to ACTH for a long period leads to the enlargement of adrenal glands and higher steroid production. Studies have demonstrated that prolonged stimulation by ACTH results in a complex interplay of gene expression changes, involving over 928 identified genes that are crucial in signaling pathways, lipid metabolism, cell proliferation, and apoptosis (Bailey et al., 2017). The increased activity of genes involved in sterol and lipid metabolism demonstrates that the pathology may result in metabolic problems that increase the risk of CVDs in patients. Researchers can use these signals to find possible treatments that help address the wide-ranging problems of the syndrome. Cushing's syndrome also leads to problems that affect people's health over the long run and their general well-being. Common symptoms in patients are weight gain, a round face, and hypertension, and if these are ignored, they may result in serious health problems. The chronic exposure to elevated cortisol levels induces profound changes in body composition, including increased fat deposition and muscle wasting, consequently leading to a decrease in functional capacity (The Rockefeller University, 2001). It is important to note that the connection between hormones and their messaging systems forms the basis for exploring chronic conditions like Cushing's syndrome. If these pathways are better understood, doctors can offer improved ways to diagnose and treat patients with this syndrome (Figure 10.18).

Test Your Knowledge

1. Name the two types of diabetes.
2. What is Cushing syndrome?

SUMMARY

When summarizing hormones and signal transduction, we should note how different signaling pathways interact with the body's responses. Hormones are responsible for passing messages between various tissues and organs, which affect numerous biological activities. The fact that these interactions are complex shows why it is important to know the molecular details of hormonal signaling. For instance, recent studies have illuminated the role of small RNAs in regulating gene expression and their interaction with phytohormones in response to environmental stressors, emphasizing how signal transduction mechanisms are not only essential for maintaining homeostasis but also for adaptation to changing conditions (Li et al., 2020). Therefore, knowing about these pathways is important for research and for creating new treatments. These hormonal pathways have effects that reach beyond biology, as they are important in the agricultural field, especially when it comes to livestock. Researchers have shown that hormonal signals play a key role in the reproductive success of dairy cattle. Variations in the expression of hormones like estradiol and progesterone demonstrate the delicate balance required for optimal fertility, which can be disrupted by stress related to increased milk production (Boer et al., 2010). Studying the ways genes are turned on and off in these processes may lead to ways to improve reproductive performance in high-producing dairy herds. Thanks to this knowledge, we can enhance livestock management and deal with matters of animal welfare and how well the animals perform. To sum up, having a thorough knowledge of the pathways of hormone action and signal transduction is necessary for both scientific and practical use. Studying these networks by combining molecular biology, genomics, and systems biology can explain their complicated interactions. Lessons learned about hormone regulation may be used to address the problems caused by changes in the environment, metabolic stresses, and health issues. Research must continue to reveal more about hormonal signaling, which will help create new ideas in areas , such as agriculture and medicine. Ultimately, this integrative perspective may lead to advancements that improve not only animal health and productivity but also human health through a better understanding of hormonal functions (Boer et al., 2010; Li et al., 2020).

Regulating the body's functions depends greatly on the connection between hormones and signal transduction. Hormones bind to certain receptors and start a series of reactions inside cells that help maintain balance in the body. These mechanisms explain the roles of endocrine signaling and also point out the importance of various transcription factors in controlling genes. For example, some recent studies have pointed out which molecular pathways are turned on by hormones, stressing the importance of receptors in regulating gene expression. They highlight that hormones play a key role in how cells interact and how the body can react to different situations. Much research has been done on how melatonin and its receptors affect the body's seasonal changes, mainly in the pars tuberalis of the pituitary gland. Since melatonin receptors are found in this region, it shows that organisms have a smart way to read light cues and control their body functions accordingly. A thorough analysis of transcriptome data has found important genes that change their activity in response to differences in photoperiod, showing how hormones help organisms adapt in different environments. Among the notable findings are changes in gene expression linked to neurogenic differentiation and cellular respiration, thereby illustrating how hormonal signals can lead to profound transcriptional changes that ultimately influence behavior and biological rhythms in response to environmental conditions (Downing et al., 2008). In addition, the Wnt signaling cascade is now recognized as a key player in hormone-related processes, mainly when it comes to tumors. For meningiomas, the way Wnt signaling and hormones interact is helping us understand what causes tumors. Even though meningiomas tend to be benign, some atypical grades can result in worse outcomes for patients. The involvement of the Wnt signaling pathway in both normal and cancerous tumors proves that hormone signaling is linked to many other important processes. This highlights the potential therapeutic implications of targeting such signaling pathways in the management of hormone-related tumors, thereby reinforcing the notion that understanding hormone signaling can pave the way for innovative treatment strategies in oncology (Kafka et al., 2016).

KEY TERMS FROM THIS CHAPTER

- Abscisic acid
- Atrial natriuretic peptide
- Dihydrotestosterone
- Estradiol
- Hormones
- Nephrotic syndrome
- Receptor binding
- Steroid hormones
- Amine hormones
- Corticotropin-releasing hormone
- Epidermal growth factor receptor
- Hormonal dysregulation
- Hypertension
- Peptide hormones
- Salicylic acid

Critical Thinking Questions

1. **Which of the following is a steroid hormone?**
   a. Insulin
   b. Glucagon
   c. Cortisol
   d. Epinephrine
2. **Which type of hormone acts via cell surface receptors?**
   a. Steroid hormones
   b. Peptide hormones
   c. Thyroid hormones
   d. None of the above
3. **Which second messenger is commonly involved in G-protein-coupled receptor (GPCR) signaling?**
   a. cAMP
   b. ATP
   c. NADH
   d. GTP
4. **Which enzyme converts ATP to cAMP in response to hormonal signaling?**
   a. Adenylate cyclase
   b. Phosphodiesterase
   c. Protein kinase A
   d. Guanylate cyclase
5. **Insulin receptor belongs to which class of receptors?**
   a. GPCR
   b. Tyrosine kinase receptor
   c. Nuclear receptor
   d. Ion channel receptor

Answers to Critical Thinking Questions

1. (c); 2. (b); 3. (a); 4. (a); 5. (b)

Short Answer Questions

1. What are hormones?
2. What is meant by signal transduction?
3. List the types of hormones.
4. What are the main mechanisms of hormone action?
5. What are the disorders caused by hormonal imbalance?

REFERENCES

1. Dzeja, P., & Terzic, A. (2009). Adenylate kinase and AMP signaling networks: metabolic monitoring, signal communication and body energy sensing. *International journal of molecular sciences, 10*(4), 1729–1772. https://doi.org/10.3390/ijms10041729 (accessed on 11th June 2025).
2. Abu-Basha, E. A. H. (2002). Arginine vasopressin-induced glucagon release: Interaction with glucose and cyclic AMP-dependent protein kinase. https://core.ac.uk/download/38896868.pdf (accessed on 11th June 2025).
3. Albrecht, C., Ardourel, M., Azcon-Aguilar, C., Balaji, B., Balestrini, R., Barker, D. G., et al. (2002). A model for the development of the rhizobia and arbuscular mycorrhizal symbioses in legumes and its use to understand the roles of ethylene in the establishment of these two symbioses. https://core.ac.uk/download/143689464.pdf (accessed on 11th June 2025).
4. Anthony, A., Avruch, J., Baird, A., Barber, B., Beugnet, B., Bhasin, B., et al. (2011). Dihydrotestosterone stimulates amino acid uptake and the expression of LAT2 in mouse skeletal muscle fibers through an ERK1/2-dependent mechanism. https://core.ac.uk/download/2780579.pdf (accessed on 11th June 2025).
5. Arend, M., Bhalerao, R. P., Boerjan, W., et al. (2007). A molecular timetable for apical bud formation and dormancy induction in poplar. https://core.ac.uk/download/55749974.pdf (accessed on 11th June 2025).
6. Armando, N. G., Dos Santos Claro, P. A., Inda, M. C., et al. (2017). Endocrinology and the brain: Corticotropin-releasing hormone signaling. https://core.ac.uk/download/159287854.pdf (accessed on 11th June 2025).
7. Audenaert, K., De Vleesschauwer, D., Höfte, M., et al. (2013). Abscisic acid promotes susceptibility to the rice leaf blight pathogen *Xanthomonas oryzae* pv. *oryzae* by suppressing salicylic acid-mediated defenses. https://core.ac.uk/download/55844481.pdf (accessed on 11th June 2025).
8. Baarendse, P. J. J., van den Brand, H., Bruggeman, V., et al. (2008). Involvement of the hypothalamic-pituitary-thyroid axis and its interaction with the hypothalamic-pituitary-adrenal axis in the ontogeny of avian thermoregulation: A review. https://core.ac.uk/download/pdf/29259797.pdf (accessed on 11th June 2025).
9. Bailey, M. A., Cairns, C., Dunbar, D. R., et al. (2017). Transcription controls growth, cell kinetics and cholesterol supply to sustain ACTH responses. https://core.ac.uk/download/322479940.pdf (accessed on 11th June 2025).
10. Boer, H. M., Veerkamp, R. F., Beerda, B., & Woelders, H. (2010). Estrous behavior in dairy cows: identification of underlying mechanisms and gene functions. *Animal : an international journal of animal bioscience, 4*(3), 446–453. https://doi.org/10.1017/S1751731109991169(accessed on 11th June 2025).
11. Biebermann, H., Cerdá-Reverter, J. M., Heyder, N., et al. (2019). Signal transduction and pathogenic modifications at the melanocortin-4 receptor: A structural perspective. https://core.ac.uk/download/227044276.pdf (accessed on 11th June 2025).
12. Bordería, A., Carrió Seguí, Á., Moreno Mariño, J., et al. (2015). Temporal aspects of copper

homeostasis and its crosstalk with hormones. https://core.ac.uk/download/71061292.pdf (accessed on 11th June 2025).

13. Bouzayen, M., Latché, A., Nath, P., et al. (2010). Mechanism of fruit ripening–Chapter 16. https://core.ac.uk/download/12042368.pdf (accessed on 11th June 2025).
14. Brucker, C., Downing, J. E. G., Head, G. M., et al. (1999). Rapid progesterone actions on thymulin-secreting epithelial cells cultured from rat thymus. https://core.ac.uk/download/16432465.pdf (accessed on 11th June 2025).
15. Choi, M. R., Della Penna, S. L., Fernandez, B. E., et al. (2014). Signaling pathways involved in renal oxidative injury: Role of the vasoactive peptides and the renal dopaminergic system. https://core.ac.uk/download/287882998.pdf (accessed on 11th June 2025).
16. Costanzo, A., & Keast, R. (2015). Is fat the sixth taste primary? Evidence and implications. https://core.ac.uk/download/pdf/30672828.pdf (accessed on 11th June 2025).
17. Gaspar, T., Kevers, C., Faivre-Rampant, O. *et al.* Changing concepts in plant hormone action. *In Vitro Cell.Dev.Biol.-Plant* **39**, 85–106 (2003). https://doi.org/10.1079/IVP2002393 (accessed on 11th June 2025).
18. Downing, A., Ando, A. S. I., Loudon, A., Ashburner, B., Bae, B., Barrett, B., Bartness, et al. (2008). Identification of melatonin-regulated genes in the ovine pituitary pars tubercles, a target site for seasonal hormone control. https://core.ac.uk/download/28967234.pdf (accessed on 11th June 2025).
19. Li, T., Gonzalez, N., Inzé, D., & Dubois, M. (2020). Emerging Connections between Small RNAs and Phytohormones. *Trends in plant science, 25*(9), 912–929. https://doi.org/10.1016/j.tplants.2020.04.004(accessed on 11th June 2025).
20. Eckardt, K. U., & Sievers, L. K. (2019). Molecular mechanisms of kidney injury and repair in arterial hypertension. https://core.ac.uk/download/222574030.pdf (accessed on 11th June 2025).
21. Freamat, M., & Sower, S. A. (2010). Functional divergence of glycoprotein hormone receptors. https://core.ac.uk/download/72049573.pdf (accessed on 11th June 2025).
22. Furman, B., Ong, W. K., & Pyne, N. J. (2010). Cyclic AMP signaling in pancreatic islets. https://core.ac.uk/download/9028568.pdf (accessed on 11th June 2025).
23. Habermann, P., Kurrle, R., Müller, G., et al. (2010). *In vitro* metabolic and mitogenic signaling of insulin glargine and its metabolites. https://core.ac.uk/download/pdf/8384842.pdf (accessed on 11th June 2025).
24. Himi, T., Kojima, T., Sawada, N., et al. (2014). Role of tight junctions in signal transduction: An update. https://core.ac.uk/download/46915996.pdf (accessed on 11th June 2025).
25. Jahn, G. A., Neira, F. J., Pennacchio, G. E., et al. (2017). Effect of hyperthyroidism on circulating prolactin and hypothalamic expression of tyrosine hydroxylase, prolactin signaling cascade members and estrogen and progesterone receptors during late pregnancy and lactation in the rat. https://core.ac.uk/download/159296141.pdf (accessed on 11th June 2025).
26. Jurca, E. M. (2011). Characterization of ROP GTPase-activated *Arabidopsis* receptor-like cytoplasmic kinases (RLCK class VI_A). https://core.ac.uk/download/11979555.pdf (accessed on 11th June 2025).

27. Kafka, A., Lechpammer, M., & Pećina-Šlaus, N. (2016). Molecular genetics of intracranial meningiomas with emphasis on canonical Wnt signaling. https://core.ac.uk/download/323071291.pdf (accessed on 11th June 2025).

28. Klingenspor, M. (Dr.), & Tups, A. (2005). Molecular and neuroendocrine determinants of seasonal body weight regulation. https://core.ac.uk/download/147498111.pdf (accessed on 11th June 2025).

29. Lee, B. (1995). Characterization of a rat clonal [beta]-cell line, RINm5F, in a passage- and morphology-dependent manner. https://core.ac.uk/download/38903386.pdf (accessed on 11th June 2025).

30. Madanu, S. (2012). The acute responses of different-sized coronary arteries to testosterone. https://core.ac.uk/download/10683771.pdf (accessed on 11th June 2025).

31. Mattila, E. (2009). Negative regulation of receptor tyrosine kinases by T-cell protein tyrosine phosphatase. https://core.ac.uk/download/197988803.pdf (accessed on 11th June 2025).

32. Mege, J. L., & Mezouar, S. (2018). Gene expression profiling of placenta from normal to pathological pregnancies. https://core.ac.uk/download/322439207.pdf (accessed on 11th June 2025).

33. Phillips, A., & Phillips, S. (2015). Recognising female sexual dysfunction as an essential aspect of effective diabetes care. *Applied nursing research : ANR*, *28*(3), 235–238. https://doi.org/10.1016/j.apnr.2015.04.007 (accessed on 11th June 2025).

34. Ząbczyńska, M., Kozłowska, K., & Pocheć, E. (2018). Glycosylation in the Thyroid Gland: Vital Aspects of Glycoprotein Function in Thyrocyte Physiology and Thyroid Disorders. *International journal of molecular sciences*, *19*(9), 2792. https://doi.org/10.3390/ijms19092792 (accessed on 11th June 2025).

35. Regad, T. (2015). Targeting RTK signaling pathways in cancer. https://core.ac.uk/download/30626046.pdf (accessed on 11th June 2025).

36. Ribeiro, A. L., Silva, A. P., Bacchetta, B., Bernheim, D., Block, D., Daya, D., et al. (2020). FGF23-klotho axis as predictive factors of fractures in type 2 diabetics with early chronic kidney disease. https://core.ac.uk/download/288958484.pdf (accessed on 11th June 2025).

37. The Rockefeller University, "Jeffrey Friedman, 2000" (2001). *Harvey Society Lectures*. 58. https://digitalcommons.rockefeller.edu/harvey-lectures/58(accessed on 11th June 2025).

38. Tups, A. (2005). Molecular and neuroendocrine determinants of seasonal body weight regulation. https://core.ac.uk/download/161970763.pdf (accessed on 11th June 2025).

39. Webster, C. M. (2019). The effects of neurosteroids such as pregnenolone sulfate and its receptor, TrpM3 in the retina. https://core.ac.uk/download/287621886.pdf (accessed on 11th June 2025).

40. Young, W. (2000). Development and application of a bioassay for follicle-stimulating hormone: A thesis presented in partial fulfilment of the requirements for the degree of Master of Science in Physiology at Massey University. https://core.ac.uk/download/148645237.pdf (accessed on 11th June 2025).

MOLECULAR BIOLOGY

11

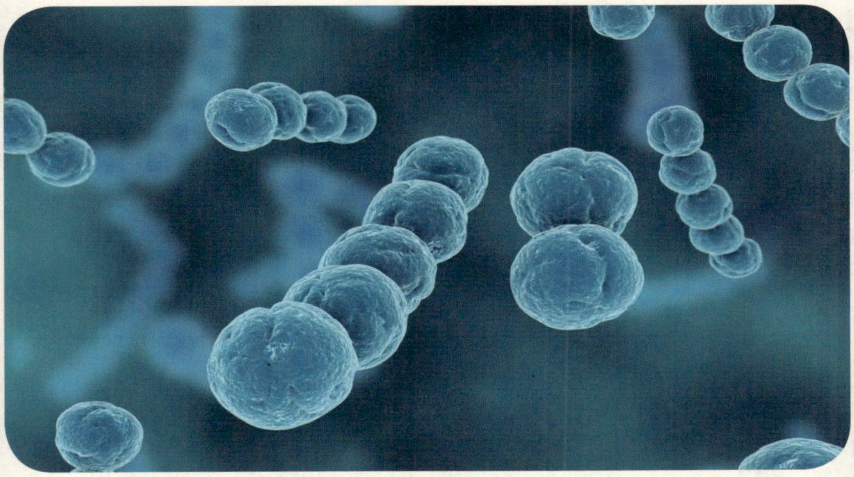

LEARNING OBJECTIVES

After studying this chapter, you will be able to:

1. Describe the structure of DNA;
2. Know the DNA replication;
3. Understand the gene expression;
4. Know the molecular techniques;
5. Describe the protein structure and function;
6. Describe the applications of molecular biology.

Introduction

Molecular biology acts as an important base for learning about the detailed processes in living organisms. Molecular biology looks at how DNA, RNA, and proteins work together to support cellular functions and the passing down of traits from one generation to another. Exploring the interactions between molecules in biology allows molecular biology to connect biology and chemistry, making it easier for students to grasp complicated concepts in an orderly way. According to recent updates in undergraduate science courses, there is now a bigger focus on combining ideas from several scientific fields. They ensure that students gain general scientific skills, which helps them see biological systems from a broader perspective. In this context, molecular biology emerges not merely as an isolated study but as a pivotal area enriched by concepts from physics and chemistry, highlighting the interconnectedness of scientific knowledge (Redish et al., 2014). In molecular biology, experiments help scientists study the many activities that happen at the molecular level. As researchers advance in their understanding of molecular interactions, they often employ exploratory experimentation (EE) to investigate hypotheses that may not yet be well-defined. This way of working helps scientists discover new things and improve current theories by carefully studying molecules. As an example, nanotoxicology shows how researchers use data science to detect and study new patterns in biology. New methods in instrumentation and data analysis help to design exploratory research for studying the complicated actions of molecules. Through this lens, molecular biology not only benefits from established theories but also contributes to shaping them as new experimental strategies emerge (Elliott et al., 2008). Also, molecular biology is important for both research and practical applications in biotechnology, medicine, and environmental science.

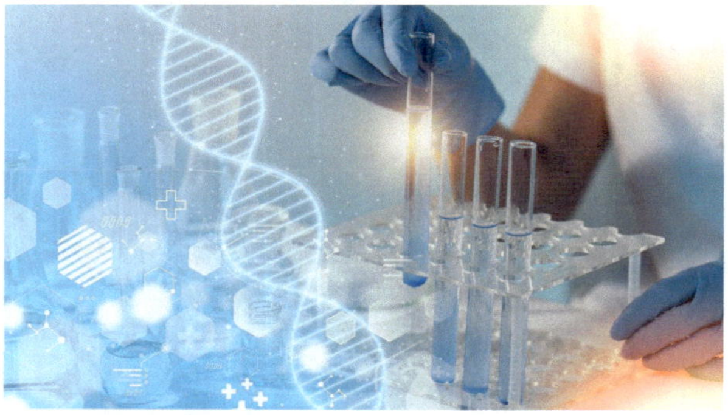

Figure 11.1. Molecular biology.

Source: https://th-i.thgim.com/public/incoming/e1qme/article67644717.ece/alternates/FREE_1200/25EPBS_MOLECULAR%20BIOLOGY.jpg.

When molecular techniques improve, they create new options for dealing with modern problems, for example, curing diseases and supporting sustainable farming. For instance, changing genetic information has resulted in gene therapy, which may be used to fix genetic disorders at the molecular level. Understanding the actions of molecules has greatly helped in the development of drugs that boost treatment results and cause fewer side effects. Molecular biology is still a key area in science because it helps to solve both present and future problems in society. When students study this area, they learn science as well as how to develop new ideas and provide answers to major global problems (Figure 11.1).

Definition and Scope of Molecular Biology

Molecular biology mainly examines the biochemical activities that control how cells work. It studies the connections between DNA, RNA, and proteins to learn how they manage the workings of living organisms. Molecular biology looks into many topics, , such as gene expression, how DNA replicates, and how cellular activities are regulated. Investigators advance their studies by using genetics and biochemistry, which helps to form a wider field that improves our knowledge of life on the molecular level. For this reason, molecular biology goes beyond old boundaries, helping us understand both simple biological activities and complicated systems in cells. Nowadays, using computational tools is a key part of molecular biology, changing the ways research is done. Because of new computational methods, scientists can now build and simulate detailed models of biological processes, helping them learn more about how molecules interact. Thanks to bioinformatics, researchers are able to analyze huge amounts of data from genomic and proteomic studies, which helps them study how genes and proteins are linked and what functions they have. What's more, programming languages, mainly Python, are now important for researchers, helping them to work with and analyze biological data. Such computational advances signify a paradigm shift in molecular biology, where the synthesis of biology and computational technology leads to new discoveries and insights into the molecular basis of life (Ekmekci et al., 2016). Moreover, molecular biology also plays a role in systems biology, as the main aim is to study biological systems as complete systems with the help of computer models. This way of modeling uses both organizational and semantic knowledge to clearly explain how biological processes happen. Ontologies are important here since they help arrange biological knowledge and support the exchange of data among various research areas. For example, the systems biology ontology (SBO) categorizes components of biological models, while the kinetic simulation algorithm ontology (KiSAO) details the algorithms used for simulating these models. This semantic layer enriches the analysis of biological datasets and enables the effective reuse of models, thus enhancing the longevity and utility of research findings (Courtot et al., 2011). With these approaches, molecular biology studies basic biology and also explores tough questions that involve several areas of biology (Figure 11.2).

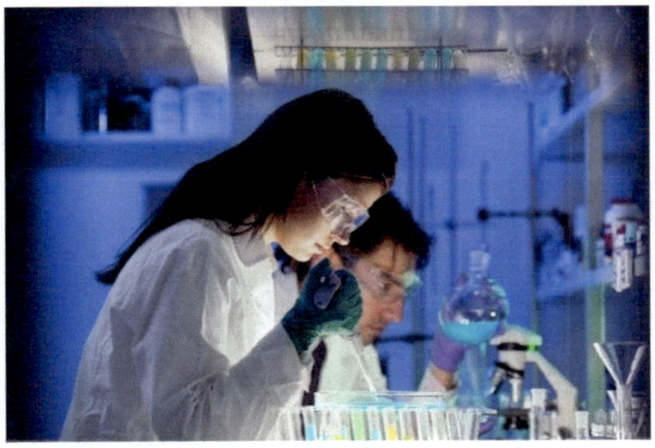

Figure 11.2. Scientists conducting molecular biology research in a laboratory setting.

Source: https://career-advice.jobs.ac.uk/wp-content/uploads/Molecular-Biology-Jobs-Profile.jpg.optimal.jpg.

Importance of Molecular Biology in Modern Science

Molecular biology plays a key role in today's science, helping us understand the basics of life. Molecular biology makes it possible to outline the complex steps involved in biological processes. It is necessary to do this mapping so that researchers can understand the molecular reasons behind diseases. Because of decoding cancer genetics, doctors can now provide treatment based on a patient's own genetic information. In addition, the findings from molecular biology are useful in agriculture and environmental science, proving how it impacts many scientific fields. Understanding how cells work at the molecular level is very important for progress in many applied fields, including biotechnology. New Zealand is one country that is strongly promoting its biotechnology industry by using its well-known agricultural resources. The government is interested in supporting innovation by using biotechnology to raise productivity and sustainability in dairy and horticulture. They are designed to help New Zealand's economy and also to make sure the country is recognized in the global biotechnology market. As molecular biology continues to drive advancements in these fields, it reinforces the importance of nurturing interdisciplinary collaboration that can spur further innovations and address contemporary challenges in agriculture and environmental stewardship (Marsh et al., 2000). Besides its importance to the economy, molecular biology has a major impact on evolution and how we see biodiversity. New ideas in evolutionary biology are now using a lot of genomic data to study how organisms adjust to their surroundings. When researchers use both molecular and cellular biology and organismic and evolutionary ideas, they can create more detailed models about evolution. By using this approach, we can see how both species and their genes help organisms to survive and thrive in different environments. Ultimately, the fusion of molecular biology with evolutionary studies highlights its essential role in unlocking the complexities of life, particularly in the context of rapid environmental changes (Arnold et al., 2013).

11.1. Structure of DNA

Learning Outcome

1. Know the double helix model and its significance;
2. Understand the nucleotide composition and base pairing;
3 Describe the chromatin structure and organization.

Because of its double helix structure, DNA is important in genetics and is both beautiful and complex. The structure has two long strands of nucleotides that are twisted together, like a ladder. Each nucleotide is composed of a phosphate group, a sugar molecule (deoxyribose), and a nitrogenous base. The nitrogenous bases, adenine, thymine, guanine, and cytosine, pair specifically (adenine with thymine and guanine with cytosine) through hydrogen bonds. It is important for replication of DNA during cell division because it helps pass on the genetic information correctly to the next generation. The special helical form of DNA gives it stability and also helps it work with proteins during transcription and translation. Analyzing genomes using computers in molecular biology depends greatly on knowing the structure of DNAs. For instance, matching DNA sequences is a basic way to understand how they are connected and plays a role in phylogenetics and evolutionary sciences. Techniques , such as those discussed by Adebiyi et al. (2009) highlight the importance of optimizing alignment, using metrics that evaluate sequence similarity to infer evolutionary relationships. Nevertheless, when the number or length of sequences rises, it takes much more time to find the best alignment. This is where methodologies , such as genetic algorithms (GAs) prove invaluable, leveraging random search strategies to enhance the efficiency of sequence alignment without sacrificing accuracy. Additionally, improvements in computational modeling have revealed how DNA's structure can be predicted, mainly when it comes to RNA arrangements and interactions. The research discussed by Drellich et al. (2016) exemplifies the significance of parametric analysis in optimizing DNA sequence alignment and RNA secondary structure prediction. Using geometric combinatorics and making models for these complex biological structures, scientists gain a detailed knowledge of how sequence variations impact the structure and function of these molecules. It is especially crucial to understand how RNA folds since this determines its ability to do important tasks in the cell. While molecular biology develops, the study of DNA's structure is still important, helping to unite theories with practical uses in genetics and biotechnology (Figure 11.3).

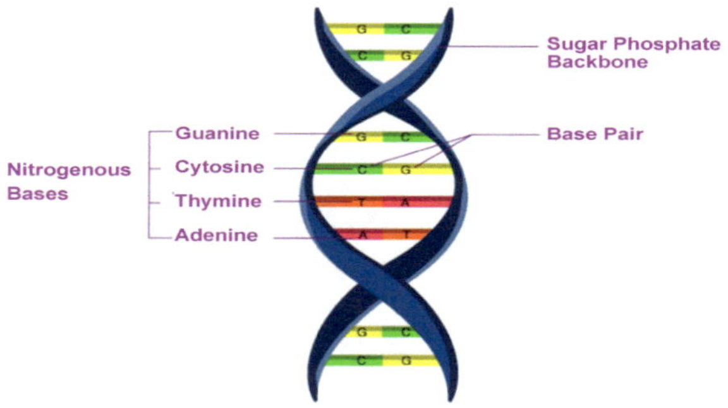

Figure 11.3. DNA diagram representing the DNA structure.

Source: https://cdn1.byjus.com/wp-content/uploads/2023/07/DNA-Structure-Updated-1.png.

11.1.1. Double Helix Model and Its Significance

The structure of DNA as a double helix, suggested by James Watson and Francis Crick in 1953, greatly contributed to the field of molecular biology by explaining the way genetic material works. The model illustrates that the two strands of nucleotides are arranged in an antiparallel way and are held by complementary pairing of adenine-thymine and guanine-cytosine. The double helix stands out for its neat structure and also for what it means for the replication and passing down of DNA. With the model, it is easier to see how nucleotide sequences store information and how this information becomes visible in the traits of an organism. Besides, this important discovery made it possible for genetic engineering and biotechnology to progress, which transformed our views on heredity and evolution. The double helix is also important in genomics, since sequencing and studying genomes are now central tasks in molecular biology. Because of its helical shape, DNA can be studied by researchers to predict how genes function, to understand how genes are controlled, and to detect genetic mutations that cause different diseases.

For example, learning about the structure of chromatin and the part played by proteins in its remodeling is possible because of the knowledge of the double helix. Analysis of recent studies points out that structural motifs in chromatin-associated proteins have similar network patterns as the ones seen in protein contact maps. Such findings, as documented in research on structural characterization and protein interactions, further underscore the relevance of the double helix in understanding gene expression and protein synthesis (Schreiber et al., 2008). Besides, the information gained from the double helix model has greatly influenced medical research, mainly in genetics. After the discovery of the DNA structure, scientists found out about Chd1 and other similar complexes that help control gene activity by organizing nucleosomes. The intricate interactions between chromatin-binding proteins and DNA underscore the biological significance of the double helix, particularly in the context of chromatin dynamics and epigenetic modifications (Ryan et al., 2011). It is clear from this that the double helix model is important for designing therapies for genetic diseases. As scientists learn more, the double helix keeps playing a key role in explaining the details of molecular biology and its usefulness in medicine and biotechnology (Figure 11.4).

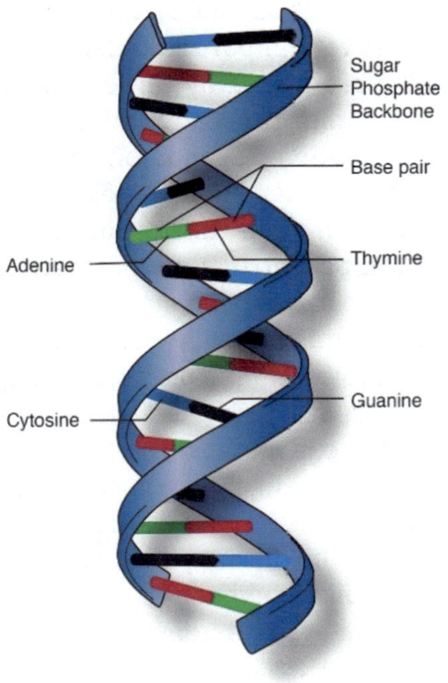

Figure 11.4. Double helix.

Source: https://cdn.storymd.com/optimized/ZoBxNMIvqM/original.jpg.

11.1.2. Nucleotide Composition and Base Pairing

The way nucleotides are arranged in DNA and RNA is important in molecular biology and affects many cellular activities , such as replicating DNA and making RNA. The four nucleotides—adenine (A), thymine (T), cytosine (C), and guanine (G)—compose the genetic material, each playing a crucial role in the fidelity of genetic information transfer. The numbers of these nucleotides are influenced by evolution and the environment, mainly in prokaryotes that live in harsh environments. Research indicates that variations in nucleotide compositions, particularly an increase in purine load (A+G content), correlate with optimal growth temperatures, emphasizing the relationship between environmental adaptation and nucleotide diversity. Through comprehensive analysis, the interplay between nucleotide composition and organismal adaptation elucidates the mechanisms by which life forms optimize their genetic material to endure fluctuating conditions, thereby furthering our understanding of evolutionary biology (Eugene et al., 2005). For the stability and integrity of nucleic acids, base pairing between nucleotides is very important. Adenine and thymine are paired by two hydrogen bonds, and cytosine and guanine are paired by three. This particular combination preserves the double helix of DNA, which allows both replication and transcription to work well. The right and accurate transfer of genetic information depends on the strong and particular way base pairs interact. Studies done lately point out that changes in nucleotide sequences can alter the frequency and stability of base pairing, which in turn influences the overall stability of the molecule. For instance, in viral genomes, compact structures promote efficient encapsulation, with a high density of base pairing fostering compactness and stability during assembly (Ben-Shaul et al., 2014). The way nucleotides are arranged and how they pair shows the essential workings behind the stability and evolution of genetic information. Apart from helping with structure, the nucleotide arrangement in DNA and the way bases pair is essential for controlling gene expression. Having particular nucleotide sequences can change how tightly transcription factors stick to DNA and how easy it is for them to reach the DNA during transcription. Also, differences in the amount of certain bases in DNA can result in biased use of codons, which may change how efficiently genes are expressed. As an illustration, in thermophilic organisms, having more A+G in their mRNA and proteins helps them work well at higher temperatures, as is shown by the relationship between the nucleotide composition and growth temperature. Understanding these relationships provides insight into how organisms adapt at the molecular level, enhancing our comprehension of molecular biology and evolutionary processes (Eugene et al., 2005) (Figure 11.5).

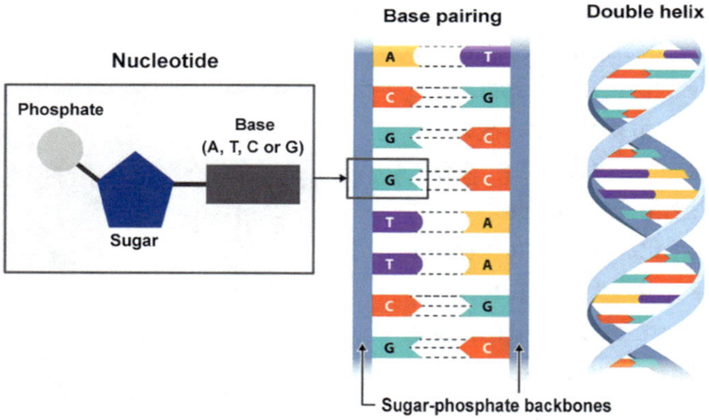

Figure 11.5. Nucleotide composition and base pairing.

Source: https://images.my.labster.com/v2/NAP/4963af1e-a76c-4f7f-b2ff-90f7b8d0a349/NAP_DNAStructure.en.x1024.png.

11.1.3. Chromatin Structure and Organization

The structure of chromatin is important for controlling gene expression and for the proper working of eukaryotic cells. DNA is wrapped around histone proteins to make chromatin, and this forms nucleosomes that look like beads on a string. Besides storing the DNA securely inside the nucleus, this structure is also important for deciding whether DNA can be accessed for transcription. By interacting with nucleosomes, chromatin remodeling complexes are able to change their positions or features, which affects how genes are expressed. The recent progress in molecular biology has pointed out that how chromatin is organized can regulate genes and, as a result, impact how cells respond to different signals and changes in the environment. Understanding these dynamics provides a glimpse into the intricate regulatory networks that underpin cellular identity and function (Bowater et al., 2012). At the molecular level, chromatin remodeling complexes, , such as the RSC (Remodeling the Structure of Chromatin) complex, are pivotal in modifying chromatin architecture. In *Saccharomyces cerevisiae*, the RSC complex is mainly explored to demonstrate how chromatin dynamics are controlled. Thanks to cryo-electron microscopy and crosslinking mass spectrometry, researchers have figured out that RSC has a firm central part and flexible arms that assist in binding to nucleosomes. This dual structure enables RSC to engage directly with both the histones and the DNA of nucleosomes, facilitating their remodeling and ultimately impacting transcription and DNA repair processes (Afonine et al., 2019). The way chromatin remodeling complexes are built at the molecular level shows that chromatin organization is both conserved and important for all species. Learning about chromatin structure and how it is organized affects health and disease a lot. Problems with chromatin remodeling can result in a range of disorders, and cancers are among them, since gene expression may become dysregulated. A disturbance in chromatin modifications can cause oncogenes to be activated or tumor suppressor genes to be turned off. For this reason, research in molecular biology should continue to find links between how chromatin works and the development of diseases. Understanding these relationships well helps scientists develop treatments that may affect chromatin-remodeling pathways to return gene function and cellular processes to normal levels. This promising avenue of research underscores the importance of chromatin structure not only in fundamental biology but also in the context of medical advancements (Bowater et al., 2012) (Figure 11.6).

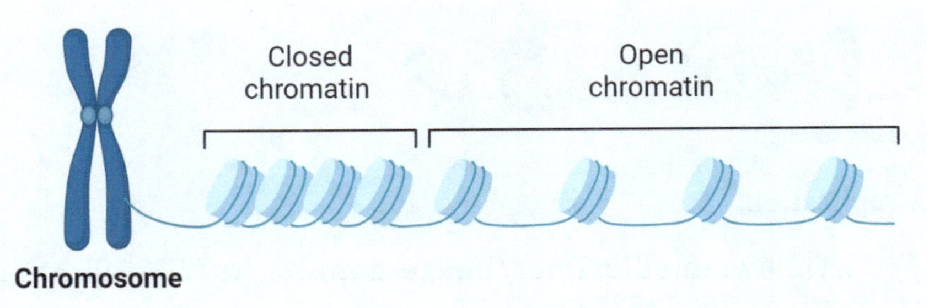

Figure 11.6. Chromatin.

Source: https://microbenotes.com/wp-content/uploads/2022/06/Chromatin.jpeg.

Test Your Knowledge

1. Who proposed the double helix model of DNA?
2. What are the four types of nucleotides?

11.2. DNA Replication

Learning Outcome

1. Understand the mechanisms of DNA replication;
2. Describe the role of enzymes in replication;
3. Understand the importance of fidelity and error correction.

The process of DNA replication is necessary for cell division to make sure the genetic material is passed correctly from parents to their offspring. It is at origins of replication on the DNA molecule that this process starts. With the strands of DNA unwinding, enzymes called DNA polymerases are able to produce new strands that match the original template. For the genetic material to stay intact, the original and the new strand must interact. Any disruption in this process can cause genomic instability, and this may increase the risk of cancer. Recent studies suggest that the formation of DNA-RNA hybrids during replication might serve as a significant source of genomic instability, complicating the fidelity of DNA replication and contributing to the pathology of various genetic disorders, underscoring the necessity of understanding the nuances of DNA dynamics in molecular biology (García-Rubioet al., 2017).

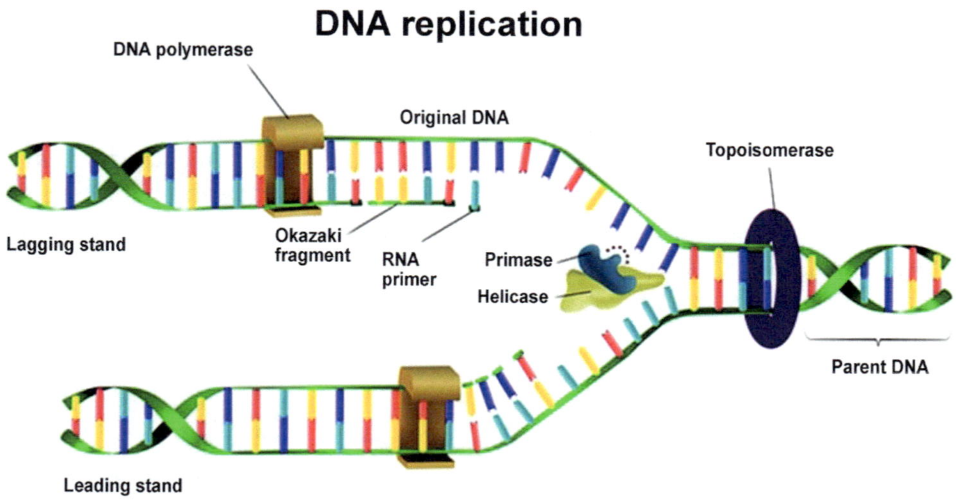

Figure 11.7. DNA replication.

Source: https://www.news-medical.net/image-handler/ts/20170531115530/ri/673/picture/2017/5/shutterstock_201778373.jpg.

Understanding how plasmid DNA is replicated adds more knowledge to molecular biology, especially in the fields of microbial genetics and biotechnology. Plasmids are DNA molecules that can replicate by themselves, and they usually contain genes that are not vital but can be helpful. Their methods of starting replication show how they are regulated in different environments, which is important for both nature and laboratory studies. Because plasmids react differently to stress inside the host, learning about their replication can make protein production more efficient. Research into the role of environmental factors in plasmid replication explains how cells can change and how this affects the regulation of genes.

Consequently, the knowledge gained from studying plasmid replication mechanisms not only advances basic molecular biology but also informs biotechnological practices, enhancing the utility of plasmids as expression vectors in genetic engineering (Wegrzyn & Wegrzyn, 2002). It is important to look at how different biological processes work together to understand DNA replication. It was mentioned earlier that the presence of DNA-RNA hybrids during replication proves how various mechanisms collaborate to maintain genome stability. Having these hybrids suggests that the cell's replication and transcription processes are not working properly, which may cause cell dysfunction. Nowadays, researchers can use DNA-RNA immunoprecipitation to properly identify and analyze the roles of these hybrids in cells. For this reason, studying how DNA replication happens means looking at the networks that handle and respond to different challenges in the genome. This multifaceted approach fosters a deeper comprehension of genetic fidelity and highlights the consequences of replication fidelity disruptions in the broader context of human health and disease (García-Rubio et al., 2017) (Figure 11.7).

11.2.1. Mechanisms of DNA Replication

For all living cells, DNA replication is key because it guarantees the accurate copying of genetic material before division. At certain places in the genome called origins of replication, proteins gather to make the pre-replicative complex. The complex consists of important enzymes, helicases that unravel the double helix, and polymerases that build new strands that match the original DNA. To avoid changes in the genome that may lead to diseases, especially cancer, the replication process must be accurate as it continues.

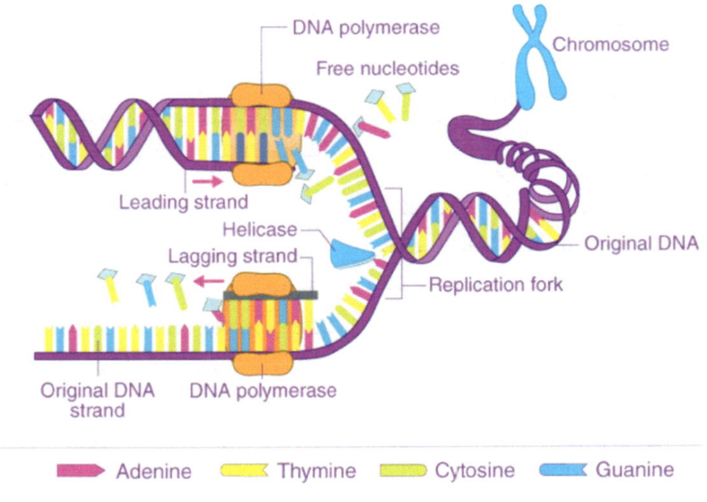

Figure 11.8. DNA replication process.

Source: https://cdn1.byjus.com/wp-content/uploads/2023/07/DNA-Replication-Process-Machinery-And-Enzymes-Updated-2.png.

Notably, DNA replication is not merely a mechanical process; rather, it embodies a highly regulated series of interactions that accommodate the structural complexities of chromatin and the presence of obstacles in the DNA template, , such as DNA-RNA hybrids, which may arise during transcription and replication (García-Rubio et al., 2017). Knowing how DNA replication happens is important since it forms the basis for understanding how cells respond to things that can disrupt DNA synthesis. For example, if DNA gets damaged, it creates a serious problem when it comes to replicating the DNA. Cells have developed ways to fix the problems they encounter. Lately, using single-molecule techniques, scientists have discovered that DNA replication is not always the same, and sometimes it can vary at the single molecule level. These insights underscore the complexity of replication as it navigates obstacles including bound proteins and chemical lesions, enhancing our grasp of how cells maintain genomic integrity in the face of adversity (Mueller et al., 2022). Also, new tools in molecular biology now enable scientists to investigate specific steps in replication with greater accuracy. By using single-molecule observation, scientists can study the role of distinct protein interactions and momentary changes in how well and accurately DNA is copied. Such advanced techniques have made it clear that DNA-RNA hybrids can either help or disrupt the normal replication process. Since these hybrids take part in transcription and replication, it is important to consider both these processes when studying molecular mechanisms. Consequently, studying these phenomena is critical for elucidating the underlying causes of genome instability and its implications in cancer and genetic disorders, ultimately enhancing our overarching understanding of molecular biology (García-Rubio et al., 2017) (Figure 11.8).

11.2.2. Role of Enzymes in Replication

The process of DNA replication depends on the careful actions of many enzymes to guarantee the correct copying of DNA. DNA polymerases, as well as other enzymes, are important in this process because they make new DNA strands by adding nucleotides that match the template strand. They act together to tackle issues , such as unwrapping the double helix and making supercoils, which might block the replication process. If these enzymes did not work, the process of sharing genetic information in cell division would be very unreliable and could cause many errors and mutations. Because enzymes are so precise, cell replication is successful and maintains the stability of the genome from one generation to another. As well as DNA polymerases, other important enzymes take part in the replication process. Helicases are important because they untangle the double-stranded DNA, which makes it possible for replication forks to appear and for the template strands to be reached. At the same time, single-strand binding proteins secure the open sections, so that DNA replication can occur without interference. Topoisomerases help by reducing the tension in front of the replication fork, which allows the process to proceed smoothly. How these enzymes work together demonstrates the complexity of the interactions needed for DNA replication and the division of chromosomes. Besides, problems with enzymes that support replication can seriously affect cell health and may make a cell more likely to develop cancer. For instance, when topoisomerases are not working correctly, sister chromatids may be tangled and the problem could last into mitosis. Such effects are associated with the development of chromosomal instability, which is a common feature of cancer. Additionally, as discussed in recent reviews, the metabolic pathways influenced by viral infections can also alter enzyme functionality, further complicating the landscape of replication fidelity and genomic integrity (Thaker et al., 2019). These insights emphasize that understanding the role of enzymes not only aids in the comprehension of basic cellular mechanisms but also highlights potential avenues for therapeutic intervention in diseases linked to replication errors, including cancer (Bartkova et al., 2014) (Figure 11.9).

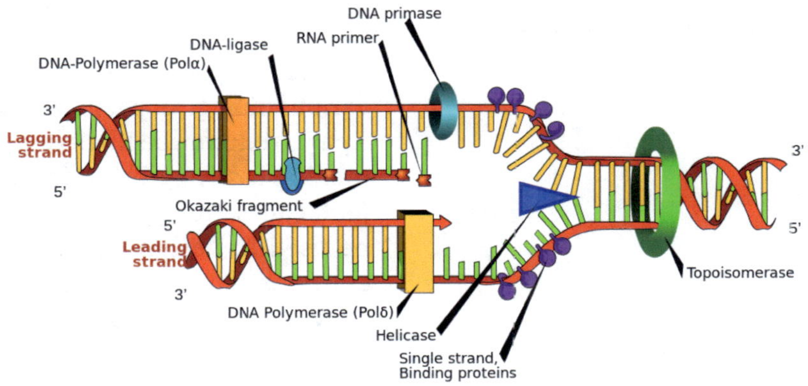

Figure 11.9. The enzymes of DNA replication.

Source: https://us-west-1.cdn.h5p.com/orgs/1290469721304332918/organization/content/1291213467038110188/images/file-601315d7cf78c.png.

11.2.3. Importance of Fidelity and Error Correction

The correctness of nucleic acid synthesis is very important for the protection of genetic information in molecular biology. Fidelity is the measure of how well DNA and RNA polymerases make nucleic acids. Errors that happen during replication and result in mutations may lead to genetic diseases or cancer. It is clear that error correction steps , such as proofreading are very important in DNA replication. They allow for finding and deleting wrong nucleotides, making sure that the final DNA is similar to the original template. Thus, maintaining a high level of fidelity is essential for preserving the stability of the genome and facilitating accurate protein synthesis, which is critical for cellular function and organismal development (Chowdhury et al., 2012). Besides proofreading, error correction involves the interaction of many molecules that help cells respond to changes. As an illustration, mismatch repair systems correct errors that happen after replication, making DNA replication more accurate. Research has shown that the destabilization of error correction complexes can lead to an increase in mutator strains, which, paradoxically, can enhance adaptation under certain stress conditions (Giraud et al., 2009). It demonstrates that sometimes, a slight decrease in accuracy in DNA copying can help produce mutations that give an advantage. The need to both adapts and stay true to their genes demonstrates a key issue in evolutionary biology. Fidelity and error correction are important in molecular biology and also affect therapeutic interventions and biotechnology. As an illustration, knowing how to correct errors can guide the development of CRISPR/Cas9 systems, as these tools depend on accurate targeting of DNA. In addition, researchers can use directed evolution to manipulate the error rates, which helps them increase the mutations and find new biomolecules with better functions.

Test Your Knowledge

1. What are the mechanisms of DNA replication?
2. What is the role of enzymes in replication?

11.3. Gene Expression

Learning Outcome

1. Understand the transcription process and regulation in molecular biology;
2. Describe the translation and the role of ribosomes;
3 Know the post-transcriptional modifications.

Gene expression is how genetic information is turned into proteins that perform several functions inside cells. Genes are controlled so that they are expressed correctly and in the right quantities. Promoters, enhancers, and repressors are important in controlling the process of transcription by RNA polymerase. Furthermore, the concept of expression quantitative trait loci (eQTLs) highlights the connection between genetic variation and gene expression levels. eQTLs are critical for understanding how non-coding genomic regions can influence the expression of nearby genes, thereby impacting phenotypic traits and disease susceptibility. As researchers delve into the complexities of gene regulation, they are increasingly reliant on computational systems biology approaches to analyze broad datasets and elucidate the intricate molecular networks that govern gene expression (Butte et al., 2016). New achievements in molecular biology have helped reveal the role of genes in health and disease. For example, eQTL studies help us discover the genetic factors linked to disease and also show how these variations are involved in changing the body's functions. Using omics data in large amounts, scientists are able to create gene networks and find out which interactions are essential. This knowledge is important for designing specific treatments because it helps researchers identify important points in the body's systems. Also, confirming predicted gene networks with computational methods strengthens the process of coming up with and testing new ideas. Through these innovative approaches, the field of molecular biology is progressively elucidating the dynamic relationships between gene expression and various biological phenomena (Butte et al., 2016). Apart from its use in biology, gene expression is making a strong mark in information security. Molecular biology's complex mechanisms can be used to design new security measures that are better than those used in computers. Since conventional cryptographic algorithms are being attacked more often, biological mechanisms of gene expression provide a special way to strengthen security infrastructure. Researchers are working on using biological information in information technology to see how real-time gene expression assays could boost the security of communication systems. The combination of molecular biology and information security shows how new methods can protect data and also brings together several scientific areas to deal with today's challenges (Figure 11.10).

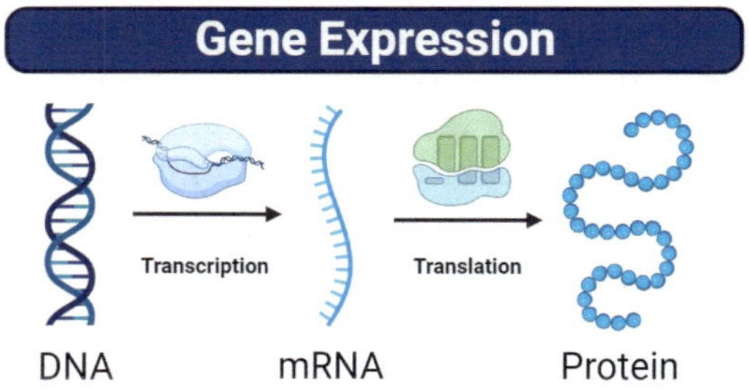

Figure 11.10. Gene expression.

Source: https://microbenotes.com/wp-content/uploads/2023/10/Gene-Expression.jpeg.

11.3.1. Transcription Process and Regulation

The creation of RNA molecules from DNA is controlled by the important process of transcription in molecular biology. The first part of this process is forming a preinitiation complex, which requires transcription factors and RNA polymerase II to go to the promoter region of the gene. While transcription goes on, RNA polymerase II attaches ribonucleotides to the DNA template, lengthening the RNA strand. The process of initiation brings together many factors to help RNA be formed accurately and efficiently. It is important to control transcription, since it enables cells to adjust how they express genes depending on what is happening around them and inside the cell. If transcription is not controlled, cells may send the wrong signals, which can lead to diseases , such as cancer or hereditary diseases, proving how important it is for transcription to keep cells healthy. When initiation and elongation are done, the process of transcription ends with the final stage of termination. When transcription ends, other processes of RNA processing start to ensure the mRNA is ready to function. Experts now believe that capping, splicing, and polyadenylation happen at the same time as transcription, so they are all part of the co-transcriptional process. Make sure that the transcript is of good quality by coupling transcription with RNA processing. If the process is interrupted, the RNA may not be exported from the nucleus or may be degraded, which stops any possible problems in the cell. The careful regulation of protein-protein interactions in cells controls the important quality control systems that help maintain the cell's health, which also affects how genes are regulated and expressed. Transcription is regulated not only at the beginning and during processing, but also by mechanisms that adjust gene expression in many ways. These two types of regulators are essential, giving a detailed control that can vary from one type of tissue to another. Enhancers help increase transcription by attaching to the promoter area, while silencers stop it from happening so there is a fine balance. Also, the activity of transcription factors that attach to these regulatory elements changes when various signaling pathways are active, which can adjust how genes are expressed in response to changes in the environment. It is important to understand how transcription regulation and cellular signaling pathways work together, since this shows how cells react to stress, differentiation, and development. Such complexities illustrate the remarkable adaptability of biological systems and the integral role of transcription regulation within the broader context of molecular biology (Hughes et al., 2019; Hidayah, 2025).

11.3.2. Translation and the Role of Ribosomes

The process of translation is a critical component of molecular biology, serving as the mechanism through which ribosomes synthesize proteins from mRNA templates. It takes place in three main stages: initiation, elongation, and termination, and every stage is carefully controlled to guarantee accuracy and efficiency. Ribosomes serve as the cellular machinery that orchestrates this complex task by providing a platform where charged transfer RNA (tRNA) molecules can match their anticodons to the codons of mRNA. Besides making proteins, ribosomes are important in regulating where and when proteins are produced within cells. As observed in studies of Caenorhabditis elegans, ribosomes can be localized to specific cellular regions, contributing to tissue-specific functions and adaptations, ultimately shaping cellular identity and response to environmental signals (Ellisman et al., 2017). Moreover, the structure of ribosomes and their functions are closely connected and can change. Recent investigations highlight the complexity of ribosomal protein (RP) composition, illustrating that ribosomes may exhibit variability in their structures based on growth conditions and the presence of mRNA during translation. It has been shown in recent studies that the stoichiometry of core RPs changes not only among different kinds of cells, for example, mouse embryonic stem cells and budding yeast, but also in response to the environment. The variety in ribosomes implies that their structure is connected to certain functions, which in turn affects how efficiently and fast proteins are produced. As ribosomes adapt to the cellular conditions, the presence or absence of specific RPs can fundamentally alter the fitness of the cell, underscoring their regulatory importance in biological systems (Slavov et al., 2014). All things considered, ribosomes are key to translation and thus play a major role in molecular biology. They work as converters, making proteins that are used in almost all cellular activities. The way ribosomes are localized and composed is controlled by regulations, which straightaway affects protein production and the health of the cell. Being aware of the many functions of ribosomes increases our understanding of basic biology and also explains how problems with translation can cause diseases , such as cancer and genetic disorders. The ongoing research into ribosomal dynamics and their implications for cellular function is crucial for developing therapeutic strategies aimed at restoring normal protein synthesis and mitigating the effects of ribosomal dysfunction on cell biology (Slavov et al., 2014; Ellisman et al., 2017) (Figure 11.11).

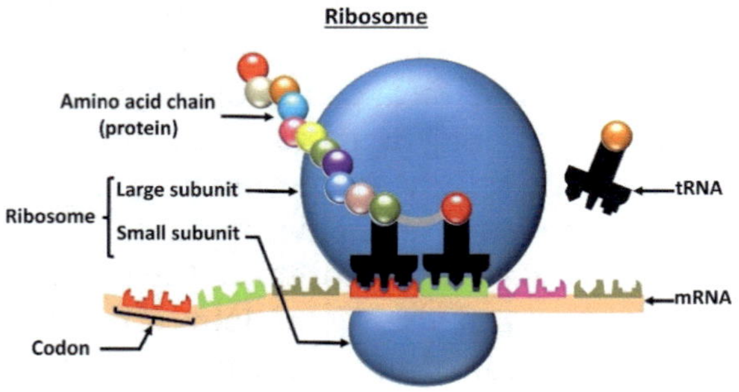

Figure 11.11. Ribosomes.

Source: https://media.beckman.com/-/media/stock-images/resource-center/images/ribosomes.jpg?rev=5ee3e98eee614975bda4fc8bd5b72747.

11.3.3. Post-Transcriptional Modifications

Gene expression is regulated precisely after transcription because of post-transcriptional modifications. These changes are adding a 5 cap, polyadenylation at the 3 ends, and splicing of introns from pre-mRNA, which together increase the stability of mRNA and allow it to be translated into proteins. The 5 end of mRNA is protected from RNase enzymes and recognized by the ribosome because of the 7-methyl guanosine cap. Adding a poly-A tail to the 3 ends of mRNA during polyadenylation makes mRNA more stable, helps it move out of the nucleus, and affects how much it is translated. These changes make sure that mRNA is ready and intact before it is translated, which improves the process of gene expression. As well as capping and polyadenylation, splicing is important for post-transcriptional regulation because it removes the introns from the pre-mRNA. Thanks to this editing, a single gene can make several protein isoforms by alternative splicing, which is needed for cells to function properly.

The splicing machinery, comprised of small nuclear ribonucleoproteins (snRNPs), recognizes specific sequences at the intron-exon boundaries to ensure accurate removal of introns and ligation of exons, which represent the coding regions of the gene. Disruptions in splicing mechanisms can lead to aberrant protein products and have been implicated in various diseases, underlining the critical importance of post-transcriptional modifications in maintaining genetic fidelity and cellular health (Bagella et al., 2013). How post-transcriptional modifications are regulated is important for understanding development, differentiation, and reactions to changes in the environment. Thanks to these changes, cells are able to respond to new conditions and keep their internal balance. In addition, problems with post-transcriptional processes have been associated with many genetic disorders and cancers, proving their importance in disease development. Epigenetic factors can also influence these modifications, as alterations in chromatin structure can impact the accessibility of genes for transcription and subsequent modifications (Bagella et al., 2013).

For this reason, studying how post-transcriptional modifications work offers new insights into molecular biology and possible treatments for diseases caused by problems in gene regulation (Figure 11.12).

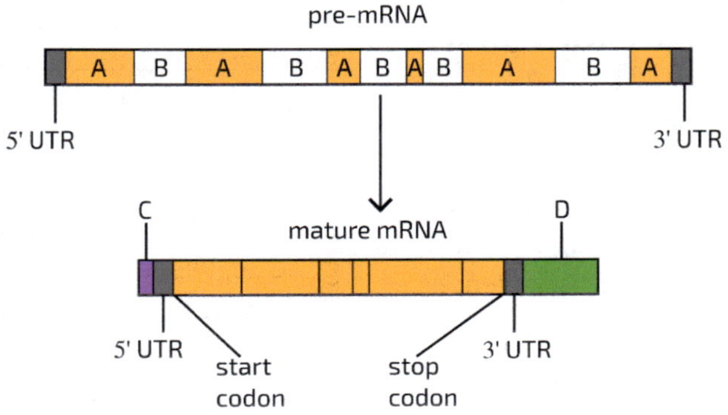

Figure 11.12. Post-transcriptional modification.

Source: https://isaacphysics.org/images/content/questions/biology/genetics/transcription/figures/Mrna_diagram.svg.

Test Your Knowledge

1. What is transcription process in molecular biology?
2. What are post-transcriptional modifications?

11.4. Molecular Techniques

Learning Outcome

1. Understand the polymerase chain reaction (PCR);
2. Know the gel electrophoresis and its applications;
3. Describe the CRISPR-Cas9 technology and gene editing.

Molecular techniques are essential for molecular biology since they help analyze, modify, and understand DNA and proteins. Such techniques allow scientists to take part in many activities, from genetic engineering to studying how cells operate. Among the most significant molecular techniques is PCR, which allows for the amplification of specific DNA sequences. This process is necessary for genetic testing, cloning, and forensic analysis since it gives enough material for further research. In addition, gel electrophoresis is used to see and separate nucleic acids by size, which is necessary for checking the outcomes of PCR and studying changes in the genes of different populations. All in all, modern biological research relies on molecular techniques, which help progress in genomics and biotechnology. Cell culture methods are also important in molecular biology since they allow controlled growth and study of cells outside the body. They make it possible for researchers to study cells and their actions in the same way, helping them learn about both healthy and unhealthy states. The first immortal cell line, HeLa cells, have played a key role in many scientific discoveries, for example, in cancer research and the making of vaccines. Cell culture techniques are also applied when studying infectious agents, as shown in studying Trypanosoma cruzi, the reason behind Chagas disease. Research utilizing cell culture provides invaluable information regarding the biology of the parasite, including responses to potential therapeutic agents, thus highlighting the vital role of molecular techniques in combating diseases and advancing medical science (Araújo et al., 2019; White et al., 2011). In addition, advanced molecular methods are applied to proteomics and metabolomics to examine proteins and metabolites inside cells. With these disciplines, it is possible to thoroughly study cellular processes and identify signs of diseases. Mass spectrometry and two-dimensional gel electrophoresis are used to study the proteome, which helps explain how proteins work and communicate with other parts of the body. Metabolomic profiling also helps explain how metabolism is affected by diseases, which might suggest new approaches for treating them. Combining these molecular methods is very important for personalized medicine since it allows treatments to be customized using a patient's biomolecular information. As a result, the combination of different molecular techniques plays a big role in helping us understand biology and create new ways to address health and disease (Figure 11.13).

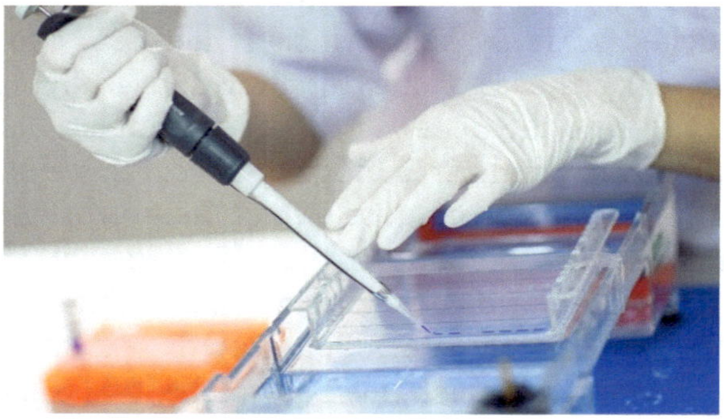

Figure 11.13. Molecular biology techniques.

Source: https://www.ncbionetwork.org/sites/default/files/styles/1280x720/public/1280x720-images/molecular-biology-techniques.jpg?itok=essPMovm.

11.4.1. Polymerase Chain Reaction (PCR)

The PCR stands as a pivotal technique within the field of molecular biology, revolutionizing how scientists analyze genetic material. PCR was invented in the 1980s and helps researchers to make millions of copies of a certain DNA sequence from just a small amount. This process is important for different uses, for example, in genetic research, forensic work, and medical diagnostics. The specificity and sensitivity in DNA detection are boosted in PCR because it relies on thermal cycling, whereas traditional methods do not. The techniques ability to target specific regions of DNA has also allowed for advancements in evolutionary biology and genetic engineering, underscoring its importance as a foundational tool in the molecular biology toolkit (Ali et al., 2022). Because PCR is now used in many areas, its influence on more than just molecular biology is more noticeable. The approach has greatly helped doctors diagnose infectious diseases and genetic disorders. PCR has allowed doctors to detect pathogens quickly, which helps them decide on the right treatment for patients. Moreover, agricultural biotechnology uses PCR to create genetically modified organisms (GMOs) that have the best traits and are more resistant and productive. The versatility of PCR exemplifies its role in addressing global challenges, from food security to public health, thereby contributing to advancements in various scientific disciplines (Dambrós et al., 2017). Also, the advancement of PCR has encouraged the growth of different types of PCR for different research purposes. Techniques , such as quantitative PCR (qPCR) enable real-time monitoring of DNA amplification, allowing for precise quantification of gene expression. Likewise, multiplex PCR allows for the amplification of several targets in a single reaction, which improves both research and clinical work. Improvements in PCR and its related techniques allow it to be used for more purposes and encourage new inventions in molecular biology. As researchers continue to refine and innovate upon this foundational method, the potential for PCR to unlock further mysteries of genetics and biology remains vast (Ali et al., 2022) (Figure 11.14).

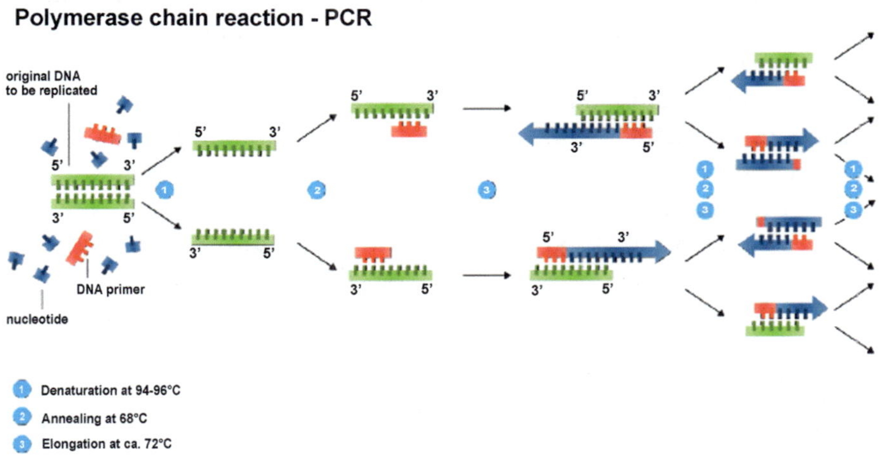

Figure 11.14. Polymerase chain reaction.

Source: https://microbeonline.com/wp-content/uploads/2016/07/Polymerase_chain_reaction.svg_.png.

11.4.2. Gel Electrophoresis and Its Applications

Separating and analyzing nucleic acids and proteins is made possible by the key technique of gel electrophoresis in molecular biology. Electric fields can be used on gel matrices with biomolecules to take advantage of the fact that molecules of different sizes and charges move differently. With this method, DNA fragments, proteins, or RNA can be precisely separated to help in their further characterization and identification. Gel electrophoresis is used in different areas like research, medical diagnostics, forensics, and biotechnology. In molecular biology, it is vital for understanding the genes of organisms and spotting genetic differences, which influences both genomics and proteomics, which depend on its clear and precise results. Gel electrophoresis is often used to study DNA for both genetic fingerprinting and diagnostics. Since this technique allows DNA fragments to be separated and seen, researchers can use it to spot genes linked to certain traits or illnesses. Thanks to DNA gel electrophoresis, Southern blotting becomes possible, making it possible to find particular sequences in a mixture. In addition, new image processing tools have made it easier to analyze the outcomes of gel electrophoresis. For example, the GELect software makes it possible to call genotypes from electrophoresis data, which speeds up analysis of many samples. This enhanced automation addresses challenges , such as lane distortion and closely migrating bands, showcasing how technology amplifies the potential of gel electrophoresis in both research and practical applications within molecular biology (Intarapanich et al., 2015). Apart from being used in nucleic acid analysis, gel electrophoresis is also important in proteomics because identifying proteins is key. With the help of two-dimensional electrophoresis, the technique separates proteins using both their isoelectric points and molecular weights. It enables scientists to find individual proteins and also learn about their interactions and modifications. Moreover, gel electrophoresis works better with immunoblotting because it helps spot particular proteins among many others. While traditional methods of protein analysis may have limitations, the advantages of gel electrophoresis in resolving complete proteins make it instrumental in advancing current and future research in proteomics (Righetti et al., 2011). Thanks to these applications, gel electrophoresis is a key technique used to study biological events and leads to progress in different areas of molecular biology (Figure 11.15).

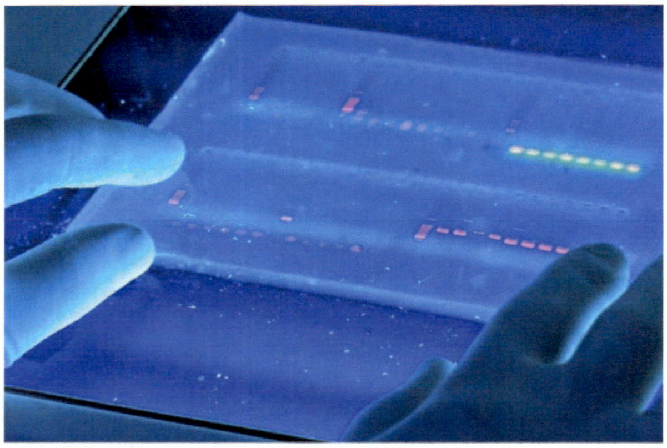

Figure 11.15. Gel electrophoresis.

Source: https://www.yourgenome.org/wp-content/uploads/2023/11/1340-Agarose_gel_with_UV_illumination_-_Ethidium_bromide_stained_DNA_glows_orange_close-up.jpg.

11.4.3. CRISPR-Cas9 Technology and Gene Editing

CRISPR-Cas9 technology has greatly changed molecular biology, mainly when it comes to gene editing. Using this method based on bacteria's immune response, scientists are able to change DNA sequences with great accuracy. Unlike before, CRISPR-Cas9 makes gene editing easier and cheaper, so more labs across the globe are using it. Specifically targeting genes helps make major progress in genetics, biomedicine, and agriculture. Besides research, CRISPR-Cas9 could be used to develop new treatments for genetic diseases and make crops more resistant to threats. Because of this, this technology changes the way we view and apply genetic manipulation in the real world. As CRISPR-Cas9 is applied more widely, it brings up important ethical issues that should be dealt with. For example, although gene editing helps address genetic problems in human embryos, it also brings up issues about the moral standing of these embryos. Editing human embryos raises difficult issues, as such procedures may not be covered by existing laws on medical malpractice since they happen at an early stage of development. The fact that laws are not clear enough points to the need for a solid ethical framework when using gene editing on people. By possibly changing our views on health and normalcy, we are also affecting the norms and values of our society. Thus, while the scientific advancements are significant, they must be balanced with a thoughtful examination of the societal responsibilities enshrined within these groundbreaking capabilities (Powell et al., 2017). Moreover, calling CRISPR-Cas9 a revolutionary technology points out that it can be used for good or bad purposes. Often, when talking about CRISPR, it is mentioned with other major inventions that have greatly influenced human abilities, for example, the Ford Model T in transportation. This way of looking at it reveals that CRISPR-Cas9 is both helpful for social progress and raises ethical questions. While those who support it point out its many benefits, those who oppose it warn about the possible risks of changing the genes of living organisms. It is important to understand CRISPR's place in society to deal with the challenges in bioethics and policymaking. Recognizing CRISPR-Cas9 as a revolutionary force necessitates that stakeholders engage in informed discussions to evaluate both its technological promise and its ethical implications (Mariscal et al., 2016) (Figure 11.16).

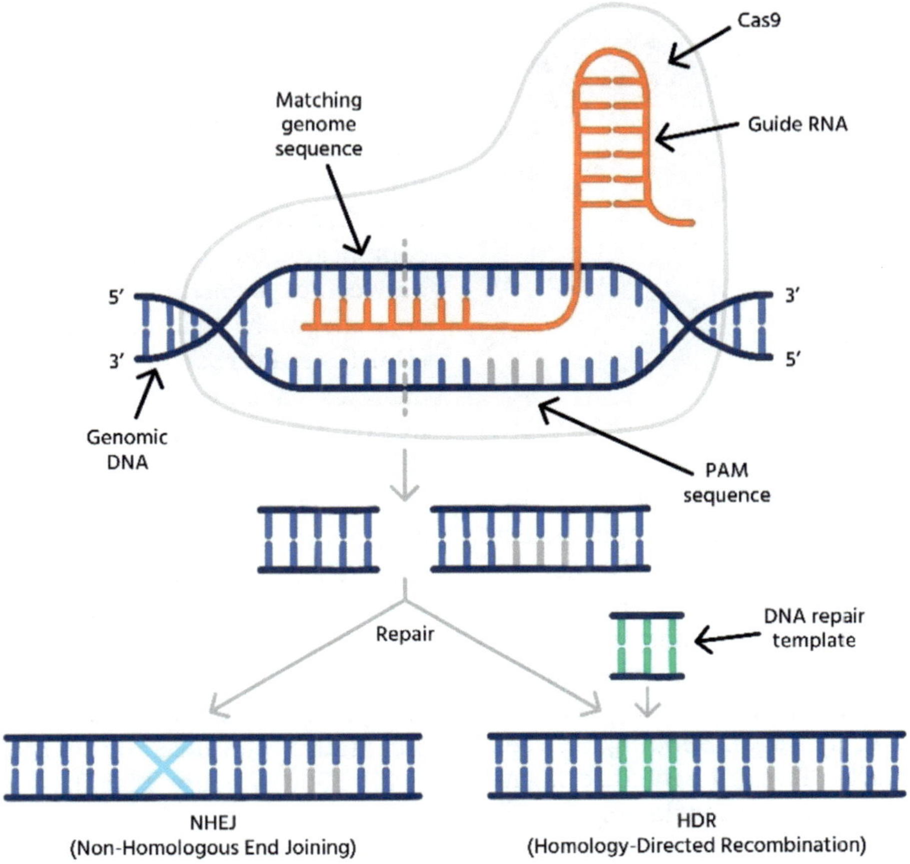

Figure 11.16. Schematic overview of CRISPR-Cas9 gene editing. In the absence of a repair template, cells will repair the break via error-prone non-homologous end joining (NHEJ), leading to functional gene disruption (gene/protein knock-out). Alternatively, a repair template can be used to introduce specific sequence changes via homologous-directed repair (HDR).

Source: https://iotasciences.com/wp-content/uploads/2024/06/CRISPR-Cas9_mechanism.jpg.

Test Your Knowledge

1. What is polymerase chain reaction (PCR)?
2. What is gel electrophoresis and its application?

11.5. Protein Structure and Function

Learning Outcome

1. Know the levels of protein structure;
2. Describe the enzyme function and kinetics;
3. Understand the role of proteins in cellular processes.

How the structure of protein relates to its function is the basis of molecular biology. Proteins consist of long chains of amino acids that bend into particular shapes, which determine what they do in the body. The activity of a protein is determined by the way its primary, secondary, tertiary, and quaternary structures are organized. The main structure is the order of amino acids, while alpha helices and beta sheets appear because of hydrogen bonding between the backbone parts. Tertiary structure is the three-dimensional form of a single polypeptide chain, and quaternary structure happens when different polypeptide chains come together. Therefore, it is important to understand how proteins get their three-dimensional shapes to know their specific roles in the body. Bioinformatics helps a lot in predicting what a protein does based on its structure. Researchers use this field to label and study proteins, using a lot of data to reach important results. Techniques , such as molecular modeling and structural alignment allow researchers to extrapolate information about uncharacterized proteins by comparing them to known structures (Manke et al., 2008). By aligning structures, researchers can find out which parts or interactions are probably kept the same in similar proteins. In addition, new computational methods, for example GAs, help to improve the way proteins are aligned. By maximizing the quality of alignment, researchers can predict evolutionary relationships and functional similarities across diverse species, broadening our understanding of protein functionality within the scope of molecular biology (Adebiyi et al., 2009). Because molecular biology is advancing, it is clear that studying proteins requires a mix of different scientific disciplines. When scientists use methods from biochemistry, genetics, and bioinformatics, they have better tools to study complicated biological issues. The collaboration between experimental methods, , such as X-ray crystallography and nuclear magnetic resonance (NMR) spectroscopy, and computational analyses leads to profound insights into protein dynamics and interactions. Information from these studies explains the basic concepts of molecular biology and also helps in designing drugs and working on synthetic biology. As researchers strive to decode the relationships between structure and function, the ongoing development of bioinformatics resources will remain crucial for interpreting vast genomic and proteomic data derived from cutting-edge techniques referenced in the literature (Manke et al., 2008) (Figure 11.17).

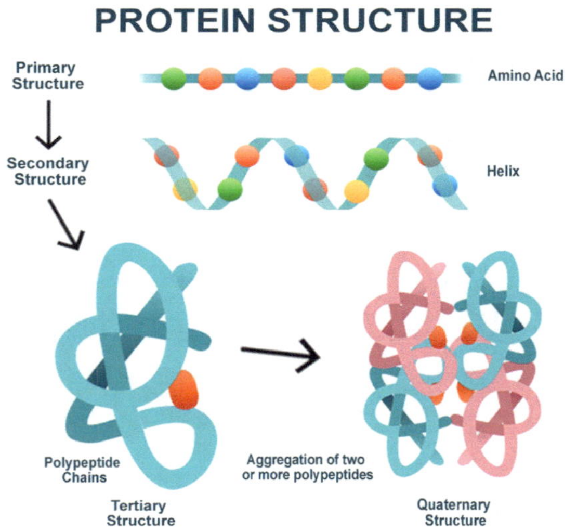

Figure 11.17. Protein structure.

Source: https://media.geeksforgeeks.org/wp-content/uploads/20220823180008/ProteinStructure.png.

11.5.1. Levels of Protein Structure: Primary to Quaternary

Proteins are understood in molecular biology mainly because of their complex structure. Protein structure goes through four different phases: primary, secondary, tertiary, and quaternary. The main structure of a protein is determined by the sequence of amino acids linked with peptide bonds. This process decides the chemistry of the area and also prepares it for forming more complex structures needed for function. Analyzing amino acid sequences through energy landscape concepts allows researchers to understand how structural configurations emerge and evolve, contributing to the principle of minimal frustration that governs biological interactions (Espada et al., 2013). So, the primary structure acts as a guide, affecting the building of the next important structures needed for biological function. Proteins in their secondary structure form alpha-helices and beta-sheets, which are held together by hydrogen bonds. The way proteins are folded is very important for their overall stability and function. Secondary structures usually appear in certain parts of the polypeptide chain and can join forces to help form motifs that help build the tertiary structure of the protein. Looking at these motifs can give clues about protein function and the effects of misfolding, which is important in diseases , such as Alzheimer's. By examining the variation of internal hydrogen bonds and hydrophobic interactions in these secondary structures, researchers can gain a deeper understanding of protein dynamics, thereby further illuminating the intricate relationships between structure and function within biological systems (Dacks et al., 2015). The quaternary structure is the last part of protein assembly, where several polypeptide chains, or subunits, interact to make a functional protein complex. Such organization is important for proteins because it helps them cooperate and be regulated. As an example, the quaternary structure of hemoglobin helps oxygen move through the blood by linking the binding sites and boosting its function. The investigation of quaternary structures extends to understanding diverse protein architectures and their evolutionary adaptations, thus employing methods , such as structural tessellation to identify repetitive motifs and their functional relationships (Espada et al., 2013). Besides, studying these structures helps us see how complicated cell functions are and why proteins are so important for life at the molecular level.

11.5.2. Enzyme Function and Kinetics

To grasp how biological processes happen at the molecular level, you need to know about enzyme function and kinetics. Enzymes help reactions happen faster by lowering the amount of energy needed, and they are not used up in the process. The way they function is very particular and depends on the concentration of their substrate, temperature, and pH. Kinetics shows us how enzymes connect with substrates to produce products. The Michaelis–Menten equation is one of the ways to describe the link between the amount of a substrate and the speed of the reaction. However, the complexity of enzyme interactions often necessitates more advanced modeling approaches that account for the multifaceted nature of biological systems, enabling researchers to predict outcomes more accurately and understand the underlying mechanisms that drive enzyme function (Priami et al., 2010). Enzyme kinetics is very important in cancer biology, mainly when it comes to the PI3K/AKT/mTOR1 signaling pathway. Since this pathway is a target for anti-cancer drugs, it shows how complex interactions between enzymes can make it hard for drugs to work properly in cells. To predict how Rapamycin or other therapies will affect a patient, one must have a good knowledge of enzyme kinetics. With kinetic modeling, findings from enzyme assays can be used to construct models that explain the ways drugs work. For example, the interplay between inhibitors and the pathways enzymatic components exemplifies how kinetic parameters can shape drug effectiveness and inform therapeutic strategies against cancer (Bown et al., 2016). Besides looking at drug interactions, studying the kinetics of enzymes often brings to light the main factors that manage cellular actions. The role of phosphatase and tensin homolog (PTEN) in modulating the sensitivity of the PI3K/AKT/mTOR1 pathway underscores the importance of incorporating all influencing factors into kinetic models. Thanks to systems biology and computational modeling, we can now see the connection between actions of a single enzyme and the whole signaling system. This way of working allows scientists to accurately predict the effects of drugs on different conditions and cell types, which improves the results of treatment. As such, exploring enzyme function and kinetics through these sophisticated modeling techniques remains essential for advancing molecular biology and its applications in personalized medicine (Bown et al., 2016) (Figure 11.18).

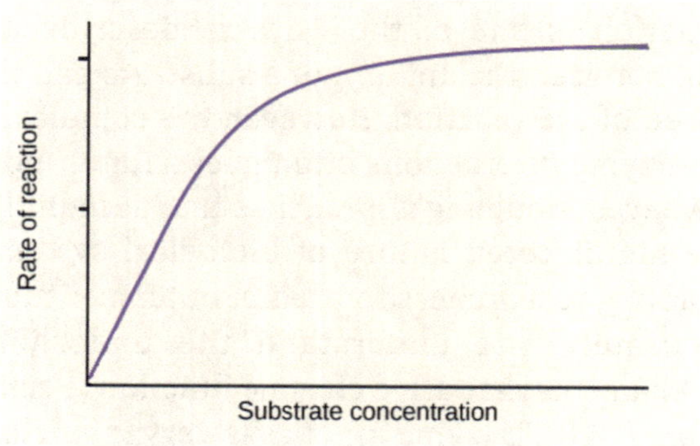

Figure 11.18. Basic enzyme kinetics graphs.

Source: https://cdn.kastatic.org/ka-perseus-images/e3a3422f253ec134f28a7a7aca27d9e08623b755.png.

11.5.3. Role of Proteins in Cellular Processes

In molecular biology, it is very important to understand that proteins help cells carry out many vital functions. Through acting as enzymes, proteins boost the rate of biochemical reactions that would take too long to complete. Having this ability is important for the metabolism, copying DNA, and other cellular activities. Besides, proteins are part of the cell's structure, helping to maintain its shape and move substances within the cell.

In addition, they are important for signaling, which lets cells react to outside factors and talk to each other. Because proteins have many functions, they are vital for keeping cells balanced and supporting the many chemical reactions needed for health and growth. Additionally, the control of protein synthesis and function is a major part of cellular activities, which points to the close relationship between genes and their protein products. Making proteins is regulated by transcription and post-transcription, so the body can adjust to different situations. For example, during stress responses or developmental changes, proteins , such as heat shock proteins (HSPs) become vital in preserving cellular integrity. According to the study on tendon disorders, HSPs known as damage-associated molecular patterns (DAMPs) are released in response to stress, helping to restore tissue homeostasis and regulate inflammatory mediators essential for recovery processes (Millar et al., 2012).

It shows that the amount of protein and its location and timing matter as much as the amount itself. Moreover, biotechnology and synthetic biology are helping to discover new uses of proteins in engineered cells. Projects like the "Building a Synthetic Cell" (BaSyC) aim to create autonomous, self-reproducing synthetic cells through the integration of various biochemical components. They increase our knowledge of cell membrane activities and how proteins play a part in its structure and functions. The study recognizes that membrane proteins are vital for cellular mechanisms, influencing everything from nutrient transport to signal transduction pathways, which are critical for cell survival and function (König, 2024). As we learn more about how proteins function in the body, new opportunities appear in medicine, biotechnology, and environmental protection, leading to important discoveries in molecular biology.

Test Your Knowledge

1. What are the four levels of protein structure?
2. What is the role of proteins in cellular processes?

11.6. Applications of Molecular Biology

Learning Outcome

1. Describe the biotechnology and genetic engineering;
2. Understand the medical applications and personalized medicine;
3. Describe the environmental and agricultural advancements.

Molecular biology is used in many areas and has greatly changed how we handle healthcare, farming, and the environment. Targeted therapies and vaccines in medicine are greatly helped by molecular biology techniques , such as gene editing and recombinant DNA technology. As an example, the CRISPR-Cas9 system has made it possible to edit genes precisely, which has helped in finding treatments for genetic disorders. In addition, synthetic biology seeks to make use of these molecular techniques to create new medicines and help treat difficult diseases. The way these developments affect each other demonstrates how molecular biology could make a real difference in medicine and disease prevention. Molecular biology is being used more often in agriculture to strengthen crops and increase their yield. With genetic modification, scientists can give one organism useful traits like the ability to resist pests and survive droughts from other organisms. As a result, farmers get better harvests and use fewer chemical pesticides, which is good for the environment. In addition, using genomic sequencing and marker-assisted selection speeds up the breeding process, so new plant varieties are developed faster to cope with climate change. Since the world's population is increasing, the use of molecular biology in agriculture helps secure food for everyone. Integrating these methods in agriculture allows farmers to adapt and face the problems they encounter on a daily basis, helping the environment. The combination of molecular biology and engineering has resulted in the field of synthetic biology, which could be very useful in different areas. When biology is considered programmable, scientists can build new organisms with special functions and use them in areas , such as cleaning up the environment and producing bioenergy. For example, scientists can design microbes to tackle environmental pollution or change waste into biofuels, proving that biotechnology can help solve important ecological problems. Besides, the fast development of the synthetic biology industry, thanks to large investments and the creation of useful tools, proves that this approach is vital. However, as the field advances, it is essential to navigate the ethical considerations and ensure that progress aligns with the foundational principles of open technology sharing and public benefit (Patel et al., 2019; Freemont, 2019) (Figure 11.19).

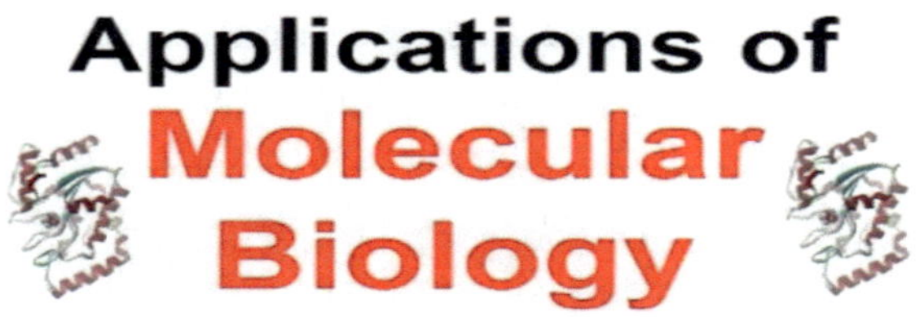

Figure 11.19. Applications of molecular biology.

Source: https://i.ytimg.com/vi/Pkmihz76a_Q/hqdefault.jpg.

11.6.1. Biotechnology and Genetic Engineering

Biotechnology and genetic engineering have greatly changed how we look at molecular biology and its uses in many sectors. The CRISPR-Cas system is leading this revolution because it can accurately modify genes. It both demonstrates the evolutionary changes in prokaryotes and marks a major advance in handling genes. Using the immune functions of bacteria and archaea, researchers have invented ways to modify DNA, which is helping to advance therapeutic interventions, farming, and other fields. As the implications of this technology continue to unfold, a comprehensive understanding of its operational mechanisms and evolutionary context becomes essential for maximizing its potential in biotechnology and genetic engineering (Bonomo & Deem, 2018). Genetic engineering in agricultural biotechnology could help plants produce more crops. Gene isolation and transfer have been studied and described in detail, mainly in model organisms. Still, to use these techniques in practice, it is important to know the molecular processes behind plant productivity. By integrating advanced approaches, , such as restriction fragment polymorphism (RFLP) as genetic markers, researchers can track specific genes that contribute to desirable traits. Moreover, finding out the molecular reasons for hybrid vigor can result in stronger and more productive crop varieties. The future of agricultural biotechnology relies on the seamless fusion of traditional breeding practices with modern genetic engineering techniques, offering a sustainable path toward enhancing food security and resilience in the face of climate challenges (Cullis, 1987). Besides, there are important ethical and regulatory issues that must be considered in biotechnology and genetic engineering. With new tools from molecular biology, people must find a way to balance progress with safety and what is right. It is important to pay attention to the public's views, rules set by authorities, and the possible outcomes of genetic manipulation to support responsible science. Because genetic engineering affects humans and the environment, everyone involved should take part in the discussion. A well-informed discourse will ultimately guide the responsible utilization of these technologies, ensuring that their implementation benefits society while minimizing potential risks (Cullis, 1987; Bonomo & Deem, 2018) (Figure 11.20).

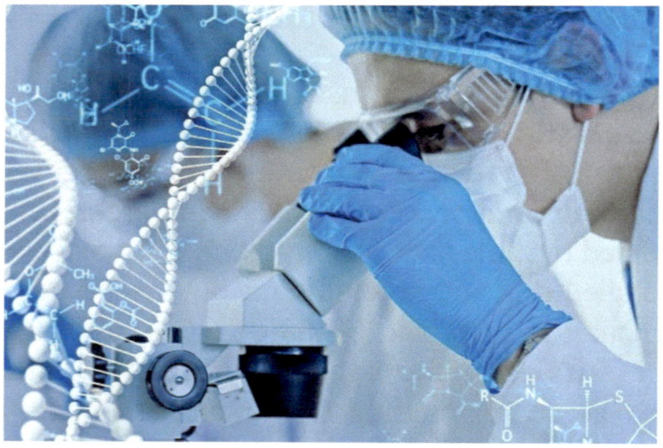

Figure 11.20. Genetic engineering.

Source: https://facts.net/wp-content/uploads/2025/04/38-facts-about-genetic-engineering-1744077156.jpg.

11.6.2. Medical Applications and Personalized Medicine

Personalized medicine has greatly changed the field of medical applications due to progress in molecular biology. Because of this, healthcare providers can adjust their prevention and treatment approaches to suit the genetic profile of every patient. Because of genomic sequencing and molecular diagnostics, scientists can now understand diseases in more detail and take better actions. Personalized medicine does not merely signify a shift in treatment but represents a paradigm change in clinical practice, embedding systems that acknowledge the complexity of human biology, as emphasized in studies on the utility and benefits of this approach in practical applications within diverse medical fields (Borro et al., 2017). The main goal of personalized medicine is to improve treatment results and reduce the risks of side effects, mainly in cancer care. When genetic and molecular data is used, clinicians can select the best treatment for a patient's tumor, which has been proven to help patients recover better. Advanced informatics tools and databases, , such as those developed by the Indiana Center for Systems Biology and Personalized Medicine, enhance this process by bridging the gap between basic research and clinical application (Wu & Cheng, 2011). Thanks to these innovative tools, it is easier to analyze a lot of data and find molecular signatures that help doctors choose the best treatment. As a result, personalized medicine helps doctors give more precise treatments and also encourages them to keep learning and adjusting their practice. Besides, personalized medicine is also related to ethics and economics, as it could influence how healthcare is available to everyone. When treatments can be chosen based on genetic and molecular details, some people who do not have access to advanced diagnostics may be left out of healthcare. Even though it has potential benefits, the unequal distribution of resources could increase the gap between people with different incomes, mostly helping those who can get proper healthcare. It is necessary to deal with these ethical issues as personalized medicine develops. Understanding the comprehensive impact of molecular techniques not only highlights their clinical significance but also emphasizes the need for inclusive policies that ensure equitable access to cutting-edge medical care, thus fostering a healthcare landscape that prioritizes the needs of all individuals (Borro et al., 2017) (Figure 11.21).

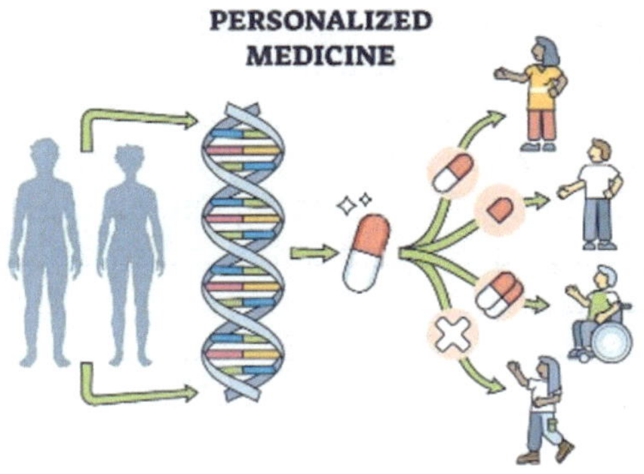

Figure 11.21. Personalized medicine.

Source: https://static.wixstatic.com/media/5cb09a_cf873955738b40a38ec043b30c03125f~mv2.jpg/v1/fill/w_550,h_388,al_c,lg_1,q_80/5cb09a_cf873955738b40a38ec043b30c03125f~mv2.jpg.

11.6.3. Environmental and Agricultural Advancements

Molecular biology has made a big difference in protecting the environment and farming, mainly through the use of genomic tools. Since biodiversity is being threatened by human actions, finding out the molecular details of various species is becoming very important. In this way, genomic data can explain the evolution of aquatic organisms, which supports better plans for saving threatened species. Using bioinformatics together with next-generation sequencing (NGS) aids in understanding the evolution of these organisms and also helps save biodiversity. By applying these technologies, researchers aim to devise solutions that mitigate the adverse effects of environmental stressors, thereby fostering a more sustainable coexistence between human needs and ecological integrity (Afiqah-Aleng et al., 2019). In farming, molecular biology greatly helps crops to withstand the effects of climate change and challenges in the environment. Innovations , such as GMOs have led to the development of crops that tolerate abiotic stresses like drought and salinity, thereby ensuring food security. Editing certain genes helps plants survive in tough environments, which helps maintain ecological balance by lessening the use of chemical substances. Moreover, analyzing plant genomes allows scientists to see which traits are helpful and can be used in breeding. As agricultural demands intensify in a changing environment, these advancements serve as vital tools for optimizing agricultural practices while maintaining ecological balance (Bhargava et al., 2023). Besides, molecular biology and environmental sciences are linked through pollinator research, especially when it comes to learning about the genetics of bees. The loss of pollinators is dangerous for farming systems that depend on them and for the health of the whole environment. Researchers in apiology are trying to find out the reasons behind the strong social behaviors and toughness of these insects at the molecular level. Through studying the genetics of bees, scientists can advise on how to save these vital pollinators. When we use this approach, we uncover more about insects in the environment and also learn how important it is to save biodiversity for agriculture and the environment. Ultimately, the advancements in molecular biology present innovative solutions to the multifaceted challenges encountered in environmental conservation and agriculture (Bhargava et al., 2023) (Figure 11.22).

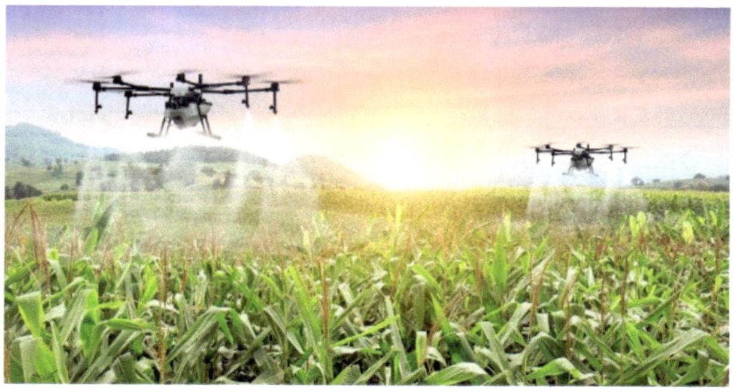

Figure 11.22. Innovation in agriculture.

Source: https://www.millerchemical.com/wp-content/uploads/2023/11/Miller-Blog-Farm-Innovations.jpg.

Test Your Knowledge

1. What is biotechnology and genetic engineering?
2. What is meant by personalized medicine?

SUMMARY

One should point out the key changes in our understanding of cells and diseases when summarizing the discussion on molecular biology. For example, recent studies that consider TRIP13 as a possible biomarker for pancreatic cancer show how combining molecular biology and bioinformatics can greatly affect research. The findings presented in the study reveal that heightened TRIP13 expression correlates with detrimental outcomes, emphasizing its significance not only as a target for early detection but also in prognostic evaluations (Afaq et al., 2024). With new discoveries in molecular biology, it is easier to see how the field can contribute to the creation of new medical treatments. Moreover, symbiotic relationships are very important for the evolution of organisms. By studying the connection between aphids and *Buchnera* sp., scientists have found how it has affected evolution for millions of years. This shows that molecular biology plays a key role in explaining genetic changes, how hosts adjust, and evolution. As evidenced by developments in genome analysis, the intricate metabolic partnership established between aphids and their symbionts showcases how symbiotic interactions can drastically alter the evolutionary pathways of species (Ham et al., 2001). The results are not limited to survival, as molecular biology appears to have the resources to study how genes and the environment affect each other. All in all, molecular biology affects many areas, including medicine and the study of evolution. Such research on TRIP13 demonstrates that scientific studies can help find better ways to diagnose and treat dangerous diseases. At the same time, the study of aphids and *Buchnera* shows how important molecular interactions are for evolutionary changes. As the area develops, using a variety of disciplines is likely to help discover solutions to today's problems in health, farming, and caring for the environment. All in all, these findings make it clear that molecular biology is vital for biological research and is used in many scientific areas.

A major focus in molecular biology is to learn about how diseases happen at the molecular level. A main study on bovine mastitis, which is an inflammation-caused disease in cattle's mammary glands, points out that it costs the dairy industry several billion dollars a year. The fact that disease susceptibility involves many factors calls for an approach that combines different areas of biology. Utilizing NGS and advanced network analysis, researchers investigated mRNA and miRNA expression profiles in immune cells during infection with *Streptococcus uberis*, illustrating the intricate molecular networks involved in disease pathology (Baker et al., 2014). The study showed that more than 3,700 genes were differently expressed in milk-isolated monocytes, which indicates major changes in immune responses when mastitis occurs. In particular, the genes that were turned on mainly worked in inflammatory pathways, showing the body's effort to resist bacterial invasion. In turn, down-regulated genes were found to play a key role in maintaining the cell's energy balance. These observations underscore the dual role of monocytes in responding to infections: amplifying inflammatory signals while simultaneously diminishing systemic metabolic functions (Baker et al., 2014). In addition, there were small changes in gene expression in blood monocytes, proving that localized infection can have effects throughout the body. Besides, the study found that specific microRNAs are involved in controlling important immune processes. Around 26 miRNAs were found only in milk-isolated monocytes, while three were found in blood-isolated monocytes, indicating the detailed control during mastitis. The results from pathway analyses revealed that the targets of down-regulated miRNAs are mainly involved in innate immunity, especially TLR signaling, suggesting they might control inflammation. On the other hand, the increased miRNAs appeared to regulate the expression of metabolic genes. As a result, the research helps us learn more about mastitis at the molecular level and also highlights the key role of miRNAs in controlling immune responses in other areas, making it easier to find new treatments.

KEY TERMS FROM THIS CHAPTER

- Agricultural biotechnology
- Double helix model
- Fidelity
- Gene expression
- Genetic material
- Molecular biology
- Polymerase chain reaction
- Supercoils
- Chromatin
- Environmental stewardship
- Gel electrophoresis
- Genetic algorithms
- Helicases
- Nucleotide composition
- Ribosomes

Critical Thinking Questions

1. **What is the primary function of DNA in the cell?**
   a. Store energy
   b. Store genetic information
   c. Catalyze chemical reactions
   d. Transport molecules
2. **Which enzyme is responsible for unwinding the DNA double helix during replication?**
   a. DNA polymerase
   b. RNA polymerase
   c. Helicase
   d. Ligase
3. **During which phase of the cell cycle does DNA replication occur?**
   a. G1 phase
   b. S phase
   c. G2 phase
   d. M phase
4. **Which repair mechanism corrects errors introduced during DNA replication?**
   a. Nucleotide excision repair
   b. Mismatch repair
   c. Base excision repair
   d. Homologous recombination
5. **What is the process by which RNA is synthesized from a DNA template?**
   a. Translation
   b. Replication
   c. Transcription
   d. Mutation

Answers to Critical Thinking Questions

1. (b); 2. (c); 3. (b); 4. (b); 5. (c)

Short Answer Questions

1. What is molecular biology and its scope?
2. Why is molecular biology important in modern science?
3. Name the four levels of protein structure?
4. What is a DNA replication process?
5. What is meant by gene expression?

References

1. E. F. Redish, C. Bauer, K. L. Carleton, T. J. Cooke, M. Cooper, C. H. Crouch, B. W. Dreyfus, B. D. Geller, J. Giannini, J. S. Gouvea, M. W. Klymkowsky, W. Losert, K. Moore, J. Presson, V. Sawtelle, K. V. Thompson, C. Turpen, R. K. P. Zia; NEXUS/Physics: An interdisciplinary repurposing of physics for biologists. *Am. J. Phys.* 1 May 2014; 82 (5): 368–377. https://doi.org/10.1119/1.4870386(accessed on 11th June 2025).

2. Ryan, D. P., Sundaramoorthy, R., Martin, D., Singh, V., & Owen-Hughes, T. (2011). The DNA-binding domain of the Chd1 chromatin-remodelling enzyme contains SANT and SLIDE domains. *The EMBO journal*, *30*(13), 2596–2609. https://doi.org/10.1038/emboj.2011.166(accessed on 11th June 2025).

3. Adebiyi, E. F., Akinyemi, I. O., & Fatumo, S. (2009). Aligning multiple sequences with genetic algorithm. https://core.ac.uk/download/12356710.pdf (accessed on 11th June 2025).

4. Afaq, F., Chauhan, S., Dhasmana, A., Dhasmana, M., et al. (2024). TRIP13's crucial role in pancreatic cancer progression. https://core.ac.uk/download/618193938.pdf (accessed on 11th June 2025).

5. Afiqah-Aleng, N., Danish-Daniel, M., Mohd Nor, S. A., et al. (2019). Applications of next-generation sequencing technologies and computational tools in molecular evolution and aquatic animals' conservation studies: A short review. https://core.ac.uk/download/286549011.pdf (accessed on 11th June 2025).

6. Afonine, P. V., Allen, K. N., Angus-Hill, M. L., Ashkenazy, H., Asturias, F. J., et al. (2019). Architecture of the chromatin remodeler RSC and insights into its nucleosome engagement. https://core.ac.uk/download/287624060.pdf (accessed on 11th June 2025).

7. Patel, A. B., Moore, C. M., Greber, B. J., Luo, J., Zukin, S. A., Ranish, J., & Nogales, E. (2019). Architecture of the chromatin remodeler RSC and insights into its nucleosome engagement. *eLife*, *8*, e54449. https://doi.org/10.7554/eLife.54449 (accessed on 11th June 2025).

8. García-Rubio, M., Barroso, S. I., & Aguilera, A. (2018). Detection of DNA-RNA Hybrids In Vivo. *Methods in molecular biology (Clifton, N.J.)*, *1672*, 347–361. https://doi.org/10.1007/978-1-4939-7306-4_24(accessed on 11th June 2025).

9. Slavov, N., Semrau, S., Airoldi, E., Budnik, B., & van Oudenaarden, A. (2015). Differential Stoichiometry among Core Ribosomal Proteins. *Cell reports*, *13*(5), 865–873. https://doi.org/10.1016/j.celrep.2015.09.056 (accessed on 11th June 2025).

10. Ali, W., Chen, Q., Deng, R., Tan, J., et al. (2022). Introduction to common molecular biological techniques used in research laboratories. https://core.ac.uk/download/541433093.pdf (accessed on 11th June 2025).

11. Araújo, L., Branco, J. C., da Silva Júnior, N. J., et al. (2019). Cell culture and maintenance of the evolutionary forms of *Trypanosoma cruzi* for studies of parasitic biology. https://core.ac.uk/download/322441572.pdf (accessed on 11th June 2025).

12. Arnold, S. J., Bejerano, G., Brodie, E. D., Hibbett, D. S., et al. (2013). Evolutionary biology for the 21st century. https://core.ac.uk/download/12174890.pdf (accessed on 11th June 2025).

13. Bagella, L. M., & Marchesi, I. (2013). Role of enhancer of zeste homolog 2 polycomb protein and its significance in tumor progression and cell differentiation. https://core.ac.uk/download/11694316.pdf (accessed on 11th June 2025).

14. Baker, M., Bryan, K., Lawless, N., Lippolis, R., et al. (2014). MicroRNA regulation of bovine monocyte inflammatory and metabolic networks in an *in vivo* infection model. https://core.ac.uk/download/45656557.pdf (accessed on 11th June 2025).

15. Bartkova, J., Baumann, C., Baxter, J., Bermejo, R., Bester, A. C., et al. (2014). "Breaking up is hard to do": The formation and resolution of sister chromatid intertwines. https://core.ac.uk/download/30611328.pdf (accessed on 11th June 2025).

16. Ben-Shaul, A., Egecioglu, D. E., Gelbart, W. M., Gopal, A., et al. (2014). Viral RNAs are unusually compact. https://core.ac.uk/download/323067057.pdf (accessed on 11th June 2025).

17. Bhargava, R., Das, D., Mishra, M. R., Pandit, P., et al. (2023). The buzz of apiology and the molecular secrets of vectors: Unraveling the genetics and physiology of insects in ecology. https://core.ac.uk/download/591404299.pdf (accessed on 11th June 2025).

18. Bonomo, M. E., & Deem, M. W. (2018). The physicist's guide to one of biotechnology's hottest new topics: CRISPR-Cas. *Physical biology*, *15*(4), 041002. https://doi.org/10.1088/1478-3975/aab6d6(accessed on 11th June 2025).

19. Borro, M., Di Sanzo, M., Fineschi, V., Frati, P., et al. (2017). Clinical applications of personalized medicine: A new paradigm and challenge. https://core.ac.uk/download/80315182.pdf (accessed on 11th June 2025).

20. Bowater, R. P., Luisi, B. F., & Wood, I. C. (2012). From beads on a string to the pearls of regulation: The structure and dynamics of chromatin. https://core.ac.uk/download/9838153.pdf (accessed on 11th June 2025).

21. Bown, J. L., Goltsov, A., Harrison, D. J., Langdon, W. B., et al. (2016). Kinetic modelling of *in vitro* data of PI3K, mTOR1, PTEN enzymes and on-target inhibitors Rapamycin, BEZ235, and LY294002. https://core.ac.uk/download/228177492.pdf (accessed on 11th June 2025).

22. Butte, A., Chatr-Aryamontri, A., Clauset, A., Joshi, A., Joshi, A., Kundaje, A. A., et al. (2016). *Detection of regulator genes and eQTLs in gene networks.* http://arxiv.org/abs/1512.05574 (accessed on 11th June 2025).

23. Thaker, S. K., Ch'ng, J., & Christofk, H. R. (2019). Viral hijacking of cellular metabolism. *BMC biology*, *17*(1), 59. https://doi.org/10.1186/s12915-019-0678-9 (accessed on 11th June 2025).

24. Xiaogang Wu, PhD and Jake Y. Chen, PhD (2011). Predictive and personalized medicine with systems biology solutions. https://core.ac.uk/download/46964267.pdf (accessed on 11th June 2025).

25. Chowdhury, D., & Sharma, A. K. (2012). Template-directed biopolymerization: Tape-copying Turing machines. http://arxiv.org/abs/1212.6827 (accessed on 11th June 2025).

26. Ciandrini, L., Romano, M. C., & Stansfield, I. (2013). Ribosome traffic on mRNAs maps to gene ontology: Genome-wide quantification of translation initiation rates and polysome size regulation. https://core.ac.uk/download/25497447.pdf (accessed on 11th June 2025).

27. Courtot, M., Juty, N., Knüpfer, C., Waltemath, D., Zhukova, A., Dräger, A., Dumontier, M., Finney, A., Golebiewski, M., Hastings, J., Hoops, S., Keating, S., Kell, D. B., Kerrien, S., Lawson, J., Lister, A., Lu, J., Machne, R., Mendes, P., Pocock, M., ... Le Novère, N. (2011). Controlled vocabularies and semantics in systems biology. *Molecular systems biology*, *7*, 543. https://doi.org/10.1038/msb.2011.77(accessed on 11th June 2025).

28. Cullis, C. A. (1987). *Biotechnology and Plant Productivity*. https://core.ac.uk/download/76311551.pdf (accessed on 11th June 2025).

29. Dacks, J. B., Dorrell, R. G., Richardson, E., Tsaousis, A. D., et al. (2015). Evolutionary cell biology: Functional insight from "endless forms most beautiful." https://core.ac.uk/download/30711862.pdf (accessed on 11th June 2025).

30. Dambrós, B. P., & Ferri, F. M. (2017). Short-course: Molecular biology applied to clinical analyzes. https://core.ac.uk/download/235132995.pdf (accessed on 11th June 2025).

31. Drellich, E., Gainer-Dewar, A., Harrington, H. A., He, Y., et al. (2016). Geometric combinatorics and computational molecular biology: Branching polytopes for RNA sequences. http://arxiv.org/abs/1509.04090 (accessed on 11th June 2025).

32. Ekmekci B, McAnany CE, Mura C (2016) An Introduction to Programming for Bioscientists: A Python-Based Primer. PLoS Comput Biol 12(6): e1004867. https://doi.org/10.1371/journal.pcbi.1004867(accessed on 11th June 2025).

33. Elliott, K. (2008). Varieties of exploratory experimentation in nanotoxicology. https://core.ac.uk/download/11921904.pdf (accessed on 11th June 2025).

34. Ellisman, M. H., Goncharov, A., Jin, Y., Noma, A., et al. (2017). Microtubule-dependent ribosome localization in *C. elegans* neurons. https://core.ac.uk/download/323064522.pdf (accessed on 11th June 2025).

35. Espada, R., Ferreiro, D. U., Parra, R. G., Sippl, M. J., et al. (2013). Detecting repetitions and periodicities in proteins by tiling the structural space. https://core.ac.uk/download/19042832.pdf (accessed on 11th June 2025).

36. Freemont, P. (2019). Synthetic biology industry–Data-driven design is creating new opportunities in biotechnology. https://core.ac.uk/download/228135116.pdf (accessed on 11th June 2025).

37. Giraud, A., Sali, A., Shaver, A. C., Li, B., Wylie, C. S., Klimov, D. K., Dekel, E., et al. (2009). Interplay between pleiotropy and secondary selection determines rise and fall of mutators in stress response. https://core.ac.uk/download/8388553.pdf (accessed on 11th June 2025).

38. Ham, R. C. H. J. van, Latorre, A., Martinez-Torres, D., et al. (2001). Molecular evolution of aphids and their primary (*Buchnera* sp.) and secondary endosymbionts: Implications for the role of symbiosis in insect evolution. https://core.ac.uk/download/pdf/29301278.pdf (accessed on 11th June 2025).

39. Hidayah, N. (2025). Regulasi transkripsi dan pasca transkripsi pada ekspresi gen. https://core.ac.uk/download/641551239.pdf (accessed on 11th June 2025).

40. Hughes, K. D., Mosley, A. L., Peck, S. A., Victorino, J. F., et al. (2019). Writing a wrong: Coupled RNA polymerase II transcription and RNA quality control. https://core.ac.uk/download/228066153.pdf (accessed on 11th June 2025).

41. Intarapanich, A., Ukosakit, K., Shaw, P. J., Kaewkamnerd, S., Tongsima, S., & Tragoonrung, S. (2015). Automatic DNA diagnosis for 1D gel electrophoresis images using bio-image processing technique. https://bmcgenomics.biomedcentral.com/track/pdf/10.1186/1471-2164-16-S12-S15?site=bmcgenomics.biomedcentral.com (accessed on 11th June 2025).

42. König, M. (2024). From lipid to life: Using simulations to connect molecular structure and

membrane function. https://core.ac.uk/download/597522258.pdf (accessed on 11th June 2025).

43. Manke, T., Roider, H., & Vingron, M. (2008). A biophysical approach to large-scale protein-DNA binding data. https://core.ac.uk/download/210658490.pdf (accessed on 11th June 2025).

44. Mariscal, C., & Petropanagos, A. (2016). CRISPR as a driving force: The Model T of biotechnology. https://core.ac.uk/download/131209784.pdf (accessed on 11th June 2025).

45. Marsh, D. (2000). Fostering innovation in a small open economy: The case of the New Zealand biotechnology sector. https://core.ac.uk/download/29195694.pdf (accessed on 11th June 2025).

46. Millar, N. L., & Murrell, G. A. C. (2012). Heat shock proteins in tendinopathy: Novel molecular regulators. https://core.ac.uk/download/9651505.pdf (accessed on 11th June 2025).

47. Mueller, S. H. (2022). Methods and applications of single-molecule fluorescence microscopy. https://core.ac.uk/download/534127367.pdf (accessed on 11th June 2025).

48. Powell, G. E., III. (2017). Embryos as patients? Medical provider duties in the age of CRISPR/Cas9. https://core.ac.uk/download/84098963.pdf (accessed on 11th June 2025).

49. Priami, C., & Zámborszky, J. (2010). BlenX-based compositional modeling of complex reaction mechanisms. http://arxiv.org/abs/1002.4065 (accessed on 11th June 2025).

50. Schreiber, G., Rahat, O., Alon, U., & Levy, Y. (2008). Understanding hydrogen-bond patterns in proteins using a novel statistical model. https://core.ac.uk/download/pdf/287637.pdf (accessed on 11th June 2025).

51. Shakhnovich, E. I., Berezovsky, I. N., Zeldovich, K. B., & Bourne, P. E. (2005). Protein and DNA sequence determinants of thermophilic adaptation. https://core.ac.uk/download/pdf/7517646.pdf (accessed on 11th June 2025).

52. Shaw, H. C. (2025). Network security via biometric recognition of patterns of gene expression. https://core.ac.uk/download/pdf/42696320.pdf (accessed on 11th June 2025).

53. Wegrzyn, G., & Wegrzyn, A. (2002). Stress responses and replication of plasmids in bacterial cells. *Microbial cell factories, 1*(1), 2. https://doi.org/10.1186/1475-2859-1-2(accessed on 11th June 2025).

54. White, B. (2011). University scholar series: Brandon White. https://core.ac.uk/download/70426279.pdf (accessed on 11th June 2025).

GENETIC DISORDERS

12

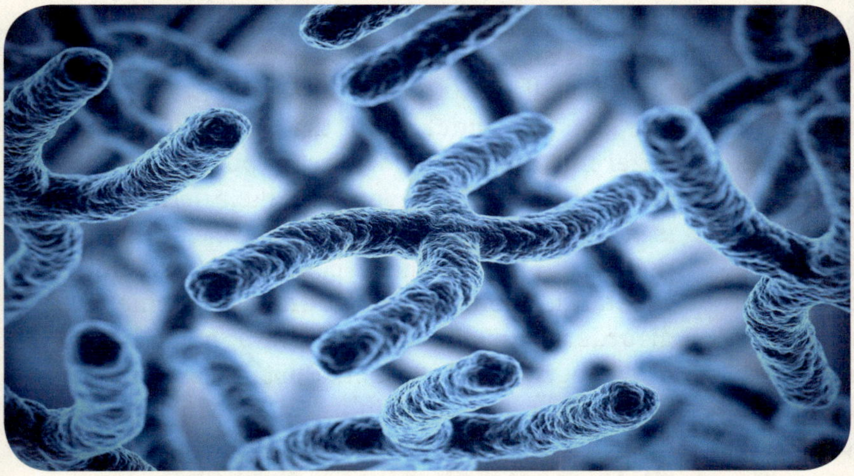

LEARNING OBJECTIVES

After studying this chapter, you will be able to:

1. Describe the types of genetic disorders;
2. Know the causes of genetic disorders;
3. Understand the symptoms and the diagnostic processes associated with genetic disorders;
4. Describe the treatment options for genetic disorders.

Introduction

Genetic disorders are many and complicated, as they are caused by different mutations in the DNA sequence. Such disorders display themselves in many forms and can influence a person's physical, mental, and developmental well-being. Improvements in genetic studies have shown that some of these disorders are passed down in families, while others happen randomly because of outside influences or genetic changes. Genetic disorders have a big impact on the patients, their families, and the healthcare system. Since genetic disorders are more common in some regions than in others, it is necessary to analyze them thoroughly to see their complete effect on the public and society. Usually, genetic disorders are separated into two categories: single-gene disorders and multifactorial disorders. A single-gene disorder is also called a Mendelian disorder, but multifactorial disorders are caused by several genes and environmental influences. It is important to make this distinction to learn about inheritance and the role of genetic counseling. Since there are many causes for multifactorial disorders, it is often hard to diagnose and treat them accurately. For instance, inborn errors of metabolism (IEMs) are a subset of genetic disorders characterized by disruptions in the enzymatic activities crucial for metabolism. The importance of early diagnosis in IEMs cannot be overstated, as timely intervention can significantly improve long-term health outcomes, highlighting the critical role of advanced screening methods in managing these conditions (Ismail et al., 2019). With advances in genetics, advanced technologies are now playing a big role in diagnosing and treating genetic problems. Thanks to genomic sequencing, we can now find gene mutations linked to these disorders and give patients personalized treatment. By leveraging untargeted metabolomics, researchers can explore a wider range of metabolic pathways, offering a more comprehensive view of metabolic disturbances that characterize various genetic disorders (Ismail et al., 2019). Even with these new developments, it is still difficult to give equal access to genetic testing and therapy to all people. Furthermore, since ethical concerns about genetic information are important, it is necessary to keep talking about them as we progress. If we look at genetic disorders using genetics, technology, and ethics, we can come up with new solutions for those affected and their families (Figure 12.1).

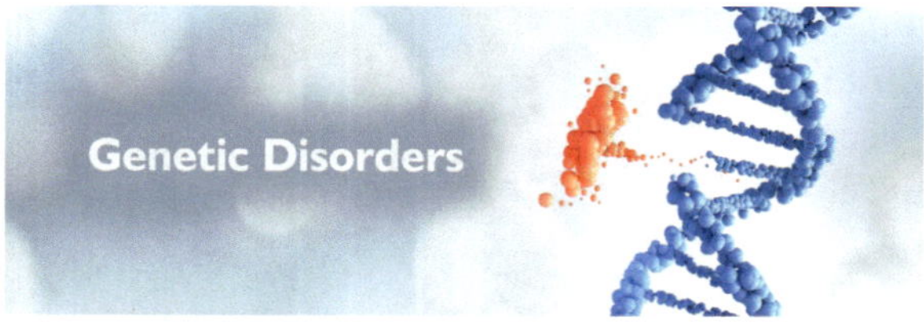

Figure 12.1. Genetic disorders.

Source: https://www.medicoverhospitals.in/images/articles/genetic-disorders.webp.

Definition of Genetic Disorders

The reason for genetic disorders is that there are abnormalities in a person's genes or chromosomes. These disorders are passed on in families by autosomal dominant, autosomal recessive, and X-linked patterns, which play a big role in their inheritance. While cystic fibrosis and sickle cell disease are caused by a single gene mutation, Down syndrome happens because of an extra chromosome 21. Genetic disorders are difficult to define because the way they present and how serious they are can be affected by both genetic factors and things happening in the environment. So, to define genetic disorders, we must look at their genetic causes as well as the medical symptoms they produce. It makes it easier to understand the ways in which different genetic disorders happen. Genetic disorders are mainly genetic, as their heritability is a key point. Twin studies have estimated the heritability of many conditions, revealing substantial genetic contributions; psychiatric disorders, for instance, show a heritability range between 40% and 80% as evidenced by recent research (Fabbri, 2022). It appears that environmental causes are important, but a major part of the variation in these disorders is due to genes. These disorders are also hard to understand because many genes can influence them by interacting with each other. This is why advanced research methods are required to study these disorders and improve the results for patients. Discoveries in genetics have greatly improved our knowledge of genetic disorders and the reasons behind them. Genome-wide association studies (GWAS) have been instrumental in identifying thousands of genetic variants associated with various psychiatric and non-psychiatric conditions, highlighting the multifactorial nature of these disorders (Stringer et al., 2015). By understanding how several risk alleles can affect someone, researchers can better predict a person's risk of certain diseases and choose better treatments. Still, there are many difficulties along the way, especially when dealing with biased data that comes from simple assumptions in genetic studies. With ongoing research, we should make sure to use genomic data along with environmental and biological aspects to design better models for handling genetic disorders (Figure 12.2).

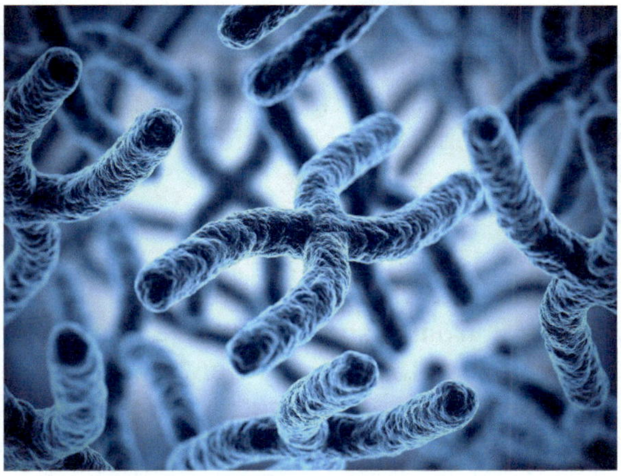

Figure 12.2. 3D illustration of human chromosomes.

Source: https://medlineplus.gov/images/GeneticDisorders_share.jpg.

Importance of Studying Genetic Disorders

Knowing about genetic disorders is essential because of their strong effect on people and the community. If genes have mutations, it can cause genetic disorders that influence the development of a person's body, mind, and feelings. By analyzing these disorders, researchers can find out how genetic changes affect a person's chances of getting certain diseases. Such research can be used to create preventative steps, early actions, and treatments that match a person's genetic makeup. So, research on genetic disorders helps advance healthcare and affects public health decisions. In addition, exploring genetic disorders greatly helps improve methods of diagnosis and treatment. Thanks to better genetic screening, conditions , such as autism and other developmental disorders can be found early, so timely help can be given to those affected and their families. As noted in discussions surrounding developmental disorders, early screening serves to identify deviations that warrant further assessment and intervention (Fernell et al., 2014). Because of this approach, genetic disorders can be managed better, and new research can help find innovative solutions, so genetic research is still very important in clinical settings. Also, learning about genetic disorders is important not only for individuals but for society as a whole. Genetic disorders cause problems that touch patients as well as their families, communities, and healthcare teams. With knowledge of what causes these disorders, researchers are able to support better healthcare systems for all kinds of people. Additionally, discourse on issues surrounding alcoholism and various genetic predispositions highlights the multidimensional factors influencing health outcomes (Sher et al., 1997). For this reason, a clear understanding of genetic disorders allows for specific actions by health authorities, schools, and lawmakers to ease their effects and improve the health of the community.

12.1. Types of Genetic Disorders

Learning Outcome

1. Describe the single-gene disorders;
2. Learn about chromosomal disorders;
3. Describe the multifactorial disorders.

Genetic disorders can be grouped into various categories, and every group is caused by basic genetic problems. Monogenic disorders are a major group, and they happen when one gene is mutated. Some of these disorders are passed on in dominant ways, while others are recessive, bringing about many different physical traits. For instance, cystic fibrosis is a typical monogenic disorder caused by changes in the CFTR gene, which results in major problems with the lungs and digestive system. The contrast demonstrates that mutations in genes can affect not only a person's health but also the health of the public, since some inherited disorders may call for special treatments and advice. Besides, knowing how monogenic disorders work helps scientists develop new treatments and medicines, making them more significant in today's medical field. Unlike monogenic disorders, polygenic disorders happen because of mutations in several genes as well as the impact of the environment. Such complications as diabetes, heart disease, and specific cancer types are examples of this since many genetic changes work together to increase the chances and seriousness of the disease. It has been found through recent studies that both our habits and the environment can affect these interactions, which shows why taking a holistic approach to health care is necessary. Also, since these disorders are caused by many factors, they are difficult to diagnose and assess using genetic testing. Since these disorders are caused by many genes, scientists must continue to study them to find better ways to stop and treat them.

Some genetic disorders happen because of chromosomal abnormalities, which may happen due to changes in their structure or number. An extra chromosome 21, as in Down syndrome, can affect both the brain and the body of the person affected. Many times, chromosomal disorders lead to extra health risks and require special help and support for education and social life. When genetic technology makes it possible to detect abnormalities earlier, it is crucial to know how these issues affect patients' treatment. It has been found through research that children who suffer from maltreatment are more likely to develop neurodevelopmental disorders. This relationship necessitates comprehensive assessments of children who exhibit multiple neurodevelopmental challenges, emphasizing the critical role of genetic and environmental factors in shaping health outcomes (Dinkler et al., 2017). Moreover, emerging studies highlight the substantial overlap between literacy problems and psychiatric disorders, indicating the intricate interplay of genetic influences in the development of diverse conditions (Angold et al., 2006) (Figure 12.3).

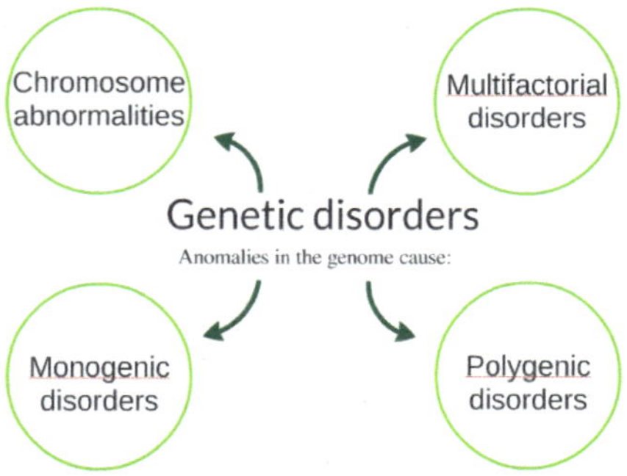

Figure 12.3. Types of genetic disorders.

Source: https://0901.static.prezi.com/preview/v2/s7uvo7eywqoatjuk6mw7wgxs3l6jc3sachvcdoaizecfr3dnitcq_3_0.png.

12.1.1. Single-Gene Disorders

These disorders are a group of genetic problems caused by alterations in only one gene. Depending on the role of the affected gene and the type of mutation, the results can be light or very serious. Cystic fibrosis and sickle cell anemia are good examples of how single-gene disorders interfere with the body's normal processes. Because they follow Mendel's laws, such disorders are easier to predict and understand within families than other types of genetic disorders. Thanks to genetic screening and counseling, people can be diagnosed early, and proper care can be given, which helps them live better lives, so it is important for both healthcare providers and patients to be educated about genetics. The causes of single-gene disorders can be quite different and may involve many cellular pathways. Pathogenic mutations may be missense, nonsense, or frameshift, and all of them can affect the way proteins function. Mutations in the CFTR gene result in cystic fibrosis since they cause the chloride channel to malfunction and disrupt how ions and fluid move in epithelial cells. In addition, some single-gene disorders happen when a mutation either stops a gene from working or causes it to produce proteins with new and usually harmful functions. Such disorders affect families and the community, leading to emotional and financial difficulties, which shows that more support is required for those who suffer. Studies are still revealing how single-gene disorders are related to overall health. Studies done recently have found that certain single-gene disorders are associated with psychiatric problems. For example, the Wolfram syndrome gene (WFS1) has been linked to mood disorders, indicating that individuals with mutations in this gene may have an increased risk for psychiatric conditions, thereby complicating their clinical management. The identification of genetic variants within the WFS1 gene that correlate with disorders , such as major depressive disorder and bipolar disorder suggests that understanding single-gene disorders may provide insights into polygenic risk factors across different medical domains (Altmäe et al., 2004). Moreover, such findings potentially contribute to a more integrated framework for addressing the complex interplay between genetic vulnerabilities and multifaceted health conditions, underscoring the necessity for continued research in the field of genetic disorders (Grotzinger et al., 2022) (Figure 12.4).

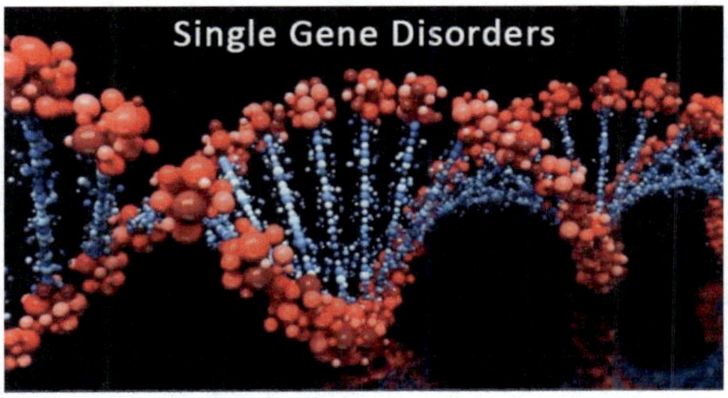

Figure 12.4. Single-gene disorders.

Source: https://www.sepalika.com/wp-content/uploads/2021/10/Single-Gene-Disorders.webp.

12.1.2. Chromosomal Disorders

When there are problems with the number or structure of chromosomes, it can seriously affect human health and growth. Some of these disorders, for example Down syndrome, result from having an extra chromosome, while others are caused by changes in the structure of chromosomes. People with these chromosomal abnormalities may experience anything from slight to serious consequences, which may include mental, physical, and health-related issues. Thanks to chromosomal microarray analysis and other advanced genetic tests, it is now simpler to find and diagnose these disorders, giving families useful information for care and support. Thus, knowing the genetic reasons for chromosomal disorders helps clinicians suggest better treatments and predictions for each patient. It has been found that genetic factors and the environment work together in the development of chromosomal disorders. Because of microarrays and next-generation sequencing (NGS), we can now find small changes in chromosomes that were not visible before. These methods have revealed a wealth of information regarding the architecture of the human genome and its variations associated with disorders like autism spectrum disorders (ASDs). In particular, chromosomal abnormalities, , such as copy number variants (CNVs), have been linked to an increased risk of developing ASDs, highlighting the importance of genetic screening in early diagnosis and intervention. The identification of these genetic biomarkers could significantly improve recurrence prediction for families and foster a more personalized approach to treatment based on specific genetic profiles (Brian et al., 2019). In addition, spotting particular changes in chromosomes affects both public health and the way diseases are managed. The increasing incidence of chronic pediatric disorders, including autism and asthma, underscores the need for ongoing research into the pathobiology of these conditions (Barzman et al., 2015). Because these diseases are caused by many different genes, using treatments that match each person's genetics could improve the results. With further study of genomic variations, their ability to signal diseases and help personalize treatment is becoming more obvious. Because of new developments in genetics and technology, healthcare workers are now able to identify the causes of chromosomal disorders and develop innovative therapies that address those causes (Figure 12.5).

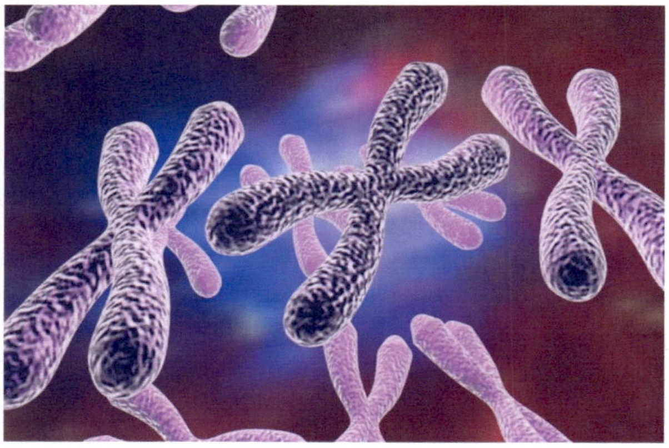

Figure 12.5. Chromosomal abnormalities.

Source: https://www.sepalika.com/wp-content/uploads/2021/10/4F5CB304976E5ACA8AD5FF03 0EB85239-1024x683-1.webp.

12.1.3. Multifactorial Disorders

These disorders are complex genetic conditions that develop because of the effects of both genetic and environmental factors. While monogenic disorders are caused by a single gene mutation, multifactorial disorders happen because of variations in several genes, all of which play a small role in influencing the phenotype. Since environmental factors can affect how genetic predisposition appears, it is usually difficult to forecast the results. It has been found that diseases , such as coronary artery disease, diabetes, and some kinds of cancer are included in this category, showing that both inherited and acquired factors can affect a person's risk of disease. It is important to realize that environmental factors can trigger multifactorial disorders along with genetic factors. Genetic factors can make a person more likely to become obese, but it is the person's diet and level of exercise that actually determine if they develop type 2 diabetes. Studies conducted recently have pointed out that making healthy lifestyle choices can help people who are at risk of such diseases. In this way, researchers hope to create strategies that focus on genetic traits and lifestyle changes, which can improve the outcome for people who may develop multifactorial diseases. It is very difficult to diagnose and treat multifactorial disorders since doctors must consider both genetic and environmental factors when caring for their patients. Genetic counseling is important for families to learn about their risks and what their genetic background means. Additionally, advancements in prenatal diagnosis methods have shown promise, particularly in identifying congenital heart defects, which may have multifactorial origins (Helner et al., 2019). Additionally, studying the growth of disorders like autism proves that both genetic and environmental factors should be taken into account. As health professionals strive to navigate the intricacies of genetic disorders, the continued study of multifactorial conditions remains essential for effective intervention and improved health outcomes (Ghosh et al., 2009) (Figure 12.6).

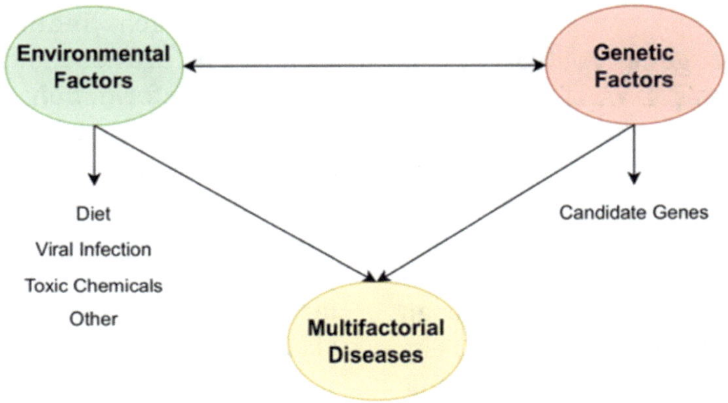

Figure 12.6. The combination of environmental factors and genetic factors is the main culprit which takes responsible for causing multifactorial diseases.

Source: https://www.frontiersin.org/files/Articles/873069/fgene-13-873069-HTML/image_m/fgene-13-873069-g001.jpg.

Test Your Knowledge

1. What is single-gene disorders?
2. What are chromosomal disorders?

12.2. Causes of Genetic Disorders

Learning Outcome

1. Describe the mutations in DNA;
2. Examine the inheritance patterns;
3. Understand the role of environmental factors in the manifestation of genetic disorders.

The main reason for genetic disorders is mutations in a person's DNA. Examples of these mutations are point mutations, insertions, deletions, and copy number variations. Although some changes may be harmless, they usually result in serious problems with how the brain functions. For instance, single-nucleotide polymorphisms (SNPs) can affect an individual's susceptibility to various diseases by altering protein function or expression levels. Furthermore, when there are big changes in chromosomes, , such as translocations or aneuploidy, it can cause Down syndrome. For this reason, it is crucial to learn about various genetic mutations, since they are responsible for a wide range of genetic disorders and their symptoms. Besides the changes in genes, the effects of both genetics and the environment are important in the development of genetic disorders. While DNA is unchanged, epigenetic modifications can still affect gene expression and therefore affect an individual's features. Problems , such as exposure to harmful chemicals or not getting enough nutrients can make the effects of genes worse. The combination of these factors points out that genetic disorders should be examined in relation to the environment as well as genetics. Therefore, it is important to consider many aspects to understand how genetic disorders develop and affect a person's health and resistance to certain diseases. New discoveries in genomics have shown that non-coding regulatory changes play a big role in genetic disorders. Traditionally, research had focused predominantly on protein-coding regions of the genome; however, recent findings underscore the significance of non-coding regions, particularly 3 untranslated regions (3UTRs). Such variants are able to affect gene activity and are very important for proper brain growth and function. As an example, research has pointed out that some non-coding variants can cause specific language impairment, autism, schizophrenia, and bipolar disorder, proving that other genetic factors are involved in these disorders. Such findings show that earlier assumptions are not enough and that non-coding regulatory information should be included in genetic studies. As the field progresses, a more nuanced understanding of genetic variations, including both coding and non-coding regions, is essential for unraveling the complex causes of genetic disorders and developing targeted interventions (Fiorentino et al., 2018; Chen et al., 2018).

12.2.1. Mutations in DNA

Changes in DNA are a basic cause of genetic variation that may greatly affect human health. There are several types of mutations, for example point mutations, insertions, deletions, and frameshift mutations, and all of them can change the normal function of genes. Although some mutations are harmless, others may result in serious genetic issues. Mutations in mitochondrial DNA are important since they mainly disrupt energy metabolism in cells. According to research, issues in the mitochondrial genome, mainly related to replication, may lead to serious mitochondrial genetic diseases that show up as various syndromes. These syndromes, , such as progressive external ophthalmoplegia and myopathy, showcase the challenges posed by mutations that disrupt critical pathways in cellular respiration and energy production (Copeland et al., 2016). Genetic disorders are also caused by changes in nuclear DNA, as well as mitochondrial DNA. They may happen because of things in the environment, mistakes in DNA replication, or genes passed down from parents. In particular, mutations in genes , such as POLG, POLG2, and others may result in hereditary diseases with mitochondrial problems and related symptoms. Mitochondrial DNA depletion syndromes demonstrate that mutations can alter cellular functions, resulting in serious effects on a person's life, mostly affecting young children. Understanding the molecular mechanisms behind these mutations is crucial for developing potential therapeutic interventions, which underscore the relevance of genetic research in addressing these disorders (Copeland et al., 2016). The results of DNA mutations affect more than just individuals' health and raise issues about genetic research and treatment for the whole community. As genetic sequencing and editing technologies grow and develop, they bring up new questions about changing human DNA. There are ethical issues about using gene editing to fix diseases that can result in unintended issues and cause unequal treatment in society. Besides, understanding mutations in DNA makes us appreciate how complex human biology is and how genes and the environment interact. As we get a better grasp of genetic disorders linked to mutations, we must make sure to focus on both scientific advancements and ethical duties, so that we can help everyone (Figure 12.7).

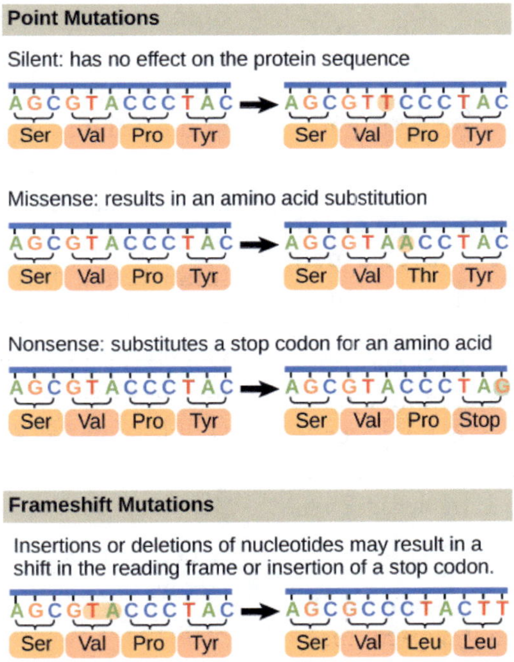

Figure 12.7. Mutations can lead to changes in the protein sequence encoded by the DNA.

Source: https://s3-us-west-2.amazonaws.com/courses-images/wp-content/uploads/sites/2318/2016/06/25204324/Types-of-Mutations.png.

12.2.2. Inheritance Patterns

It is necessary to understand how genetic disorders can move from parents to their children. Mendelian genetics explains how traits are passed on in families by showing the roles of dominant and recessive alleles. Still, in multifactorial inheritance, several genes and environmental influences interact to shape a person's traits. Such patterns play a key role in causing genetic disorders, so it is important to use genetic counseling and risk assessment. Knowing about dominant and recessive inheritance helps scientists find out the reasons behind someone getting a disorder, which leads to better treatments and therapies. Epigenetics plays a major part in inheritance by making sure traits are displayed without changing the DNA sequence.

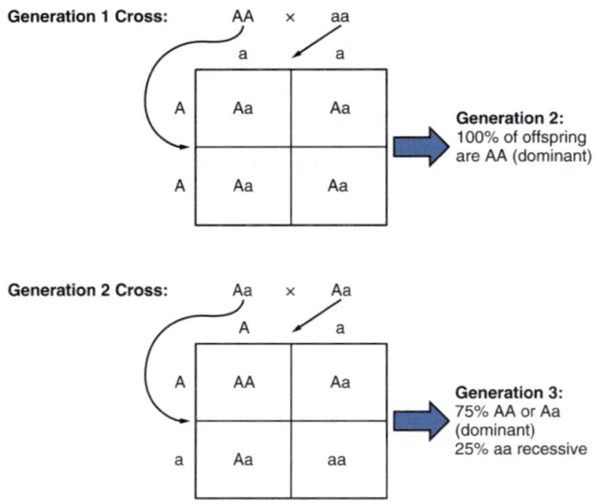

Figure 12.8. In the formation of gametes, it is equally likely that either one of a pair alleles from one parent will be passed on to the offspring. This figure follows the possible combinations of alleles through two generations following a first-generation cross of homozygous dominant and homozygous recessive parents. The recessive phenotype, which is masked in the second generation, has a 1 in 4, or 25%, chance of reappearing in the third generation.

Source: https://s3-us-west-2.amazonaws.com/courses-images-archive-read-only/wp-content/uploads/sites/403/2015/04/21032028/2924_Mendelian_Pea_Plant_Cross.jpg.

Such changes as DNA methylation and histone modifications, known as epigenetic modifications, may be passed down to future generations, affecting how genes are expressed. It has been found that the environment parents experience may change their children's genetic predispositions using epigenetic mechanisms. If parents go through stressful situations, it can bring about epigenetic changes that may continue to influence the health of their descendants. This phenomenon indicates the importance of a broader understanding of inheritance patterns beyond classical genetics, as it highlights how life experiences can imprint on the genome, thus influencing evolutionary processes in potentially Lamarckian ways (Lacal & Ventura, 2018). Moreover, the study of genetic disorders , such as sickle cell disorder (SCD) illustrates the practical implications of inheritance patterns in public health and education. Since SCD is becoming more common in specific groups, it is important to focus on genetic screening and inform the public. People's knowledge and opinions about SCD seem to influence their decision to take part in genetic screening. Studies have pointed out that there are gaps in the public's understanding, so it is important to educate more people about the inheritance of SCD, its carriers, and the health risks involved. This highlights that the understanding of genetic inheritance not only possesses theoretical significance but also practical ramifications that can shape healthcare strategies and ultimately, improve health outcomes in affected populations (Eboh et al., 2006) (Figure 12.8).

12.2.3. Environmental Factors

A combination of environmental and genetic factors usually leads to the appearance of genetic disorders. It has been suggested by different studies that the environment can either make genetic problems worse or lessen their impact. The severity and the way genetic disorders appear can be affected by pollutants, not having enough nutrients, and social and economic factors. At this time, environmental factors play a bigger role in mood and behavior because the brain is going through important changes. Because of this relationship, it is important to look at both genes and the environment when trying to understand genetic disorders. Efforts to implement integrative approaches that address these environmental factors may significantly reduce the prevalence and impact of such disorders, highlighting the necessity for targeted preventive strategies in public health initiatives (Bolton et al., 2013). In addition, the importance of genetics should not be underestimated, especially when it comes to genetic disorders. The nutrition of a person during pregnancy and early childhood can play a big role in how their brain and body develop. Evidence indicates that poor nutrition can bring about epigenetic changes that may increase someone's risk of neurodevelopmental disorders. In particular, if a mother lacks important nutrients, if her child is exposed to heavy metals, or if there are poor dietary habits during the early stages of life, it may increase the chance of autism spectrum disorder and attention-deficit/hyperactivity disorder. As such, understanding how nutritional factors influence genetic expression and development is critical, advocating for early nutritional interventions that could alleviate potential developmental issues (Cernigliaro et al., 2024). Besides what we eat, psychosocial influences in the environment are important for the development of genetic disorders. Genetic traits may be more or less visible depending on family relationships, experiencing trauma, and the financial situation of a person. A poor psychosocial environment can cause stress, which may affect gene expression by epigenetic means. As an illustration, going through adverse childhood experiences has been shown to cause mental health issues and may have a strong effect on how the brain develops. Both environmental factors and genetics must be considered to get a full understanding of genetic disorders. By focusing on improving the quality of the environment children are raised in, from supportive family structures to access to healthcare and education, it becomes possible to mitigate the adverse effects that often accompany genetic predispositions (Bolton et al., 2013).

Test Your Knowledge

1. What are the 4 forms of DNA mutations?
2. What is the interplay of environmental factors and genetic predispositions?

12.3. Symptoms and Diagnosis

Learning Outcome

1. Understand the common symptoms of genetic disorders;
2. Describe the diagnostic techniques for genetic disorders;
3. Understand the role of genetic counseling.

It is very important to know the symptoms and the ways doctors diagnose genetic disorders for their proper management and treatment. The way symptoms appear can change a lot, depending on the particular mutation present in the genes. For example, people with epilepsy could have different seizures, problems with cognitive function, and various EEG features that identify their electro-clinical syndrome. With the help of these electro-clinical signs, doctors can identify different types of epilepsy and design the best treatment strategies. By focusing on distinct symptoms and associated EEG patterns, healthcare providers can employ a more personalized approach that considers not only the physiological aspects but also the cognitive and developmental consequences associated with the disorder as emphasized in current literature (Verrotti et al., 2011). Diagnosing genetic disorders is not easy because it is often accompanied by many difficulties. The reliance on standardized diagnostic criteria, as outlined in the diagnostic and statistical manual of mental disorders (DSM), highlights a significant advancement in ensuring consistency in mental health diagnoses. On the other hand, some experts question the system because it is not always able to define disorders clearly, especially due to new discoveries in genetics. Although the DSM-IV includes guidelines for consistent diagnoses, it may not give enough space for clinical insight because it mainly focuses on existing disorders and not enough on new evidence from genetics and neuroscience. This limitation can hinder progress in achieving more valid and nuanced diagnoses, which are imperative for the effective treatment of individuals with genetic disorders (Andrews et al., 2010). In addition, using genetic testing in healthcare can help improve the accuracy of diagnosing genetic problems. With the help of genomic medicine, it is now possible to find genetic mutations that cause certain conditions and make diagnoses more precise. For instance, people who display symptoms of some genetic syndromes can be helped by genetic testing, which can explain the reasons for their symptoms and suggest appropriate care. This way of thinking helps to explain the disorder's causes better, which enhances the accuracy of treatment plans. As scientists and doctors keep studying how genetics and symptoms are connected, there is hope that diagnoses will become more accurate and treatments more successful in dealing with genetic disorders (Figure 12.9).

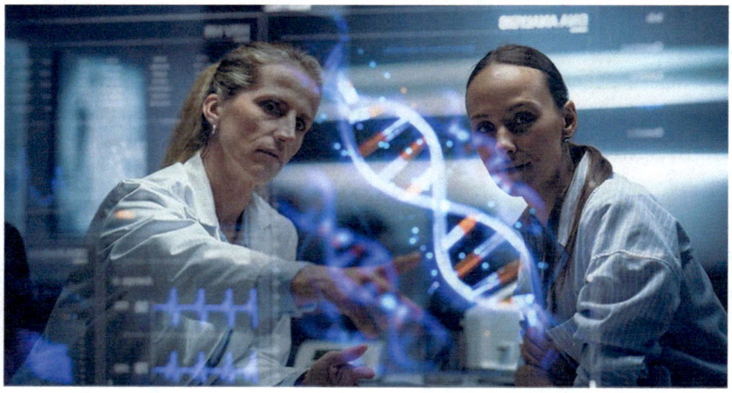

Figure 12.9. Researchers analyzing genetic data through an interactive digital interface.

Source: https://servier.com/wp-content/uploads/2025/02/servier-diagnostic-odyssey-genetic-history.png.

12.3.1. Common Symptoms of Genetic Disorders

Genetic disorders usually cause several common symptoms that can seriously affect a person's physical, mental, and emotional health. Depending on the disorder and its genetic factors, these symptoms may differ a lot, but they usually involve delayed growth, unusual body features, and a higher risk of health problems. Often, genetic disorders lead to special facial traits or changes in body structures, showing how genetics and physical features are related. In the end, recognizing these common symptoms is very important for early action, which can help improve a person's quality of life. Along with physical signs, genetic disorders commonly cause psychological symptoms that make it harder to diagnose and treat them. For instance, Huntingtons disease and some anomalies in chromosomes have been linked to both mental and emotional problems. Genetic conditions may cause emotional symptoms that are affected by both biology and the social and psychological environment of a person. Research indicates that psychometrically defined mental health phenotypes, as opposed to traditional summation scores, can provide more profound insights into the complexity of these symptoms, revealing patterns that enhance our understanding of genetic disorders and their impacts on mental health (Brown et al., 2015). It is made more difficult to manage genetic disorders because the current systems , such as the DSM-IV have their own limitations. While this manual was designed to standardize diagnostic criteria and improve interrater reliability, it has struggled to accommodate the diverse and multifaceted nature of mental health symptoms stemming from genetic disorders (Andrews et al., 2010). With researchers acknowledging that genetic factors play a big role in psychiatric diseases, it is obvious that both correct diagnosis and successful treatment depend on using an integrated method. Using this approach would encourage experts from different fields to cooperate and discover similar symptoms, which would help in providing suitable care for those with genetic disorders (Figure 12.10).

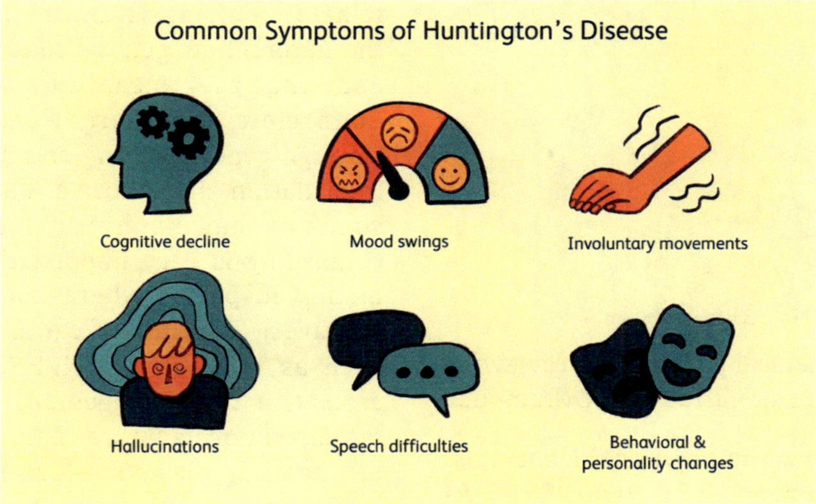

Figure 12.10. Symptoms of Huntington's disease.

Source: https://www.verywellhealth.com/thmb/vg9yhp33xSqEqyW2SHQhS6BH69c=/1500x0/filters:no_upscale():max_bytes(150000):strip_icc()/huntingtons-disease-symptoms-5091956-Final-c6e5d478c42945b593bafa65d9408e23.jpg.

12.3.2. Diagnostic Techniques

Genetic disorders are identified and treated with the help of important diagnostic methods. While karyotyping and Sanger sequencing have been helpful in spotting chromosomal and single-gene issues, they are not fast enough for all needs, so new methods in genomic medicine are required. Recent developments in NGS technologies offer a robust alternative, allowing for a more comprehensive analysis of genetic variants across the genome. Sequencing several genes at the same time with NGS helps reveal the complicated genetic causes of disorders, which enhances the accuracy of diagnosis. Moreover, combining how a patient looks with their genetic information is important for properly diagnosing congenital heart defects and other genetic problems, which helps doctors choose the best treatment for each person. The importance of early and accurate diagnosis cannot be overstated, especially regarding IEMs and congenital disorders. A lot of these conditions must be treated right away to avoid permanent harm. For example, newborn screening mostly uses tests that check for a few conditions, so there is a chance of getting false results. On the other hand, untargeted metabolomics looks like a promising development in diagnosing IEMs. By analyzing many metabolites at once, this approach could find several changes in the metabolism at the same time. With this extensive screening, doctors may find more metabolic disorders and improve how accurately they diagnose them, as stated in recent studies.

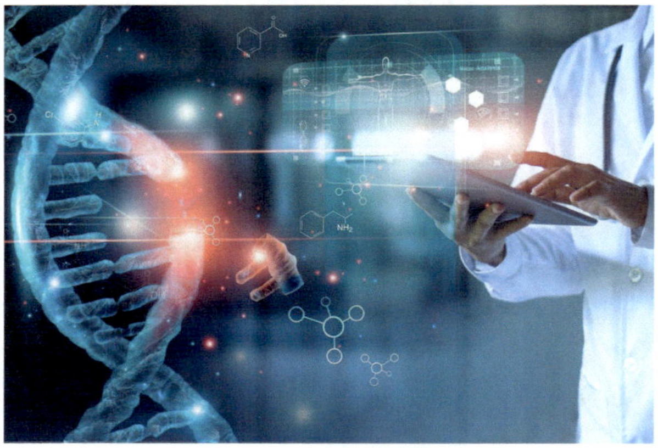

Figure 12.11. A medical professional reviewing digital genomic data alongside a 3D DNA model.

Source: https://imageio.forbes.com/specials-images/imageserve/1150397417/DNA-molecule/0x0.jpg?format=jpg&crop=3656,2438,x670,y0,safe&width=960.

Using untargeted methods in diagnostic frameworks may significantly change how genetic disorders are found and managed, ensuring quick action by clinicians. Using a combination of different strategies increases the success of current diagnostic approaches. For instance, clearly identifying the different forms of congenital heart defects is important for finding out their genetic reasons. Using both whole-exome sequencing and transcriptome analysis can provide more information about the links between genes and their effects. It is important to create biobanks and join forces in research to help these advances. Having such infrastructure would help gather top-quality biological samples from specific groups of patients, which would lead to better integration of molecular, phenotypic, and genotypic data. All in all, perfecting these diagnostic approaches is key to the progress of precision medicine, helping people with genetic disorders by highlighting important advances in research for CHDs and IEMs (Figure 12.11).

12.3.3. Role of Genetic Counseling

Genetic counseling is very important for dealing with the difficulties related to genetic disorders. It helps individuals and families know about the nature, how genetic conditions are passed, and what they mean by giving information. Counselors are there to help patients go through genetic testing and make sense of the information they receive. For example, when someone has nephrotic syndrome, genetic counseling is very important for their family, mainly in places where many people marry relatives. The identification of mutations, , such as those in the NPHS2 gene, not only assists in the management of the condition but also informs future reproductive decisions, emphasizing the counselor's role in facilitating informed decision-making and reducing the incidence of hereditary renal diseases in affected communities (Almukhtar et al., 2024). Besides providing facts, genetic counseling gives emotional support to people and their families who are unsure about genetic disorders. Talking about the emotions linked to genetic testing, , such as fear, anxiety, or guilt, is possible with the help of a counselor. In the context of disorders like maturity-onset diabetes of the young (MODY), patients may grapple with the implications of their genetic predispositions not only for themselves but also for their offspring. Counselors can help relieve the mental stress of families by explaining the possible impacts and results of genetic conditions. This supportive role is crucial, as the emotional ramifications of a genetic diagnosis can have lasting impacts on family dynamics and individual well-being (Bińczyk et al., 2024). In addition, when genetic counseling is part of healthcare, more people can use genetic services and they become more effective. Because genetic testing is becoming more common, thanks to new technology and more people knowing about it, the need for skilled counselors is also on the rise. Genetic counseling that works well can result in a quicker diagnosis and special treatment plans for genetic disorders. Those who are affected by genetic mutations may get advice on how to change their lifestyle, monitor their health, and use possible treatments. With genetic counseling, patients can make better health decisions and learn how to handle their genetic issues. Thus, the role of genetic counseling is integral to enhancing clinical care and promoting public health in the realm of genetic disorders (Almukhtar et al., 2024) (Figure 12.12).

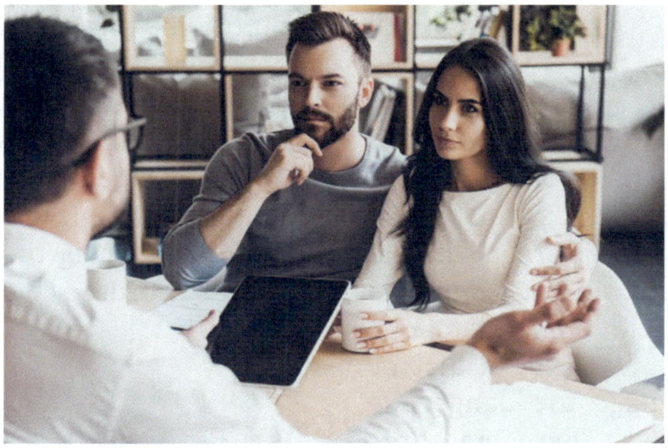

Figure 12.12. Genetic counseling.

Source: https://www.sepalika.com/wp-content/uploads/2021/10/shutterstock_431851987.webp.

Test Your Knowledge

1. What techniques are used to detect genetic disorders?
2. What is the role of genetic counselling?

12.4. Treatment Options

Learning Outcome

1. Understand the role of medical management in addressing the complexity of genetic disorders;
2. Describe the role of gene therapy in addressing genetic disorders;
3. Understand the lifestyle and supportive care requirements for individuals affected by genetic disorders.

Treatment for genetic disorders is designed according to the disorder, its level of severity, and what the individual requires. Usually, these approaches involve changing a person's habits and medicines that help deal with the symptoms of the disorder. Patients with some metabolic issues are advised to follow a special diet or take supplements to manage the dangerous metabolites in their bodies. These measures are very important, but they usually form just one part of a complete treatment plan. With the growth of genetics, more doctors are using personalized medicine in treating patients. Genetic profiling makes it possible to give each patient a treatment that matches their genes, so the treatment is more effective and patients have better outcomes. Gene therapy, a new treatment, has been made possible by the progress in biotechnology. Gene therapy tries to correct or replace genes that cause genetic disorders, providing a more lasting answer to the problem. In some inherited retinal diseases, using gene therapy has helped restore vision for a number of patients. Even so, there are issues with applying gene therapy, for example, ethical questions, high costs, and the requirement for ongoing research. The breadth of possibilities offered by gene therapy underscores the potential to redefine the landscape of treatment options for genetic disorders, shifting focus from merely managing symptoms to addressing their underlying causes (Ismail et al., 2019). In addition to gene therapy, pharmacological interventions have also expanded, particularly for IEMs. Usually, IEMs are caused by a lack of certain enzymes, which results in the buildup of toxic substances. Therefore, doctors can now use enzyme replacement therapies to help the body get the missing enzymes and restore balance. Besides, new drug approaches , such as substrate reduction therapy focus on lowering the amount of harmful metabolites produced, giving patients more treatment choices. The new developments point to the importance of having full newborn screening, as it allows for early detection of IEMs and better treatment. Ongoing research into untargeted metabolomics shows promise in enhancing screening processes and potentially identifying new therapeutic targets for IEMs, further advancing the treatment landscape for genetic disorders (Woodie et al., 2009) (Figure 12.13).

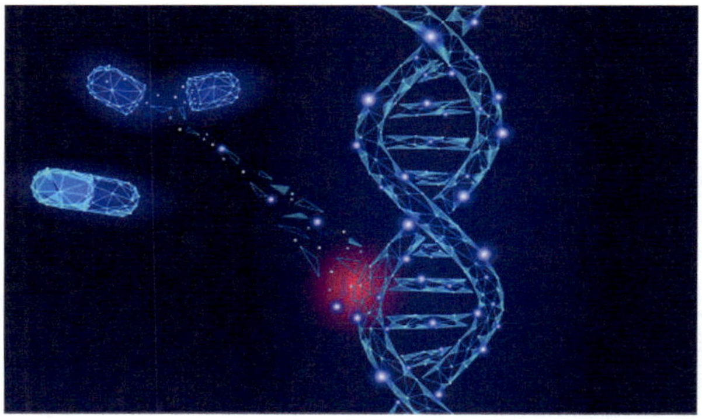

Figure 12.13. Treatment in genetic disorders.

Source: https://geneticsinindia.com/blog/wp-content/uploads/2020/08/genetic-disorders.jpg.

12.4.1. Medical Management

Treating genetic disorders requires medical management since the treatment plan has to be customized for each person's genes and the symptoms they experience. This way of treating patients is important since genetic disorders can be very different in how severe they are and which body systems they affect. As an example, metabolic disorders could require you to change your diet, whereas cystic fibrosis may call for inhalation treatments or the use of enzymes. Genetic counseling should be part of medical care because it helps patients and families understand how the disorder is inherited and what to do about it. Being involved in their care helps patients stick to the treatments, which improves their health and well-being. Taking care of the patient's psychological needs is a key part of managing genetic disorders. Many patients with these disorders tend to feel very anxious and depressed because of the problems they face, including the lasting effects of their condition. So, it is common for effective management to include psychological therapies, especially for children, since being emotionally strong helps them stick to treatment and feel better. Cognitive-behavioral therapy and similar evidence-based treatments have been proven to ease the psychological effects of chronic illnesses in children, showing that a team approach is necessary in medical care. This holistic perspective also aligns with recent findings that underscore the necessity of addressing mental health as a protective factor against the deterioration of physical health in children with genetic disorders (Storey & Smith, 2008). Additionally, progress in technology and research keeps improving the ways medical professionals handle genetic disorders. For instance, gene therapy is now used to fix the genes responsible for some genetic diseases. With CRISPR, and other gene editing technologies, it is now possible to directly treat genetic disorders that could not be managed before. It is also important to mention that data analytics plays a key role in managing patients, since analyzing health data all the time helps determine how well treatments work and what the long-term results will be. This integration of cutting-edge technology not only enhances the precision of medical management but also supports ongoing research efforts aimed at developing novel therapeutic strategies tailored to genetic disorders (Kitsiou et al., 2013) (Figure 12.14).

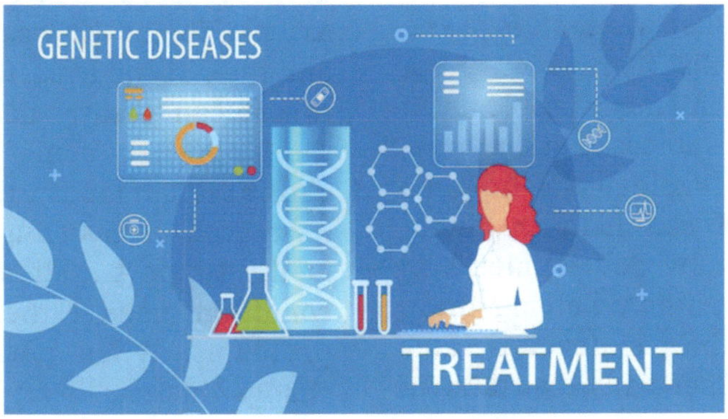

Figure 12.14. Genetic disease medical treatment.

Source: https://img.freepik.com/premium-vector/genetic-disease-medical-treatment-flat-style_81522-4796.jpg.

12.4.2. Gene Therapy

Gene therapy is a new method that helps fix or replace genes that are responsible for various hereditary problems. Gene therapy tries to solve the main causes of these disorders by inserting helpful genes into patients' cells, instead of just treating their symptoms. Innovative methods , such as adeno-associated virus (AAV) vectors and lipid nanoparticle-encapsulated mRNA have been pivotal in advancing gene therapy. Thanks to these technologies, it is now possible to reach cells that were thought to be inaccessible. Gene therapy marks a key change in how genetic disorders are handled, suggesting that it can address the problem for a long time rather than just ease the symptoms. Gene therapy research has mainly shown how it can be used to treat rare genetic disorders, since there are usually not many options for treating them. One important progress is the creation of therapies that work on functional haploinsufficiency, which is a common reason for many rare diseases. Since traditional therapies only manage symptoms, gene therapy gives a new way to deal with these genetic problems. Promising studies and clinical trials underscore the versatility of gene therapy, showcasing its adaptability across a range of disorders, including mucopolysaccharidoses (MPS) and other hereditary conditions. In particular, the refinement of both AAV and mRNA technologies enhances their suitability for therapeutic applications, providing hope for patients who have historically faced limited medical options and poor prognoses due to the nature of their genetic conditions (Bara-Ledesma et al., 2025). When we look forward, gene therapy for genetic disorders shows great promise, but also comes with many problems. At present, gene therapy is subject to strict rules, and it is necessary to consider the immune system's reactions, which can make treatment less effective. Even so, new developments in AAVs and mRNA are gradually solving these issues, making it possible to develop safer and better therapies. Especially, the arrival of enzyme replacement therapy (ERT) and substrate reduction therapy that can cross the BBB is a key sign of new targeted treatment options. When more research is completed, the use of new gene therapies in clinical care could change how genetic disorders are managed, making it possible to cure them instead of only treating their symptoms. Such a paradigm shift emphasizes the need for continued investment in research and development to fully harness the power of gene therapy (Chról et al., 2025) (Figure 12.15).

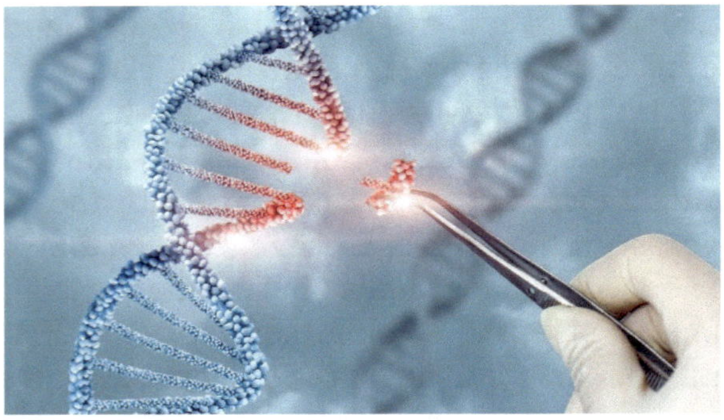

Figure 12.15. Gene therapy.

Source: https://cdn.mos.cms.futurecdn.net/97QX5fRoqwVAQD5cZ6nPoa.jpg.

12.4.3. Lifestyle and Supportive Care

It is very important to understand how to support people with genetic disorders to improve their general well-being. Taking care of these disorders involves medical help as well as attention to what patients eat, their feelings, and their social lives. Receiving advice on what to eat can greatly help with symptoms and the progress of some genetic conditions since eating certain foods can prevent complications. Furthermore, involving both families and peers in the support system helps people with the condition manage their emotional and social problems. When patients make such wide changes in their lifestyle, they are better able to take care of their health and remain strong in the face of their illness. Psychosocial interventions are part of supportive care and help people with genetic disorders deal with mental health problems. Adolescents are more likely to face depression and anxiety, especially when the stressors linked to their conditions are added. It appears that psychoeducational interventions help patients gain insight into their conditions and offer them useful strategies to manage them. They help families notice signs of illness and talk about them, as well as support their relatives in helpful ways. It is necessary to see how lifestyle affects mental health, so we can help people by focusing on both their emotional and physical well-being. As a result of these efforts, people can develop a stronger approach to care that looks after both their mental and physical well-being. It is very important for healthcare professionals to assist patients with genetic disorders by helping them make healthy changes and providing support. Treatment plans should be created by clinicians who join forces with dietitians, mental health specialists, and genetic counselors to address the specific problems of patients. Thanks to this model, care plans are made to fit each person's preferences and medical requirements. Any intervention used should be based on solid research and should be able to change with the wide variety of genetic disorders and their symptoms. Healthcare providers should also be aware of the newest developments in supportive care to help patients and their families. Therefore, making sure care providers and patients communicate well can improve the health and quality of life of people with genetic disorders and help build a better care environment.

Test Your Knowledge

1. What is the role of medical management?
2. What is a technique that can be used to treat genetic disorders?

SUMMARY

The findings from recent research on genetic disorders show that these conditions are not simple and have many aspects. It is becoming obvious that genetic disorders are not only problems within the body's biological systems. According to recent studies, some neurological disorders, for example schizophrenia, might actually have features that are helpful rather than harmful. It goes against the common belief that all genetic differences always lead to harm. Instead, the evidence shows that some strange physical features linked to genetic disorders play a role in the overall workings of an individual's body. This shift in understanding requires a re-evaluation of how we approach diagnosis, treatment, and societal perceptions of mental disorders and conditions of genetic origin (Garson, 2010). Besides, there are ethical concerns about genetic testing in minors that make the topic of genetic disorders more difficult to discuss. European guidelines point out that predictive and presymptomatic testing should be done when medical treatments can benefit a person's health. Yet, doctors' reluctance to perform such tests on children highlights the many aspects of genetic disorders and their possible effects on a person's life. It is clear from studies that there are big differences in how countries advise genetic testing for children, suggesting that cultural and ethical issues are present and need to be handled with care. As practitioners grapple with best practices, the need for standardized protocols coupled with flexibility to accommodate individual circumstances becomes paramount (Marie et al., 2009). To sum up, dealing with genetic disorders requires knowledge of science and medicine as well as dealing with ethical, social, and psychological matters. Looking at genetic conditions as either harmful or beneficial brings up new ways to explore and manage them. If we make sure more people understand the effects of genetic disorders, we can support better treatment and raise compassion among the public. With the progress of research, it will be necessary for scientists, clinicians, and ethicists to keep discussing future policies and educational systems that address the challenges and opportunities of genetics. As a result, people with genetic disorders can get the help and care they need, which is suited to their own situations.

It is important to realize that prenatal genetic testing plays a big role in understanding genetic disorders. New technologies have made it possible to detect health problems early, which has greatly improved health results. A recent study highlighting the use of a Delphi process to evaluate relevant questions for health technology assessments (HTA) showcases this shift. By systematically gathering expert opinions, the study established a framework for determining which aspects of new prenatal genetic tests should be prioritized, creating a meaningful dialogue around essential questions in the field (Freeman et al., 2005). Therefore, it becomes more important for professionals to work together in genetic testing, which helps stakeholders make better decisions about genetic disorders and the related care. In addition, understanding genetic disorders can be improved by looking into neurodevelopmental disorders, for example, schizophrenia. It has been found that craniofacial dysmorphology may indicate brain dysmorphogenesis, which helps researchers learn more about the genetic conditions involved. By employing genetically modified mouse models, researchers can analyze how targeted disruptions of specific genes relate to physical manifestations of these disorders (Bowman et al., 2017). Besides discovering new genetic traits, these studies show how genetic factors are related to development and, in a controlled environment, suggest ways to prevent or treat diseases. Thanks to new methods , such as geometric morphometrics, examining genetic disorders becomes easier. With these methods, researchers can analyze facial features in mutant animals and find out more about the structure-related impacts of genetic changes. For instance, utilizing mutant mice with disruptions in genes linked to schizophrenia has provided compelling evidence of the relationship between genetics and observable phenotypes (Bowman et al., 2017). By studying this way, we can discover how genetic disorders occur, which may not be visible in people. They help the field move ahead, adding important improvements to both diagnosis and treatment approaches in genetics.

KEY TERMS FROM THIS CHAPTER

- Adeno-associated virus
- Chromosomal disorders
- Down syndrome
- Genetic counseling
- Genetic heterogeneity
- Karyotyping
- Multifactorial disorders
- Schizophrenia
- Autism spectrum disorders
- DNA sequence
- Gene therapy
- Genetic disorders
- Huntingtons disease
- Medical management
- Next-generation sequencing

Critical Thinking Questions

1. **Which of the following is an example of an autosomal dominant disorder?**
   a. Cystic fibrosis
   b. Huntington's disease
   c. Sickle cell anemia
   d. Hemophilia
2. **What is the genetic basis of Down syndrome?**
   a. Trisomy 13
   b. Trisomy 21
   c. Deletion on chromosome 5
   d. Monosomy X
3. **Sickle cell anemia is caused by a mutation in the gene encoding:**
   a. Myoglobin
   b. Hemoglobin
   c. Collagen
   d. Keratin
4. **Which of the following disorders is caused by a single gene mutation?**
   a. Turner syndrome
   b. Tay-Sachs disease
   c. Klinefelter syndrome
   d. Down syndrome
5. **Hemophilia is primarily caused by:**
   a. Autosomal recessive mutations
   b. X-linked recessive mutations
   c. Autosomal dominant mutations
   d. Chromosomal deletions

Answers to Critical Thinking Questions

1. (b); 2. (b); 3. (b); 4. (b); 5. (b)

Short Answer Questions

1. What are genetic disorders?
2. Why is it important to learn about genetic disorders?
3. Name the 3 types of genetic disorders.
4. What are the causes of genetic disorders?
5. What are the symptoms of genetic disorders?

REFERENCES

1. Grotzinger, A. D., Mallard, T. T., Akingbuwa, W. A., Ip, H. F., Adams, M. J., Lewis, C. M., McIntosh, A. M., Grove, J., Dalsgaard, S., Lesch, K. P., Strom, N., Meier, S. M., Mattheisen, M., Børglum, A. D., Mors, O., Breen, G., iPSYCH, Tourette Syndrome and Obsessive Compulsive Disorder Working Group of the Psychiatric Genetics Consortium, Bipolar Disorder Working Group of the Psychiatric Genetics Consortium, Major Depressive Disorder Working Group of the Psychiatric Genetics Consortium, ... Nivard, M. G. (2022). Genetic architecture of 11 major psychiatric disorders at biobehavioral, functional genomic and molecular genetic levels of analysiws. *Nature genetics*, *54*(5), 548–559. https://doi.org/10.1038/s41588-022-01057-4 (accessed on 11th June 2025).
2. Almukhtar, S. E., & Hamed, T. M. (2024). Next generation sequencing reveals mutation patterns and prevalence of inherited renal disease in Erbil City. https://core.ac.uk/download/640070156.pdf (accessed on 11th June 2025).
3. Altmäe, S., Hallast, P., Heinaste, E., Koido, K., et al. (2004). Polymorphisms in wolframin (*WFS1*) gene are possibly related to increased risk for mood disorders. https://core.ac.uk/download/611943547.pdf (accessed on 11th June 2025).
4. Hyman S. E. (2010). The diagnosis of mental disorders: the problem of reification. *Annual review of clinical psychology*, *6*, 155–179. https://doi.org/10.1146/annurev.clinpsy.3.022806.091532 (accessed on 11th June 2025).
5. Angold, A., Arnold, L. E., Banaschewski, T., Maughan, B., Byrne, M., Carroll, J., Craig, T. K. J., et al. (2006). Literacy and mental disorders. https://core.ac.uk/download/49099.pdf (accessed on 11th June 2025).
6. Bara-Ledesma, N., Fabregate, M., Gómez del Olmo, V., López Rodríguez, A., et al. (2025). Advances in gene therapy for rare diseases: Targeting functional haploinsufficiency through AAV and mRNA approaches. https://core.ac.uk/download/644661203.pdf (accessed on 11th June 2025).
7. Barzman, D., Hutton, J., Ji, H., Lin, S., et al. (2015). Pediatric asthma and autism—genomic perspectives. https://core.ac.uk/download/323070690.pdf (accessed on 11th June 2025).
8. Bevan Jones, R., Jones, I., Simpson, S., Smith, D., et al. (2017). Psychoeducational interventions in adolescent depression: A systematic review. https://core.ac.uk/download/132211505.pdf (accessed on 11th June 2025).
9. Bińczyk, W., Brzozowska, P., Dróżdż, O., Lissak, M., et al. (2024). Re-diagnosis of diabetes mellitus type 1 to maturity-onset diabetes of the young type 2 (*MODY 2*) in a 26-year-old male: A case report. https://core.ac.uk/download/620863094.pdf (accessed on 11th June 2025).
10. Bolton, P., Collins, P. Y., Jordans, M., March, D., Muñoz, M., Patel, V., Patel, V., et al. (2013). Reducing the burden of depression in youth: What are the implications of neuroscience and genetics on policies and programs? https://core.ac.uk/download/42631341.pdf (accessed on 11th June 2025).
11. Bose, S., Burg, M. B., Caldecott, K. W., Chu, G., Digweed, M., Fernandez-Capetillo, O., Fousteri, M., et al. (2010). DNA repair: Disorders. https://core.ac.uk/download/2717477.pdf (accessed on 11th June 2025).

12. Bowman, A. W., Katina, S., O'Tuathaigh, C. M. P., Waddington, J. L., et al. (2017). Translational genetic modelling of 3D craniofacial dysmorphology: Elaborating the facial phenotype of neurodevelopmental disorders through the prism of schizophrenia. https://core.ac.uk/download/132211200.pdf (accessed on 11th June 2025).

13. Brian, J., Bryson, S. E., Buchanan, J. A., D'Abate, D., et al. (2019). Predictive impact of rare genomic copy number variations in siblings of individuals with autism spectrum disorders. https://core.ac.uk/download/323067913.pdf (accessed on 11th June 2025).

14. Brown, A., Demirkan, A., Green, A. E., Voight, B. F., Minica, C. C., Goldberg, D. P., Goldberg, D. P., et al. (2015). Psychometric precision in phenotype definition is a useful step in molecular genetic investigation of psychiatric disorders. https://core.ac.uk/download/30612906.pdf (accessed on 11th June 2025).

15. Bufford, R. K. (1988). Mental disorders. In *Counseling and the Demonic* (Chap. 6). https://digitalcommons.georgefox.edu/cgi/viewcontent.cgi?article=1009&context=counselingandthedemonic (accessed on 11th June 2025).

16. Cernigliaro, F., Correnti, E., D'Agostino, S., Lo Cascio, S., Marchese, F., Nardello, R., Pitino, R., et al. (2024). Prenatal nutritional factors and neurodevelopmental disorders: A narrative review. https://core.ac.uk/download/638998389.pdf (accessed on 11th June 2025).

17. Sher, K. J., Johnson, J. L., Schuckit, M. A., Jacob, T., & Chassin, L. (1997). A critical analysis of COA research. *Alcohol health and research world, 21*(3), 258–264. (accessed on 11th June 2025).

18. Chen, X. S., Devanna, P., Fisher, S. E., Francks, C., Gajewski, D., Gialluisi, A., Ho, J., et al. (2018). Next-gen sequencing identifies non-coding variation disrupting miRNA-binding sites in neurological disorders. https://core.ac.uk/download/491496512.pdf (accessed on 11th June 2025).

19. Chról, M., Dzikowska, I., Gronowicz, G., Homa, M., et al. (2025). Advancements in the treatment of mucopolysaccharidoses: From established therapies to gene therapy. https://core.ac.uk/download/646080076.pdf (accessed on 11th June 2025).

20. Copeland, W. C., & Young, M. J. (2016). Human mitochondrial DNA replication machinery and disease. https://core.ac.uk/download/60582847.pdf (accessed on 11th June 2025).

21. Dinkler, L., Gajwani, R., Gillberg, C., Lichtenstein, P., et al. (2017). Maltreatment-associated neurodevelopmental disorders: A co-twin control analysis. https://core.ac.uk/download/74230270.pdf (accessed on 11th June 2025).

22. Eboh, W., Millan, J., & van Teijlingen, E. (2006). Knowledge and attitudes towards sickle cell disease screening: A study of members of the UK Sickle Cell Society. https://core.ac.uk/download/75067.pdf (accessed on 11th June 2025).

23. Fabbri, C. (2022). Genetics in psychiatry: Methods, clinical applications and future perspectives. https://core.ac.uk/download/591964328.pdf (accessed on 11th June 2025).

24. Ismail, I. T., Showalter, M. R., & Fiehn, O. (2019). Inborn Errors of Metabolism in the Era of Untargeted Metabolomics and Lipidomics. *Metabolites, 9*(10), 242. https://doi.org/10.3390/metabo9100242(accessed on 11th June 2025).

25. Fiorentino, A., Gialluisi, A., Gialluisi, A., Jacobsen, A., Quinlan, A. R., Tebbenkamp, A. T., Conne, B., et al. (2018). Next-gen sequencing identifies non-coding variation disrupting miRNA-binding

sites in neurological disorders. https://core.ac.uk/download/491496512.pdf (accessed on 11th June 2025).

26. Freeman, K., Hyde, J., Osipenko, L., et al. (2005). Emerging prenatal genetic tests: Developing a health technology assessment (HTA) framework for informed decision-making. https://core.ac.uk/download/105293.pdf (accessed on 11th June 2025).

27. Garson, J. (2010). Schizophrenia and the dysfunctional brain. https://core.ac.uk/download/131210931.pdf (accessed on 11th June 2025).

28. Ghosh, S., Koch, M., Rao, M. R. A. N., Shobha, S., et al. (2009). Assessment of metabolic parameters for autism spectrum disorders. https://core.ac.uk/download/pdf/87213.pdf (accessed on 11th June 2025).

29. Helner, N., Makukh, H., Prokopchuk, N., Sharhorodska, O., et al. (2019). Medical genetic counseling of women with congenital heart diseases of fetus. https://core.ac.uk/download/301580705.pdf (accessed on 11th June 2025).

30. Kitsiou, A., Caforio, A. L. P., Porta-Sanchez, A., Vahanian, A., Iung, B., Carrera, C., Szymanski, C., et al. (2013). *ESC core curriculum for the general cardiologist* (2013). https://core.ac.uk/download/55756305.pdf (accessed on 11th June 2025).

31. Lacal, I., & Ventura, R. (2018). Epigenetic Inheritance: Concepts, Mechanisms and Perspectives. *Frontiers in molecular neuroscience, 11*, 292. https://doi.org/10.3389/fnmol.2018.00292(accessed on 11th June 2025).

32. Plass, A. M. C., Bloch, M., Borry, P., Benjamin, C., Julian-Reynier, C., Anionwu, E. N., European Societies, et al. (2009). Testing the children: Do non-genetic health-care providers differ in their decision to advise genetic presymptomatic testing on minors? A cross-sectional study in five countries in the European Union. https://core.ac.uk/download/16415066.pdf (accessed on 11th June 2025).

33. Reemtsen, B., Finn, J. P., Alejos, J., Touma, M., Touma, M., Halnon, N., Nelson, S. F., et al. (2017). A path to implement precision child health cardiovascular medicine. https://core.ac.uk/download/323077346.pdf (accessed on 11th June 2025).

34. Fernell, E., Wilson, P., Hadjikhani, N., Bourgeron, T., Neville, B., Taylor, D., Minnis, H., & Gillberg, C. (2014). Screening, intervention and outcome in autism and other developmental disorders: the role of randomized controlled trials. *Journal of autism and developmental disorders, 44*(8), 2074–2076. https://doi.org/10.1007/s10803-014-2070-5(accessed on 11th June 2025).

35. Pamela Storey and Marjorie Smith(2008). *Methods and Approaches to Improving the Emotional Health and Well-Being of Children: A Briefing Paper Concerning Interventions to Prevent Internalizing Disorders*. Thomas Coram Research Unit, Institute of Education, University of London . https://core.ac.uk/download/pdf/82102.pdf (accessed on 11th June 2025).

36. Stringer, S. (2015). *Breaking the Code: Statistical Methods and Methodological Issues in Psychiatric Genetics*. https://core.ac.uk/download/489662083.pdf (accessed on 11th June 2025).

37. Verrotti, A., Castaldo, R., Ferretti, A., Ianniello, F., Chiarelli, F., et al. (2011). "Electro-clinical syndromes" with onset in pediatric age: The highlights of the clinical-EEG, genetic and therapeutic advances. https://core.ac.uk/download/54438866.pdf (accessed on 11th June 2025).

INDEX